Clinical
Orthodontics
Current Concepts, Goals and Mechanics

Clinical Orthodontics

Current Concepts, Goals and Mechanics

Second Edition

Ashok Karad BDS, MDS, M ORTH RCS(EDIN)
Director Smile Care – India
Diplomate, Indian Board of Orthodontics
Private Practice, Mumbai, India
Past Chairman, Indian Board of Orthodontics
Past Editor-in-Chief, The Journal of Indian Orthodontic Society
INDIA

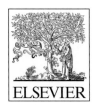

ELSEVIER
A division of
Reed Elsevier India Private Limited

Clinical Orthodontics: Current Concepts, Goals and Mechanics, 2e
Karad

ISBN: 978-81-312-3739-7
eISBN: 978-81-312-3740-3
epub ISBN: 978-81-312-3848-6

Notices

Knowledge and best practice in this field are constantly changing. As new research and experience broaden our understanding, changes in research methods, professional practices, or medical treatment may become necessary.

Practitioners and researchers must always rely on their own experience and knowledge in evaluating and using any information, methods, compounds, or experiments described herein. In using such information or methods they should be mindful of their own safety and the safety of others, including parties for whom they have a professional responsibility.

With respect to any drug or pharmaceutical products identified, readers are advised to check the most current information provided (i) on procedures featured or (ii) by the manufacturer of each product to be administered, to verify the recommended dose or formula, the method and duration of administration, and contraindications. It is the responsibility of practitioners, relying on their own experience and knowledge of their patients, to make diagnoses, to determine dosages and the best treatment for each individual patient, and to take all appropriate safety precautions.

To the fullest extent of the law, neither the Publisher nor the authors, contributors, or editors, assume any liability for any injury and/or damage to persons or property as a matter of products liability, negligence or otherwise, or from any use or operation of any methods, products, instructions, or ideas contained in the material herein.

Please consult full prescribing information before issuing prescription for any product mentioned in this publication.

The Publisher

Published by Reed Elsevier India Private Limited
Registered Office: 305, Rohit House, 3 Tolstoy Marg, New Delhi-110 001
Corporate Office: 14th Floor, Building No. 10B, DLF Cyber City, Phase II, Gurgaon-122 002, Haryana, India

Sr Content Strategist: Nimisha Goswami
Managing Editor: Anand K Jha
Project Manager: Prasad Subramanian
Project Coordinator: Isha Bali
Manager - Publishing Operations: Sunil Kumar
Sr Production Executive: Ravinder Sharma
Sr Cover Designer: Milind Majgaonkar

Laser Typeset by GW India
Printed and bound in India at EIH Limited – Unit Printing Press, IMT Manesar (Haryana).

Dedicated
to

My wife Vaishali and daughter Tanushka

Without their love, support, sacrifice and continued encouragement,
this project could not have been completed

Foreword

Clinical Orthodontics: Current Concepts, Goals and Mechanics by Dr Ashok Karad is a comprehensive and well-written text. Most importantly, the thrust of this work is centred around the key word in the subtitle 'Current'. It is vigorously integrated into all biomechanical, diagnostic and treatment planning areas of the text.

This robust document is intelligently structured with 17 comprehensive chapters by a dynamic group of world-class clinicians, researchers and teachers who clearly discuss the cutting-edge concepts and technologies of their respective areas of expertise.

Dr Karad has done an outstanding job of editing this text into a valued resource that belongs to the bookshelves of all orthodontists who are interested in, and involved, with structuring their professional careers to comply with contemporary clinical concepts, goals and mechanics.

I unreservedly recommend this book to clinicians, academics and postdoctoral students. It is a worthy text.

John J Sheridan DDS, MSD
Professor, Department of Orthodontics
Jacksonville University, Florida, USA

Contributors

A Bakr M Rabie BDS, PhD, MSC, CERT ORTHO, FHKAM (DENTAL SURGERY), FCDSHK ORTHODONTICS, HON FDS RCS (EDIN)
Oya Body Shaping Clinics Limited
10th floor, Baskerville House, 13 Duddell Street, Central, Hong Kong

Ashok Karad BDS, MDS, M ORTH RCS (EDIN)
Director Smile Care – India
Diplomate, Indian Board of Orthodontics
Private Practice, Mumbai, India
Past Chairman, Indian Board of Orthodontics
Past Editor-in-Chief, The Journal of Indian Orthodontic Society
India

Barry H Grayson DDS
Associate Professor of Surgery (Orthod)
New York University Langone Medical Center
Institute of Reconstructive Plastic Surgery
USA

Chester H Wang BSC (MATHS-COMPUTER SC)
Dolphin Imaging
9200 Eton Avenue,
Chatsworth, CA 91311
USA

Fernando de la Iglesia DDS, MS, PhD
Associate Professor
Department of Orthodontics
International University of Catalonia,
Spain

Hitesh Kapadia DDS, PhD
Craniofacial Center,
Seattle Children's Hospital,
4800 Sandpoint Way NE,
Seattle, WA 98102
USA

Kazumi Ikeda DDS
Private Practice and Director
Roth/Williams Center for Functional Occlusion
Japan

Karen Moawad BSC
Amrita University
Bainbridge Island,
WA 98110
USA

Ki Beom Kim, DDS, MSD, PhD
Associate Professor
Department of Orthodontics
Center for Advanced Dental Education
Saint Louis University
3320 Rutger Street
Saint Louis, MO 63105

Larry W White DDS, MSD, FACD
Diplomate
American Board of Orthodontics
Adjunct Assistant Professor
Texas A&M, Baylor College of Dentistry
USA

Lisa Randazzo BA (LIT -CREATIVE WRITING/MINOR IN COMMUNICATIONS)
Dolphin Imaging
9200 Eton Avenue,
Chatsworth, CA 91311
USA

NR Krishnaswamy MDS, M ORTH RCS (EDIN), DIP NB
Professor and Head
Department of Orthodontics
Ragas Dental College and Hospital
Chennai
India

Prasanna K Shivapuja BDS, MDS, DDS, MS
Diplomate
American Board of Orthodontics
Private Practice
Roseville, Michigan
USA

Pradip R Shetye DDS, MDS
Assistant Professor of Plastic Surgery (Craniofacial Orthodontics)
New York University Langone Medical Center
Institute of Reconstructive Plastic Surgery
USA

P Emile Rossouw BSC, BCHD, BCHD (HONS-CHILD DENT), MCHD (ORTHO), PhD, FRCD(C)
Professor
Department of Orthodontics
University of North Carolina School of Dentistry
USA

Ratnadeep Patil BDS PCAD (USA)
Director
Smile Care – India
Program Director (India) CDE
New York University College of Dentistry
Associate Fellow
American Academy of Implant Dentistry
Diplomate
International College of Oral Implantologists
USA

Ricky W K Wong BDS, M ORTH, PhD, M ORTH RCS (EDIN),
    FRACDS, FHKAM, CDSHK (ORTHOD)
Department of Dentistry Maxillofacial Surgery,
United Christian Hospital,
Kowloon, Hong Kong

Sung-Hoon Lim, DDS, MSD, PhD
Professor
Department of Orthodontics
School of Dentistry
Chosun University
303 Pilmun-daero, Dong-gu
Gwangju, Korea

Yanqi Yang BDS, M ORTH RCS (EDIN), PhD
Clinical Assistant Professor in Orthodontics
Faculty of Dentistry
The University of Hong Kong
Hong Kong

Preface

This is indeed an extraordinary period in the orthodontic profession and it gives me a great feeling to be a part of this chosen field of interest, experiencing the enormous benefits and professional satisfaction that I enjoy while practising orthodontics. Over the last few years, Orthodontics has taken tremendous strides through expanding knowledge and improved technology. This has resulted in ever increasing levels of excellence in treatment accomplished with greater efficiency than was thought possible even a decade ago. The profession has witnessed many substantial contributions in the form of scientific and research articles, textbooks etc. to form an enormous body of information available today. This is truly a result of hard work and great vision of many clinicians, researchers and teachers who have accepted the challenge and gone beyond it.

I have been overwhelmed by the positive response to the first edition of this book from a wide cross-section of practising orthodontists, teachers and postgraduate students. These generous comments assured me that the book was a valuable addition to the learning experience, citing among other things the evidence-based approach to clinical orthodontics presented in an easy-to-learn format. Perhaps the most notable contribution of the first edition to the field was its content format, evidence-based and clinically useful information. This coupled with research and clinical innovations proliferated over the last few years and the need to update certain key areas of modern orthodontic practice has led me to undertake the challenge of a new edition. The second edition of this book has been built on the strengths of its predecessor. It certainly was a challenge to develop this edition that would capture the excitement of this era and the new dimensions in orthodontic practice that have been generated through continued research and innovation; however at the same time, to keep the volume optimal in order to use it effectively as a reference guide.

The organization of the text and presentation of the subject material have been based on its theme 'Current Concepts' – dealing with a systematic approach to diagnosis, treatment planning, treatment sequencing and the execution of treatment in diverse clinical situations; 'Goals' – redefining orthodontic treatment goals in accordance with the current understanding of the science; and 'Mechanics' – highlighting newer methods, unbiased approach and refined mechanics to produce high-quality results.

In the development of a project of this magnitude, leading world-class clinicians, researchers, teachers and authors having different professional, academic and research backgrounds and interests have delivered cutting-edge information in their respective chapters. Various chapters in this text covering a wide array of current clinical topics demonstrate the principles and techniques that are universally applicable in orthodontics. The concepts, treatment goals and individual treatment modalities can be applied to any technique and are easily adaptable. No book can completely cover all aspects of a discipline; however, I feel I have incorporated useful areas in the field, and done necessary upgrades to the existing chapters and added new chapters that are critical for balanced composition of the text, adhering to the core philosophy, organization and objectives of this book.

The intention of the book is not to present an exhaustive review and analysis of the research literature; rather it is structured to present clinical material with the relevant literature that is evidence-based, in a concise but complete manner. The author and contributors, have of course, made every effort to ensure that the contents of this book comply with the state-of-the-art at the time of publication; and sincerely hope that this combined effort will help orthodontic professionals to serve their patients better.

Ashok Karad

Acknowledgements

This book is the culmination of years of rich clinical and teaching experience to provide the optimal body of information as a part of comprehensive reference in clinical orthodontics. It is impossible for any one professional or even a group of professionals, to stay abreast with all the diverse developments taking place at such a rapid pace. Good books are the result of teamwork, and an author must draw upon the skills and expertise of many colleagues and friends. I profusely thank the contributors already listed, who without fail, responded constructively and enthusiastically to my queries and found time to deliver extraordinary chapters, true to the theme of the book.

I would also like to thank Dr John J Sheridan for taking time from his busy schedule to share his wisdom and experience in the 'Foreword' to this book.

As this edition of the book is built on the strengths of its predecessor, I sincerely thank Ms Arlene Fernandes, Dr Vishal M. Dhanjani and Dr Vijay Bagul for their significant contribution to the first edition.

A special acknowledgement is due to Dr (Mrs) Vaishali Karad for her contribution towards lateral cephalometric tracings, analyses and several sketches in my chapters. The preciseness of this book is no small measure due to her attention to detail.

My sincere thanks to Dr Ratnadeep Patil, who collaborated with me on one of the chapters and his clinical assistance in rendering perio-restorative work in many of our patients requiring interdisciplinary treatment. I thank Prof Shailesh Deshmukh for his valuable inputs. Many thanks to Dr Clarence Bryk and Dr Ravi Anthony from the Department of Orthodontics, University of Texas Health Science Center at San Antonio Dental School, USA, for their help crucial to the development of this book. I personally thank Dr Shankar Iyer for his continuous encouragement and support.

I extend my gratitude to entire team of Elsevier for recognizing the impact this topic imposes on the average orthodontic professional, and for their usual careful handling of the publication and maintaining their standards of excellence. I especially thank Mrs Nimisha Goswami, Senior Content Strategist, who throughout this project has been available to advise and encourage. Her professional vision has been a valuable contribution to this manuscript. She is the force who kept me on track and always moving forward. I want to thank our Managing Editor, Mr Anand Kumar Jha, who worked tirelessly, and with admirable patience, and coordinated the production of this new volume with remarkable speed.

Finally, I am indebted to many extraordinary patients and families who have undergone treatment at our centre to achieve long-term functional and aesthetic solutions to their problems. Mere listing of the names is most inadequate expression of my indebtedness to all those who made this prodigious effort possible.

Contents

Detailed Contents

Prologue

Ashok Karad

CURRENT STATUS OF ORTHODONTIC PROFESSION

Advances in diagnostic technology, changing treatment concepts and philosophies, appliance design innovations and subsequent exponential growth of practices to include diverse patient populations have transformed the face of orthodontics over the past several years. It was towards the end of the nineteenth century the great evolutionary process in orthodontics commenced. A clearer conception of orthodontic problems was gained principally through the careful application of fundamental principles by such dedicated workers as Farrar, Guildford, Jackson, Case and Angle. Angle's final achievement, the edgewise appliance, was the culmination of many years of effort and many different appliance designs attempting to position the teeth according to his 'line of occlusion'. Since the time modern orthodontics gathered momentum under the leadership of Edward H Angle more than 100 years back, basic and clinical research and innovative technology have been instrumental in getting the orthodontic profession to its present level.

Orthodontics is a dynamic and changing field. Advances in science and technology are taking place at a rapid pace. As newer technologies are being introduced, their integration into a busy practice can take a lot of time, energy and money. A few of these new technologies include temporary anchorage devices (TADs), the use of fixed appliances with fully customized bracket prescriptions, cone beam computed tomography (CBCT), sophisticated treatment planning for patients in need of orthognathic surgeries, periodontal bone engineering, new protocols for improved treatment efficiency, interdisciplinary treatment for complex dentofacial problems, corticotomies to accelerate tooth movement, control of adverse effects of orthodontic treatment, laser surgery, and lingual orthodontics. However, there is very little standardization across orthodontic practices on the degree of exposure to new techniques. For example, some clinicians take routine 3-D radiographs on each and every patient, while others advocate them only as deemed necessary, and some do not consider them at all.

Many of these newer techniques are being gradually incorporated into private practices. As these new technologies do not always provide solutions to complex problems in patients, and are likely to bring associated new risks and uncertainties; individual training, diagnostic acumen and therapeutic skills of the orthodontic professional become critical.

DIAGNOSIS AND IMAGING

Diagnosis in orthodontics, like in other disciplines of dentistry and medicine, is a scientific procedure to generate objective, relevant and accurate information of patient's problem and its synthesis that helps the clinician to plan appropriate treatment strategy. Is this diagnostic process driven by innovations? Until 1931, orthodontic diagnosis was performed using clinical examination, study models and facial photographs. However, after the introduction of Broadbent–Bolton cephalometer in 1931, the orthodontic profession witnessed several cephalometric analyses, significantly contributing to the extensive study of human craniofacial growth and its impact on the way diagnoses were established. Both lateral and frontal cephalometric analyses enabled the clinician to identify various components contributing to the development of sagittal, vertical and transverse problems in the dentofacial complex. This further enhanced the ability of both the orthodontist and the maxillofacial surgeon to treat patients with skeletal problems to produce outstanding results that are aesthetic and functionally efficient.

Diagnostic capabilities in orthodontics have been improved drastically along with advances in computer technology. Current concepts in the multifaceted aspects of diagnosis have been based on an in-depth analysis of soft tissues and their considerations in treatment planning. Aesthetic needs of patients are always on the rise in both medical and dental fields, and orthodontics is no exception. With a great majority of patients visiting orthodontic offices for enhancement of appearance, the goal of maximizing facial aesthetics has forced the orthodontist to revisit fundamental concepts of art and beauty. Contemporary orthodontics has certainly made valuable progress in considering both aesthetics and function as priorities in orthodontic treatment. This has resulted in a major emphasis shift formerly based on the dental and skeletal components to the one that is currently based on the soft tissue aspects.

Recent advances in imaging technology have further provided clinicians with a documented view of craniofacial and dental structures before, during and after treatment, enhancing the clinician's diagnostic capabilities and also facilitating the patient's understanding of a problem and outcome of the treatment procedure. This certainly made a significant impact on doctor–patient interaction, making the patient a partner in the treatment planning process. This new technology is digital, resolving the limitations of film photographs and radiographic records offering numerous options to the practitioner.

Cone-beam computed tomography represents a significant advantage in imaging capabilities, replacing conventional two-dimensional radiographic images with three-dimensional data sets, with only a small increase in radiation. Three-dimensional images of the craniofacial anatomy of a patient can be used with advanced application software for diagnosis and development of treatment plans.

RESEARCH AND MATERIAL SCIENCE

The rapid advances in orthodontic research and the sophistication at the molecular level of science have generated enormous body of literature and new knowledge in the last 10 years. This has resulted in a new terminology and language, quite often little understood by the practising orthodontist. To understand the mechanism, by which various orthodontic treatment procedures can be explained, the clinician is required to have a sound knowledge of biological aspects. As the focus of current continuing education programs is on training the mind and intellect, as well as superior manual skills, it is equally important to acquire the methodological skills to assess the treatment outcomes of alternative treatment strategies. Evidence-based approach ensures that clinical decisions are based on the best available information, derived from integrating relevant clinical research, basic sciences and clinical experience.

Orthodontists are dependent on a variety of devices that are made from a large array of biomaterials possessing qualities of nontoxicity, high purity, good strength, hydrolytic stability, sterilizability, etc. The end of the nineteenth century was marked by the scarcity of adequate orthodontic materials suitable for orthodontic work. This was followed by major developments in metallurgy, analytic and organic chemistry and metal treatment, as well as the emergence of new plastic, all leading to the first mass-produced orthodontic consumables way back in the 1960s. Technological advances in biomaterials such as metals, ceramics and organic polymers, as well as their combinations, have also graced the profession over the last few years. The orthodontic practitioner today has a much more powerful and sophisticated array of appliances, better materials and a much greater understanding of the issues of biocompatibility. Improvements of the morphology, structure and mechanical properties of adhesives and bonding with conventional and acid-etching technique, archwires, elastomeric modules, and ceramic and metal brackets have significantly contributed to increased treatment efficiency and reduced chair time.

CLINICAL ORTHODONTICS AND PRACTICE MANAGEMENT

Several fundamental conceptual changes and newer trends in the orthodontic profession clearly signify alterations of traditional emphasis that have gradually emerged over the past decade or so. The existing clinical practice has emphasized the broader scope of various orthodontic procedures to encompass children in primary and mixed dentition through adolescence and also including all aspects of adult orthodontic treatment. Orthodontic treatment was universally considered to be easier when it was limited to children and adolescent patients since these patients tend to have intact, nonworn dentitions associated with optimal periodontal health. Levelling and alignment of teeth and good occlusal interdigitation were the primary treatment goals. However, function does not improve automatically if the teeth are simply aligned within the dental arches with the molars in Angle Class I relationship. Recognizing that orthodontic procedures are meant to be therapeutic and not just cosmetic, these goals were later redefined to include functional aspects of occlusion to improve the posttreatment health of the patient's stomatognathic system with lasting effect.

Traditionally, the correction of sagittal discrepancy was considered a common goal for both the patient and the orthodontist. However, a large proportion of clinical situations are not a single entity and are often associated with significant skeletal and dental imbalances in all three planes of space – sagittal, vertical and transverse. The current thinking makes every specialist familiar with and be able to critically analyse biologic, biomechanic, diagnostic and therapeutic concepts in clinical orthodontics. This has drawn clinician's attention to the fact that an emphasis should be placed on careful and complete diagnosis of various components of malocclusion and their interaction, appropriate treatment mechanics based on sound biomechanical principles, a continued diagnostic monitoring during treatment and a careful step-by-step accomplishment of the treatment objectives.

Lack of compliance in all age groups, especially in the adolescent population, has been a matter of concern for the practising orthodontists, having significant impact on the treatment outcome. The serious consequences of poor patient compliance have been well appreciated by most clinicians, which have shown its increasing trend over the years. Recognizing this aspect of clinical practice, the current orthodontic practice incorporates treatment designs and appliance systems that depend minimally on patient cooperation. This has led to the emergence of many new techniques and a variety of appliances available to the clinician to treat the noncompliant patient.

Anchorage control in fixed orthodontic treatment is considered one of the most important factors influencing treatment results. For planning efficient treatment mechanics and to avoid undesirable or detrimental effects on anchor units, it is critical to have a secure and stable anchorage. Compromised anchorage, especially in adult malocclusions characterized by missing teeth, poor periodontal health, etc. is often recognized as the limiting factor in achieving optimal results. With the limited anchorage potential in such cases and acceptance problems associated with conventional intraoral and extraoral aids, several implant anchorage systems have been introduced to provide absolute orthodontic anchorage. These exciting innovations that are developing at a rapid pace are constantly offering new treatment options for previously untreatable clinical situations.

For generations, most specialists have concentrated exclusively on their own speciality. The boundaries between various dental disciplines have become more and more sharply drawn over the last few years. Recently, an increased awareness of malocclusion, aesthetic appliances and functional benefits of orthodontics have all played an important role in making orthodontic treatment popular in adult population. With the explosive growth and advances in various dental disciplines, there has, on the contrary, been a drawing together on the level of maximizing treatment results in adult compromised dentition by combining orthodontic, periodontic and restorative principles and ways of thinking. Adult orthodontic patients have different problems like excessive tooth wear, missing teeth, restored teeth, periodontally compromised teeth, etc. which demand some alteration in treatment strategy. The most efficient and effective care in such individuals is coordinated by an interdisciplinary team where providers of the critical elements of the care have special training, expertise and experience. In addition, these team members comprising essentially of orthodontist, periodontist and restorative dentist have learned to benefit from one another's expertise.

Stability of the orthodontic result, an area of great concern to every clinician, at least partially depends on the way the cases have been finished. In current scenario marked by advances in treatment mechanics, there is hardly a separate stage of complicated wire bending to fine-tune the tooth positions; rather, it is a gradual progression towards fi nishing. In the management of a routine orthodontic case, the clinician defi nes finishing goals at the beginning of treatment and continues to focus on them till the fi nishing stage, in order to achieve them with appropriate treatment mechanics. Finishing goals are essentially defi ned for optimal aesthetics, good function of the stomatognathic system, normal periodontal health and long-term posttreatment stability.

In the past, every orthodontist spent years for learning how to be an excellent clinician, with less effort on understanding the business principles of practice. In an effort to grow and prosper, most orthodontic practices today plan on treating more number of patients, which cannot be accomplished with traditional methods of management. Recognizing that extraordinary service, profi tability and high level of patient satisfaction are key elements in managing an ideal orthodontic practice, attempts are being made to modify or discard the systems that are not effi cient and effective. Modern orthodontic practices are trying to adopt a management style that can optimize available technology, can refine work systems, has effective staff management principles and has efficient treatment protocols for high-quality treatment results and service.

APPLIANCE INNOVATIONS

Innovations in orthodontic appliance systems, archwires, bonding and imaging have dramatically improved clinical efficiency, patient acceptance, profitability and level of patient satisfaction. Over the years, the orthodontic bracket design has undergone a series of evolutionary changes from the initial brackets used by Dr Angle, to the twin bracket, to the preadjusted edgewise bracket introduced by Dr Larry Andrews and now to the self-ligating brackets. Preadjusted edgewise appliances in their current variations are probably the most significant advancement in orthodontic appliance design providing great benefits to orthodontists in all stages of treatment, especially during finishing and detailing. Self-ligating brackets is a magnificent step forward in the effi cient and effective treatment of orthodontic patients.

Lingual orthodontic therapy is now much more widely used for its undisputable aesthetic, biomechanical and therapeutic advantages. In the past, some patient-related problems like tissue irritation, speech difficulties and occlusal interferences and certain operator-related problems like bonding, archwire placement and ligation were associated with lingual appliance system. However, continued research in this field over the last few years has led to several improvements in the original lingual appliance, and a variety of new lingual appliance systems are now available. The current lingual appliances are much more refined to address these associated problems and offer great promise in clinical practice. The development of newer brackets, introduction of superelastic archwires and refi nements in laboratory procedures have all contributed to the way lingual orthodontics is practiced today, making it easier and more comfortable for both doctors and patients. With the advances in computer technology like Computer Aided Designing and Manufacturing, one signifi cant development that is making its presence felt is the use of mass- produced customized orthodontic appliances – both labial and lingual. These innovations significantly improve the convenience and comfort for both patients and orthodontists as they customize treatment on an individual basis.

These changing trends in the profession are certainly having a great impact on the way orthodontics is practiced today. Though basic and clinical research and innovative technology will continue to drive orthodontic advances in the future, it is author's firm belief that the area that has great potential to influence the profession in the future will be 'individualized diagnosis and customized care' to ensure that all aspects of patient care are carefully matched and optimized.

Craniofacial Growth: A Clinical Perspective

Ashok Karad

Majority of the problems that are encountered by the orthodontist in a day-to-day clinical practice, are related to growth. The difficulty in dealing with such problems may involve a failure on the part of the orthodontist to diagnose a growth and development problem or a poor patient cooperation in which the orthodontist is not given the chance to solve the problem, or it may be a growth pattern that is beyond the control of both the patient and the orthodontist. It is, therefore, essential that the clinician gives due importance to the significance and assessment of craniofacial growth while dealing with variety of clinical situations. The orthodontic practitioner must realize that the facial pattern is not constant; it is changed during growth and is also changed by orthodontic treatment. The treatment planning process must involve proper prediction of future growth and response to treatment, which requires better understanding of facial growth. This helps the clinician to institute optimal treatment to the patient. When jaws grow, they move and carry the dentition with them. If the amount and the direction of the movement of both the jaws as a result of growth is the same, the occlusion remains unchanged. However, disproportionate growth leads to the development of a new relationship of jaws to each other. This change in jaw relationships is often associated with compensatory tooth movements in one or both the jaws. Differential growth can occur anteroposteriorly, vertically or transversely. As the changes in the face and dentition continue throughout life, the clinician must consider both the immediate outcome of the treatment and the long-term stability and the benefits of the treatment as important goals.

For better understanding of the craniofacial growth, it is important to know the sites or the location of the growth and the type of growth occurring at that location. The growth of the craniofacial complex that is relevant to the orthodontic professional can be divided into following areas:

- The cranial base
- Maxilla
- The mandible
- Dental arches

CRANIAL BASE

The cranial base is essentially a midline structure in which the bones are formed initially in a cartilage and later transformed to bone by endochondral ossification. The changes in the cranial base take place primarily as a result of endochondral growth, mainly at various synchondroses (Figs 1.1 and 1.2). As ossification proceeds, bands of cartilage called *synchondroses* remain between the centres of ossification, which subsequently get converted into bone. The midline cranial base contains four primary cartilaginous sutures or synchondroses: the intersphenoidal sutures close by birth, the intraoccipital synchondrosis closes around 5 years of age, the spheno-ethmoidal synchondrosis closes around 6–7 years of age and the spheno-occipital synchondrosis closes by 13–15 years of age.

As the sphenoethmoidal synchondrosis closes by 6–7 years of life, the segment of the anterior cranial base — designated as the planum sphenoidale — becomes relatively stable, early in life.[1] Therefore, this area is usually used for cephalometric superimpositions to evaluate the changes in the face due to either growth or treatment. The sella–nasion (SN) plane is frequently used as a reference plane in order to more accurately determine the

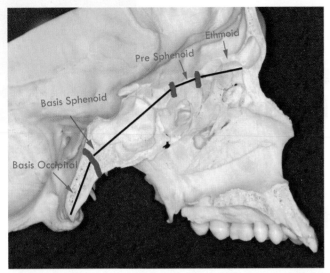

Figure 1.1 Sagittal section of the skull showing the cranial base and the approximate location of important growth sites.

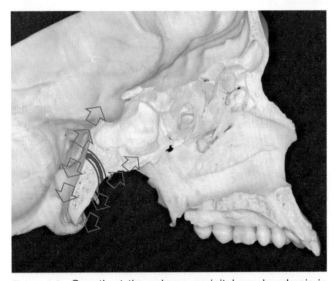

Figure 1.2 Growth at the spheno-occipital synchondrosis in which the maturing cartilage cells extend in both directions away from the centre as a part of endochondral ossification occurring at both margins. It contributes to the increase in length of this area of the cranial base.

changes occurring in the facial structures. The distance between sella and nasion normally increases by approximately 1 mm per year from 6 to 16 years of age. Another frequently used reference plane is nasion–basion plane. The distance between nasion and basion increases by approximately 1.7 mm per year between 6 and 16 years of age. After the closure of the spheno-occipital synchondrosis, any changes occurring either in the length or in the flexure of the cranial base are as a result of remodelling or surface deposition or resorption.[2]

Though there are minor opening and closing movements in the cranial base angle, this angle is relatively stable for most part. The average cranial base angle is approximately 130°. Obtuse or open cranial base angles are usually associated with a more backward position of the mandible and hence a Class II type of facial pattern. A more acute or closed cranial base angle is normally associated with a more forward position of the mandible and hence a Class III type of facial pattern. The sagittal growth centre — the spheno-occipital synchondrosis — is located in the region of the posterior cranial base, and the growth changes in this area determine the position of the fossa. A large angle between the anterior and posterior cranial bases, measured cephalometrically as N-S-articulare (Ar), indicates a posterior position, and a small angle indicates an anterior position of the fossa. The mean value is 123° ±5° (Fig. 1.3). This deviation in the position of the fossa is often compensated by the length of the ascending ramus. If there is no compensatory growth of the ascending ramus, this leads to either retrognathic or prognathic facial profile. Because the glenoid fossa determines the posterior/superior limit of the mandible, it holds important implications for mandibular displacement. Björk[3] indicated that the distance between the fossa and the nasion increases by 7.5 mm between 12 and 20 years of age when the landmark Ar is used. As a result of the elongation of the posterior cranial base, the fossa and the temporal bone are displaced inferiorly and posteriorly.[4] It was observed that the glenoid fossa was displaced between 1.8 and 2.1 mm posteriorly and between 1.0 and 1.8 mm inferiorly, and it demonstrated greater posterior and inferior displacement during adolescence than during childhood.[5] Therefore, during the treatment planning process for skeletal correction, the clinician should consider posterior fossa displacements to be added to any existing

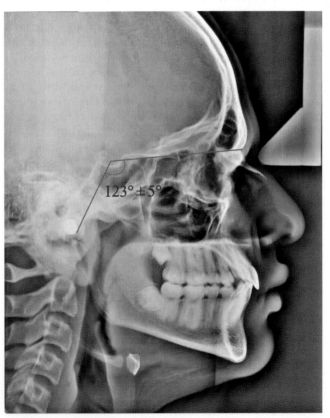

Figure 1.3 Diagrammatic representation of changes in the cranial base angle.

anterior discrepancies and future growth deficiencies. Another important growth change that occurs in the cranial base is the remodelling that takes place in the anterior cranial fossa. This brings about a forward displacement of the frontal bone and the nasal area.[6]

MAXILLA

The maxillary complex is surrounded by a system of sutures, such as zygomaticomaxillary, frontozygomatic, sphenopalatine and pterygomaxillary. The maxilla mainly grows by bone apposition at the sutures that connect the maxilla to the cranium and the cranial base and by surface remodelling (Fig. 1.4). Björk[7] in his implant study carried out to evaluate the changes in the growth direction of the nasomaxillary complex between 7 and 19 years of age and observed that the maxilla grew in a downward and forward direction at an angle of approximately 51° to the anterior cranial base (S–N plane) with a very large range of 0–82° (Fig. 1.5). This variation explains the fact that the maxilla would grow primarily in a horizontal direction in some patients, while it would grow primarily in a vertical direction in others. It has been observed that during the first decade of life, the maxillary growth proceeds normally in a horizontal direction, while during the second decade of life, it proceeds in a more vertical direction.[7]

The displacement and remodelling changes play an important role in the growth of the maxilla.[6] The horizontal displacement of the maxilla is primarily due to remodelling expansion within the middle cranial fossa. Also, deposition of bone on the posterior aspect of the maxilla, in the area of tuberosity, allows it to keep pace with the forward displacement of the frontal and nasal bones (as a result of expansion of the anterior cranial base) and to accommodate for the eruption of the permanent molars. The maxillary length changes are shown in Table 1.1. The vertical displacement of the maxilla occurs primarily by growth and expansion of the eyeballs and the nasal septum. The growth of the cartilaginous nasal

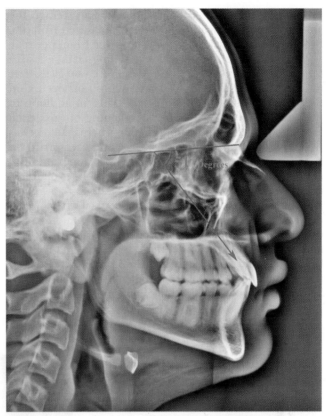

Figure 1.5 The growth of the nasomaxillary complex from 7 to 19 years of age moves it downward and forward at an average angle of 51° with the cranial base.

Table 1.1   Maxillary length changes (MM)*

Age	Males	Females
6	83	81
8	85	83
10	88	85.5
12	92.5	89
14	96.5	92
16	100	93.5

*Longitudinal observations made in a patient ST at ages 6, 8, 10, 12, 14 and 16; measured from Co (Condylion) to ANS (a point on the lower curvature of the anterior nasal spine where the vertical thickness is 3 mm)

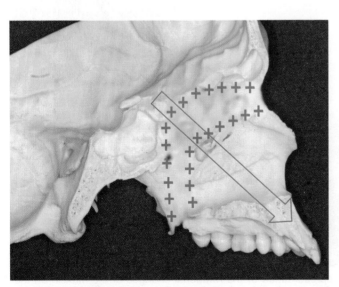

Figure 1.4 Sagittal section of the skull showing downward and forward displacement of the maxilla.

septum, especially the vomer and the perpendicular plate of the ethmoid, carries the nasomaxillary complex downward and forward.[1] At birth, the nasal septum is made up entirely of cartilage and extends down to lie within the U-shaped vomer in the vomerine groove. During the first year of life, ossification begins in the perpendicular plate of the ethmoid. By 3 years of age, ethmoid reaches the vomer, and by 10 years of age, it is in contact. After this period, the downward growth of the upper face occurs primarily by the process of apposition. On an average, the amount of this vertical displacement measured from the S–N plane to the palatal plane is just over 1 mm per year.

The maxilla, as a result of remodelling changes, takes on periosteal deposits of bone on all of its surfaces. The most significant amount of bone deposition occurs on the posterior aspect of the maxilla. This, in addition to the lateral deposits, allows for lengthening of the dental arch and eruption of the upper teeth. The palate receives periosteal deposits on its oral surface and is resorbed on its nasal surface. In addition to these horizontal and vertical growth changes, the maxilla can undergo rotational change (Fig. 1.6). The maxilla can rotate in a downward and forward direction anteriorly, as occurs in the anterior deep bite case, or it can rotate in an upward and forward direction, as occurs in anterior open bite case. The amount and the direction of these rotational changes can be determined by the angle between the S–N plane and the palatal plane or by the angle of inclination (AM Schwarz) between the Pn line (perpendicular from N')

and the palatal plane. The posterior end of the hard palate does not seem to be subjected to influence by Class III elastics.[8] However, the maxillary molars may be encouraged to grow downward away from the palatal plane. Anterior end of the hard palate is easily influenced by Class II elastics and extraoral anchorage.[9] Growth at the intermaxillary and interpalatine sutures, contributing mainly to the maxillary width, occurs during the first 5 years of life.

MANDIBLE

Compared with the growth of the maxilla, both endochondral and periosteal activities play an important role in growth of the mandible. For years, the condylar cartilage was considered a primary growth centre, acting in a manner similar to the epiphyseal growth plate of a long bone. However, histologically, the condylar cartilage is quite different from the cartilage of the epiphyseal

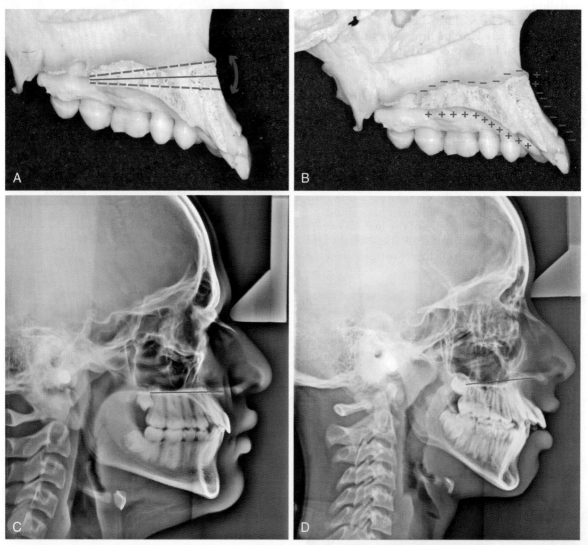

Figure 1.6 Rotational changes in the maxilla. **(A)** Diagrammatic representation of the rotational changes of the maxilla on the sagittal section of the skull. **(B)** Surface remodelling changes at the nasal floor, the roof of the mouth and the anterior surface below the anterior nasal spine. **(C)** Normal orientation of the palatal plane. **(D)** The palatal plane is tipped upward anteriorly.

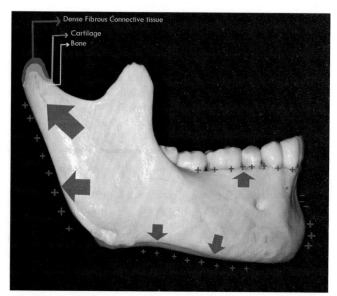

Figure 1.7 Surface remodelling changes in the mandible. Diagrammatic representation of the unique growth mechanism of the mandibular condyle showing both interstitial and appositional proliferations.

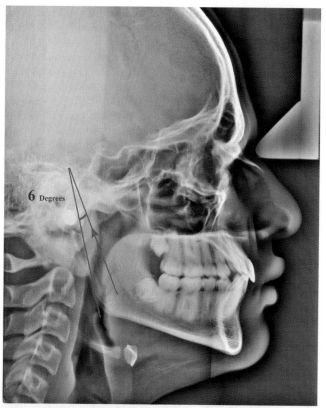

Figure 1.8 Directional changes in the growth of the mandibular condyles from 7 to 19 years of age.

growth plate. The mandible is a unique bone that grows in many different ways. It should not be considered a single growth entity but rather different entities, mainly at condyle and ramus, corpus, posterior alveolar process and anterior alveolar process. Other than condyle, all other areas of the mandible are formed and grow by direct surface apposition and remodelling (Fig. 1.7).[6]

Björk[10] provided an excellent information on the growth of the mandible with his implant studies. These studies revealed that average direction of condylar growth was 6° anterior to a line drawn tangent to the posterior border of the ramus (Fig. 1.8). This emphasized the distinct curvature in the direction of condylar growth. He observed condylar growth of 3 mm per year during the childhood period, a slight decrease to prepubertal minimum, followed by an adolescent spurt peaking at 5.5 mm per year at approximately 14.5 years of age. Baumrind et al[1] observed that condylar growth remains relatively constant between 8.5 and 15.5 years for both treated and untreated patients. The results of another study showed that the condyle grew between 0.8 and 1.3 mm posteriorly and between 9.0 and 10.7 mm superiorly over the 4-year period.[5] The vertical condylar growth was approximately nine times greater than the posterior condylar growth. Boys showed significantly greater superior condylar growth during adolescence than during childhood.

The average individual experiences resorption below the ramus and deposition of bone below the symphysis. These two changes by themselves would tend to increase the gonial angle. The anterior aspect of the chin is generally unaffected and chin prominence occurred by horizontal growth and some resorption at point B. Due to extensive and variable remodelling changes on the inferior border of the mandible, it is considered unsuitable to be used as a reference plane. Björk stated that the four areas in the mandible that are most suitable for the purpose of superimposition are the tip of chin, the inner

cortical surface of the inferior border of symphysis, the mandibular canal and the lower contour of the third molar germ from mineralization to root formation.

The posterior growth of the condyle and the posterior border of the ramus contribute to the elongation of the mandibular corpus and the primary displacement of the mandible. Table 1.2 shows growth changes in the mandibular length. The mandible also undergoes secondary displacement as a result of the enlargement of the middle cranial fossa. However, this is not as pronounced as that of the maxilla since the middle cranial fossa growth is mostly localized anterior to the

Table 1.2   Mandibular length changes (MM)*

Age	Male	Females
6	98	96
8	103.5	101
10	107	106
12	112	112
14	119.5	116
16	126	118

*Longitudinal observations made in a patient ST at ages 6, 8, 10, 12, 14 and 16; measured from Co (Condylion) to Gn (Gnathion).

condyles. On the average, ramus height increases by 1–2 mm per year and body length increases by 2–3 mm per year.[12]

The mandible also undergoes rotational change due to the rotation that occurs in the core of the jaw, called *internal rotation*, and due to surface bone remodelling and alterations in the rate of tooth eruption leading to *external rotation*[13] (Fig. 1.9). The internal rotation essentially consists of rotation around the condyle (matrix rotation, 25%; Fig. 1.9A) and rotation centred within the body of the mandible (intramatrix rotation, 75%; Fig. 1.9B). The combination of internal and external rotations results into the overall change in the orientation of the jaw. In majority of the individuals, the core of the mandible, the bone that surrounds the inferior alveolar nerve, rotates during growth in a manner that tends to decrease the mandibular plane (MP) angle (up anteriorly and down posteriorly).

The compensatory surface changes (external rotation) do not allow proportionate decrease in the MP angle as a result of the forward rotation of the core of the mandible. In the average individual, during childhood and adolescence, approximately 15° of internal rotation (forward rotation), as observed normally, results into just 3°–4° of decrease in MP angle due to compensatory 11°–12° of external rotation (backward rotation). This compensatory external rotational change is considered to be due to resorption at the posterior part of the lower border of the mandible and due to the apposition at the anterior part of the lower border.

DENTAL ARCHES

The growth of the maxillary and mandibular alveolar bone is significantly influenced by the presence and eruption of the teeth. Alveolar processes undergo selective remodelling changes through bone deposition and resorption. The facial height is increased primarily due to the vertical growth of the maxillary and the mandibular alveolar processes, which in turn is determined by the eruption of the teeth.

As mentioned earlier, the growth of the alveolar processes is influenced by the presence and the eruption of the teeth. After the eruption of teeth, the progression of the primary dentition to the permanent dentition has an impact on dental arch length, circumference and intercanine and intermolar widths[14] (Fig. 1.10). In the maxillary arch, there is an increase in the intercanine width by an average of 6 mm between 3 and 13 years of age and by an average of 1.7 mm between 13 and 45 years of age.[14] The intermolar width in the primary dentition increases by 2 mm between 3 and 5 years of age. The inter-first-molar width increases by 2.2 mm between 8 and 13 years of age, and by 45 years of age, it decreases by 1 mm.

In the mandibular arch, the intercanine width increases by approximately 3.7 mm and then decreases by 1.2 mm between 13 and 45 years of age.[14] There is an increase in intermolar width of 1.5 mm between 3 and 5 years of age. An increase in inter-first-molar width of 1 mm between 8 and 13 years of age is followed by a decrease of 1 mm by 45 years of age.[14] Certain changes in the mixed and permanent dentition, like uprighting of the incisors and the loss of the leeway space, result in decrease in the arch length.

HORIZONTAL AND VERTICAL GROWTH INTER-RELATIONSHIP

It has been recognized that the growth at the mandibular condyles brings the chin forward, not downward, nor downward and forward. Then, how does the chin move downward and forward or downward and backward? It is only when the vertical growth increments of facial growth begin to influence the condylar growth through occlusal contact that a downward and forward/backward direction of the chin is produced. Therefore, the final vector of growth of the chin is a resultant of the interaction between horizontal growth (condylar growth) and vertical growth (vertical growth of molars). If the condylar growth is greater than the vertical growth in the molar region, there is counterclockwise rotation of the mandible with a resultant horizontal change in

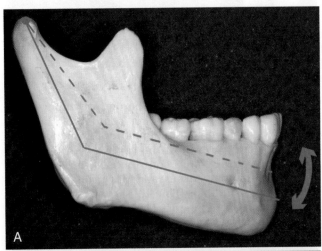

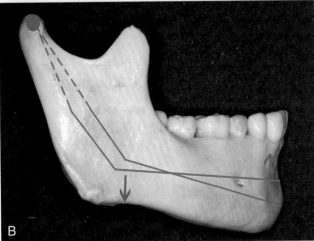

Figure 1.9 Internal rotation of the mandible. **(A)** Rotation around the condyle (matrix rotation). **(B)** Rotation within the body of the mandible (intramatrix rotation).

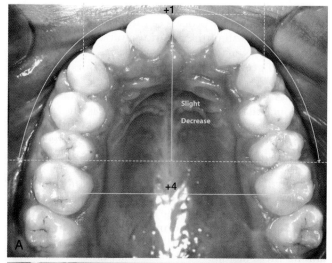

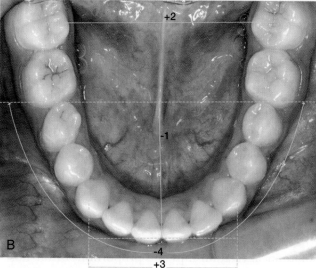

Figure 1.10 Dimensional changes (in millimetres) in dental arches between 6 and 18 years of age. **(A)** Maxillary arch changes. **(B)** Mandibular arch changes.

3. Growth of the mandibular posterior alveolar processes leads to the movement of molars towards the occlusal plane.

It should be remembered that, in a patient with clockwise rotation of the mandible, an excessive vertical growth would not help to reduce the ANB angle and also the correction of Class II molar relationship. However, it does facilitate the correction and retention of overbite.[15] On the other hand, counterclockwise rotation of the mandible associated with excessive condylar growth moves the pogonion forward, increases the facial angle, flattens the MP and tends to increase the overbite. In patients showing this type of growth pattern, it is difficult to correct the overbite and retain it. Therefore, molar height plays an important role in controlling the vertical position and, to some extent, the anteroposterior position of the chin.

It is evident from the above discussion that the clinician must have deep understanding of these five principal growth increments — condylar growth, anteroposterior growth at nasion, the vertical growth of the corpus of the maxilla, vertical growth of the maxillary alveolar process and the vertical growth of the mandibular alveolar process — and the impact of their interaction on the chin position and outcome of the treatment. For the normal expression of the growth and the behaviour of the mandible, the condylar growth should equal the total of other four growth increments[15] (Fig. 1.11). The

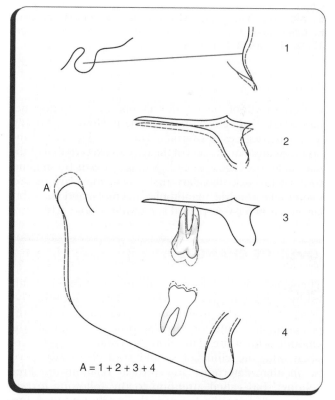

Figure 1.11 Growth increments. In an individual with average facial growth, Condyle **(A)** should be equal to combined increments at nasion **(1)**, maxilla **(2)**, maxillary dentition **(3)**, and mandibular dentition **(4)**.

the chin position and a less increase in anterior facial height. The greater change in this relationship leads to deep bite. However, if the vertical growth in the molar region is greater than the growth at the condyles, the mandible rotates clockwise with a resultant vertical change in the chin position (less horizontal change) and an increased anterior facial height. The greater change in this relationship causes open bite.

Fred Schudy[15] pointed out that the following vertical growth increments contribute to an increase in facial height:

1. Growth at nasion and in the corpus of the maxilla increases the distance between the nasion and the anterior nasal spine and the movement of the maxillary molars and posterior nasal spine away from the SN plane.
2. Growth of the maxillary posterior alveolar processes causes the maxillary molars to move away from the palatal plane.

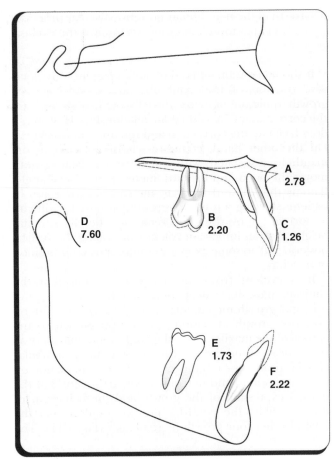

Figure 1.12 Average growth (in millimetres) of A, maxilla; B, maxillary first molar; C, maxillary incisor; D, condyle; E, mandibular first molar and F, mandibular incisor, from 12 to 15 years (a 3-year period).

vertical growth of the anterior alveolar processes does not have a significant effect on facial height. However, it results in varying degrees of overbite. The vertical growth of the posterior alveolar process of the maxilla exceeds that of the mandible from age 8 to 14.[16] Average growth (in millimetres) of maxilla, maxillary first molar, maxillary incisor, mandibular condyle, mandibular first molar and mandibular incisor in a 3-year period is shown in Figure 1.12.

OVERBITE CHANGES

The growth of the jaws plays an important role in establishing varying degrees of overbite. The relationship between the condylar growth and the vertical growth of the posterior and anterior alveolar processes controls the amount of overbite. Therefore, to control deep bite or open bite, the clinician should control growth increments that determine this vertical relationship. Fred Schudy[17] has called attention to the following growth increments that are relevant to the overbite relationship.

1. The mandibular condyles
2. The body of the maxilla, having effect of lowering the palatal plane

3. Posterior alveolar process of the maxilla
4. Posterior alveolar process of the mandible
5. Vertical growth of the anterior alveolar process of the maxilla
6. Vertical growth of the mandibular incisors

As mentioned earlier, the vertical growth of the body of the maxilla and maxillary molars has the effect of pushing the mandible downward and backward through occlusal contact, influencing the overbite. The downward growth of the maxillary molars significantly exceeds the downward growth of maxillary incisors (by almost 2:1). Of all the six growth increments, the movement of maxillary incisors downward and away from the palatal pane is the smallest, while the mandibular incisor growth is perhaps the greatest and most variable.[17] The vertical growth of the mandibular molars plays a minor role among these factors.

FACIAL SOFT TISSUE GROWTH

Establishing optimal facial aesthetics is the primary goal of orthodontic treatment. As the position of the underlying hard tissues influences the morphology of the overlying facial soft tissues, it is essential for the clinician to have adequate knowledge of the soft tissue components of the face. In addition to this, the soft tissues of the face undergo significant changes throughout life due to growth, maturation and ageing; this information plays an important role in orthodontic diagnosis and treatment planning.

Nasal growth

Anatomical relationships and proportions of the nose, lips and chin largely determine the configuration of the face. The balance and harmony among these components is essential for the pleasing soft tissue facial profile. This is influenced by both growth and orthodontic treatment. In addition to understanding the changes that occur due to orthodontic treatment, the clinician should have knowledge about the amount and the direction of growth of the soft tissue elements of the face.

The projection of the 'dorsal hump' is increased due to the rotation of the upper nasal dorsum upward and forward (counterclockwise) between 6 and 14 years of age.[18] The lower dorsum growth changes are related to vertical and horizontal skeletal patterns in the lower face, with clockwise rotation of the lower dorsum in vertically growing individuals. In females, the nasal projection remains virtually constant from 12 to 17 years of age, while in males, it shows a continued greater rate of growth with a resultant greater degree of nasal prominence at age 17.[19] Several studies have pointed out that the nose grows downward and forward[20,21] (Fig. 1.13). Both males and females experience proportionally more growth in the vertical dimension than the anteroposterior projection of the nose. In males, a spurt of growth occurs between 10 and 16 years of age with its peak from 13 to 14 years.[20] The females show comparatively a steadier growth curve, with small percentage of subjects showing a nasal growth

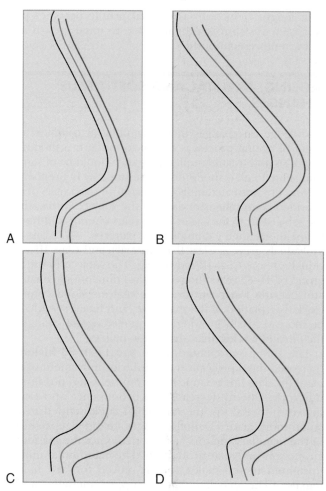

Figure 1.13 Nasal growth **(A)** Class I male. **(B)** Class I female. **(C)** Class II male. **(D)** Class II female.

Table 1.3 Length and height of the nose

	Nose Length		Vertical Height of Nose	
Age	Male	Female	Male	Female
6	42.2	40.8	35	33.2
8	45.0	43.2	37.8	34.8
10	47.7	46.1	39.8	37.2
12	50.3	49.8	42.0	40.1
14	53.0	52.2	44.2	42
16	57.8	55.1	46.4	43.6

spurt around the age of 12 years. The majority of growth in length of the nasal bones takes place before the age of 10 years, but the soft tissues continue to grow downward and forward along with the maxillary complex.[22] The growth changes in length and height of the nose are shown in Table 1.3.

Growth changes in the lip length and thickness

The upper lip rapidly increases in length from approximately 1 to 3 years of age, with a reduction in the rate of incremental growth between 3 and 6 years of age.[20] From age 6 onward, a progressive increase in lip length continues till age 15. Most of the maxillary lip length is achieved by age 14 in females and by age 18 in males. The mandibular lip length growth continues longer than the maxillary lip length growth in females, which is completed by age 16.[23] The incremental growth is greater in males than in females, which is not entirely completed by age 18. The changes in the lower anterior facial height due to vertical skeletal and dentoalveolar growth are usually concluded before completion of vertical lip growth, with comparatively more growth of the lower lip than the upper lip.[24] Similar to many aspects of facial growth, the vertical growth of the lips is age and gender related.

The upper lip thickness increases in both males and females between 1 and 14 years of age, which continues in males beyond age 14.[20] The upper lip thickness increases more in the vermilion region than in the part of the lip overlying point A. This change is proportional to the increase in length of the lip. In a similar manner, an increase in the thickness of the lower lip is greater in the vermilion region than at pogonion and point B. The upper lip thickness in females is at its maximum by 14 years of age and remains the same till age 16, with lip thinning afterward.[23] In males, the upper lip thickness is at its maximum by 16 years of age, with lip thinning afterward. The lower lip thickness in both males and females is generally concluded by 15 years of age.[23]

The chin growth

The soft tissue chin thickness in females from 7 to 9 years of age is 11.7 mm, which increases by 1.6 mm up to age 17, whereas in males, it is 10.8 mm from age 7 to 9 and shows an increase of 2.4 mm up to age 17.[19] This results in similar soft tissue chin thickness of 13.3 mm in both males and females at the age of 17 years.

POST-TREATMENT CRANIOFACIAL GROWTH

In this chapter, the discussion on craniofacial growth so far has been related to actively growing individuals who constitute a large portion of the average orthodontic patient population. However, a portion of growth that usually occurs after orthodontic treatment can influence the long-term stability of a treated case. Therefore, for comprehensive and successful treatment of the growing child, every clinician should have knowledge about this 'terminal growth' of the craniofacial complex. George Schudy[25] studied 74 orthodontically treated Caucasians to analyze the effects of post-treatment terminal growth on dentition and deeper basal structures (Fig. 1.14). He suggested that the typical terminal growth is characterized by a decrease in SN–MP, SN–occlusal plane and the gonial angle. The mandible moves forward more than the maxilla, and the

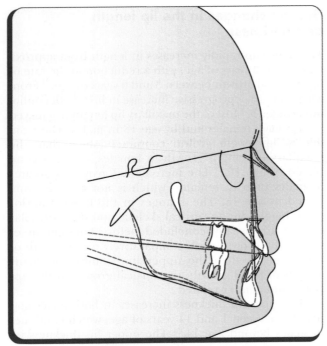

Figure 1.14 Terminal growth changes seen between 14 years 4 months and 19 years 7 months.

condylar growth proceeds in a predominantly vertical direction. The maxillary first molar moves forward more than the mandibular first molar. The upper incisors usually tip forward during the terminal phase of jaw growth. Post-treatment mandibular rotation, expressed by decreased SN–MP angle and lingual movement of lower incisor teeth, contribute to the overbite relapse and

arch length reduction. The facial profile becomes progressively less convex primarily due to nasal growth and forward movement of the chin.

AGEING: SKELETAL AND SOFT TISSUE CHANGES

Knowledge on changes in the dentofacial complex as a result of ageing process is crucial to modern orthodontic diagnosis and treatment planning and should be of significant value to all orthodontists. The study by Behrents[26] involving 113 untreated individuals from 17 to 83 years of age provided comprehensive data on the subject. In his study, the subjects from the age of 17–41 years (young adulthood) maintained their craniofacial patterns — Class II individuals grew as Class II individuals, and Class III individuals grew as Class III individuals. The subjects in the age group of 41–83 years showed vertical dimensional changes and became less protrusive. The males showed counterclockwise rotation of the mandible, and females tended to be more vertically growing. The percentage of change in the females was less than that in the males.

The soft tissue changes from age 17 to 83 included increased nasal projection and inferior movement of the nasal tip. The lips became less prominent and positioned inferiorly. Due to decreased lip prominence and lowering of the nasal tip, the nasolabial angle tended to become more acute. Dental changes included uprighting of the maxillary incisors and protrusion of the mandibular incisors in female group only. The mandibular molars uprighted in the males, and it moved forward in the females. The maxillary molars tipped mesially in the males, and it uprighted in the females.

CONCLUSION

Orthodontics influences jaw position, brings about changes in the position of teeth, and facial profile in patients who are changing themselves due to growth and ageing process. In other words, orthodontist has a moving target. Fundamental to the treatment provided for young patients is an understanding of how their faces are changing while under orthodontic care.

The knowledge of growth and development distinguishes orthodontists from many other dental practitioners. Patient demand for straight and beautiful teeth and a pleasant smile has never been greater. This has led many clinicians to invest

considerable time, effort and money mastering various treatment techniques and procedures. While this is certainly commendable, it should be recognized that moving teeth efficiently in their desired positions is one aspect; but making them last long in their final positions, and function in harmony with the rest of the masticatory system are another important aspects. With a broad knowledge of dental, skeletal and soft-tissue facial growth and development, the clinicians will be able to manage their cases successfully, and will also be able to communicate better with patients and parents about orthodontic treatment.

REFERENCES

1. Knott VB. Changes in the cranial base measures of human males and females from age 6 years to early adulthood. Growth 1971; 35:145–158.
2. Hight JR. The correlation of spheno-occipital synchondrosis fusion to hand-wrist maturation. Am J Orthod 1981; 79:464–465.
3. Björk A. Cranial base development. Am J Orthod 1955; 41:198–225.
4. Baumrind S, Korn EL, Isaacson RJ, et al. Superimpositional assessment of treatment-associated changes in the temporomandibular joint and the mandibular symphysis. Am J Orthod 1983; 84:443–465.
5. Buschang PH, Santos-Pinto A. Condylar growth and glenoid fossa displacement during childhood and adolescence. Am J Orthod Dentofacial Orthop 1998; 113:437–442.
6. Enlow DH. Facial growth. 3rd edn. Philadelphia: WB Saunders; 1990.
7. Björk A. Sutural growth of the upper face studied by the implant method. Acta Odontol Scand 1966; 24(2):109–127.
8. Schudy FF. Vertical growth versus anteroposterior growth as related to function and treatment. Angle Orthod 1964; 34(2):75–93.
9. Ricketts RM. The influence of orthodontic treatment on facial growth and development. Angle Orthod 1960; 30:103–133.
10. Björk A. Variations in the growth of the human mandible. Longitudinal radiographic study by the implant method. J Dent Res 1963; 42(suppl 1):400–411.
11. Baumrind S, Ben-Bassat Y, Korn EL, et al. Mandibular remodeling measured on cephalograms I. Osseous changes relative to superimposition on metallic implants. Am J Orthod Dentofacial Orthop 1992; 102:134–142.

12. Riolo ML, Moyers RE, McNamara JAJr, et al. An atlas of craniofacial growth. Ann Arbor: University of Michigan, Center for human growth and development; 1974.

13. Björk A, Skieller V. Normal and abnormal growth of the mandible: a synthesis of longitudinal cephalometric implant studies over a period of 25 years. Eur J Orthod 1983; 5:1–46.

14. Bishara SE, Jakobsen JR, Treder J, et al. Arch width changes from 6 weeks to 45 years of age. Am J Orthod Dentofacial Orthop 1997; 111:401–409.

15. Schudy FF. The rotation of the mandible resulting from growth: its implications in orthodontic treatment. Angle Orthod 1965; 35(1):36–50.

16. Schudy FF. Vertical growth versus anteroposterior growth as related to function and treatment. Angle Orthod 1964; 34(3):75–93.

17. Schudy FF. The control of vertical over bite in clinical orthodontics. Angle Orthod 1968; 38(1):19–39.

18. Buschang PH, Ronald De La Cruz, Anthony D. Viazis, Arto Demirjian et al. Longitudinal shape changes of the nasal dorsum. Am J Orthod Dentofacial Orthop 1993; 103:539–543.

19. Genecov JS, Sinclair PM, Dechow PC. Development of the nose and soft tissue profile. Angle Orthod 1990; 60(3):191–198.

20. Subtelny JD. Longitudinal study of soft tissue facial structures and their profile characteristics, defined in relation to underlying skeletal structure. Am J Orthod 1959; 45:481–507.

21. Chaconas SJ. A statistical evaluation of nasal growth. Am J Orthod 1969; 56:403–414.

22. Manera JF, Subtelny MD. A cephalometric study of the growth of the nose. Am J Orthod 1961; 47:703–705.

23. Mamandras AH. Linear changes of the maxillary and mandibular lips. Am J Orthod 1988; 94:405–410.

24. Vig PS, Cohen AM. Vertical growth of the lips: a serial cephalometric study. Am J Orthod 1979; 75:405–415.

25. Schudy GF. Post-treatment craniofacial growth: its implications in orthodontic treatment. Am J Orthod 1974; 65(1):39–57.

26. Behrents RG. Growth in the aging craniofacial skeleton: craniofacial growth series. Ann Arbor: University of Michigan; 1985.

2 Diagnosis and Treatment Planning

Ashok Karad

Advances in diagnostic technology, appliance design innovations and expansion of practices to include diverse patient populations have transformed the face of orthodontics over the past several years. These have resulted in ever increasing levels of well-conceived efficient and customized care, while simultaneously increasing the challenge of designing a treatment plan appropriate for each individual patient. Accurate diagnosis is a key element in the design of any successful treatment plan.

Diagnosis in orthodontics, like in other disciplines of dentistry and medicine, is the recognition of abnormal conditions, the practical synthesis of the diagnostic information that helps the clinician to plan an appropriate treatment strategy. A well-designed questionnaire for patient interview, numerous clinical observations, individual findings and analysis of relevant diagnostic records are essential to establish a correct diagnosis. It is a scientific procedure and does not offer any scope for individual opinion or judgment. The information generated must be objective, relevant and accurate.

This information is sourced from patient history—both dental and medical examinations, clinical examination and functional analysis. As a part of a routine examination, it is supplemented with the findings of the analysis of various diagnostic records, like lateral cephalometric analysis. Certain cases may require further examination

methods or specialized diagnostic records to generate additional information about a specific area. These various individual findings must be properly synthesized to result into a summary of the most important findings, devoid of any insignificant information having no relevance to the treatment. The clinician's ability to interpret and synthesize the relevant data is a key to establish comprehensive diagnosis. Improper or inaccurate diagnosis is often caused by insufficient information or predetermined decisions made in an effort to adapt the case to a particular type of treatment modality.

This requires that the practitioner should also have adequate knowledge about the craniofacial growth and its clinical implications as discussed in Chapter 1.

DIAGNOSTIC INFORMATION

The first step in the assessment of orthodontic patients is to generate relevant diagnostic information to establish accurate diagnosis and formulate a treatment plan. It is important to consider the improvement of patient's physical and emotional well-being as a part of a successful orthodontic treatment outcome. A sound knowledge of normal anatomy, growth and development is essential to recognize various dentofacial deformities.

The goals of diagnostic and treatment planning process are threefold:

1. To identify various elements of malocclusion and their contribution to the development of a problem
2. To define the nature of the abnormality with an emphasis on exploring the possible aetiological factor
3. To formulate a treatment plan based on the specific needs and desires of the patient

Patient interview (Questionnaire)

The patient interview is often the first formal interaction between the patient and the orthodontist. Patient's general personal information and demographic data should be recorded to facilitate efficient communication between the patient and the office. The patient interview essentially consists of family history and patient history. The goal is to understand the development of the problem to institute appropriate therapeutic procedures and eliminate early causative factors. The author considers the patient's chief complaint or concern as the most important ingredient of patient interview process, as it provides valuable information on whether the patient is seeking functional improvement, aesthetic improvement or both. It also helps in designing a treatment strategy that should ideally incorporate the specific needs and desires of the patient.

A family (genetic) history is aimed at gathering some valuable information about certain malocclusions and other abnormalities present in members of the same family. A data pertaining to the history of orthodontic treatment for any siblings of the patient and either or both parents and the nature of their problems should be recorded. It should be noted that relatively a large number of craniofacial abnormalities are inherited and transmitted through a dominant gene, while in cases of cleft lip and palate, it is mostly through a recessive gene. During the course of interaction, it is common to have a patient or a parent respond that a close relative had a severe problem that required surgery.

Patient's history should include any postnatal trauma, the manner of feeding and nutritional disturbances. Inquiries should be made with respect to the child's general development, like the initiation of walking and talking and the eruption of the first deciduous tooth. It is important to explore the possibility of having any abnormal habits, like digit sucking and mouth breathing. Relevant information regarding allergies, medications, previous hospitalizations or traumatic injuries should be carefully recorded. While taking patient history, psychological aspects of orthodontic treatment should be discussed with the patient to determine motivation and attitude towards treatment, treatment result expectations, patient compliance, etc. Such information is extremely useful to estimate future cooperation during treatment. Medical history of the patient forms an important part of the diagnostic information as it can indicate compromising factors that need special attention during treatment.

In patients with diabetes mellitus, it is essential to get blood glucose level under control prior to orthodontic treatment.[1] Plaque control is critical in such patients as they are more prone to develop tooth decay and periodontal breakdown. Diabetes-related microangiopathy can occasionally occur in the periapical vascular supply, resulting in unexplained odontalgia, sensitivity on percussion, pulpitis or even a loss of vitality in sound teeth.[2,3] The clinician should be alert to this phenomenon and should regularly check the vitality of teeth involved, especially when treatment is carried out for a prolonged duration. In adult patients with diabetes, it is important, prior to orthodontic treatment, to obtain a full-mouth periodontal examination including probing depth, plaque and gingivitis scores to determine the need for specific periodontal treatment. Deviations from appropriate diet and the scheduled insulin injections will result in distinct changes in the serum glucose level.[4] Hypoglycaemic reactions might occur more often in these patients. Type I diabetes mellitus is more often encountered in younger patients who frequently come for orthodontic treatment. For such patients, it is advisable to schedule long duration appointments in the morning hours, and the patient is advised to eat a usual meal and take required medication.

Orthodontic patients with bleeding disorders present two main challenges to the orthodontist: risk of viral infection (hepatitis and HIV) and risk of excessive bleeding. Treatment planning in such patients should incorporate reduction in the duration of treatment and nonextraction treatment whenever possible. Any gingival or mucosal irritation should be avoided; therefore, bonding of molar tubes is preferred over placing bands on the molars. In painful situations, it is better to prescribe acetaminophen with codeine, if required, and avoid aspirin. In case of gingival bleeding, 25% zinc chloride should be applied.

Patients with HIV infection are in an immunodeficient state and are more susceptible to infections. Therefore, necessary precautions should be taken to avoid cross-infections. Case history pertaining to the past and current medications should be obtained, and its relevance to the orthodontic treatment should be assessed. Low dosage of corticosteroids (1 mg/kg body weight) decreases tooth movement by suppressing osteoclastic activity.[5] However, high dosage of corticosteroids (15 mg/kg body weight) increases osteoclastic activity, producing more rapid tooth movement and subsequent relapse.[6] Therefore, it is advisable to avoid use of corticosteroids during orthodontic treatment.

As there are more and more adults seeking orthodontic treatment, it is important to know the impact of use of bisphosphonates, used in the treatment of osteoporosis and malignancies, on orthodontic treatment. Certain procedures, like extractions and placement of miniscrews for skeletal anchorage, should be avoided.[7]

Clinical examination

Orthodontic complications almost always arise from errors in diagnosis and not from failures in implementation of the proposed treatment plan. The clinical findings, therefore, become the basis of diagnostic procedures to establish accurate diagnosis. The goals of clinical examination are as follows:

1. To assess aesthetics, teeth and jaw relationships, hard and soft tissue pathology and jaw function
2. To determine the type of diagnostic records required
3. To determine the need for treatment

Natural head position

To record accurate clinical findings, the clinician should first determine the reference position of the patient in which the examination is carried out. For this purpose, it is appropriate to use the natural head position (NHP) in which the patient carries himself or herself in everyday life.[8,9] In this position, the patient is instructed to sit upright and look straight ahead into the horizon or directly into a mirror mounted on the wall. This establishes a true horizontal line, parallel to the floor, where pupils of the eyes are centred in the middle of the eyes (Fig. 2.1). It is based on the line of vision when the patient looks straight ahead, and it is related to the natural body posture and alignment with the cervical column.[10] This position has shown reproducibility within the clinically acceptable variation of 4° as compared to the variability of 26° of FH plane and SN plane.[9, 11] NHP radiograph is obtained with the patient in the cephalostat looking straight ahead into a mirror and ear rods placed directly in front of the tragus with light contact with the skin to stabilize head in transverse plane. The patient should also be observed from the side to make sure that the pupil is in the middle of the eye. It should be noted that the lateral cephalostat ear rods alter the position of the head and neck during postural recordings.[12] The patient should be comfortable and relaxed. The nose piece is then placed to establish third light contact with the skin, which secures the patient in NHP.

Extraoral examination

Cephalic and facial type

Extraoral examination should be carried with the patient in NHP. This essentially consists of an assessment of the facial structures and the shape of the head. The shape of the head can be determined by the measurements derived from the cephalic index (Fig. 2.2). It is based on the anthropological measurements of the width and the length of the head.

$$\text{Cephalic index} = \frac{\text{Maximum head width}}{\text{Maximum head length}}$$

- Dolichocephalic (long skull): less than 75.9
- Mesocephalic: 76.0–80.9
- Brachycephalic (short skull): 81.0–85.4

An assessment of facial frontal and profile view is essential in order to have a comprehensive understanding of the patient's aesthetic characteristics.[13] The facial type should be established from measurements derived from the proportional relationship of height and width of the face. The facial height and the width are determined by the distance between nasion and gnathion and bizygomatic width, respectively.

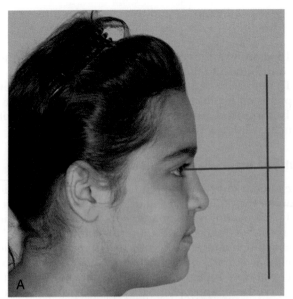

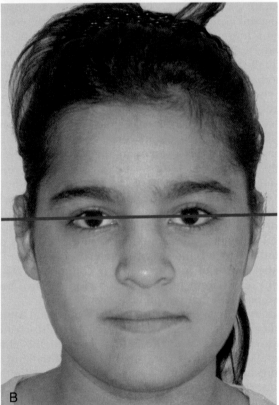

Figure 2.1 Natural head position. **(A)** The patient is looking straight ahead with the true horizontal coinciding with the line of vision and parallel to the floor. The pupils of the eyes are centred in the middle of the eyes. **(B)** The 'true vertical' is perpendicular to the floor and the 'true horizontal' (passing through the pupils).

$$\text{Facial index} = \frac{\text{Facial height (Nasion} - \text{Gnathion)}}{\text{Bizygomatic width (zy} - \text{zy)}}$$

- Euryprosop: 79.0–83.9
- Mesoprosop: 84.0–87.9
- Leptoprosop: 88.0–92.9

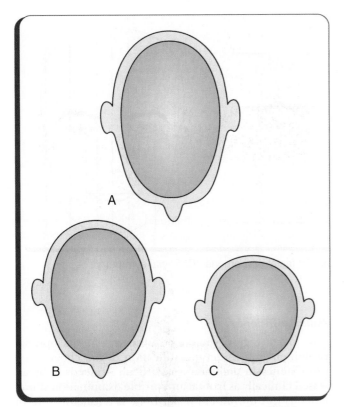

Figure 2.2 Cephalic type. **(A)** Dolichocephalic. **(B)** Mesocephalic. **(C)** Brachycephalic.

least maintaining the facial index. Also, it has been generally recognized that the form of the facial morphology has a certain relationship to the type of the archform. In a broader sense, expansion treatment modality is usually considered in borderline crowding cases of a broad facial type, while extractions are preferred in long face types.

Frontal facial examination

Frontal view of the face is evaluated to determine vertical and horizontal proportions and symmetry, as any abnormality in proportion or asymmetry significantly contributes to the impaired facial aesthetics. In a patient with harmonious facial morphology, the height of the upper face determined by the distance between the hairline and the glabella (supraorbital ridges) should equal the height of the mid-face (measured between the supraorbital ridges to the base of the nose) and should also equal the height of the lower face (distance between the base of the nose and the chin)[14] (Fig. 2.4A & B). Within the lower one-third of the face, the distance between the base of the nose and the stomion should be half the distance from the stomion to the chin. Usually, the forehead is considered to be narrow or wide based on its relationship to the bizygomatic width.

In a bilateral symmetric face, the true vertical or the mid-line passes through the middle of the forehead, tip of the nose, the lips and the chin, perpendicular to the true horizontal (the line of vision) and divides the face into right and left equal halves (Fig. 2.4C). Horizontally, the frontal face extending from left eye to right eye may be divided into three equal thirds: right and left eye widths and the nasal width. Also, the alar base (width of the base of the nose) should approximately equal the interinner canthal distance, and the width of the mouth should equal the distance between irises.[14] At this stage of facial examination, it is important to evaluate facial and dental midlines for any deviation. A slight amount of facial asymmetry is common and may be considered 'normal'. However, any gross facial asymmetry usually warrants further functional assessment for any

The average facial index in males is 88.5 ±5.1, and in females, it is 86.2 ±4.6. The facial index below normal is brachyfacial face type, indicating a broad and round face. The normal range facial index suggests that the face type is mesofacial, having average facial skeleton. If it is above normal, it is dolichofacial face type, indicating a long and narrow face due to high facial skeleton (Fig. 2.3). This has a high significance in treatment planning as orthodontic treatment mechanics should be directed towards normalizing or at

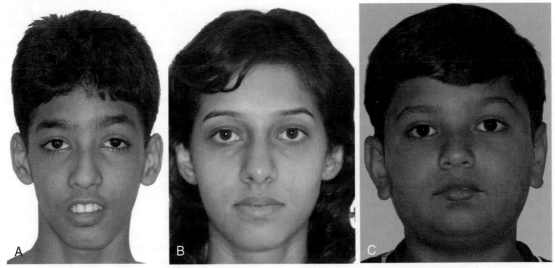

Figure 2.3 Facial type. **(A)** Dolichofacial. **(B)** Mesofacial. **(C)** Brachyfacial.

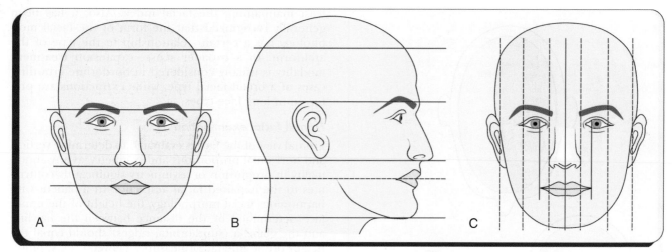

Figure 2.4 Frontal facial examination. **(A** and **B)** Vertical facial proportions. **(C)** Facial symmetry.

deviations during various mandibular movements and also a skeletal examination with a posteroanterior cephalogram. Such evaluation provides fairly good information to the clinician for the overall facial appearance and proportionality.

Profile facial examination

Examination of the facial profile of the patient is carried out to assess the jaw relationships and soft tissue drape, both anteroposteriorly and vertically. It is imperative that the patient is relaxed with the head oriented in the NHP. Variations in the configuration of the forehead have been observed according to age and gender and are genetically and ethnically determined. The lateral contour of the forehead can be flat, protruding or oblique. Patients with steep forehead generally tend to have more prognatic dental bases than those with flat forehead.

While assessing the facial profile, the clinician should consider vertical facial proportions (Fig. 2.5A) and the relationship between two vertical lines—one from the glabella to the base of the upper lip and the other from the base of the upper lip to the most prominent point on the chin. This establishes whether the face is convex, straight or concave (Fig. 2.5B). A convex angle indicates a Class II skeletal relationship, and a concave angle indicates a Class III skeletal relationship. The profile angle, however, only indicates the spatial relationship between the jaw bases relative to each other. Any deviation from the normal may be due to a disparity in absolute size, position or both. The facial divergence is determined by the inclination of the lower face relative to the forehead. Therefore, the possible line, normally straight and suggestive of an orthognathic profile, may slope anteriorly (anterior divergence) or posteriorly (posterior divergence). An inclination of MP should be clinically assessed by placing a scale or any instrument handle along the lower border of the mandible. A steep angulation indicates a high MP angle and usually a vertical growth direction. A nearly horizontal angulation indicates a low MP angle and generally a horizontal growth direction.

Malar sufficiency

The malar region should be observed for its optimal prominence. A direct quantification of the cheek bone prominence in millimetres is difficult. It needs to be assessed clinically as frontal and profile examination simultaneously. A prominent malar bone is a usual feature of an extreme case of horizontal grower (Fig. 2.6A). Malar insufficiency is usually seen in an individual with maxillary retrognathism (Fig. 2.6B).

Examination of nose

Morphological characteristics of the nose play an important role in the aesthetic appearance of the face (Fig. 2.7A). To get an overall estimate of nasal proportion, the clinician should assess the ratio of the nasal width to the nasal height (GL-Sn), which should be 70%.[15] Various anatomical parts of the nose, their analysis, interaction and role in nasal aesthetics and their contribution to an overall facial profile appearance may be evaluated with soft tissue cephalometric analysis. However, clinical examination should assess contour of the bridge and tip of the nose. The size, shape and width of the nostrils and position of the nasal septum should be assessed to determine an impairment of nasal breathing.

The nasolabial angle, formed by intersection of columella and upper lip tangent, should be in the range of 90°–120° (Fig. 2.7B). Its morphology is a function of several anatomic features. An acute nasolabial angle is an indication of procumbency of maxilla, while obtuse nasolabial angle is produced by maxillary retrusion. When facial profiles are compared between males and females, female profiles with smaller noses are more aesthetically pleasing, and it is ideal for females to have less prominent noses and for males to have more prominent ones in relation to their chins.[13]

Examination of lips

The purpose of this clinical examination is to assess the configuration of the lips, which includes lip length, thickness, competence and posture. It is performed when the patient is in a relaxed position and the lips are

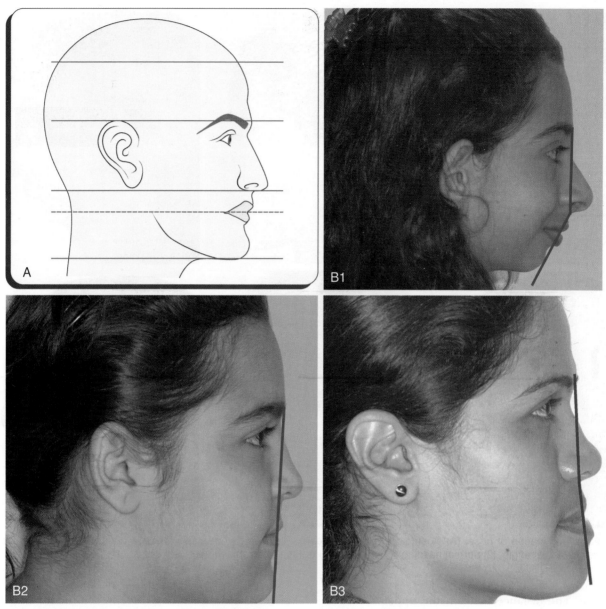

Figure 2.5 Profile facial examination. **(A)** Vertical facial profile proportions. **(B)** Profile types: (1) convex profile, (2) straight profile and (3) concave profile.

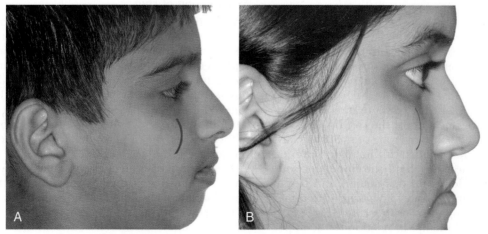

Figure 2.6 Cheek bone prominence. **(A)** Malar sufficiency. **(B)** Malar insufficiency.

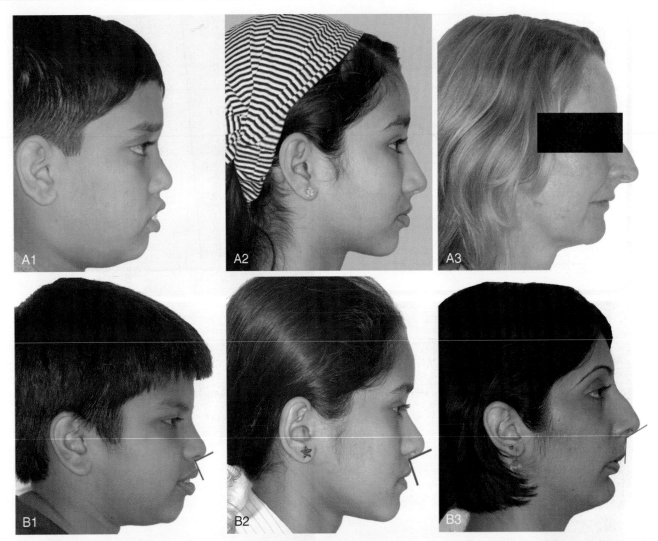

Figure 2.7 Examination of nose. **(A)** Nose sizes: (1) small noses, (2) average nose and (3) large nose. **(B)** Nasolabial angles: (1) acute nasolabial angle, (2) normal nasolabial angle and (3) obtuse nasolabial angle.

in repose. The distance between the upper and lower lips when in repose should ideally be 2–3 mm. If this distance is increased, the lips are considered to be incompetent (Fig. 2.8A). Under normal circumstances, the length of the upper lip measures one-third, and the lower lip and the chin measure two-thirds of the lower facial height. Incompetent lips could be due to either short upper lip or lips of normal length but everted as a result of incisor protrusion. The average upper lip length is 22 ±2 in males and 20 ±2 in females. A short upper lip results in incompetence of lips in the absence of incisor procumbancy. Ethnic characteristics do influence the lip protrusion. However, apart from this, lip protrusion is influenced by the configuration of underlying bony structures, thickness of the soft tissues, position of the anterior teeth and the tone of the orbicularis oris muscle. At rest, in patients with increased overjet, the lower lip is positioned behind the upper incisors. This situation causes lower lip dysfunction and is self-aggravating as the trapped lower lip pushes the upper teeth forward, increasing the overjet further (Fig. 2.8B). The vertical position of the lips in relation to the upper incisors should be assessed when the patient is in repose

(at rest) and on smiling. Ideally, the incisor display at rest should be 2–4 mm. On smiling, a gingival display of 1–3 mm is considered to be more aesthetic. It should be noted that with increasing age, the incisal display tends to reduce.

Examination of chin

The configuration of the chin plays an important role in facial aesthetics. It should be assessed in patient's NHP and relaxed facial musculature. The chin contour is evaluated with respect to the lower lip position and the configuration of the mentolabial fold (Fig. 2.9). It is influenced by underlying bony structure and thickness and tone of the mentalis muscle. The chin position, both anteroposterior and vertical, is determined by the growth of the condyle, the displacement of the glenoid fossa and the vertical growth of the molar teeth.

The mentolabial sulcus in an average individual is shallow and follows a gradual S-shaped curve (Fig. 2.10). A deep mentolabial sulcus is abnormal and is seen in case of reduced anterior facial height and lower anterior proclination. Abnormal muscle activity of the chin, observed clinically as puckering of skin over chin—golf ball chin,

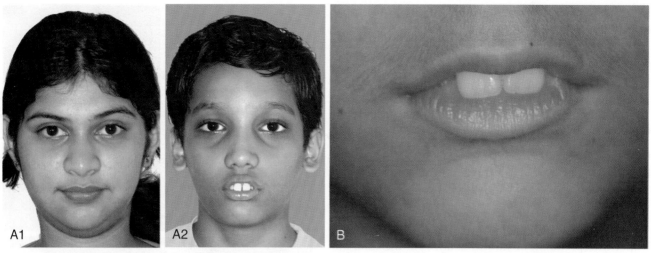

Figure 2.8 Examination of lips. **(A)** Lip competency: (1) competent lips and (2) incompetent lips. **(B)** Lower lip-trap.

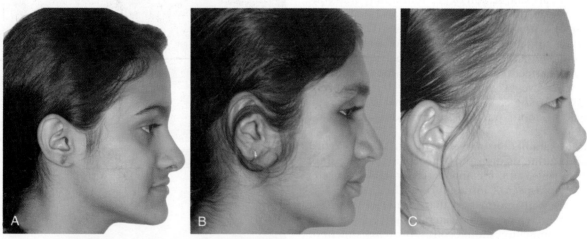

Figure 2.9 Assessment of chin. **(A)** Prominent chin. **(B)** Normal chin. **(C)** Deficient chin.

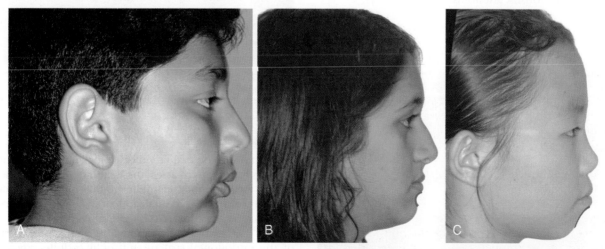

Figure 2.10 Mentolabial fold configuration. **(A)** Deep mentolabial sulcus. **(B)** Normal mentolabial sulcus. **(C)** Shallow mentolabial sulcus.

is suggestive of hyperactive mentalis. This may cause ret-roclination of mandibular incisors.

Another important factor that needs to be considered during an examination of facial profile is the determination of facial height. An increased or a decreased lower facial height, identified as long and short faces, presents the ultimate challenge to the orthodontist. The malocclusions that are associated with these distinct facial types are some of the most difficult treatment problems.

Intraoral examination

The findings of intraoral examination are the basis of diagnostic procedures. The goals of this part of clinical examination are: (1) to recognize individual teeth malpositions, and intra-arch and interarch relationships; (2) to detect any abnormality or pathology of soft tissue. Proper interpretation of various analyzes at the time of establishing a diagnosis requires that these findings are accurately recorded, which serve as the foundation for treatment decisions. Intraoral clinical examination essentially consists of the examination of hard and soft tissues. Clinical examination of the dentition should consist of an assessment of the dental status and an accurate recording of dental and occlusal anomalies (Fig. 2.11). It is important to determine the number of teeth present and the number of teeth missing and also the presence of supernumerary teeth. The maxillary and the mandibular dental arches are examined separately for archforms, symmetry, crowding of teeth, interproximal spacing, rotations, ectopic tooth positions, arch width and palatal depth (Fig. 2.12).

Clinical examination of the occlusion should record molar and canine relationships, interincisal relationship, overjet, overbite, anterior and posterior crossbites, etc. An important aspect of intraoral clinical examination is to reveal relevant information that cannot be obtained from the plaster models and lateral cephalogram. The soft tissue examination should consist of an assessment of tongue in relation to its size and posture; a gingival assessment pertaining to the gingival type, like thick-fibrous, thin-fragile, anterior gingival architecture and mucogingival lesions; an assessment of frenal attachments and an examination of tonsils, adenoids, etc. (Fig. 2.13).

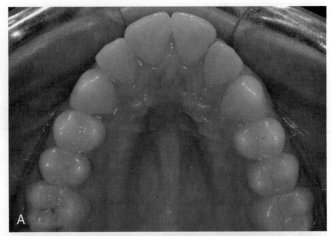

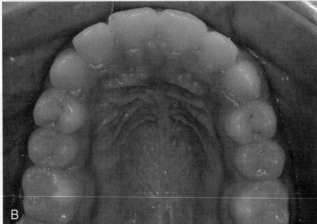

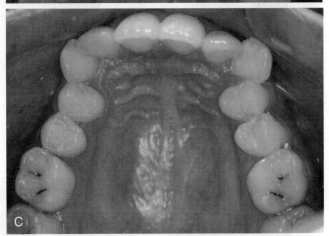

Figure 2.12 Maxillary archforms. **(A)** Narrow. **(B)** Ovoid. **(C)** Square.

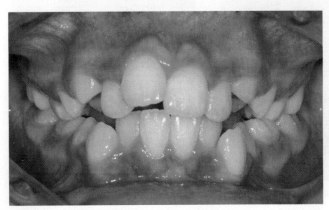

Figure 2.11 Severe malocclusion.

Evaluation of oral health

In addition to the evaluation of skeletal and dental anomalies, it is important to assess the health of oral hard and soft tissues. Orthodontic treatment should only be commenced following improved dental and oral health. A thorough dental caries or pulpal pathology evaluation is an important part of the orthodontic examination. Clinical examination of the periodontal structures should include gingival inflammation, the amount of attached gingiva, existing or potential mucogingival problems, etc. (Fig. 2.14).

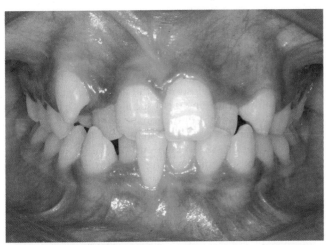

Figure 2.13 Mucogingival lesion in the region of mandibular right central incisor.

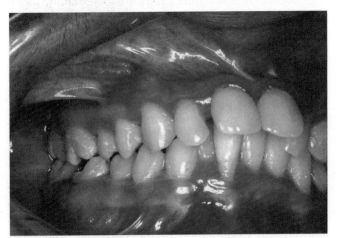

Figure 2.14 Compromised periodontal health.

Functional examination

Clinical examination of various components of the craniofacial complex in static relationship should be followed by the analysis of functional units of the masticatory system. The goals of this examination are directed towards the aetiologic evaluation of abnormality and the determination of type of orthodontic therapy. Modern orthodontic diagnosis and treatment planning should include three most important areas of functional analysis.[16]

1. Examination of the postural rest position of the mandible and the interposed freeway space
2. Examination of the temporomandibular joint (TMJ) function
3. Examination of orofacial function

Assessment of the postural rest position of the mandible

The primary goal of the functional analysis is to assess the mandibular position as determined by the musculature

(Fig. 2.15). The rest position of the mandible is influenced by the head and body posture. Therefore, it must be determined in an NHP, which can be reproduced easily. To determine this position, the patient is requested to repeat selected consonants. The letter 'M' or 'C' can be used, based on the fact that the mandible usually returns to postural rest. Alternatively, the patient can be requested to lick his or her lips first and then swallow to allow the mandible to return to the postural rest position. If the clinician is not being able to get the consistent postural rest position, another approach is to make careful observations as the patient talks or swallows as he or she has no idea of what is being examined.

Once the postural rest position of the mandible is determined, it can be registered by different methods. Extraorally, it is possible to make direct caliper measurements on the patients profile. The distance between the two points, e.g. nasion and menton, is measured in both postural rest and habitual occlusion. The difference between the two measurements determines the interocclusal space. The cephalometric method is considered to be most reliable in providing successful results. It consists of obtaining three lateral cephalograms at three different positions: the first in the postural rest, the second in the initial contact of the teeth and the third in the habitual occlusion. The movement from the postural rest to the initial contact records the hinge movement of the condyle

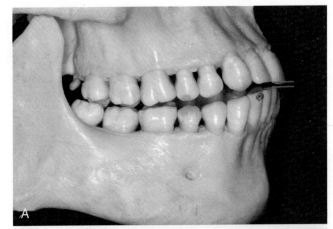

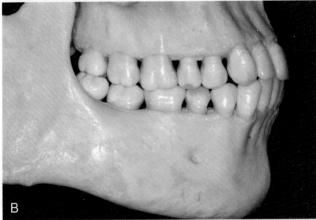

Figure 2.15 Functional examination. **(A)** Mandibular position at rest and interocclusal space. **(B)** Habitual occlusal position.

in the vertical plane, while the movement from the initial contact to the habitual occlusion is the sliding or translatory action in the sagittal plane. In orthodontic diagnosis, the clinician should assess the path of closure of the mandible from postural rest to habitual occlusion in sagittal, vertical and transverse planes.

Assessment in the sagittal plane

In the sagittal plane, it is important to know whether the movement of the mandible from the rest position to occlusion is pure hinge movement, partly hinge with anterior sliding or partly hinge with posterior sliding component (Fig. 2.16). This should be assessed in sagittal discrepancies, like Class II and Class III malocclusions.

1. Class II malocclusions

a. Class II malocclusions without functional disturbance, therefore, exhibiting pure hinge movement of the condyle in the fossa, with path of closure of the mandible straight upward and forward from the postural rest to occlusion, are considered to be true Class II malocclusions.
b. The path of closure from the rest position to occlusion in some Class II malocclusions may be upward and backward — a posterior shift, indicating a combined rotary and sliding movement. This functional Class II appears to be more severe than it actually is.

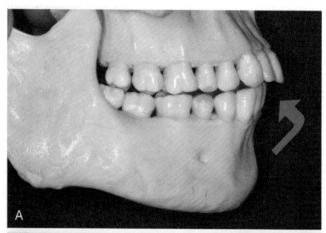

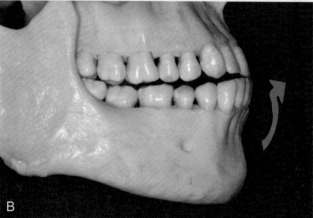

Figure 2.16 Mandibular path of closure. **(A)** Abnormal functional pattern with posterior sliding into the occlusal position. **(B)** Anterior sliding into the occlusal position.

c. Class II malocclusions with upward and forward displacement of the mandible upon closure appear to be less severe than they actually are.

2. Class III malocclusions

a. A straight path of closure of the mandible with a hinge-type condylar movement is associated with a true Class III malocclusion without functional component.
b. In patients with severe mandibular prognathism, the path of closure may be upward and backward — an anterior postural resting position. The mandible slides posteriorly into the position of maximum intercuspation, masking the true sagittal dysplasia.
c. The path of closure of the mandible characterized by an anterior displacement with rotary and translatory action of the condyle from postural rest to habitual occlusion is associated with pseudo-Class III malocclusion.

Assessment in the vertical plane

This assessment is of significant value in determining therapeutic potential of functional appliances in the management of deep overbite cases. The amount of interocclusal clearance between the true deep overbite and the pseudo-deep overbite problems can be a distinguishing factor. The true deep overbite, associated with a large interocclusal clearance and caused by infraocclusion of the posterior segments, has good prognosis with functional appliance therapy. The pseudo-deep overbite problem, associated with a small or normal interocclusal clearance due to normal eruption of the posterior teeth, has poor prognosis with functional appliances. The discrepancy is mainly caused by overeruption of the incisors, which requires intrusive mechanics on the incisor teeth with fixed appliances.

Assessment in the transverse plane

The clinical examination of the transverse functional relationships is carried out by assessing the path of closure of the mandible from postural rest to habitual occlusion. This can be done by observing the position of mandibular midline as the mandible moves from the postural rest to occlusion.

In patients with pseudo-crossbite, the midline shift of the mandible is observed only in the occlusal position, while in postural rest, the midlines are coincident and well centred. This clinical situation is usually caused by tooth guidance. In patients with true-crossbite, due to a true asymmetric facial skeleton, the midline deviation is observed in both habitual occlusion and postural rest position.

This part of the functional examination provides valuable information related to the indications and contraindications for use of functional appliances and the prognosis.

Examination of the TMJ

The functional analysis must include the examination of TMJs and associated structures to assess normal or abnormal joint function; clicking, pain and dysfunction are characteristic features of pathologic TMJs. During the TMJ examination of the patient, the clinician should look for the following:

1. Any 'clicking' noises
2. Possible sore muscles

3. Mandibular deviation on opening and closing
4. Signs of any parafunctional habits
5. Overall stress-level status of the patient

The key to understanding temporomandibular disorders is the differential diagnosis of the joint (internal derangement) as against the muscle pathology (myofascial pain) or the combination of the two.[17,18]

Any joint noise, like clicking or crepitus, may be diagnosed during anteroposterior or eccentric movements of the mandible with the use of a stethoscope or digital palpation. The joint clicking is differentiated as initial, intermediate, terminal and reciprocal clicking.[16] Initial clicking is associated with retruded condyle position in relation to the disc. Intermediate clicking is observed in patients with uneven condylar and articular disc surfaces. Terminal clicking is a sign of the condyle being moved too far anteriorly, in relation to the disc, on maximum jaw opening. Reciprocal clicking is observed during opening and closing and is suggestive of incoordination between displacement of the condyle and disc. Any crepitus joint sound, observed as a cracking sound, indicates a rough condyle, disc or eminence surface. It occurs as a result of direct, long-term bone contacts between the fossa and the condyle.[18]

Palpation of the TMJ and the musculature should be performed for possible pain or sore muscles in the neck and mouth area. During opening and closing jaw movements, the TMJs may be palpated to reveal any pain on pressure. Palpation of muscles involved in mandibular movements is considered a significant part of the clinical examination. The lateral pterygoid and the masseter muscles should be palpated and examined bilaterally on every orthodontic patient, and any palpatory tenderness should be recorded.

The opening and closing movements of the mandible should be evaluated for any deviation or the extent of these movements. The mandible usually tends to deviate towards the side of an anteriorly dislocated disc. Uncoordinated zigzag movements occur as a result of asynchronic pattern of muscle contractions. Under normal circumstances, the patient should be able to open the mouth anywhere between 35 and 45 mm. Quite often, the patient cannot open the mouth, a situation called a *closed lock*, due to the displaced disc interfering with mouth opening. However, on some occasions, the patient cannot close the mouth — a situation called *open lock* — as the posteriorly displaced disc may not allow the condyle to return to its position in the fossa.[19,20] If the joints demonstrate excessive mobility or hypermobility, it should be recorded in order to avoid overstretching the already compromised ligaments.[18]

The patient should also be examined for any signs of bruxism and clenching. It is usually night time clenching that, in many individuals, results in morning headaches. The patient's occlusion should be analyzed during various border excursions of the mandible for any prematuries or deflective contacts. This is because at the end of the orthodontic treatment, the patient should be left with a healthy masticatory musculature and good functional occlusion in centric, lateral excursive and protrusive movements.

Examination of orofacial function

A thorough analysis of all possible functions or dysfunctions of stomatognathic system is a part of modern orthodontic diagnosis and treatment planning. Any deviation in normal function may be a primary aetiologic factor in the development of a malocclusion. During the early stages of development, a child may develop unphysiologic reflex actions along with the normal physiologic reflex activities, which when prolonged may contribute to the development of a discrepancy. The resultant deformation of structures leads to the adaptive functional activity that may persist even after the disappearance of the original causative factor, e.g. thumb sucking habit. The functional examination to identify the abnormal functional aspects of stomatognathic system requires a detailed evaluation of the tongue, lips, swallowing, breathing, etc.

Examination of the tongue

The examination should essentially include an assessment of the tongue function, posture, size, etc. The abnormal tongue function, like tongue thrust, plays an important role in aetiopathogenesis of malocclusions (Fig. 2.17). This can be either a primary causative factor as a result of retained infantile deglutitional pattern or other abnormal pressure habits or a secondary or an adaptive to an existing abnormal skeletal or dentoalveolar pattern. The tongue thrust may be present in the anterior region, usually associated with anterior open bite, and in the lateral region, associated with the development of lateral open bites, or it can be a complex in nature, where occlusion is supported only in the molar region.

The tongue posture should be examined clinically with the mandible in postural rest position. The posture and the shape can be narrow and long, protracted or retracted, spread laterally and shortened, flat or arched, etc. The recognition of the type of tongue dysfunction is extremely important not only for determining its effect or associated deformity but also for generating useful information in designing the treatment strategy.

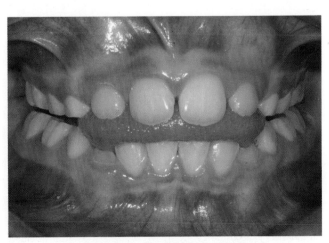

Figure 2.17   Tongue-thrust habit.

Deglutition

The functionally balanced or mature somatic swallow should take place without contracting the muscles of facial expression, the tongue inside the mouth and the teeth momentarily in contact. Abnormal swallowing is caused by retained infantile swallow or tongue thrust. The visceral or infantile swallow, found during the first few years of life, is gradually replaced by somatic or mature swallow as proprioception causes tongue postural and functional changes. Under normal developmental pattern, the functionally balanced or mature swallow is established between 2 and 4 years of age.

Examination of respiration

The clinical examination should incorporate an evaluation of respiration to determine the mode of breathing. An impaired nasal breathing represents a dysfunction of the orofacial musculature and interferes with the normal development of the dentition and orthodontic treatment. Patients with oronasal breathing typically present with constricted upper arch, deep palate, crossbite, poor oral hygiene and gingival hyperplasia. In patients with mouth breathing, the case history provides details regarding recurrent diseases of the upper air passages; the evaluation reveals low tongue posture and disturbed function, and the lip seal is usually inadequate.

Speech and malocclusion

Speech problems are quite often associated with severe malocclusion in some patients. The presence of certain abnormalities of teeth and jaws interferes with the normal production of certain sounds, thereby making the pronunciation of some words difficult or impossible (Table 2.1). Patients with impaired speech may require orthodontic treatment to correct abnormalities of teeth and jaws contributing to speech pathology, prior to effective speech therapy.

Diagnostic records and their analysis

It is essential to obtain high-quality, uncompromised diagnostic records for further evaluation of teeth and oral structures, occlusion and facial and jaw proportions. These records consist of study models and occlusal records, facial and intraoral photographs and radiographic records. The diagnostic records document the patient's pretreatment condition and provide additional information required to establish accurate diagnosis.

Study models

For the evaluation of the occlusion, a set of plaster study models should ideally display all teeth and alveolar processes. This requires that the impression is well extended into the labial/buccal and lingual sulci by producing maximum displacement of soft tissues. Also, for better visualization of asymmetries in the archform and tooth positions, models should be trimmed with a symmetric base. Poor quality study models do not offer adequate valuable diagnostic information.

It is important to obtain an occlusal record by registering the patient's wax-bite in habitual occlusion. The clinician should make sure that a gross discrepancy does not exist between this position and the retruded cuspal position. A sagittal discrepancy of 1–1.5 mm is of little significance; however, a discrepancy of greater magnitude or lateral shifts should be carefully recorded by obtaining centric relation (CR) bite registration.

Study model analysis is a three-dimensional evaluation of the maxillary and mandibular dental arches, the occlusion and the determination of the degree of malocclusion.

It must be correlated with other important diagnostic criteria, like cephalometric analysis and radiographic analysis. Certain relationships between arch width, length and mesiodistal tooth material have been expressed by various indices of Pont, Linder, Harth and Korkhaus. In modern orthodontic diagnosis, these methods are generally considered to be of minimal diagnostic value; however, they are still widely used in most of the orthodontic practices and institutions.

Archform analysis

1. The maxillary arch width in the premolar and molar regions should be assessed to determine, if it is narrow, normal or broad. These values depend on the combined mesiodistal widths of the four upper incisors (SI).

Pont Index

$$\text{Maxillary arch width (premolar region)} = \frac{\text{SI} \times 100}{80}$$

$$\text{Maxillary arch width (molar region)} = \frac{\text{SI} \times 100}{64}$$

$$\text{Linder and Harth modification} = \frac{\text{SI} \times 100}{85} \text{ and } \frac{\text{SI} \times 100}{64}$$

for the arch width in premolar and molar regions, respectively

The values thus obtained indicate the ideal values of premolar and molar widths. The actual measured values of the interpremolar (mesial occlusal pit of first premolars on either side) and intermolar (mesial occlusal pit of first molar on either side) widths are compared to the ideal values to conclude whether the arch is narrow, normal or broad.

Table 2.1 Occlusal traits and speech	
Occlusal relationship	**Associated speech problem**
Increased overjet	Distortions of / S / sound
Class III	Misarticulation of / f /, / V /
Anterior openbite	Defective speech sounds of / S /, / Z /, / th /
Maxillary anterior spacing	Distortions of / S /, / Z / sounds due to lisp
Irregular anterior teeth and palatal displacement of maxillary incisors	Difficulty in production of / t /, / d/ sounds

2. To assess the adequacy of the arch perimeter from molar to molar, to accommodate an existing tooth material or to assess the degree of discrepancy, Carey's analysis for the mandibular arch and arch perimeter analysis for the maxillary arch are used.

The arch length mesial to the first molars is measured by using soft brass wire that is placed on the occlusal surfaces over the contact points and the incisal edges. This is the measured arch length. The total tooth material is calculated by adding the individual mesiodistal widths of the teeth mesial to the first molars.

When the measured arch length and the total tooth material are compared, if the discrepancy is less than 2.5 mm, the case should be treated nonextraction; if it is between 2.5 and 5 mm, second bicuspids should be extracted; and if the discrepancy is above 5 mm, first bicuspids are extracted.

3. To assess basal arch width and length of the maxilla and to determine the treatment modality, extraction or expansion, based on the degree of dental arch width, Ashley Howe's analysis is used.

$$\text{Ashley Howe's index} = \frac{\text{CFD} \times 100}{\text{TTM}},$$

where CFD is the canine fossa distance and TTM is the total tooth material.

If the ratio is less than 37%, extractions are required to resolve the discrepancy; if it is between 37% and 44%, the case is borderline; and if the ratio is more than 44%, no extractions are required.

Bolton's tooth ratio analysis

This is used to identify any occlusal misfit that is caused by interarch tooth-size incompatibility. By studying the ratios of total mandibular versus maxillary tooth size and anterior mandibular versus maxillary tooth size, one may estimate the overbite and overjet relationships likely to be obtained after treatment is finished. As the location and magnitude of tooth material excess is identified by this analysis, it helps guide the treatment planning to produce better posterior occlusion and incisal relationship. The procedure is as follows:

$$\text{Overall ratio} = \frac{\text{Sum of widths of mandibular 12 teeth}}{\text{Sum of widths of maxillary 12 teeth}} \times 100$$

An overall ratio of 91.3 $\pm$0.26 is considered ideal.

If the overall ratio is more than 91.3, then mandibular tooth material is excessive.

$$\begin{matrix}\text{Amount of} \\ \text{mandibular} \\ \text{tooth excess}\end{matrix} = \begin{matrix}\text{Sum of} \\ \text{mandibular} \\ \text{12 teeth}\end{matrix} - \frac{91.3 \times \text{Sum of} \\ \text{maxillary 12 teeth}}{100}$$

If the overall ratio is less than 91.3, then maxillary tooth material is excessive.

$$\begin{matrix}\text{Amount of} \\ \text{maxillary} \\ \text{tooth excess}\end{matrix} = \begin{matrix}\text{Sum of} \\ \text{maxillary} \\ \text{12 teeth}\end{matrix} - \frac{\text{Sum of mandibular} \\ \text{12 teeth} \times 100}{91.3}$$

Similarly, an anterior ratio is computed for the six anterior teeth in either arch.

$$\begin{matrix}\text{Anterior} \\ \text{ratio}\end{matrix} = \frac{\begin{matrix}\text{Sum of widths of} \\ \text{mandibular 6 anteriors}\end{matrix}}{\begin{matrix}\text{Sum of widths of} \\ \text{maxillary 6 anteriors}\end{matrix}} \times 100$$

An anterior ratio of 77.2 $\pm$0.22 is considered ideal.

If the anterior ratio is more than 77.2, then mandibular anterior tooth material is excessive.

$$\begin{matrix}\text{Mandibular} \\ \text{anterior} \\ \text{tooth excess}\end{matrix} = \begin{matrix}\text{Sum of} \\ \text{mandibular} \\ \text{6 anteriors}\end{matrix} - \frac{77.2 \times \text{Sum of} \\ \text{maxillary 6 anteriors}}{100}$$

If the anterior ratio is less than 77.2, then maxillary anterior tooth material is excessive.

$$\begin{matrix}\text{Maxillary} \\ \text{anterior} \\ \text{tooth excess}\end{matrix} = \begin{matrix}\text{Sum of} \\ \text{maxillary} \\ \text{6 anteriors}\end{matrix} - \frac{\text{Sum of mandibular} \\ \text{6 anteriors} \times 100}{77.2}$$

Ideal ratio will give ideal overbite and overjet relationship, provided the angulations and the labiolingual thickness of the teeth are correct.

When planning treatment, if there is maxillary anterior excess, proximal stripping of anteriors may be considered. If there is mandibular anterior excess, extraction of a lower incisor or proximal stripping may be considered.

Mixed dentition analysis

Mixed dentition analysis is useful to estimate the size of unerupted permanent teeth to calculate the space available. The information procured assists treatment planning in cases with intra-arch discrepancy (crowding, rotations, etc.) and in those requiring interarch occlusal adjustments.

Despite numerous suggested methods, they basically fall into two types:

1. Methods involving measurements from radiographic images
2. Methods involving use of prediction tables, for example, Moyers' prediction tables and Staley–Kreber graph.

Each method has its disadvantages and advantages. Accuracy, ethnic variations and ease of application need to be prime considerations while selecting a method. The author finds the following two methods to be reasonably accurate, easy and clinically useful.

1. Measurement of teeth on radiograph: A good quality, undistorted periapical radiograph is essential. The magnification on the radiograph can be accounted for by simply measuring another erupted tooth and applying the following proportionality equation:

$$\frac{\text{Actual width of primary molar}}{\text{Radiographic width of primary molar}}$$
$$= \frac{\text{Actual width of unerupted premolar}}{\text{Radiographic width of unerupted premolar}}$$

This method can be used in either arches and in all ethnic groups.

2. Tanaka and Johnston method: The width of the lower incisors is used to estimate the width of the unerupted canines and premolars. The method has a slight bias towards overestimating the unerupted tooth sizes.

Tanaka and Johnston Prediction Values:*

One-half of the mesiodistal width of the four lower incisors + 10.5 mm = estimated width of mandibular canine and premolars in one quadrant

One-half of the mesiodistal width of the four lower incisors + 11.0 mm = estimated width of maxillary canine and premolars in one quadrant

*(From Tanaka MM, Johnston, LE. J Am Dent Assoc 1974; 88:798). No radiographs or reference tables are required. Hence, it is very convenient.

Radiographic records

Radiographic records and their analysis form an integral part of orthodontic diagnosis. A routine clinical examination should be followed by obtaining necessary radiographs to confirm certain clinical findings and to generate additional information to establish an accurate diagnosis. As a part of routine examination, two types of radiographic records are required: panoramic, periapical and occlusal views to provide information regarding the condition of the teeth, bony structures, abnormal position of teeth, etc. and cephalometric radiographs to evaluate malocclusion with respect to facial proportions, components involved and their inter-relationships (Fig. 2.18).

Radiologic examination

A panoramic radiograph is valuable for orthodontic evaluation at any age. It provides a broader spectrum of views sufficient enough to show any pathologic lesions and supernumerary or impacted teeth. Trabecular pattern, bone loss, caries, developmental status of the teeth, etc. can be easily assessed, and the areas that require a detailed view with intraoral periapical radiographs can be identified. It is certainly a valuable tool for the screening examination to generate adequate information for the clinician to make crucial initial decisions. A series of intraoral periapical radiographs is essential for an adult patient with periodontal disease. For patients with impacted teeth or malposed unerupted teeth, intraoral occlusal radiograph is indicated to determine their exact location. For children and adolescents, bitewing radiographs may be required for a thorough assessment of interproximal caries. The basic principle of radiologic examination is to obtain maximum information with a minimum radiation exposure.

Cephalometric analysis

An analysis of the lateral cephalometric radiograph is one of the valuable tools used in orthodontic diagnosis and craniofacial research. With the help of various linear and angular measurements, both sagittally and vertically, it is possible to localize the malocclusion,

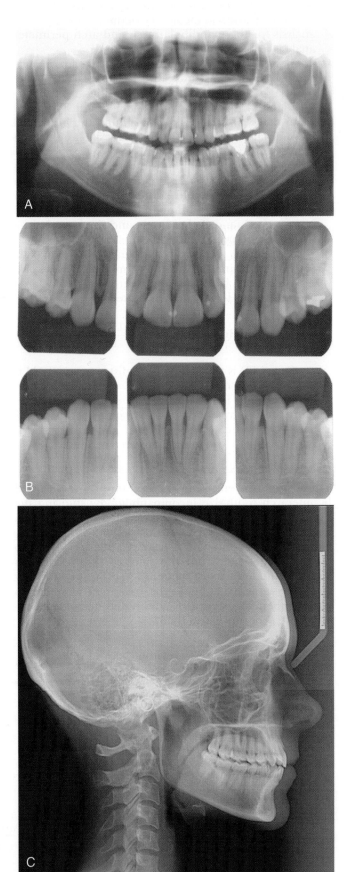

Figure 2.18 Radiographic records. **(A)** Orthopantomogram. **(B)** Intraoral periapical radiographs. **(C)** Lateral cephalogram.

assess the configuration of the facial skeleton, ascertain the extent of jaw bases and their inter-relationship, assess the soft tissue morphology, identify the growth pattern and direction, evaluate the axial inclination of incisors, analyze the post-treatment changes and define the treatment possibilities and limitations. As a clinician, it is important not to establish the diagnosis solely based on the lateral cephalometric analysis as it lacks information on certain important criteria, like transverse discrepancies, functional relationships and soft tissue dynamics.

Clinical examination is useful in assessing the facial proportions and jaw relations along with the soft tissue drape in all three planes of space. However, accurate quantification of size, position and orientation of the jaws, teeth and the soft tissues is possible only with cephalometric assessment. The information generated from cephalometric analysis helps in pinpointing the problem areas, which is essential in arriving at accurate diagnosis and establishing a detailed treatment plan. In fact, the data, on numerous occasions, also helps predict the prognosis for a case.

The basic cephalometric points required to analyze various components of the craniofacial complex are shown in Figure 2.19.

Systematic approach to cephalometric analysis should include assessment of:

- Cranial base
- Skeletal maxilla
- Maxillary dentoalveolar region
- Mandibular dentoalveolar region
- Skeletal mandible
- Maxillomandibular relation
- Soft tissues of the face

Cranial base assessment

Growth of the cranial base, though appears to be remote from the orthodontist's primary concern, influences the height and depth of the upper face and position of the upper teeth during orthodontic treatment (Fig. 2.20, Table 2.2). It is essential to assess the anterior and middle cranial fossa length (1,2) and flexure (3,4). Since the anterior and middle cranial fossae are related to the maxilla and the mandibular ramus, respectively, when they are of average length, an average length of the maxilla and the mandibular ramus is normal and expected. When the cranial fossae are shorter or longer, a corresponding change in the maxilla or ramus height may be considered normal. A greater flexure of the cranial base

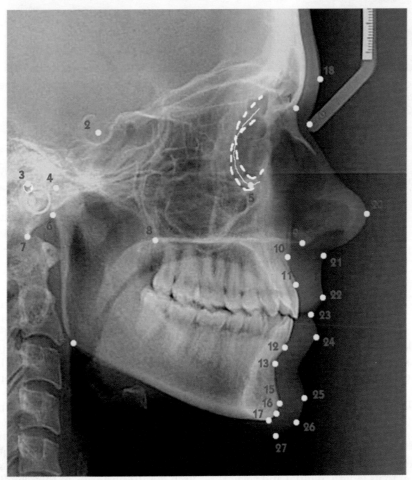

Figure 2.19 Cephalometric points. 1. N, hard tissue nasion; 2. S, sella; 3. Po, porion; 4. Co, condylion; 5. Or, orbitale; 6. Ar, articulare; 7. Ba, basion; 8. PNS, posterior nasal spine; 9. ANS, anterior nasal spine; 10. A, point A; 11. Pr, prosthion; 12. In, infradentale; 13. B, point B; 14. Go, gonion; 15. Pg, hard tissue pogonion; 16. Gn, hard tissue gnathion; 17. Me, hard tissue menton; 18. G, glabella; 19. N', soft tissue nasion; 20. P, pronasale; 21. Sn, subnasale; 22. Ls, labrale superior; 23. St, stomion; 24. Li, labrale inferius; 25. Pg', soft tissue pogonion; 26. Gn', soft tissue gnathion; 27. Me', soft tissue menton.

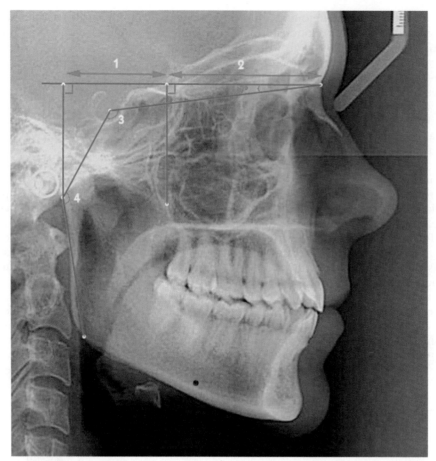

Figure 2.20 Cranial base. 1. Effective length of middle cranial fossa (distance between Ar and Ptm when projected on the HP), 2. Effective length of the anterior cranial fossa (distance between Ptm and N along the HP), 3. Saddle angle (N-S-Ar), 4. Articular angle (S-Ar-Go). The HP is a constructed horizontal plane at 7° to the SN plane.

Table 2.2   Cranial base assessment

No	Parameters	Mean female	Mean male
1	Ar-Ptm	32.8 ± 1.9 mm	37.1 ± 2.8 mm
2	Ptm-N (parallel to HP)	50.9 ± 3.0 mm	52.8 ± 4.1 mm
3	Saddle angle (N-S-Ar)	123°± 5°	
4	Articular angle (S-Ar-Go)	143°± 6°	

or smaller saddle angle will lead to an increased predisposition to skeletal Class III relationship despite normal-sized maxilla and mandible. Similarly, a decreased cranial base flexure or larger saddle angle will lead to greater probability of a Class II jaw relationship, even if the jaws are of normal size.

Maxillary skeletal assessment

The skeletal component of the maxilla should be carefully assessed in relation to its length, sagittal and vertical positions and rotational pattern (Fig. 2.21, Table 2.3). After determining the effective maxillary length (3,4), the clinician should evaluate its sagittal position relative to the cranium (1,2), as even a normal-sized jaw may be

protrusive or retrusive, if it is positioned anteriorly or posteriorly. The cephalometric assessment should include the identification of vertical component contributing to the malocclusion, as it influences the sagittal jaw position. Therefore, the vertical position of the maxilla (5,6) and the inclination of the palatal plane (7) should be evaluated.

Maxillary dentoalveolar assessment

The inclination and position of the dental units in each jaw should be assessed relative to the facial plane and the jaw base itself (Fig. 2.22, Table 2.4). The anteroposterior extent of the maxillary alveolar process relative to the cranial base should be determined (1). To differentiate a skeletal problem from a dental problem, it is critical to assess the inclination and sagittal position of the maxillary incisors relative to both the maxillary skeletal base and the cranium (2–5). The vertical position of the incisal edge and the first molar cusp tip relative to the nasal floor should be assessed to identify any dentoalveolar excess or deficiency (8,9). An assessment of the dental arch length posterior to the maxillary first molar is done to evaluate the amount of alveolar arch length available for molar distalization mechanics. This analysis is done relative to the pterygomaxillary fissure (7) and is useful when contemplating maxillary molar distalization.

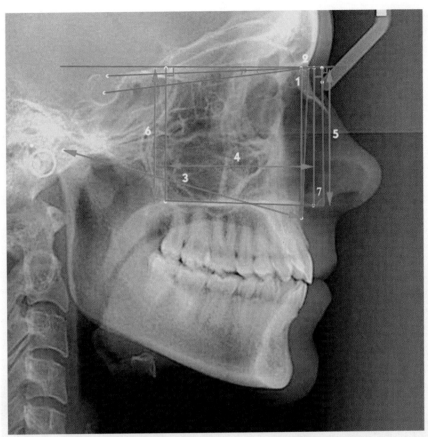

Figure 2.21 Maxillary skeletal. 1. SN-A, 2. Horizontal distance from N to A (parallel to the HP), 3.Effective maxillary length (Co-point A), 4.Effective length of palate (distance between PNS-ANS parallel to the HP), 5. Distance between N and ANS (perpendicular to HP), 6. Distance between N and PNS (perpendicular to HP), 7. J angle—angle between palatal plane and perpendicular to N-Se passing through N'.

Table 2.3 Maxillary skeletal assessment

No	Parameters	Mean female	Mean male
ANTEROPOSTERIOR			
1	SNA (Steiner's)	82°	82°
2	N to A (parallel to HP) (Burstone)	0 ± 3.7 mm	2 ± 3.7 mm
3	Effective maxillary length (Co-A) (McNamara)	91.0 ± 4.3 mm	99.8 ± 6.0 mm
4	PNS-ANS (Burstone)	52.6 ± 3.5 mm	57.7 ± 2.5 mm
VERTICAL			
5	N-ANS (perpendicular to HP)	50.0 ± 2.4 mm	54.7 ± 3.2 mm
6	N-PNS (perpendicular to HP)	50.6 ± 2.2 mm	53.9 ± 1.7 mm
7	Angle of inclination (Pn-Pal) (Schwarz)	85°	85°

Mandibular dentoalveolar assessment

The clinician should determine the anteroposterior extent of the mandibular alveolar process in relation to the cranium (Fig. 2.23, Table 2.5) (1). The inclination and horizontal position of the mandibular incisors are analyzed with respect to jaw base and facial plane (A-Pog) (2–4). The vertical position of the incisors and molars is evaluated relative to the MP to ascertain dentoalveolar excess or deficiency (5,6). The proper assessment of mandibular dentoalveolar segment is of significant value to determine its role in development of a problem and to identify associated dental compensations.

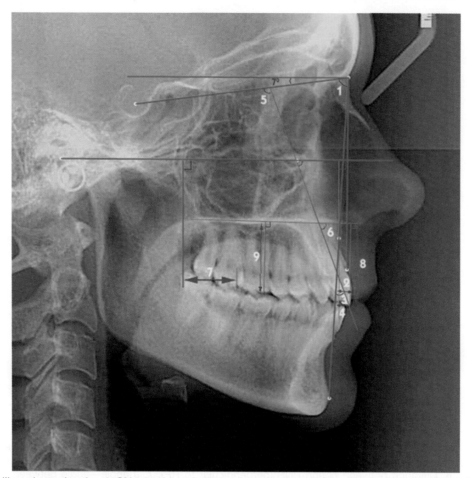

Figure 2.22 Maxillary dentoalveolar. 1. SN-prosthion, 2. Upper incisor axis to NA (inclination) and horizontal distance from most labial aspect of upper incisor to NA, 3. Horizontal distance from upper incisor to A-vertical (perpendicular from FH through point A), 4. Horizontal distance from upper incisor edge to A-Pog line, 5. Angle between upper incisor axis and SN plane (inner angle), 6. Angle between upper incisor axis and palatal plane, 7. Horizontal distance between Ptv (perpendicular to FH through distal most point on pterygomaxillary fissure) to distal aspect of upper first molar, 8.Upper incisor edge to nasal floor (NF) (perpendicular distance to NF), 9.Upper first molar mesiobuccal cusp tip to NF (perpendicular distance to NF).

Table 2.4   Maxillary dentoalveolar assessment

No	Parameters	Mean female	Mean male
ANTEROPOSTERIOR			
1	SN-prosthion	84°	84°
2	Incisor to NA (Steiner's)	22°	22°
		4 mm	4 mm
3	Incisor to A-vert (McNamara)	4–6 mm	4–6 mm
4	Incisor to A-Pg (Down's)	−1 to +5 mm	−1 to +5 mm
5	Incisor to SN plane (Jarabak's)	102°± 2°	102°± 2°
6	Incisor to Pal plane (Schwarz)	70°± 5°	70°± 5°
7	Molar to Ptv (Ricketts)	Age + 3 mm	Age + 3 mm
VERTICAL			
8	Upper incisor-NF (perpendicular to NF)	27.5 ± 1.7 mm	30.5 ± 2.1 mm
9	Upper molar-NF (perpendicular to NF)	23.3 ± 1.3 mm	26.2 ± 2.0 mm

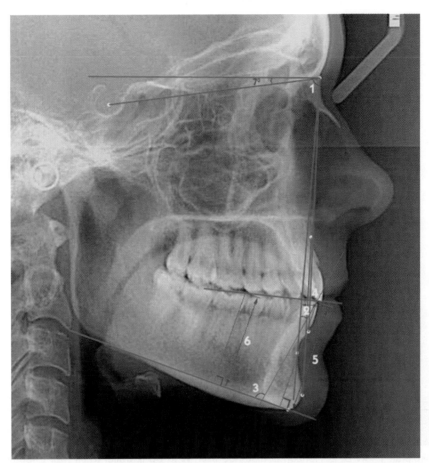

Figure 2.23 Mandibular dentoalveolar. 1. SN-infradentale, 2. Lower incisor axis to NB (angle) and horizontal distance from most labial aspect of lower incisor to NB, 3. Angle between lower incisor axis and mandibular plane (MP), 4. Horizontal distance from lower incisor edge to A-Pg plane, 5. Lower incisor edge to MP (perpendicular distance to MP), 6. Lower first molar mesiobuccal cusp tip to MP (perpendicular distance to MP).

Table 2.5   Mandibular dentoalveolar assessment

No	Parameters		Mean female	Mean male
ANTEROPOSTERIOR				
1	SN-infradentale		81°	81°
2	Incisor to NB (Steiner's)		25°	25°
			4 mm	4 mm
3	Incisor to MP (Tweed)		90° ± 5°	90° ± 5°
4	Incisor to A-Pg (Ricketts)		1 ± 2 mm	1 ± 2 mm
VERTICAL				
5	Lower incisor to MP (perpendicular to MP)		40.8 ± 1.8 mm	45.0 ± 2.1 mm
6	Lower molar to MP (perpendicular to MP)		32.1 ± 1.9 mm	35.8 ± 2.6 mm

Mandibular skeletal assessment

A cephalometric evaluation of the mandible should involve the analysis of its morphologic and positional variations (Fig. 2.24, Table 2.6), in addition to the evaluation of the effective length of the body (3,4), chin (5) and vertical ramus (9); the sagittal mandibular position should be assessed relative to the cranium (N) (1) and the facial plane (N-Pg) (2). The gonial angle configuration (10) is another important parameter that gives a fair indication of morphologic growth pattern of the mandible. The assessment of the inclination of the mandibular base relative to the cranium is done using various reference planes (6–8).

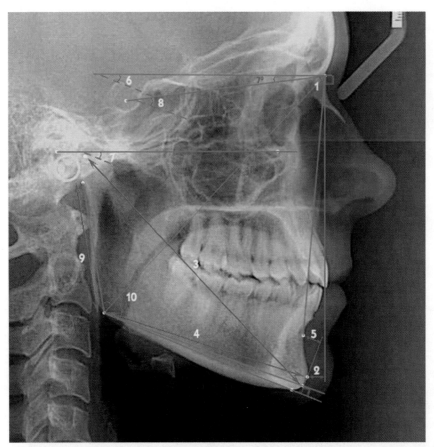

Figure 2.24 Mandibular skeletal. 1. SN-B, 2. Horizontal distance from N to Pg (parallel to HP), 3. Effective mandibular length (Co-Gn), 4. Length of mandibular body (Go-Pg), 5. Horizontal distance from point B to Pg (parallel to MP), 6. MP-HP (angle), 7. Angle between FH and MP, 8. Angle between SN plane and Go-Gn, 9. Length of mandibular ramus (Ar-Go), 10. Gonial angles — upper gonial angle (Ar-Go-N), lower gonial angle (N-Go-Gn), total gonial angle (Ar-Go-Gn).

Table 2.6   Mandibular skeletal assessment

No	Parameters	Mean female	Mean male
ANTEROPOSTERIOR			
1	SN-B (Steiner's)	80°	80°
2	N to Pg (parallel to HP) (Burstone)	–6.5 ± 5.1 mm	–4.3 ± 8.5 mm
3	Effective mandibular length (Co-Gn) (McNamara)	120.2 ± 5.3 mm	134.3 ± 6.8 mm
4	Go-Pg	74.3 ± 5.8 mm	83.7 ± 4.6 mm
5	B-Pg	7.2 ± 1.9 mm	8.9 ± 1.7 mm
VERTICAL			
6	MP-HP (angle)	24.2° ± 5.0°	23.0° ± 5.9°
7	FMA (FH-MP) (Tweed's)	25°	25°
8	SN-Go-Gn (Steiner's)	32°	32°
9	Ar-Go	46.8 ± 2.5 mm	52.0 ± 4.2 mm
10	Gonial angle		
	Upper	52°–5°	52°–5°
	Lower	70°–5°	70°–5°
	Total	130° ± 7°	130° ± 7°

Maxillomandibular relation

After the maxilla and mandible have been assessed individually, it is critical to evaluate their relationship to each other (Fig. 2.25, Table 2.7) (1–3,8,10,11). It is the relative position of the jaws to each other that determines a Class I, Class II or Class III malocclusion and facial types.

The lower anterior face height (4) is a representation of the sum of the anterior dentoalveolar heights of the two jaws and skeletal base inclination. The facial convexity (5) is determined by the relative position of the cranium (N), maxilla and mandible to each other. To predict the probable direction and pattern of future facial growth, the

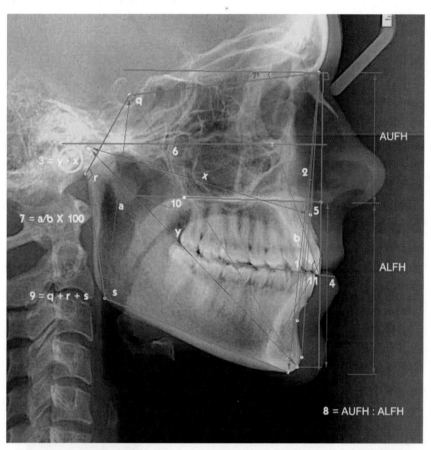

Figure 2.25 Maxillomandibular relation. 1. Distance between point A perpendicular (AO) and point B perpendicular (BO) on occlusal plane, 2. A-N-B, 3. y(Co-Gn) –x (Co-point A), 4. Distance between ANS and Gn (perpendicular to HP), 5. N-A-Pg (angle), 6. Angle between FH plane and S-Gn, 7.Posterior facial height (S-Go)/anterior facial height (N-Me) x 100, 8. Anterior upper facial height (vertical distance from N to ANS): anterior lower facial height (vertical distance from ANS to Me), 9. Saddle angle (N-S-Ar) + articular angle (S-Ar-Go) + gonial angle (Ar-Go-Gn) = Björk's sum, 10. Angle between palatal plane (ANS-PNS) and mandibular plane, 11. Inner angle between long axes of upper and lower incisors.

Table 2.7   Maxillomandibular relation

No	Parameters	Mean female	Mean male
1	Wits AO/BO appraisal	0 mm	–1 mm
2	ANB (Steiner's)	2°	2°
3	Maxillomandibular differential (McNamara)	29.2 ± 3.3 mm	34.5 ± 4.0 mm
4	ANS-Gn (perpendicular to HP)	61.3 ± 3.3 mm	68.6 ± 3.8 mm
5	Angle of convexity (Down's)	–8.5 to +10°	–8.5 to +10°
6	Y-axis (Down's)	53°–66°	53°–66°
7	Jarabak's ratio	58–64%	58–64%
8	AUFH:ALFH	45:55%	45:55%
9	Björk's sum	396°± 3°	396°± 3°
10	Palatal plane – mandibular plane	25°	25°
11	Interincisal angle (Down's)	130°–150°	130°–150°

growth axis (*Y*-axis) (6) and facial pattern (Jarabak's ratio) (7) should be assessed. The cranial base flexure, glenoid fossa inclination and gonial angle of the mandible together provide valuable information in the prediction of the growth pattern, horizontal or vertical, of the jaws (9).

Soft tissue analysis

As the orthodontic treatment influences the position of teeth and jaws, which in turn influences the morphology of the overlying facial soft tissues, the evaluation of the soft tissue components of the face plays an important role in diagnosis and treatment planning (Figs 2.26 and 2.27, Table 2.8).

1. The nose morphology, position and size, though cannot be directly influenced by orthodontic or orthopaedic intervention, have a significant bearing on the overall facial appearance. Hence, its various parameters demand careful evaluation (1,3).
2. The nasolabial angle (2) is determined by the tip of the nose and the prominence of the upper lip. The assessment of a deviation from normal nasolabial angle should be done by individual evaluation of either factors by drawing a true horizontal line through sub-nasale. Nasolabial angle helps determine prominence of the upper dental units and upper lip and is an important factor to be considered when contemplating amount of anterior dental retraction.
3. The length of the lips (6) influences the incisal show at rest and during function (smiling). This is a very critical factor in designing anterior intrusion and retraction mechanics.
4. The assessment of the overall maxillary and mandibular prominence (jaws, teeth and soft tissue drape) plays an important role in planning sagittal orthodontic or orthopaedic correction (7,8).
5. The upper lip thickness and strain factor, if any, should be calculated (9,10). Thicker lips follow tooth movement less closely as compared to thin lips. The upper lip strain needs to be eliminated by equivalent incisal retraction for the lips to assume normal form and thickness.
6. The prominence of the lips is assessed relative to various reference lines (11–16). Appropriate lip prominence is essential for good facial balance.

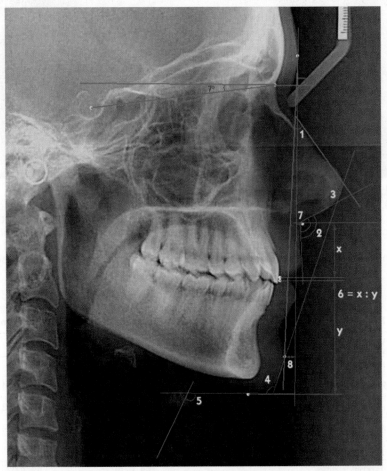

Figure 2.26 Soft tissue assessment 1: 1. Angle between G-Pg' and line along axis of radix of nose, 2. Nasolabial angle — angle between columella tangent and upper lip tangent at subnasale. It is divided into two by a postural horizontal line passing through subnasale. 3. Nasomental angle — angle between E-line and line along axis of radix of nose. 4. Mentocervical angle— angle between E-line and tangent to submental area. 5. Angle between tangent to submental area and neck tangent. 6. Upper lip length *(x)* (subnasale to stomion superior): lower lip length *(y)* (stomion inferior to soft tissue menton). 7. Horizontal distance from G perpendicular (perpendicular to HP through glabella) to subnasale. 8. Horizontal distance from G perpendicular to soft tissue pogonion.

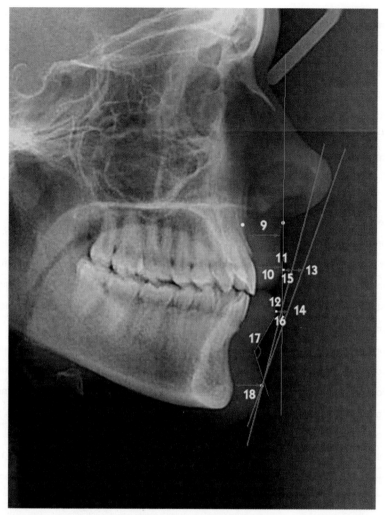

Figure 2.27 Soft tissue assessment 2: 9. Upper lip thickness — horizontal distance from a point on the outer alveolar plate 2 mm below point A on to the outer border of the upper lip, 10. Upper lip strain — horizontal distance from vermilion border of the upper lip to the labial surface of the maxillary central incisor (this measurement should be within 1 mm of the upper lip thickness. If it is lesser, the lips are considered to be strained), 11. Upper lip prominence — horizontal distance from labrale superior to Sn-vertical (true vertical passing through Sn), 12. Lower lip prominence — horizontal distance from labrale inferius to Sn-vertical, 13. Horizontal distance from E-line to upper lip, 14. Horizontal distance from E-line to lower lip, 15. S-line to upper lip, 16. S-line to lower lip, 17. Mentolabial angle — angle between lower lip tangent and chin tangent at deepest point in soft tissue mentolabial sulcus, 18. Soft tissue chin thickness — distance between the bony and soft tissue facial planes (i.e. Pg to Pg').

Diagnostic process

The entire process of orthodontic diagnosis and treatment planning involves recognition of the various characteristics of malocclusion, defining the nature of the problem and its aetiology and designing a treatment strategy based on the needs and desires of the individual patient. The diagnostic procedure begins with the patient interview and the initial examination; however, the diagnostic process is focused on the synthesis of relevant diagnostic information and its proper interpretation to establish an accurate diagnosis. The patient interview and the initial examination quickly capture the attention of the clinician to formulate an initial diagnosis, which then guides the practitioner to carry out relevant detailed examination and analysis of records to establish a final diagnosis (Fig. 2.28).

The goal of the diagnostic process is to synthesize the relevant diagnostic information and its proper interpretation to produce a comprehensive but concise list of patient's problems. This should ultimately help the clinician to design a rational treatment plan that maximizes benefit to the patient. It is important to derive a problem list from the diagnostic information and prioritize it according to the patient's needs and desires. The patient's concern and the chief complaint are essential components of this process.

DEFINING TREATMENT GOALS

Malocclusion or abnormalities of the teeth is not a disease; therefore, patient's problems do not result from disease but rather from abnormal growth and development. This

Table 2.8   Soft tissue assessment

No	Parameters	Mean female	Mean male
1	Nasofacial angle (O'Ryan et al) G-Pg'–line along axis of radix of nose	30–5°	30–5°
2	Nasolabial angle (McNamara)	102° ± 8°	102° ± 8°
	Columella tangent to postural horizontal (Scheideman et al)	–25°	–25°
	Upper lip tangent to postural horizontal (Scheideman et al)	–85°	–85°
3	Nasomental angle (O'Ryan et al) E-line–line along axis of radix of nose	120°–32°	120°–32°
4	Mentocervical angle (O'Ryan et al) E-line–tangent to submental area	110°–20°	110°–20°
5	Submental-neck angle (O'Ryan et al) Submental tangent – neck tangent	121°	126°
6	Upper lip length: lower lip length (Sn-Stms:Stmi-Me')	1:2	1:2
7	Maxillary prominence (G perpendicular to Sn) (Legan and Burstone)	6 ± 3 mm	6 ± 3 mm
8	Mandibular prominence (G perpendicular to Pg') (Legan and Burstone)	0 ± 4 mm	0 ± 4 mm
9	Upper lip thickness (Holdaway's)	14–16 mm	14–16 mm
10	Upper lip strain (Holdaway's)	13–14 mm	13–14 mm
11	Upper lip prominence (Ls to Sn-vert) (Bell et al)	1–2 mm	1–2 mm
12	Lower lip prominence (Li to Sn-vert) (Bell et al)	–1 to 0 mm	–1 to 0 mm
13	Upper lip to E-line (Rickett's)	–4 ± 2 mm	–4 ± 2 mm
14	Lower lip to E-line (Rickett's)	–2 ± 2 mm	–2 ± 2 mm
15	Upper lip to S-line (Steiner's)	0	0
16	Lower lip to S-line (Steiner's)	0	0
17	Mentolabial angle (Bergman's)	122° ± 11.7°	122° ± 11.7°
18	Chin thickness (Holdaway's)	10–12 mm	10–12 mm

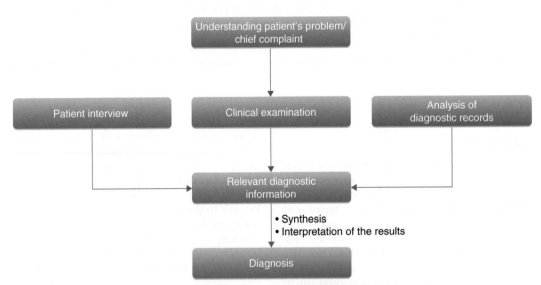

Figure 2.28   The diagnostic process.

has a potential influence on patient's physical and mental health. Orthodontic treatment should now be viewed more clearly as a health service dedicated to improve the patient's life by enhancing dental and jaw functions and dentofacial aesthetics. Once patient's diagnostic information is synthesized into dental, skeletal, functional and soft tissue profile, the orthodontic treatment goals should be clearly defined. A common mistake made by the clinician at this stage is to establish treatment goals based on a specific treatment mechanics or the appliance system.

This approach diminishes the scope of available solutions for patient's individual problems. The diagnostic information, especially the clinical examination, must reveal what the patient desires to gain from the treatment, and it must be included in the treatment goals and in the final treatment plan. In order to provide a high-quality orthodontic care to our patients, it is essential to define treatment goals comprehensively as follows:[21-23]

1. Static occlusal goals
2. Stomatognathic function
3. Optimal dentofacial aesthetics
4. Normal periodontal health
5. Post-treatment stability

Static occlusal goals

Achieving proper occlusal relationship of maxillary and mandibular teeth at the conclusion of orthodontic treatment has been a fundamental goal of any treatment plan. Angle[24] proposed his most famous key to occlusion as a guide to orthodontic diagnosis and treatment planning. It was based on the sagittal relationship of the maxillary permanent first molar to the mandibular permanent first molar. Since the occlusal problems exist in all three planes of space—sagittal, transverse and vertical, the contemporary orthodontic diagnosis must include a three-dimensional assessment of these abnormalities and establishment of goals accordingly. Andrew's[25] six keys to occlusion, which he developed by studying untreated ideal occlusions, constitute well-defined goals for static dental alignment. It is important to establish treatment goals for each individual tooth with respect to its best-fit, both anatomically and functionally, and achieve them with appropriate treatment mechanics. Proper alignment of maxillary and mandibular teeth, well-coordinated archforms, levelled marginal ridges, proper position of contact points, three-dimensional position of individual teeth and the maximum intercuspation of posterior teeth are some of the important static occlusal goals.

Stomatognathic function

a) Dynamic occlusal relationships

In addition to the above-mentioned static occlusal relationships that at least partially contribute to the stability of a treated case, the clinician should expand the scope of these goals to include the neuromuscular and bony structures of the temporomandibular joint (TMJ). This requires a careful consideration of mainly three areas of functional occlusion: centric relation (CR), anterior guidance and stability of posterior tooth arrangement. CR of the mandible is a superior limit position of the condyles in

the fossae, with the mandible centred and at its most closed position.[22] The essence of optimal TMJ form and function is considered the 'seated condylar position', which is defined as superior, anterior and mid-sagittal (centred transversely).[26] This should represent an idealized treatment goal. It is important to achieve stable CR of the mandible with maximum intercuspation of the teeth at this position. In the intercuspal position and retruded contact position, the mandible should be situated in the same sagittal plane; the distance between the two positions being less than 1 mm. When the mandible is in CR, all the teeth must occlude in maximum intercuspation. The occlusal scheme that is most successful in preventing occlusal problems in patients over a long period of time is the mutually protected occlusion.[27] In the absence of other problems, mere presence of centric occlusion–centric relation (CO–CR) discrepancy by itself is not an indication for treatment. However, if there is sufficient cause to treat, the treatment goal should be to achieve the physiologic position of the condyles as determined by the musculature in a superior-anterior fossa position, with the maximum intercuspation of the teeth taking place in this position.

As soon as the mandible moves out of centric closure, the maxillary and mandibular anterior teeth should work against each other to separate or disclude the posterior teeth. This anterior guidance is determined by the position of the maxillary and mandibular anterior teeth and their relationship to each other. The lingual surfaces of the upper anteriors should provide harmonious glide path to disclude posteriors during the protrusive excursion of the mandible.

During the mandibular lateral excursions, the maxillary and mandibular canines work against each other and form the main gliding inclines to provide gentle lateral lift, with no lateral interferences on the balancing side. Under certain situations when maxillary cuspid is missing, the mandibular cuspid can be made to work satisfactorily with a maxillary bicuspid. If more teeth than the cuspids on working side are allowed to contact in lateral excursions, uneven wear is likely to occur because each tooth is at a different distance from the rotating condyle and, therefore, moves on a different arc.[28] Therefore, in order to achieve the optimal functional occlusion, the following criteria should be carefully observed.

1. Stable CR—condyles in a seated position
2. Maximum intercuspation of teeth in CR position
3. Relaxed healthy musculature
4. When molars are in occlusion, the anteriors are in a very close approximation but do not touch
5. The mandibular anteriors engage the lingual surfaces of the opposing maxillary anteriors immediately with the protrusive mandibular movement
6. During the lateral mandibular excursive movements, cuspids are in the best position to provide the main gliding inclines, with no interferences on the balancing side.

Acceptable goals for centric occlusion (CO)—CR discrepancy for orthodontic cases are as follows:

• Anteroposterior 1 mm
• Vertical 1 mm
• Transverse less than 0.5 mm

Occlusal disharmonies cannot be studied in the functioning mouth because the muscles and nerve reflexes, often called *neuromuscular avoidance mechanism*, protect the teeth by overriding the joint's guidance.[29] Records taken in the seated condylar position and mounted on the articulator allow the joint and tooth relationships to be evaluated without interferences from the neuromuscular avoidance mechanism. In the process of diagnosis, in order for the clinician to recognize the potential or existing problem cases, it is necessary to know the signs and symptoms of occlusal disharmony. Some of the signs and symptoms of occlusal interferences[22] include the following:

1. Excessive tooth mobility
2. Occlusal wear
3. TMJ sounds
4. Limitation of opening or movement
5. Myofascial pain
6. Contracture of the mandibular musculature
7. Some types of tongue-thrust swallow

b) Orofacial function

The traditional approach to orthodontic treatment planning has been directed towards the achievement of hard tissue goals, while contemporary principles of treatment planning place an emphasis on the soft tissue assessment and management. However, when it comes to defining orthodontic treatment goals, the focus has been on planning tooth movements to achieve ideal occlusal relationships and aesthetics, almost ignoring the goals for stomatognathic function. It is important to understand a relationship between anatomic form and physiologic function and the effects of abnormal functional influences on dentofacial structures and growth.

The clinician should define goals related to the functional criteria that exist in the soft tissue relationships to the teeth. This includes the ability of the patient to achieve adequate lip closure after orthodontic treatment.[30] The assessment of lip dysfunctions should be done in relation to the configuration and functioning of the lips, and if present, appropriate measures should be taken to eliminate non-nutritive sucking habits, including the visual evidence of mentalis muscle hyperactivity.

The abnormal pressure habit, like thumb sucking, generally interferes with normal eruption of incisors and promotes excessive eruption of posterior teeth. This habit should be corrected prior to the initiation of orthodontic therapy to make sure that there are no abnormal influences that bring about displacement of teeth. Restoration of normal tongue function and teeth-together swallowing pattern should be the integral parts of treatment goals. As the chronically impeded nasal breathing represents a dysfunction of the orofacial musculature, the patient should be examined carefully to identify the mode of respiration. If abnormal function is detected, a suitable plan should be instituted to encourage nasal breathing to promote normal development of the dentition and efficient orthodontic treatment.

Optimal dentofacial aesthetics

Achievement of optimal facial aesthetics is the primary goal of orthodontic treatment. The aesthetic benefits of orthodontic treatment are the most universally recognized by both patients and practitioners.[31,32] Orthodontic diagnosis and treatment planning have become more sophisticated and scientific, and the emphasis should be placed on soft tissue analysis and its influence on treatment planning. This information should help the clinician to define treatment goals for a well-proportioned, balanced and harmonious soft tissue profile at the conclusion of treatment. The relationships of nose, lips, chin and facial soft tissue dynamics are important considerations. A comprehensive soft tissue evaluation of the patient's facial frontal and profile view should provide valuable information for better understanding of the patient's aesthetic characteristics. This ensures that the patients are treated to their soft tissue/facial aesthetic goals and not just to the cephalometric norms. It should be emphasized that the facial aesthetic goals are not compromised for a good occlusion. The patient's facial aesthetic is determined by the inter-relationships and proportions of nose, upper and lower lips and the chin. Those goals can be outlined as follows:

- Establishing normal configuration of the lips, which is assessed by lip length, width and curvature
- Normal nasolabial angle
- Normal lip protrusion, which is influenced by the soft tissue thickness, position of the anterior teeth and the underlying bony structures
- Establishing normal configuration of the soft tissue chin, which is influenced by the thickness and tone of the mentalis muscle
- Normal chin position is also determined by the morphology and the craniofacial relationship of the mandible

One of the most important aesthetic goals of orthodontic treatment pertaining to the soft tissue dynamics of face is to achieve a 'balanced smile'. There is no universal ideal smile. The orthodontic treatment should be aimed at achieving the perfect smile that is characterized by the maxillary anterior dentition following the curvature of the lower lip, the corners of the lips that are elevated to the same height (symmetrical), the bilateral negative spaces that separate the teeth from the corners of the lips and displaying appropriate position of the teeth and normal gingival architecture.[33,34]

The ideal facial aesthetics require the following:

1. Nasolabial angle of 90°–110°
2. Strong chin—90° soft tissue facial plane
3. Gonial angle of 120°–5°
4. Lower facial height of 55% of total face height from nasion to menton
5. Competent lips
6. No lip strain on closure of lips

Other desirable features include the following:

1. Vermilion border of upper lip showing one-third of upper central incisor crown
2. Full smile showing entire upper central incisor and 1–2 mm of attached gingiva
3. Lips should be contained within the nose-chin line (Ricketts)
4. Optimal upper incisor torque
5. Mesial convergence of upper central and lateral incisors

For attractive faces, a range for facial profile analysis (Powell) is as follows:

1. Soft tissue facial plane angle—90°
2. Nasofrontal angle—115°–30°
3. Nasal projection—30°–40°
4. Nasolabial angle—90°–110°
5. Nasomental angle—120°–32°
6. Mentocervical angle—80°–95°

Periodontal health

One of the prime goals of orthodontic treatment is to achieve optimal periodontal health. This includes the preservation and minimum treatment-induced deterioration of hard and soft tissues of the periodontal apparatus. In post-orthodontic treatment, the patient should not show signs of gingival recession, fenestration, dehiscence, periodontal pockets, root resorption or unusual pattern of attrition or crown wear facets. The orthodontist should make a careful assessment of patient's existing periodontal condition and the potential for bone loss or gingival recession during orthodontic tooth movement. An evaluation of the periodontal soft tissues should include an assessment of oral hygiene, areas of mucogingival tension, frenum pulls, amount of attached gingiva, etc. Of paramount importance is the amount of attached gingiva—both height and labiolingual thickness.

The following procedures, directly or indirectly, promote better periodontal health:

- Proper alignment of teeth to facilitate oral hygiene maintenance
- Proper proximal contacts to prevent food lodgment and impaction
- Parallelism of roots that promotes sufficient bone between the roots, which is generally considered to provide greater resistance to periodontal bone loss, if patient develops periodontal disease in the future
- No premature contacts in maximum intercuspation and during various mandibular excursions to prevent tooth mobility, periodontal damage, etc.
- Proper positioning of teeth in the cancellous bone between labial and lingual cortical plates to prevent gingival recession
- Normal interincisal relationship to prevent redevelopment of deep bite and subsequent stripping of gingival tissue either from the palatal aspect of maxillary incisors or from the labial aspect of mandibular incisors
- Controlling the magnitude of orthodontic force levels, as the application of heavy forces over a period of long time contributes to the external root resorption
- Elimination of pretreatment bony defects by controlled force eruption or uprighting of teeth
- Effective oral hygiene maintenance protocol by the patient

Post-treatment long-term stability

Long-term stability of tooth positions achieved after orthodontic treatment should be the primary goal of every orthodontic treatment plan. It is an area of great concern to the orthodontic profession and greatly influences the treatment plan. Many of the post-treatment changes in the dentition, like deepening of overbite, increased overjet, relapse of treated Class II relationship and crowding of the maxillary and the mandibular incisors, are being considered mainly due to post-treatment growth changes. The post-treatment growth significantly contributes to the lingual movement of mandibular incisors leading to deepening of overbite, loss of arch length and lower incisor crowding. Other post-treatment changes, like anterior open bite and interdental spacing and changes in a single rotated tooth, are considered primarily due to local factors, such as persistent habits, inability of the periodontal fibres to reorganize and lack of adaptability of the soft tissues.

As mentioned earlier, achievement of static and dynamic occlusal goals, optimal periodontal health and bone support as guidelines to finish orthodontic cases to the highest standards at least partially contribute to the stability. In addition to this, the clinician should consider anticipated post-treatment growth and local factors in the planning of active treatment and retention protocol to enhance long-term stability.

ORTHODONTIC TREATMENT PLANNING

Proper treatment planning depends on accurate diagnosis, which in turn requires objective, relevant and accurate information, patient data and an analysis of various records. It is important to understand that both the treatment planning process and the delivery of orthodontic care involve much more than the simple process of bonding brackets to the teeth and following a predetermined sequence of archwires. The treatment must be dictated by the individual patient's problem and diagnosis.[35] Orthodontic treatment planning process is illustrated in Figure 2.29. The goal-based treatment planning provides a guide for the techniques and mechanics used in the delivery of orthodontic care. The entire process of treatment planning is influenced by many factors.

Factors influencing treatment planning

Growth

Presence or absence of the growth is frequently a significant factor in selection of a treatment plan. Facial growth occurs in a downward and forward direction, and its presence is usually a positive factor in resolution of many adolescent malocclusions. Several treatment modalities, like headgear or functional appliances, rely on this growth as a part of orthopaedic treatment for stable correction of skeletal discrepancies. Orthodontic treatment mechanisms influenced by growth are not available for the adult patient. The natural eruption of teeth along with the vertical growth of the alveolar bone provides many treatment options to the clinician, as controlling the vertical dimension significantly contributes to occlusal correction. The growing patients present with significant potential for adaptability of stomatognathic system, which allows a variety of biomechanical choices, like the

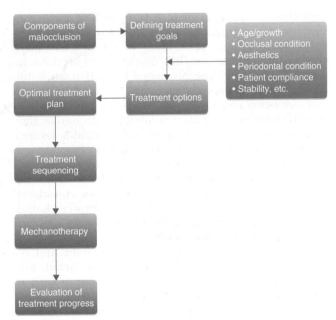

Figure 2.29 Treatment planning process.

use of Class II elastics. The ageing process appears to result in changes in the biologic system of the teeth and alveolar process.[36] It alters the ability of the fibroblast to produce collagen.[37] Since there is minimal skeletal adaptability and no growth in adult patients, orthodontic treatment is dependent on tooth movement to achieve entirely desired results unless surgical procedures are used for the underlying skeletal disharmonies. In planning a tooth movement, the clinician must recognize that the growing patients exhibit predictable and rapid rate of tooth movement, especially during eruptive stages when permanent root development is not yet completed.[38] Adult orthodontic patients are at no greater risk for orthodontically induced root resorption on the average; however, they exhibit more severe root resorption than in adolescent patients.[39]

Location of discrepancy

One of the key factors influencing the treatment planning process is the location of the problem within the dentofacial complex. Since orthodontic treatment affects many structures of the craniofacial complex, like teeth, supporting structures, maxillary and mandibular basal bones, TMJs and facial structures, the clinician must define treatment goals for these areas in order to establish an effective treatment plan.

- If there is only occlusal problem, this can be addressed by orthodontic tooth movement alone, at any time, or by occlusal equilibration.
- If the problem is dentoalveolar in nature, effective measures may be taken even after cessation of growth. Treatment procedures in this area are indicated, if compensation of the underlying skeletal discrepancy is required.
- If the discrepancy is confined to the skeletal bases (skeletal malocclusion), the treatment should influence the facial sutures and TMJs, and it is possible only during the periods of active growth. In non-growing

patients, changes in the abnormal skeletal relationships can be achieved with surgical intervention.

Existing discrepancy

Proper assessment of various elements contributing to the existing discrepancy to determine the complexity of a problem is essential for treatment planning. There are many clinical entities that contribute to the complexity of a problem and its management, and it is not possible to include every clinical entity to determine the severity of discrepancy. The American Board of Orthodontics developed the discrepancy index (DI) based on those disorders that represent most conditions that orthodontists treat.[40] The target disorder elements chosen to make up the DI are measurements of overjet, overbite, anterior open bite, lateral open bite, crowding, occlusion, lingual posterior crossbite, buccal posterior crossbite, ANB angle, IMPA and SN-Go-Gn angle. Other conditions that influence the treatment complexity are missing or supernumerary teeth, ectopic eruption, transposition, anomalies of tooth size and shape, CO–CR discrepancies, skeletal asymmetry and excess curve of Wilson. It has been generally recognized that more severe the case, the more complex the treatment and more difficult to treat. However, the degree of difficulty is somewhat subjective and a matter of perception. Some clinical situations that are considered difficult by some clinicians might be perceived as relatively easy to treat by others. This is usually due to differences in diagnostic approach, appliances used, overall approach to treatment and training.

Functional assessment

The importance of functional analysis in the examination of different clinical situations has been universally recognized. Equally important is the understanding of its significance in treatment planning. The movement of the mandible is hinge-like as it changes from the rest to the occlusal position. The postural rest position of the mandible can be either anterior or posterior to the habitual occlusal position. The functional disorder is more serious than the findings of the occlusal examination. Any abnormality in mandibular position resulting in transposition should be eliminated in order to assess the full extent of the discrepancy. The path of closure of the mandible and condylar position in the fossa should be evaluated properly. Intermaxillary relationships and the rest position can only be changed during active growth with functional appliances.

The assessment of lip configuration in relation to incisor relationship and angulation plays an important role in treatment planning. For example, lip dysfunction in patients with skeletal Class II relationship will have much more serious consequences due to the presence of unfavourable relationship of the maxillary and mandibular skeletal bases. The abnormal outcome of the assessment of tongue position and function should be considered in the final treatment plan. The elimination of tongue dysfunction determines the treatment outcome and its potential stability. The clinician must assess the upper airway patency to determine the mode of breathing. Enlarged adenoids that may be distinguished in the radiograph often lead to reduced patency of upper respiratory passages and oral breathing. The final treatment plan should incorporate the necessary measures to establish nasal breathing and teeth-together swallowing pattern.

Aetiological assessment

Once the abnormality has been located in the dentofacial complex based on the clinical examination and analysis of diagnostic records, and functional relationships have been determined, the orthodontist should draw some conclusions to the cause of the problem. The orthodontic treatment plan for any malocclusion must include the elimination of the aetiological factor. There are many causative factors that contribute to the development of malocclusion and dentofacial deformity. In some patients, the aetiology of some characteristic malocclusions appears to be almost genetic in nature, while in others, it is a result of some environmental influences. Certain malocclusions are developed as a result of disturbances of dental development, like congenitally missing teeth, malformed and supernumerary teeth, interference with tooth eruption due to sclerotic bone or heavy fibrous gingiva and ectopic eruption. Sometimes, improper guidance of eruption either due to early loss of primary teeth or due to functional shifts of the mandible while permanent teeth are erupting leads to the development of a problem.

Some kind of a trauma to the teeth in children during their formative years and childhood jaw fractures due to falls and impacts cause severe mandibular deficiency requiring surgical correction in about 5% of affected patients.[41] It is also interesting to note that about 75% of children with early condylar process fractures have normal mandibular growth and, therefore, do not contribute to the development of malocclusion.[42] The functional influences, like thumb sucking, tongue-thrusting and mouth-breathing habits, affect dentofacial development leading to a deformity. Whatever may be the aetiological factor, the diagnostic process should guide the clinician to identify it, and its elimination should become an integral part of a well thought-out treatment plan.

Patient compliance

Patient compliance is one of the determinants of the use of various treatment options that are available in modern orthodontic practice. Lack of compliance in the present orthodontic patient population has been a major concern for the orthodontists. Over the few years, the percentage of patients exhibiting poor compliance has been increased tremendously, with only about 10% demonstrating excellent compliance.[43] It is the author's experience that both patients and their families misrepresent, generally overestimate, the extent of compliance. The clinician must be aware of the fact that the patient compliance usually decreases when longer duration treatment is required.[44] Therefore, patient compliance should be given due importance in the treatment planning process, and appropriate measures should be designed and explained at the time of case presentation.

Patient compliance may be improved by many ways:

1. Patient motivation: The ability to motivate a patient to comply is an essential ingredient of successful outcome of orthodontic therapy.

2. Reduction of treatment duration: A well-defined treatment goal must be defined before the execution of treatment plan to prevent unnecessary, prolonged treatment that may 'burn out' the patient subsequently.

3. Involvement of patient and parent in treatment decision: The orthodontist must make every effort to involve the patient and the parent in the treatment decision and emphasize the importance of high levels of patient cooperation as per the specific needs of the patient.

4. Lastly, it would be prudent for the clinician to consider that the patient will demonstrate diminished compliance over a period of time and, therefore, design treatment plans and mechanics that minimize the need for compliance.

Dentofacial aesthetics

The aesthetic benefits of orthodontic treatment have been universally recognized by both patients and orthodontists. In majority of cases, patients seek orthodontic treatment primarily because of aesthetic concerns, and the influence of orthodontic treatment in attaining aesthetic improvements should neither be understated nor be overemphasized during the treatment planning process. This is because any discrepancy in aesthetic treatment outcome and patient expectations leads to patient dissatisfaction. In patients with significant anterior teeth crowding due to severe maxillary and mandibular arch length discrepancies, alignment of teeth with orthodontic treatment plays an important role in achieving an attractive smile. This can be accomplished by:

- Non-extraction treatment approach:
  - Incisor advancement
  - Transverse expansion
  - Molar distalization
  - Interproximal stripping
- Extraction approach: Bicuspids are extracted to gain adequate space. Another commonly featured aesthetic problem is excessive teeth and gingival display upon smile.[45] The treatment considerations for excessive incisor show depend on the aetiological reasons. The maxillary incisors may be intruded with intraoral intrusion arches. The detorqued maxillary incisors should be adequately torqued or advanced. If it is due to soft tissue defect, short philtrum, V-Y cheiloplasty may be performed. In adults, if it is associated with vertical maxillary excess, surgical impaction of the maxilla using LeFort I osteotomy is useful. On the other hand, patients also express their concern over inadequate incisor show. Orthodontic torquering, or retraction of flared maxillary incisors, increase in adequate crown length by various dental procedures, soft tissue surgical procedure (direct or indirect lip lift) for long philtrum, and maxillary downgraft using LeFort I osteotomy for vertical maxillary deficiency are some of the treatment options to deal with this problem.

The lip position is influenced by the relative protrusion or retrusion of incisors and is considered to be the determinant of extraction or non-extraction treatment decision.[46] It is important to consider that the increase in size of nose and chin is usually more than the soft tissue lip thickness changes over a period of time.[47] Lip projection is a function of: (a) protrusion or retrusion of teeth, which can be resolved by incisor retraction or advancement, (b) maxillomandibular protrusion or retrusion, which can be addressed by orthopaedic correction at early age or surgical intervention in adults and (c) lip thickness, which is influenced by patient age, ethnicity, etc.

Patient motivation and expectations

Patients seeking orthodontic treatment show different motivation levels at different age groups.[48] Since adult patients themselves make their decision to undergo orthodontic treatment, they may be considered internally motivated.[49] These highly motivated patients may be more compliant during the course of treatment contributing to the success of treatment outcome. The areas of patient satisfaction and happiness are highly sensitive and extremely important in orthodontic practice. The practising orthodontist must be prepared to assess certain influencing factors, like patient expectations and psychological well-being of the patient. Aesthetic benefits of orthodontic treatment have been universally recognized. Even for those patients who choose to undergo orthodontic treatment primarily for the improvement of function, aesthetic concerns play a major role. The successful correction of patient's abnormal clinical entities along with the achievement of functional goals does not always ensure patient satisfaction, if it has compromised aesthetic relationships. The clinician should identify the reasons for seeking orthodontic treatment as unrealistic patient expectations may lead to poor satisfaction with the final outcome. The key factor here is to make sure that the treatment results are aligned with the patient expectations, which need to be incorporated into treatment planning process.

Periodontal condition

Orthodontic treatment involves the use of light, continuous forces to bring about a controlled tooth movement in a predetermined direction. During this period, it is a basic requirement to maintain an optimal periodontal health to avoid any unfavourable response from the supporting structures of the teeth. During the treatment planning process, abnormal findings pertaining to the periodontal health revealed during the careful clinical examination should guide the clinician to incorporate appropriate measures in the final treatment plan to restore its normal health. It is critical to assess the potential impact of planned tooth movement on the tooth-supporting tissues. If the patient has experienced bone and attachment loss leading to tooth migration or extrusion, orthodontic treatment is recommended to improve the prognosis of such periodontally compromised teeth.[50] Reduced periodontal attachment consequent to disease requires that the orthodontic force systems are modified to produce desired force magnitudes to induce predictable tooth movement without any damage to the periodontium. As a result of an attachment loss, the centre of resistance of a tooth also shifts apically causing a great tendency for the tooth to tip.[51] It must be recognized that in the absence of plaque, orthodontic tooth movements do not induce gingivitis; however, in the presence of plaque, the same may produce marginal bone loss.

Another important aspect to be considered in the treatment plan is the type of bone through which the tooth is moved. An excessive tooth movement, especially in a labiolingual direction that displaces the root through the cortical bone, results in a fenestration. Therefore, the clinician has to be more careful in planning torque movements, especially in the incisor and canine region and in the maxillary premolars and molars where the labial cortical bone plate is considered thinner than at the lingual aspect. The bone fenestration effect is seen in the region of the apical part of the root, while the bone dehiscence involves marginal bone loss on the facial aspect of the root.

Rapid maxillary expansion (RME) produces most favourable outcome, if carried out at young ages when sutures are not closed. Research studies on palatal suture closure have shown large individual variations with age.[52] RME used in patients with fully or partially closed sutures or orthodontic overexpansion usually results in tipping of buccal segment teeth leading to a marginal bone resorption.

Retention and stability considerations

Retention and stability of an orthodontically treated case has been the area of great concern to the profession since the inception of this speciality. Ideally, retention planning to ensure better stability should begin with diagnosis and treatment planning. During the treatment planning process, the practising clinician should identify the areas of potential relapse, define goals for tooth positions for better stability, design appropriate treatment mechanics to achieve these goals and establish individualized retention protocol. It is important to distinguish physiologic recovery and relapse as two separate entities. Orthodontically treated patient typically shows post-treatment changes that are related to the treatment and those that are considered to be normal developmental changes as part of the ageing. Elimination of causative factors for the development of malocclusion plays an important role in preventing recurrence. Tooth-supporting structures, both hard and soft tissues, must be given sufficient time to reorganize around newly positioned teeth. Occlusal goals must be defined and achieved with proper finishing procedures, as the proper occlusion with good intercuspation is a potent factor in holding the teeth in their corrected position.[53] The archform, particularly in the lower arch, should not be permanently altered. Root parallelism at the extraction sites should be achieved and verified radiographically before appliance removal. As the time for formation of mineralized bone increases with advancing age, it is important to consolidate teeth after movement and prolong the retention period. Periodontal considerations, extraction decisions and retention regimens play a vital role in the achievement and maintenance of an optimal result.[54]

Therefore, the secret of successful planning of retention and long-term stability lies in the consideration of malocclusion-specific, treatment-specific and adult-specific principles in the treatment planning process.

Growth prediction

The ability to forecast or predict dentofacial growth is perhaps the most essential and integral part of contemporary clinical orthodontics. There are several elements the clinician has to deal with in the prediction of craniofacial changes: the direction, the magnitude, the timing, the rate of change and the effects of treatment. The growth changes in the face are complex and demonstrate a great degree of individual variations, but how predictable are these variations that are considered to be normal, in the growth of the face?

In a broader perspective, the growth prediction can be accomplished by three basic methods: longitudinal, metric and structural.

Longitudinal method of growth prediction

This method evaluates an individual over a period of time to determine the pattern of growth and age-related individual peculiarities. Tweed[55] used this approach on his growing patients by advocating two lateral cephalograms, 12–18 months apart, to assess the skeletal facial changes. The limitation of this approach to growth prediction is that it is accurate only when it is performed retrospectively and not prospectively. Also, the growth pattern is not constant, and the pattern of growth recorded at a juvenile age may well have changed by adolescence. Therefore, it should not be considered an accurate method of predicting future dentofacial changes.

Metric approach to growth prediction

This method of growth prediction uses a single radiograph to measure different structures that are then related to future growth changes. It is based on statistical information on average growth increments derived from a normative sample to be added to the recorded actual facial dimensions of the patient. The goal is to estimate the statistically probable future facial dimensions of the patient.

Structural approach to growth prediction

Björk[56] developed a structural method for the prediction of mandibular growth direction by using metallic implants. This method involves the recognition of specific structural morphological features in the mandible that would help to identify future growth trends. Björk[57] considered seven areas on a single cephalogram to predict mandibular rotation:

1. The inclination of the condyle (with vertical condylar growth, the mandibular rotates forward)
2. The curvature of the mandibular canal (the more curved the canal is, the more forward mandibular rotation will be)
3. Inclination of the symphysis (if it is inclined lingually, the mandible will rotate forward)
4. Shape of the lower border of the mandible (the forward rotator has concave lower border as against the convex, or notched, lower border of the backward rotator)
5. The interincisal angle (more acute in forward rotators)
6. The intermolar angles (more acute in forward rotators)
7. The anterior lower face height

Later, Skieller et al[58] found that, of these original signs, four of the variables—mandibular inclination, intermolar angle, the shape of the lower border and inclination of symphysis—when combined gave the best prognostic estimate of 86% of mandibular growth rotation.

Treatment options

In designing a treatment plan, it is an important step to select the appropriate treatment strategy to resolve the discrepancy. There are several general treatment options available, which need to be carefully explored and evaluated before finalizing on the modality of choice. As stated earlier, the treatment plan should be individualized— tailored to individual patient needs. This guides the clinician to make sure that the potential treatment option is carefully assessed and fits with the general treatment goals. One of the common mistakes made by the orthodontist is to design a treatment strategy instinctively based on a quick impression of whether the patient needs extractions or not. It requires a great deal of flexibility on part of the clinician to examine all the rational possibilities to formulate the successful treatment plan.

Early treatment

The optimal timing of treatment of the various problems in growing patients remains a controversial issue. In author's opinion, the two-phase treatment—an interceptive phase carried out during the mixed dentition and corrective phase in the permanent dentition—should not only optimize oral health, function, aesthetics and stability but also justify the time, cost and resources involved. The variability in initial clinical conditions and treatment response and differences among the orthodontic professionals concerning treatment beliefs, goals and even skills significantly contribute to the complexity in determining the relative merits of these two treatment approaches. The early treatment approach provides the clinician with more treatment options, better use of growth potential and less need for en masse tooth movement, torque and dental compensations in the second phase of treatment.

The leeway space can provide adequate space to align and accommodate crowded teeth in majority of patients.[59] The combined mesiodistal widths of the deciduous canine and first molar are the same as the combined mesiodistal diameters of the permanent canine and first premolar, and the space gain represents only the 'E' space.[60] The 'E' space can be accomplished by using passive appliances, such as holding arches in the late mixed dentition stage. The transpalatal arch is used in the mixed dentition to produce molar rotations, changes in root torque, transverse molar changes, etc.

Early arch development can be achieved by the use of lip bumper and rapid palatal expansion (RPE) treatments to induce spontaneous expansion of dental arches. It has been reported that both arch length and width are increased with lip bumper therapy.[61,62] Interestingly, the largest amount of post-retention irregularity was observed in a group of mixed dentition patients whose treatment involved more than 1 mm of arch length expansion.[63] It then guides the clinician to limit the lip bumper therapy to a 1-mm increase in arch length. This can be fairly established after 3–6 months of use of lip bumper.[62]

Orthodontic expansion, produced by removable expansion appliances or fixed appliances, is primarily a dentoalveolar in nature due to buccal movements of posterior teeth. An excessive expansion leads to a buccal tipping of crowns and a lingual tipping of the roots of the posterior teeth. This occlusal change along with the presence of the cheek musculature forces provides instability to the achieved expansion. On the other hand, RME produces orthopaedic expansion, affecting the underlying skeletal components rather than by the movement of teeth through alveolar bone. This method separates the mid-palatal suture where new bone is deposited to establish the integrity of the mid-palatal suture in 3–6 months.[64]

In the management of Class II malocclusions, the use of extraoral appliances produces an orthopaedic effect that is important for patients with maxillary prognathism. The results of extraoral appliance use, when compared between patients in the early and late mixed dentition stage, showed a 1-mm greater orthopaedic effect in the younger group.[65]

The use of functional appliances in patients with Class II malocclusions characterized by mandibular retrognathism, with the intent to stimulate mandibular growth, has been advocated. The use of Functional Regulator (FR-II) appliance demonstrated an age-dependent mandibular growth response, showing more mandibular growth in patients older than 10.5 years (4.0 mm/year) than that observed in younger group (less than 10.5 years, exhibiting a mandibular growth of 3.2 mm/year).[66]

The appropriate time for the optimal use of space maintaining (holding arches) and various functional appliances is not clear. However, it is author's experience that treatment goals can be accomplished in majority of the patients when treatment is initiated in the late mixed dentition stage of development. This treatment approach also reduces the prolonged duration of treatment and the increased cost associated with the treatment that is started in the early mixed dentition stage.

Treatment modalities that are commonly used in the early intervention of Class III malocclusion include the reverse pull headgear along with RPE and chin cup therapy. The face mask therapy is very effective in patients with maxillary deficiency. It is important for the clinician to know that the face mask therapy does not normalize growth; treated patients resuming a Class III growth pattern characterized by deficient maxillary growth is considered to be the main cause for post-treatment relapse.[67] In patients with Class III malocclusion characterized by excessive mandibular growth, the use of chin cup is believed to alter the mandibular form and retardation of condylar growth. It has been suggested that the chin cup must be worn by the patient till growth is complete, if meaningful results are to be expected.

Early orthodontic treatment specifically designed to reduce overjet can affect the incidence of maxillary incisor trauma in children. Early intervention is of significant value for the management of tooth eruption disturbances in patients with ectopic eruption, presence of mesiodens, canine impactions, etc. It also has psychological benefits, and there is strong evidence to suggest that children who received early orthodontic treatment have higher self-esteem and more positive childhood experience than those who did not receive it.

Extraction and non-extraction

Extraction of teeth has been a most reliable and widely practiced method of gaining space to resolve intra-arch discrepancy. However, introduction of other methods of gaining space, early treatment, growth modification therapy, better anchorage control and changing aesthetic standards for a fuller face and profile, have all contributed to the non-extraction approach. The decision of extraction or non-extraction can be difficult in many circumstances, and there are several factors that govern the decision-making process. The degree of intra-arch crowding is one of the parameters to determine the need for extractions. Equally important is to predict the effect of subsequent treatment on lip protrusion and soft tissue profile. In a general sense, the more severe pretreatment crowding, the more likely that extractions are required to gain adequate space to resolve discrepancy. The modern orthodontic treatment planning should be individualized since every patient varies morphologically and functionally. Therefore, the specific amount of crowding may require extractions in one patient; however, the same may not warrant extractions in another. The author considers nasolabial angle as one of the determinants of extraction therapy. If a patient has obtuse nasolabial angle, it is not appropriate to retract the lip further. Extractions are required, if the teeth are severely proclined, which does not allow the patient to achieve adequate lip seal during swallowing. The impact of sagittal movement of incisors on the lip position is also influenced by the morphology of lips. It should be noted that thinner, incompetent lips respond more dramatically to incisor position change than do thicker and competent lips.

If mandibular incisors are likely to be advanced as a part of non-extraction treatment plan, the periodontal condition, especially the width and thickness of attached gingiva, should be considered. In a patient with signs of gingival recession, or thin or deficient attached gingiva associated with mandibular anterior teeth, the labial positioning of such teeth is likely to cause progression of the condition.[68] It may be advisable to reconsider extraction therapy or place a gingival graft prior to treatment in such cases. The resolution of moderate crowding in patients with deep overbite, upright incisors and a convergent skeletal profile should be managed with non-extraction treatment approach as the extraction therapy will require retraction of already upright teeth and greater movements of roots to achieve normal tooth angulations.

Surgical and nonsurgical treatment

The presence or absence of skeletal components contributing to the malocclusion and the amount of growth remaining for a given patient influence the surgical or nonsurgical treatment decision. In a growing patient, there are many nonsurgical treatment options available to achieve desirable treatment goals. Several orthopaedic appliances are used to resolve skeletal discrepancies in Class II and Class III malocclusions. Obviously for adult patients, these nonsurgical, orthopaedic treatment options are not possible due to the absence of growth potential.

If surgical intervention is the treatment of choice, when should it be performed? Is it before or after the completion of growth? Surgical correction before the completion of growth is certainly a controversial issue. There is no scientific evidence to support that surgery performed at an early age creates a normal environment to promote favourable growth.[69] Surgical correction of abnormal skeletal bases, carried out at an early stage of development, does not contribute to the improvement of abnormal growth pattern.[69,70]

In a mild to moderate Class II patient, it is possible to achieve normal occlusal relationships with a combination of favourable growth and well-designed treatment mechanics. However, it is unlikely that a patient with very severe skeletal abnormalities and unfavourable growth pattern will suddenly grow normally and establish normal relationships of various components involved. Most believe that surgery should not be attempted before the completion of growth.

Dentofacial aesthetics is probably one of the common reasons why patients opt for surgical intervention. Surgical treatment produces dramatic facial changes in patients with certain sagittal discrepancies, like increased facial convexity, and vertical discrepancies, like increased lower facial height, which are not possible through orthodontic tooth movement alone.[71,72]

Therefore, when it comes to making a treatment option decision, the clinician should fully explore the best surgical and nonsurgical options and weigh advantages and disadvantages of each procedure and its impact on aesthetics, function and stability.

Orthopaedic and orthodontic treatment

It has been universally recognized that abnormal growth is responsible for a high percentage of malocclusions, both sagittally and vertically. The goal of orthopaedic treatment is to correct existing or developing skeletal imbalances to improve the orofacial environment at an early stage of development. Therapeutically-induced neuromuscular and skeletal adaptations in the craniofacial complex initiated during the mixed dentition stage can be achieved using variety of functional appliances. Quite often, the differential growth between the maxilla and the mandible—mandible growing faster than maxilla—contributes significantly to the improvement of occlusal relationships in Class II malocclusion. Does this mean that Class II malocclusions in growing patients are self-correcting? It is author's experience that in spite of this differential growth, the occlusion still remains the same as a result of maxillary teeth compensation by downward and forward movements. The key to control and correct this discrepancy is to hold the maxillary teeth and prevent them from displacing downward and forward by using headgears or orthopaedic appliances. Also, in growing Class II individuals, mandibular growth can be enhanced; however, there is little evidence to support that the growth of the mandible can be restrained by using chin cup in growing Class III individuals.[73]

Class III malocclusion is one of the most difficult malocclusions to treat in mixed dentition stage. Early treatment with orthopaedic facial mask, ideally initiated at the time of eruption of maxillary central incisors, produces the most dramatic results in the shortest period of time. The early intervention of Class III malocclusion does not necessarily eliminate the need for orthognathic surgery, especially in patients with significant skeletal imbalances and a family history of Class III malocclusion.

Treatment sequencing

Establishing a 'sequenced-treatment mechanics plan' based on the specific tooth movement goals is essential for a smooth and efficient treatment progress. After the formulation of final treatment plan, the practitioners must be precise in outlining the steps of treatment and the rationale for these steps. In most patients, the treatment mechanics used to achieve a particular goal will also help in the correction of another problem.[74]

In a routine orthodontic treatment, the posterior crossbites should be corrected first prior to addressing other problems. The gross correction of asymmetries may be accomplished easily before the complete bonding is done. However, in some cases, it is mandatory to achieve intra-arch alignment of teeth to facilitate correction in both the maxillary and mandibular arches, especially if elastics are going to be used. Typical treatment sequencing in patients with deep overbite involves initial alignment of teeth followed by intrusion of incisors. Overbite correction usually precedes the closure of extraction spaces; however, in some cases, simultaneous intrusion and retraction of incisors can be accomplished. In non-extraction treatment approach, the maxillary molars can be distalized using fixed distalizing modules to gain adequate space and accomplish molar correction. This will be followed by the stabilization of molars in their new positions, intrusion of incisors, distal drifting of bicuspids, bonding of mandibular arch and progressing to finishing and detailing (Fig. 2.30). The above-mentioned couple of examples demonstrate the fact that the treatment sequencing should be individualized, should not follow a set pattern and should be based on the specific tooth movement goals.

The concept of treatment sequencing in the management of patients with interdisciplinary treatment approach is little different and more complex. An interdisciplinary dentofacial therapy is the ultimate utilization of the expertise and skills in the various disciplines of dentistry.[75] It involves a team of various specialists, like orthodontist, prosthodontist and periodontist with active communication among themselves throughout treatment, from the diagnosis and treatment planning stages through to the completion of active treatment and into the retention phase. The primary goal of treatment sequencing here is to organize the sequence of various treatment procedures provided by different specialists into a logical order so that each intervention performed by one of the specialists from the interdisciplinary team facilitates the next in order.[76] Interdisciplinary treatment typically involves a sequence of disease control (periodontal, periapical infections), correction of structural malrelationships, correction of periodontal defects, restorative therapy and maintenance of optimal oral health.

Evaluation of treatment progress

After the execution of final treatment plan, it is an important step to closely monitor the treatment progress. Active orthodontic treatment phase, the duration of which is estimated and defined at the beginning of

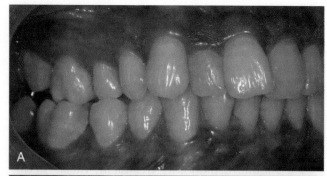

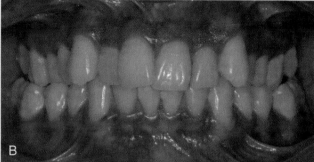

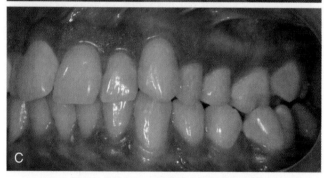

Figure 2.30 Treatment sequencing. Intraoral photographs of a 28-year-old male patient showing **(A)** maxillary and mandibular anterior crowding, **(B)** bilateral posterior crossbite and **(C)** labially placed maxillary canines. The proposed treatment sequencing for this patient is correction of bilateral posterior crossbite; bilateral distalization of maxillary molars; stabilization of maxillary molars in their new positions, while simultaneous differential retraction of bicuspids (also to address evident anterior midline shift) and intrusion of incisors; mandibular arch bonding; alignment and levelling; finishing and detailing of dentition and placement of retainers.

treatment and the same is communicated to the patient, involves a series of procedures and events; the goal of every practitioner is to make sure that it proceeds smoothly and efficiently. This is often influenced by many factors, like efficiency of orthodontic appliances and their clinical management by the doctor, keeping regular appointments by the patient and reinforcement of oral hygiene protocol by the orthodontic office. It is a good practice to continue to focus on certain specific treatment goals, like planned tooth movements or skeletal movements, and roughly estimate the time frame by which these goals are expected to be met in order to have total control of progress throughout treatment.

If, for example, maxillary molar distalization therapy with fixed distalizing module has been implemented to gain space in the maxillary arch, its progress should be monitored to check, if the molar is being moved distally in a predetermined direction. Certain associated untoward movements, like palatal movement of molars, should be detected early and the force direction should be altered promptly to avoid unnecessary delays. Quite often, in spite of careful formulation of treatment plan, treatment does not always proceed as planned, especially for patients in whom growth or cooperation is expected. Decalcification of the enamel surface mainly due to poor patient compliance is associated with fixed orthodontic appliance therapy.[77,78] Therefore, appropriate measures should be instituted to prevent the development of white spot lesions and ensure proper treatment progress. An initial inaccurate diagnosis may sometimes lead to the changes in treatment direction. These unexpected revisions of treatment plan are generally expected by the patient, if the possibilities are defined and explained at the beginning of treatment. The goal of any good orthodontic treatment plan is to make sure that the decision-making process is complete before the treatment is executed. Progressive evaluation and reevaluation of treatment progress will only help the clinician intercept and reverse untoward events, if any, as they appear rather than allowing them to become big problems leading to a significant extension of overall treatment time. This will also ensure good patient experience and higher levels of patient satisfaction.

CONCLUSION

Diagnosis in orthodontics, like in other disciplines of dentistry and medicine, is the recognition of abnormal conditions, the practical synthesis of the diagnostic information that helps the clinician to plan an appropriate treatment strategy. It is essential to have a sound knowledge of normal anatomy and craniofacial growth to recognize various dentofacial deformities; and high-quality, uncompromised diagnostic records for further evaluation of teeth and oral structures, occlusion and facial and jaw proportions.

The entire process of orthodontic diagnosis and treatment planning involves recognition of the various characteristics of malocclusion, defining the nature of the problem and its aetiology and designing a treatment strategy based on the needs and desires of the individual patient. Once patient's diagnostic information is synthesized into dental, skeletal, functional and soft tissue profile, the orthodontic treatment goals should be clearly defined. Proper treatment planning depends on accurate diagnosis, which in turn requires objective, relevant and accurate information, patient data and an analysis of various records. Establishing a 'sequenced-treatment mechanics plan' based on the specific tooth movement goals is essential for a smooth and efficient treatment progress and treatment outcome.

REFERENCES

1. Bensch L, Braem M, VanAckerK, et al. Orthodontic treatment considerations in patients with diabetes mellitus. Am J Orthod Dentofacial Orthop 2003; 123:74–78.

2. Firkin D, Ferguson J. Diabetes mellitus and the dental patient. NZ Dent J 1985; 81:7–11.

3. Geza T, Rose L. Dental correlations for diabetes mellitus. In: Rose LF, Kaye D, eds. Internal medicine for dentistry. 2nd edn. St. Louis: Mosby; 1990. 1153.

4. Van Venrooy JR, Proffit WR. Orthodontic care for compromised patients: possibilities and limitations. J Am Dent Assoc 1985; 111:262–266.

5. Ong CK, WalshL J, Harbrow D, et al. Orthodontic tooth movement in the prednisolone – treated rat. Angle Orthod 2000; 70(2): 118–125.

6. Ashcraft MB, Southard KA, Tolley EA. The effect of corticosteroid induced osteoporosis on orthodontic tooth movement. Am J Orthod Dentofacial Orthop 1992; 102:310–319.

7. Graham JW. Bisphosphonates and orthodontics. J Clin Orthod 2006; 40(7):425–428.

8. Moorrees CFA, Kean MR. Natural head position, abasic consideration in the interpretation of cephalometric radiographs. Am J Phys Anthropol 1956; 16:213–234.

9. Viazis AD. A cephalometric analysis based on natural head position. J Clin Orthod 1991; 25:172–182.

10. Solow B, Tallgren A. Head posture and craniofacial morphology. Am J Phys Anthropol 1976; 44:417–436.

11. Solow B, Siersbaek-Nielsen S, Greve E. Airway adequacy, head posture, and craniofacial morphology. Am J Orthod 1983; 86: 495–500.

12. Greenfield B, Kraus S, Lawrence E, et al. The influence of cephalostatic ear rods on the positions of the head and neck during a postural recordings. Am J Orthod Dentofacial Orthop 1989; 95:312–318.

13. Lines PA, Lines RR, Lines CA. Profile metrics and facial esthetics. Am J Orthod 1978; 73:648–657.

14. Proffit WR. Orthodontic diagnosis: the development of a problem list. In: Proffit W, ed. Henry fields. Contemporary orthodontics. St. Louis: Mosby; 1986; 123–167.

15. Stella JP, Epker BN. Systematic esthetic evaluation of the nose for cosmetic surgery. Oral Maxillofac Surg Clin North Am 1990; 2:273–287.

16. Graber TM, Rakosi T, Petrovic A. Functional analysis. In: Graber TM, Rakosi T, Petrovic A, eds. Dentofacial orthopedics with functional appliances. St. Louis: Mosby; 1985. 111–149.

17. Williamson EH. Occlusion and TMJ dysfunction. J Clin Orthod 1981; 15:393–410.

18. Okeson JP. Management of temporomandibular disorders and occlusion. 2nd edn. St. Louis: Mosby; 1989.

19. Williamson EH. Occlusion and TMJ dysfunction. J Clin Orthod 1981; 15:333–350.

20. Williamson EH. Occlusion: understanding or misunderstanding. Angle Orthod 1976; 46:86–93.

21. Karad A. Excellence in finishing: current concepts, goals and mechanics. J Indian Orthod Soc 2006; 39:126–138.

22. Roth RH. Functional occlusion for the orthodontist. J Clin Orthod 1981; 1:32–50.

23. Mclaughlin RP, Bennett JC. Finishing with the preadjusted orthodontic appliance. Semin Orthod 2003; 9:165–183.

24. Angle EH. Malocclusion of the teeth. 7th edn. Philadelphia: S.S. White; 1907.

25. Andrews LF. The six keys to normal occlusion. Am J Orthod 1972; 63:296–309.

26. Okeson JP. Management of temporomandibular disorders and occlusion. 3rd edn. St. Louis: Mosby; 1993.

27. Stallard H. Organic occlusion. In: Parone BW, ed. Oral rehabilitation and occlusion, section II, topic 9. San Francisco: University California; 1972.

28. Huffman RW, Regenos TW. Principles of occlusion. London: H and R press; 1973.

29. Roth RH. The maintenance system and occlusal dynamics. Dent Clin North Am 1976; 20:761–788.

30. Burstone CJ. Lip posture and its significance in treatment planning. Am J Orthod 1967; 53:262–284.

31. Breece GL, Nieberg LG. Motivations for adult orthodontic treatment. J Clin Orthod 1986; 20:166–171.

32. Shaw WC, Rees G, Dawe M, et al. The influence of dentofacial appearance on the social attractiveness of young adults. Am J Orthod 1985; 87:21–26.

33. Ahmad I. Geometric considerations in anterior dental esthetics: restorative principles. Pract Periodont Aesthet Dent 1998; 10(7): 813–822.

34. Janzen E. A balanced smile: a most important treatment objective. Am J Orthod 1977; 72:359–372.

35. Chaconas SJ. Orthodontic diagnosis and treatment planning. J Oral Rehabil 1991; 18:531–545.

36. Norton LA. The effect of aging cellular mechanisms on tooth movement. Dent Clin North Am 1988; 32:437–446.

37. Sodek J. A comparison of the rates of synthesis and turnover of collagen proteins in adult rat periodontal tissues and skin using microassay. Arch Oral Biol 1977; 22:655–665.

38. Musich DR. Assessment and description of the treatment needs of adult patients evaluated for orthodontic therapy. Part I, II, III. Int J Adult Orthodon Orthognath Surg 1986; 1(1):55–67,1(2): 101–107,1(4):251–274.

39. Mirabella AD. Risk factors for apical root resorption of maxillary anterior teeth in adult orthodontic patients. Am J Orthod Dentofacial Orthop 1995; 108:48–55.

40. Cangialosi TJ, Riolo ML, Owens SEJr, et al. The ABO discrepancy index: a measure of case complexity. Am J Orthod Dentofacial Orthop 2004; 125:270–278.

41. Proffit WR, Vig KW, Turvey TA. Early fracture of the mandibular condyles: frequently an unsuspected cause of growth disturbances. Am J Orthod 1980; 78:1–24.

42. Lund K. Mandibular growth and remodeling process after mandibular fractures. Acta Odontol Scand 1974; 32(suppl 64).

43. Michaud PA, Frappier JU, Pless IB. Compliance in adolescents with chronic disease. Arch Fr Pediatr 1991; 48:329–336.

44. Blowey DL, Hébert D, Arbus GS, et al. Compliance with cyclosporine in adolescent renal transplant recipients. Pediatr Nephrol 1997; 11:547–551.

45. Peck S, Peck L, Kataja M. The gingival smileline. Angle Orthod 1992; 62:91–100.

46. Drobocky OB, Smith RJ. Changes in facial profile during orthodontic treatment with extraction of four first premolars. Am J Orthod Dentofacial Orthop 1989; 95:220–230.

47. Nanda RS, Meng H, Kapila S, et al. Growth changes in the soft tissue facial profile. Angle Orthod 1990; 60:177–190.

48. Varela M. Impact of orthodontics on the psychologic profile of adult patients: a prospective study. Am J Orthod Dentofacial Orthop 1995; 108:142–148.

49. Breece GL, Nieberg LG. Motivation for adult orthodontic treatment. J Clin Orthod 1986; 20:166–171.

50. Melsen B. Adult orthodontics: factors differentiating the selection of biomechanics in growing and adult individuals. Int J Adult Orthodon Orthognath Surg 1988; 3:167–177.

51. Haskell BS, Spencer WA, Day M. Auxiliary springs in continuous arch treatment: part 1. An analytical study employing the finite-element method. Am J Orthod Dentofacial Orthop 1990; 98: 387–397.

52. Persson M, Thilander B. Palatal suture closure in man from 15 to 35 years of age. Am J Orthod 1977; 72:42–52.

53. Kahl-Nieke B, Fischbach H, Schwarze CW. Postretention crowding and incisor irregularity – a long-term follow-up evaluation of stability and relapse. Br J Orthod 1995; 22:249–257.

54. Melsen B, Agerbaek N, Markenstam G. Intrusion of incisors in adult patients with marginal bone loss. Am J Orthod Dentofacial Orthop 1989; 96:232–241.

55. Tweed C. Clinical orthodontics, vol.1. St.Louis: Mosby; 1966. 13–29.

56. Björk A. The face in profile. Sven Tandlak Tidskr 1947;40.

57. Björk A. Prediction of mandibular growth rotation. Am J Orthod 1969; 55:585–599.

58. Skieller V, Björk A, Linde-Hansen T. Prediction of mandibular growth rotation evaluated form a longitudinal implant sample. Am J Orthod 1984; 86:359–370.

59. Arnold S. Analysis of leeway space in the mixed dentition, Master's thesis. Boston: Boston University; 1991.

60. Moyers RE, vander Linden FPGM, Riolo ML, et al. Standards of human occlusal development. Monograph 5. Craniofacial Growth Series. Ann Arbor: Center of Human Development, The University of Michigan; 1976.

61. Osborn WS, Nanda RS, Currier GF. Mandibular arch perimeter changes with lip bumper treatment. Am J Orthod Dentofacial Orthop 1991; 99:527–532.

62. Bergersen EO. A cephalometric study of the clinical use of the mandibular labial bumper. Am J Orthod 1972; 61:578–602.

63. Little RM, Reidel RA, Stein A. Mandibular arch length increase during the mixed dentition: postretention evaluation of stability and relapse. Am J Orthod Dentofacial Orthop 1990; 97:393–404.

64. Haas AJ. The treatment of maxillary deficiency by opening the mid-palatal suture. Angle Orthod 1965; 65:200–217.

65. Wieslander L. Early or late cervical traction therapy of Class II malocclusions in the mixed dentition. Am J Orthod 1975; 67:432–439.

66. McNamara JA Jr, Bookstein FL, Shaughnessy TG. Skeletal and dental relationships following functional regulator therapy on Class II patients. Am J Orthod 1985; 88:91–109.

67. Turley P. Managing the developing Class III malocclusion with palatal expansion and face mask therapy. Am J Orthod Dentofacial Orthop 2002; 122(4):349–352.

68. Artun J, Krogstad O. Periodontal status of mandibular incisors following excessive proclination. Am J Orthod Dentofacial Orthop 1987; 91:225–232.

69. Washburn MC, Schendel SA, Epker BN. Superior repositioning of the maxilla during growth. J Oral Maxillofacial Surg 1982; 40:142–149.

70. Huang CS, Ross RB. Surgical advancement of the retrognathic mandible in growing children. Am J Orthod 1982; 82:89–103.

71. McNeil RW, West RA. Severe mandibular prognathism: orthodontic versus surgical orthodontic treatment. Am J Orthod 1977; 72:176–182.

72. Sinclair PM. Orthodontic consideration in adult surgical orthodontic cases. Dent Clin North Am 1988; 32:509–528.

73. Sugawara J, Asano T, Endo N, et al. Long-term effects of chin cap therapy on skeletal profile in mandibular prognathism. Am J Orthod Dentofacial Orthop 1990; 98:127–133.

74. Lindauer SJ. Orthodontic treatment planning. In: Nanda R, Kuhlberg A, eds. Biomechanics in clinical orthodontics. Philadelphia: WB Saunders, 1996; 23–49.

75. Roblee RD. Interdisciplinary dentofacial therapy. In: Roblee RD, ed. Interdisciplinary dentofacial therapy – a comprehensive approach to optimal patient care. Quintessence publishing, Printed in Singapore, 1994; 17–43.

76. Spear FM, Kokich VG, Mathews DP. Interdisciplinary management of a patient with a skeletal deformity. Adv Esthet Interdiscip Dent 2005; 1(2):12–18.

77. Årtun J, Brobakken BO. Prevalence of carious white spots after orthodontic treatment with multibonded appliances. Eur J Orthod 1986; 8:229–234.

78. Øgaard B. Prevalence of white spots lesions in 19-year-old: a study on untreated and orthodontically treated persons 5 years after treatment. Am J Orthod Dentofacial Orthop 1989; 96:423–427.

Digital Imaging in Orthodontics

3

Lisa Randazzo and Chester H Wang

Imaging is a key tool in the practice of orthodontics, providing clinicians with a documented view of craniofacial and dental structures before, during and after treatment. Photography and dentistry are forever bonded in history by Alexander Wolcott, a New York City dentist who invented the camera in 1839 (Fig. 3.1). In 1840, he opened the world's first commercial photography studio; this was also the year the world's first dental journal was printed (Fig. 3.2). In 1850, this same journal—the *American Journal of Dental Science*—published before-and-after photographs of a dental procedure, marking the birth of a new frontier in diagnosis and treatment planning (Fig. 3.3 A and B).[1] The introduction of X-rays in 1895 further revolutionized orthodontics by allowing the visualization of hidden anatomy.

One hundred years later, digital imaging technology would resolve the limitations of film photo and radiograph records, while paving the way for the three-dimensional data sets that are revolutionizing the practice of orthodontics. The digital format offers exponential benefits in terms of diagnostic and treatment planning capabilities: The ability to manipulate and enhance data; collect and collate data for the purpose of establishing norms; integrate with other digital data to create a composite patient profile; and store, organize and share records instantly are some obvious advantages of digital imaging in comparison to film. As we write, digital technology continues to advance at an alarming rate. In this chapter, we will explore the applications of digital photography and radiography in orthodontics, and what this technology holds for the future.

DIGITAL CLINICAL PHOTOGRAPHY

An advantage of digital photographs over traditional film is the ability to take countless photos at no extra cost. This is especially significant when taking clinical photos at the initial exam, given that multiple choices of angles and poses give the clinician more information for evaluation. Other advantages of digital photos include immediate viewing with option of deleting; image integrity not compromised with age, dust or scratches; zero film processing costs; easy storage, retrieval, duplication and transmission.[2] Staff can routinely take a standard set of facial and intraoral photographs in mere minutes. The images can then be reviewed on a computer monitor and, using simple image management software, can be

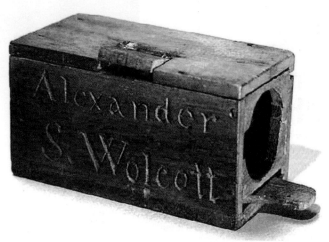

Figure 3.1 Alexander S. Wolcott's patent model for a daguerreotype camera with concave reflector was the first US patent for a photographic invention. (image © National Museum of American History, Smithsonian Institution).

THE

AMERICAN JOURNAL

OF

Dental Science.

PUBLISHED UNDER THE AUSPICES OF THE

American Society of Dental Surgeons.

VOLUME X.—1849–50.

EDITORS:

CHAPIN A. HARRIS, M. D., D. D. S.

AMOS WESTCOTT, M. D., D. D. S.

WILLIAM H. DWINELLE, M. D., D. D. S.

BALTIMORE:

ARMSTRONG & BERRY,

PHILADELPHIA: LINDSAY & BLAKISTON.

JOHN W. WOODS, PRINTER.

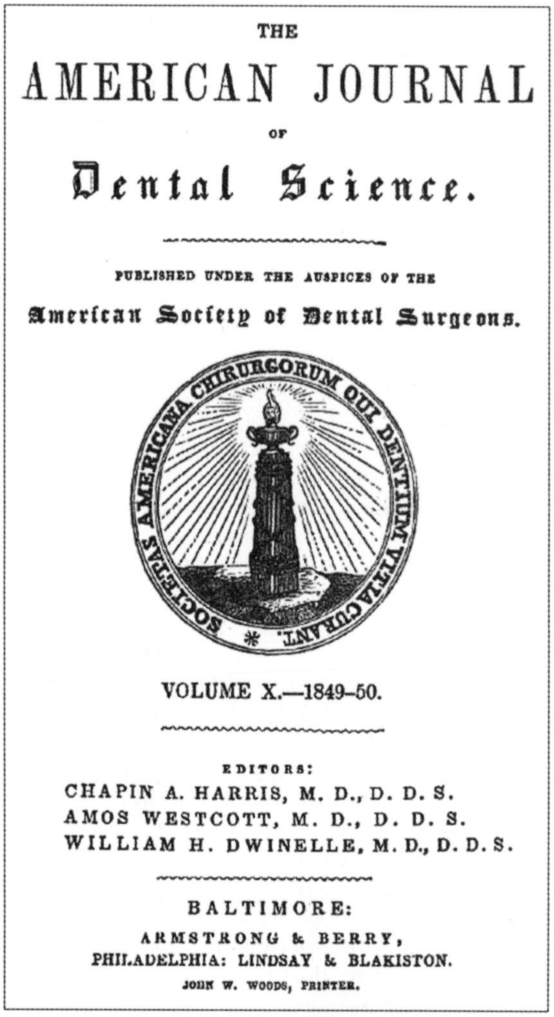

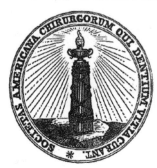

Figure 3.2 The world's first dental journal, *The American Journal of Dental Sciences*, published under the auspices of the American Society of Dental Surgeons. (Image courtesy: The University of Michigan Dental Library).

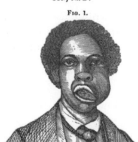

172 *Resection of Superior Maxillary Bone.* [April,

ARTICLE V.

Resection of the Left Superior Maxillary Bone. By R. THOMPSON, M. D.

FIG. 1.

Fig. 1. An engraving from a daguerreotype before the operation.

The subject of this operation, Joseph Day, a young man, aged twenty years, about five years ago had an attack of pain in the second molar tooth of the left superior maxillary bone, which he believed to be nothing more than ordinary tooth-ache. The tooth, soon becoming loose, was removed; after which, within a very few days, he discovered, protruding from the place previously occupied by the tooth, a small projection or tumor, which, though it grew but slowly, was deemed of sufficient importance to demand attention. His parents accordingly consulted, from time to time during the progress of the case, several physicians, without obtaining any important relief, or definite opinion as to its nature. During the first three years of its

A

178 *Resection of Superior Maxillary Bone.* [April,

every anticipated end, until the parts were deemed sufficiently contracted and firm to admit of the adaptation to the parts of a metallic palate and porcelain teeth, which were devised and constructed in a most masterly manner by one of our excellent dentists, Wm. E. Ide, M. D., of this city, whose skill and execution have restored to the individual the power of mastication on the left side of his mouth, and improved his voice so as to leave a stranger unadvised of his previous misfortune, while it assures us of the importance, in view of both the utility and beauty, of the highly improved profession of Dental Surgery.

FIG. 4.

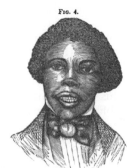

Fig. 4. An engraving from a daguerreotype after the dental operation by Dr. Ide.

REMARKS.—Before entering upon the operation, I informed my patient of my intention as to the use of chloroform—stated that my purpose was *not* to induce a perfect suspension of consciousness, but to have him

B

Figure 3.3 The very first before-and-after photographs of a dental procedure to be published: Article V, Resection of the left superior maxillary bone, by R. Thompson, M.D., Vol. X. 1849–50; 172–179. (Image courtesy: The University of Michigan Dental Library).

quickly edited, cropped, aligned, rotated, saved and printed in only a few minutes (Fig. 3.4).[3]

Most current digital cameras will interface nicely with third party image management software. There exists software packages designed especially for the dental professional that offer image organization and patient search capabilities, while also integrating with other technologies commonly found in an orthodontic office.

A typical digital imaging system for standard clinical photography consists of a camera, computer, image management software and a colour printer (Fig. 3.5). Colour inkjet technology is preferred over laser because of superior colour replication.[4] Most 3-megapixel cameras work well for viewing images on a computer screen or monitor, enlarging up to 4 by 5 inches, which is suitable for a variety of needs including presentations, lectures and printing. Digital cameras can be easily purchased through retailers online. Packages are also available from specialized camera dental supply companies that offer technical and setup assistance as well as accessories, such as intraoral mirrors and lip retractors.[3]

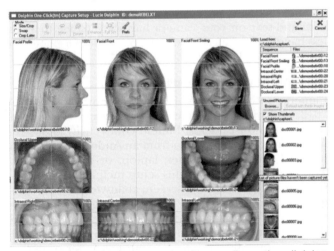

Figure 3.4 Image management software allows the clinician to quickly review, edit, align and otherwise manipulate images on the computer screen for diagnosis and record-keeping. (Image courtesy: http://www.dolphinimaging.com).

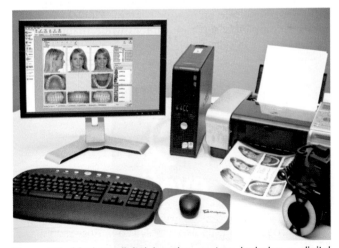

Figure 3.5 Modern digital imaging system includes a digital camera, a computer, a colour printer and an image management software. (Image courtesy: http://www.dolphinimaging.com).

TIPS FOR CAPTURING THE PERFECT DIGITAL CLINICAL PHOTOGRAPH

Quality digital photos are contingent on the protocol of capturing a set of images. It is advised to experiment with different camera settings, document the findings and refine them over time. The basic settings that should be experimented with are aperture, lens speed, zoom factor, capture distance, flash lighting, and ambient lighting. Experts advise to reduce camera settings to 'medium' or 'small' resolution in order to produce a 3–5 megapixel image. Larger images will serve no diagnostic advantage, and will slow down all aspects of any management system. Other factors to consider when designing a photo capture protocol:

- Dedicate an area with a controlled environment void of variable ambient light, such as provided by windows
- Utilize occlusal mirrors and cheek retractors to manipulate lighting and avoid shadowing (Fig. 3.6)
- Use a pure background colour, such as white or blue and an adjustable chair with a rotating seat; height adjustment is important to accommodate patients of different heights and sizes (Fig. 3.7)
- Use a ring flash for intraoral photos to avoid shadowing especially on intraorals (Fig. 3.8)

The American Board of Orthodontics has dictated and documented detailed photograph requirements for case report submissions of both facial and intraoral photographs. Standards for capturing digital dental photos have been developed by entities, such as Olympus America and the American Academy of Cosmetic Dentistry.

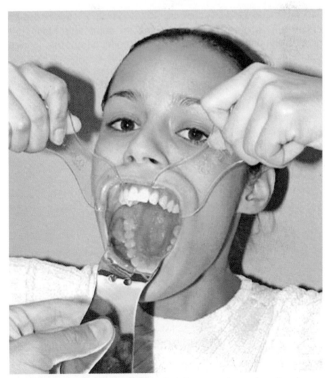

Figure 3.6 Utilizing cheek retractors and occlusal mirrors help increase visibility of crucial anatomy when taking intraorals. (Image courtesy: http://www.dolphinimaging.com).

Because the protocols have been rigorously tested and refined, these standards provide an excellent guide for orthodontic staff and laboratory technicians.[5] Ideally, a customized protocol should be developed by the individual practice to accommodate the specific needs of that practice, and then followed uniformly for each patient photo sequence.[4]

ALTERNATE IMAGE CAPTURE AND MANAGEMENT: WIRELESS TETHERED PHOTOGRAPHY (FIG. 3.9)

WiFi connectivity can be added to your digital camera via a secure digital (SD) memory card—which combines a WiFi transmitter with onboard memory. An SD card streamlines the image management process by eliminating the need to manually transfer the photos from your camera to your desktop or laptop computer. The SD card will automatically transmit all new digital photos over your in-office WiFi zone to a designated folder in your computer, so they can be loaded directly into your practice management programme. Some of the benefits of a WiFi system include less wear-and-tear on your camera hardware (since there is less handling); reduced downtime of waiting for photos to upload; and reduced staff involvement.[6]

Built-in WiFi for remote capture and control

Cameras with built-in WiFi became available in early 2012, and within a couple of years became a standard feature in most cameras. Built-in connectivity allows remote control of the camera from an Android or iOS app installed on your computer, laptop, or mobile device. The many capabilities of this setup include: instant preview on a high-resolution screen; ability to remotely trigger the camera's shutter; online sharing of images directly from camera; and wireless transfer of images to a designated folder on your computer. In short, remote software apps allow you to use your computer or device as a control panel for your camera.[7,8]

Detachable lens as WiFi access point (Fig. 3.10)

In late 2013, Sony introduced a new lens-style camera that is meant to attach to a smart phone with the intent to transform the phone into an upscale camera. The lens can also act as a completely separate camera while maintaining a

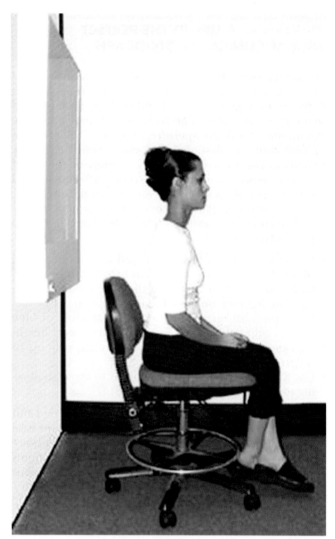

Figure 3.7 A pure background and an adjustable chair that rotates will assist in uniformity among clinical photos. (Image courtesy: http://www.dolphinimaging.com).

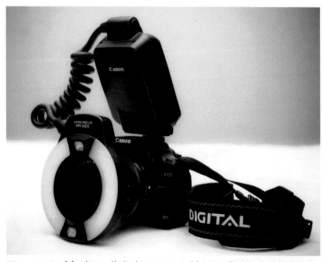

Figure 3.8 Modern digital camera with ring flash. (Image courtesy: http://www.dolphinimaging.com).

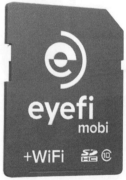

Figure 3.9 The EyeFi Mobi Digital (SD) memory card with built-in WiFi. (Image courtesy: Eye-Fi Inc).

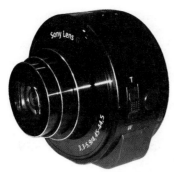

Figure 3.10 The Sony Cyber-shot QX10 detachable lens camera. (Image courtesy: http://dolphinimaging.com).

wireless connection to the smartphone, allowing the phone to be used as viewing pane and control panel.[9] The benefits of this setup, especially in orthodontics, would be the ability to more efficiently capture photos of hard-to-reach locations, such as intraorals.

Digital impressioning systems for intraoral data capture (Fig. 3.11)

Digital impressions, CAD/CAM, 3D printing

The ultimate goal of a dental impression is to obtain an accurate negative copy of the teeth and interocclusal

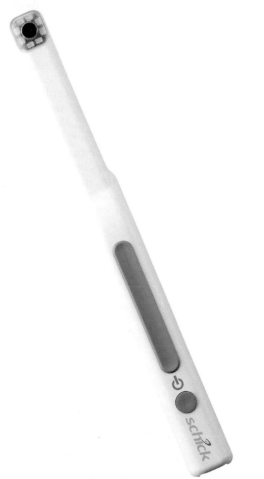

Figure 3.11 USBCam4 intraoral camera from Schick by Sirona. (Image courtesy: Sirona Dental, Inc).

relationship, from which to build a precise replica of the dentition for the purpose of creating restorations. Dentists began using elastomeric materials to create impressions—from which they made gypsum models—beginning in 1937, when Sears introduced agar as an impression material for crown preparations.[10] In the 1980s, dental impressioning digital scanners were introduced. These hand-held scanners captured virtual 3D images of teeth that could be used to fabricate restorations.[11]

3D printing was first used in dentistry in the 1980s with the separate contributions of three pioneers of CAD/CAM systems. These include Dr. Moermann, who developed the Sirona CEREC® product which employed a digital impression system that feeds the obtained digital data directly into a milling system capable of carving out the restoration from ceramic or resin blocks.[12] In the late 2000s, more advanced digital impressioning systems and 3D printing technology made possible a far broader application of CAD/CAM beyond crowns and overlays. Progressive practices are already using the integration of these technologies to streamline the entire diagnostic, treatment planning and treatment process.

Restoration fabrication is not the only application of intraoral digital impressioning. Newer digital impressioning systems, such as iTero®, use an intraoral scanner to capture data for the purpose of creating study models, completely bypassing the need for traditional PVS impressions. The data sets gathered from intraoral scanning systems can be used to create both stereolithographic and three-dimensional digital models, and have been determined to be a valid and reproducible method for measuring distances in a dentition.[13] The scanners are being used by both doctors and staff, with typical scanning time being reported less than 10 minutes for the entire process. These digital files have lots of uses—they can be easily archived; imported to systems, such as SureSmile® and Invisalign®; and merged with a patient's CBCT scan as part of their comprehensive record.

COMMUNICATION: CASE PRESENTATION, PATIENT EDUCATION, AND MARKETING

The inherent versatility of digital images allows for a single image to have multiple uses. An image stored in a patient record, for example, can also be placed in a communication to a referring doctor (Fig. 3.12), emailed, printed and given to the patient to take home, and/or placed in a presentation program, such as PowerPoint or Keynote. This ability to improve communication through visualization empowers the clinician in his relationships with both patients and colleagues. It has been proven that patients more readily accept treatment when they understand their conditions (Fig. 3.13).[14]

Pre- and post-treatment images can serve as powerful marketing tools. The ability to create an electronic presentation of your most attractive treatment outcomes to loop on a monitor as a patient waits in the lobby or consultation room is a productive use of otherwise empty time.[15] Further, these same images can be used to create advertisements for placement in local media, such as newspapers, magazines, or even television spots to promote your practice.

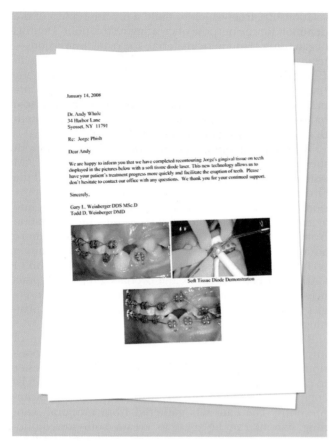

Figure 3.12 Digital records can easily be dropped into letters to patients and referrals for enhanced communication. (Image courtesy: Dr Gary and Dr Todd Weinberger, Plainview, New York).

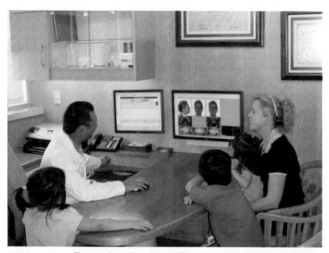

Figure 3.13 Easy visualization offered by digital technology allows the orthodontist to easily convey conditions and treatment to patients and parents. (Image courtesy: Chang Orthodontics, Los Alamitos, California).

COMPUTERIZED CEPHALOMETRY: TRACING, SUPERIMPOSITION, AND TREATMENT PLANNING

Cephalometry is the system of measuring the bones of the cranium for purposes of scientific analyzes. Introduced in 1931 by BH Broadbent (Fig. 3.14), cephalometry has

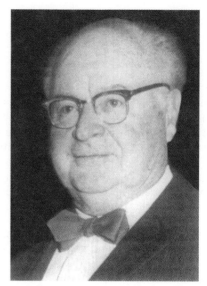

Figure 3.14 B.H. Broadbent, father of cephalometrics. (Image courtesy: Journal of Clinical Orthodontics).

been a vital tool in orthodontics. Practitioners rely on this system to diagnose, treatment plan, and monitor changes resulting from treatment and growth.[16] Because each cephalometric measurement is primarily based on distances, angles and ratios amongst established landmarks within the cranium, the precise—and consistent—identification of these landmarks is of great value to the practitioner.

Tracing and analysis

The manual performance of a single cephalometric tracing and analysis is time consuming, and its accuracy is contingent on many variables (Fig. 3.15). Initial variables include exposure settings and developing techniques that can affect the integrity of the cephalogram and subsequently the quality of the tracing. Sources of error in the manual process include the inherent magnification of radiographic film, hand-tracing, measuring, recording

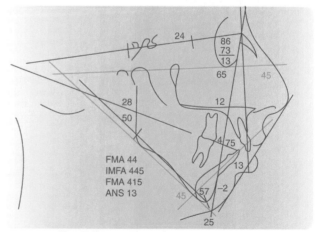

Figure 3.15 Traditional cephalometric tracing done by hand. (Source: Reprinted with permission from eMedicine.com, 2009; http://emedicine.medscape.com/article/839645-overview).

and landmark identification. Further, there is the additional risk of misreading the measurements that were obtained manually. Computerized cephalometric analysis programs, on the other hand, automate both the data acquisition and analysis processes while reducing user error. In a comparative study of the reliability of computerized cephalometric analysis programs versus manual tracing, there was found to be no statistically significant difference between manual tracing and the computerized programs.[17] The ability to digitally enhance and/or correct for chemical and/or exposure errors immediately renders the cephalogram viable for tracing, while also eliminating the need for a second exposure.[18]

Cephalometric computer programs often contain hundreds of analyzes, any number of which can be performed simultaneously under the direction of the operator. This instantaneous access to such a large spectrum of data enhances the clinician's ability to make a more accurate diagnosis, while also saving countless hours of labour (Fig. 3.16).[19]

Superimposition and treatment planning

The process of superimposing cephalometric tracings inherently contains a margin of variability when aligning traced structures. This error correlates to the consistency and quality of each cephalogram, augmented by the skill of the operator in detecting key structures. While a finely tuned X-ray capture protocol and years of practice on the part of the operator greatly to reduce this phenomenon, the margin of error still remains. Further accuracy can be improved with digital technology by using specialized software on imported digital versions of the radiographs. This method greatly improves the user's ability to uniformly orient the images and their structures in a series of time points. Using this combination of technology greatly minimizes the need for additional exposure of X-ray. [20]

GROWTH/TREATMENT PREDICTION AND VISUAL TREATMENT OBJECTIVE (VTO)

Establishing a visual treatment objective serves multiple purposes for the orthodontist. Fundamentally, its purpose is to forecast both the patient's growth, when applicable, and the anticipated influence of treatment to create an estimated outcome. The VTO allows the orthodontist to treatment plan more effectively by keeping his goal in sight, so to speak, and also helps him communicate that goal to the patient and colleagues.[21] In the larger picture, the VTO serves to facilitate dialogue between the patient and clinical team regarding aesthetic expectations, while helping to guide the clinician toward the desired result.[22] In this sense, the VTO serves as not only a treatment planning tool, but also as an education and communication tool. Patients are more likely to accept treatment when they are able to visualize the outcome up front, and understand how treatment will affect them on a day-to-day basis as well as within the broader scheme of their lifespan.

In summary, the VTO accomplishes the following:

- Predicts craniofacial growth based on individual morphogenetic pattern (Fig. 3.17)
- Analyzes the soft tissue profile
- Graphically, plans the optimum soft tissue facial profile for the specific patient
- Determines optimum tooth re-positioning, especially incisors and molars
- Helps determine total arch length discrepancy while considering 'cephalometric correction' (Fig. 3.18)

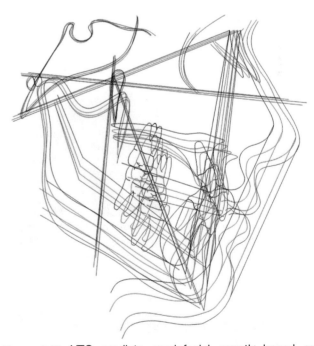

Figure 3.17 VTO predicts craniofacial growth based on designated norms by superimposing tracings from different time points; Bolton Growth program is shown here. (Image courtesy: Dolphin Imaging & Management Solutions http://www.dolphinimaging.com).

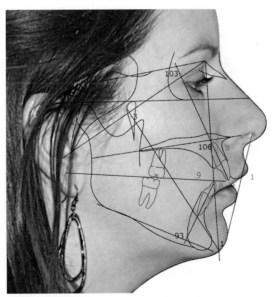

Figure 3.16 Automated cephalometric tracing programs afford the clinician the instant access to hundreds of analyzes. (Image courtesy: http://www.dolphinimaging.com).

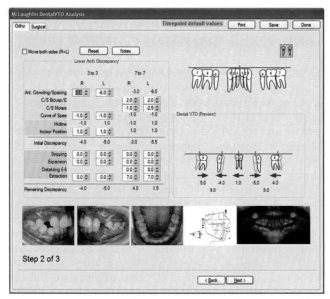

Figure 3.18 Automated VTO programs can help the clinician determine total arch length discrepancy while considering cephalometric correction. (Image courtesy: Dr Richard P. McLaughlin, San Diego, California).

- Aids in determining between extraction and non-extraction treatment
- Helps determine which teeth to extract
- Assists in planning treatment mechanics
- Provides a visual goal for which to strive during treatment (Fig. 3.19)[23]

Growth prediction

Growth prediction plays a critical role in creating a reliable VTO.[21] Curiosity about craniofacial growth and development was the motivation behind the development of cephalometry, which was introduced by Broadbent in an attempt to chart the course of a normal growing child.[24] The first attempts at prediction can be dated to 1937, when he suggested that, on average, the face grows downward and forward along a straight line.[21] Before computerized cephalometrics was introduced in the 1970s, the method of growth prediction evolved from the logical act of extending the orientation pattern of the original cephalogram, to the more individualized practice of comparing two serial cephalograms, observing a growth 'trend,' and applying it to a future time frame. Neither of these methods was reliable due to the fact that a patient does not always follow his/her original growth pattern. Still, growth prediction remained a mainstay in the orthodontic treatment planning armamentarium.

Computerized prediction and planning

The modern concept of the VTO is most often attributed to Dr. Robert M. Ricketts (Fig. 3.20) and his work on computerized cephalometry with Rocky Mountain Orthodontics Data Services®, RMO® Inc, Denver, CO in the mid-1970s (Fig. 3.21). Incidentally, the term was actually coined by Reed A. Holdaway (Fig. 3.22) in 1971 while engaged in research on soft tissue analysis and its use in orthodontic treatment planning. Creating a VTO from a computerized cephalogram affords the clinician the opportunity to instantly build a customized treatment plan. A typical automated VTO program requires the operator to digitize the cephalogram by inputting the landmarks (Fig. 3.23). If appropriate, the program will apply an algorithm calculated from generalized growth averages to produce a tracing that represents the expected growth of the patient during a given amount of time.[21] Often the operator will be presented with multiple analyzes to choose from. The program uses the specific algorithm to produce

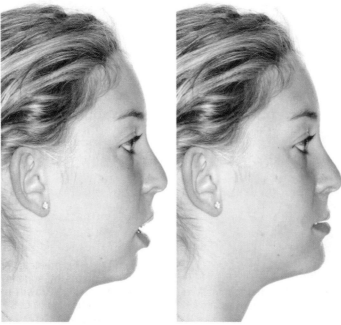

Figure 3.19 Images of pretreatment and simulated treatment (using VTO software). (Image courtesy: http://www.dolphinimaging.com).

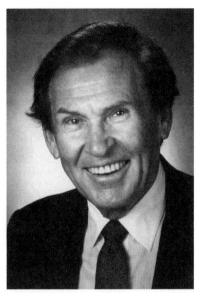

Figure 3.20 Dr Robert M. Ricketts is known for his work on computerized cephalometry with Rocky Mountain Orthodontic Data Services®, RMO® Inc, Denver, CO (Photo by Rick Mueller Photography, Scottsdale, Arizona, 1992. Image courtesy: the American Association of Orthodontists).

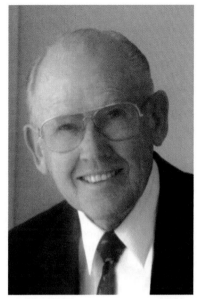

Figure 3.22 Reed A. Holdaway coined the term *visual treatment objective* in 1971 while engaged in research on soft tissue analysis and its use in orthodontic treatment planning.

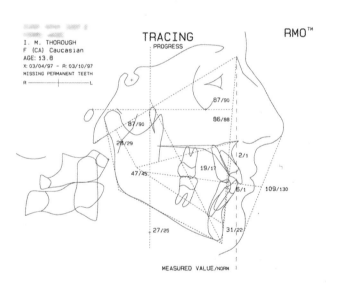

Figure 3.21 A tracing from Rocky Mountain Orthodontic Data Services®, RMO® Inc, Denver, CO one of the first computerized cephalometric tracing systems. (Image courtesy: Rocky Mountain Orthodontics Data Services®, RMO® Inc., Denver, CO).

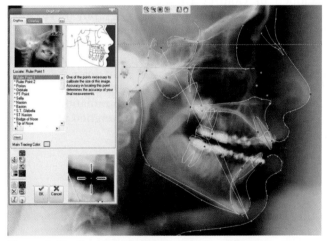

Figure 3.23 Sophisticated yet simple software programs allow the clinician to digitize the cephalogram by inputting landmarks. (Image courtesy: http://www.dolphinimaging.com).

biomechanics and allowing the clinician to conduct tasks, such as morphing soft tissue images to illustrate the anticipated aesthetic outcome.[23]

THREE-DIMENSIONAL RADIOGRAPHY: WHY CONE BEAM COMPUTED TOMOGRAPHY (CBCT)?

The goal of imaging in orthodontics is to document the craniofacial anatomy at a given time point during treatment and, as applicable, growth. Orthodontists in the past, in utilizing two-dimensional radiographs, have been trained to compensate for the inherent limitations of projecting three-dimensional structures in a two-dimensional medium. Unfortunately, these compensations are characterized by a margin of error directly related to the 'guess work' involved in the

guidelines for tooth positioning and recommendations regarding procedures and modalities—such as extraction or anchorage—which might be needed to achieve the desired goal. The computerized VTO is dynamic and interactive, taking into account both growth and

task itself.[18] The volumetric (three-dimensional) data produced by computed tomography (CT) offers spatial reality in addition to the discrimination of many types of tissues including bone, teeth, nerves and soft tissue. So, while medical CT, which generates three-dimensional data sets, resolves many of the limitations of 2D radiography, it is costly and emits far too large a dose of radiation than is acceptable for the serial imaging required by orthodontics and other dental specialties (Fig. 3.24).

The introduction of cone beam computed tomography (CBCT) in the late 1990s was able to answer the need for a low-radiation, volumetric data set that delivers exponentially more information than the traditional dental 2D imaging series. Ten years of utilizing CBCT within the medical field has proven it especially useful for the spectrum of dental specialties, prompting a paradigm shift within the dental disciplines that has not been witnessed since the invention of the camera and dental X-rays.

History of CBCT

Computerized scanning technology has been used in medicine for diagnostic purposes since the 1970s. Developed by Godfrey Hounsfield (Fig. 3.25) for EMI Laboratories, computed axial tomography (CAT) technology allowed clinicians the first glimpse of hidden anatomy as it exists in true spatial reality.[25] The ability to construct three-dimensional images of crucial internal anatomy of interest was a giant leap forward in medical diagnostic capabilities: In the circumstances of critical medical conditions, the high radiation dose was considered a negligible risk when weighed against the

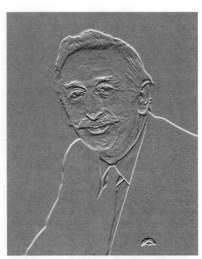

Figure 3.25   Godfrey N. Hounsfield was an engineer at EMI Laboratories in England when he invented computed axial tomography technology. (Image courtesy: http://www. dolphinimaging.com).

benefit of discovery. Unfortunately, it was not a viable solution for routine dental imaging.

Cone beam computed tomography

The need for a three-dimensional scanning technology that would emit significantly less radiation led to the development of cone beam computed tomography (CBCT). CBCT technology differentiates itself from CAT technology in the shape, or trajectory, of the beam used to capture the image. The CAT uses a 'fan-shaped beam' to take multiple individual slices, which are later reconstructed to form a three-dimensional composite image. On the other hand, the 'cone-shaped beam' is able to capture the entire object with one quick scan, translating to a far lower dose of radiation (Fig. 3.26). While this method sacrifices some image integrity in terms of contrast resolution, the fast scan time minimizes motion artifacts and provides more than enough data for certain medical uses, specifically dental imaging.[26]

The first CBCT scanner was built in 1982 and developed for use in angiography at the Mayo Clinic.[27] It was not until 1999 that the NewTom 9000 CBCT unit (Fig. 3.27) was developed specifically for dental use by Quantitative Radiology in Verona, Italy (Fig. 3.28). In 2001, the first unit arrived in the United States, and by 2003 more than 500 units had been sold by five different manufacturers. The rapid pace of development continues to deliver more affordable models, leading to a growing prevalence that some predict will translate to the standard of care in the very near future (Fig. 3.29).

Spatial reality

Volumetric data provides immensely more information than traditional 2D records, and does so in a 1-to-1 image-to-reality ratio.[28] This allows the practitioner to examine and evaluate conditions without the burden, or margin of error, associated with accommodating for magnification and distortion. The magnification

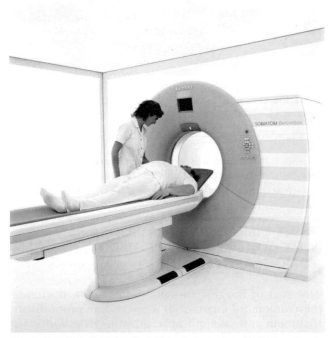

Figure 3.24   Modern medical CT unit: Somatom Definition. (Image courtesy: Siemens Technikkommunikation, Munich, Germany http:// w1.siemens.com/innovation/en/news_events/innovationnews/ innovationnews_articles/medical_solutions/a_new_dimension_in_ computed_tomography.htm).

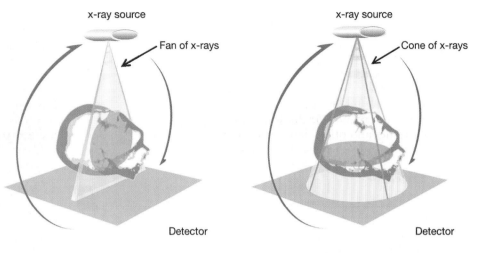

Figure 3.26 Computed axial tomography projects a fan-shaped beam to capture the image, whereas cone beam computed tomography uses a cone-shaped beam. (Illustration by Ardy Ho, 2009. Image courtesy: http://www.dolphinimaging.com).

Fan Beam CT   **Cone Beam CT**

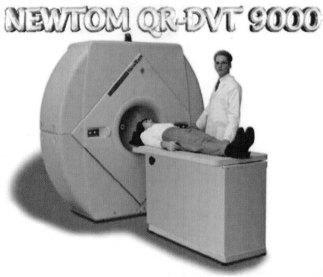

Figure 3.27 The NewTom 9000 was the first CBCT unit developed exclusively for dental use. (Image courtesy: DDI Imaging Centers, Sacramento, California).

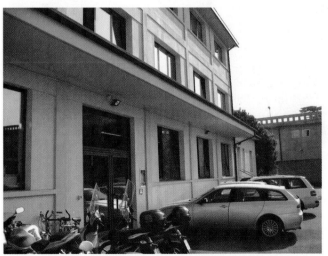

Figure 3.28 The unpretentious exterior of the birthplace of CBCT: Quantitative Radiology in Verona, Italy, developer of the NewTom 9000. (Image courtesy: http://www.dolphinimaging.com).

distortion produced by conventional X-rays is a result of the geometrical phenomenon that occurs when a three-dimensional object is projected on a two-dimensional recording plane.[29]

Witnessing anatomy in true spatial perspective removes the guesswork inherent in the analysis of conventional radiography. Further, features imbedded in 3D software allow for the exact measurement of anatomy (Fig. 3.30), making possible the precise location of pathologies, such as bone cysts, various stages of erosion, and secondary arthritis (Fig. 3.31). A volumetric data set can show the physical relationship of anatomical parts and provides the actual measurement of their relationship. For example, it is possible to measure the width of each tooth to help with the arch length calculation for orthodontic purposes. In addition to measuring distances, cephalometric landmarks can be accurately identified on hard and soft tissues—in three dimensions.[30] Although, a lot more research, data gathering, and product development are necessary before orthodontists may utilize these techniques to fully take advantage within their daily practice.

Point of view

The added dimension of volumetric data opens a window that remains closed in traditional 2D imaging: being able to view anatomy from all angles and in three dimensions allows the clinician to view and identify previously hidden conditions (Fig. 3.32). In addition to clearly identifying supernumeraries and impactions, this also allows for the serial tracking of expanding or contracting lesions, and accurately anticipating the progress of infectious lesions.[31] The ability to manipulate volumetric data sets has enabled practitioners to assess anatomy from previously impossible angles, such as viewing the occlusion from the back of the patient's head into the oral cavity (Fig. 3.33).[32]

Specialized 3D dental software programs are also able to display and measure the airway volume of the oropharyngeal airway and sinuses, enabling the clinician to calculate the most restricted areas within these areas

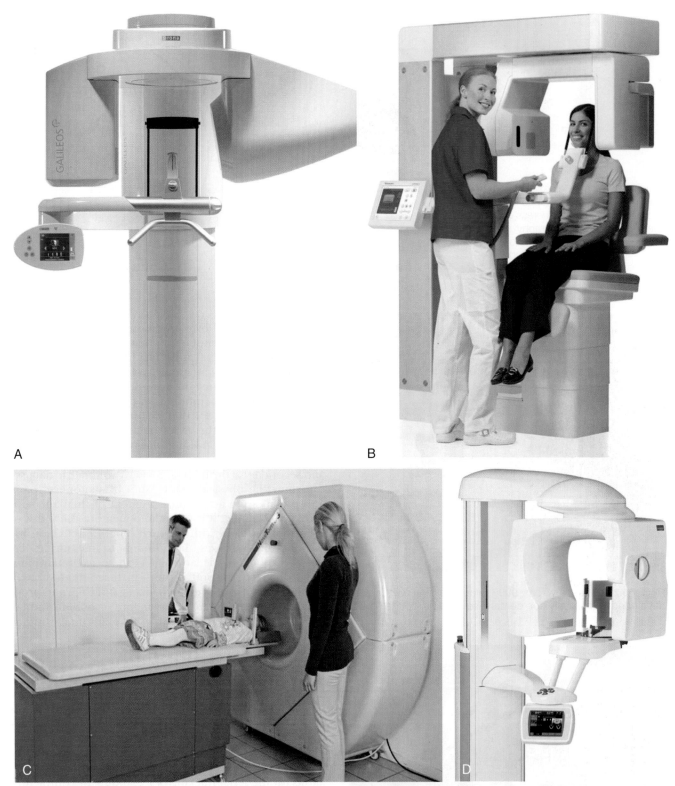

Figure 3.29 Several current CBCT units. **(A)** GALILEOS by Sirona. **(B)** Scanora 3D by Soradex. **(C)** NewTom 3G by AFP Imaging. **(D)** Promax by Planmeca.

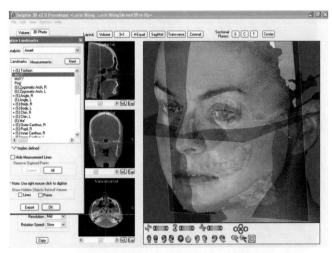

Figure 3.30 Tools embedded in 3D software allow the clinician to measure anatomy and thereby determine the precise location of pathologies. (Image courtesy: http://www.dolphinimaging.com).

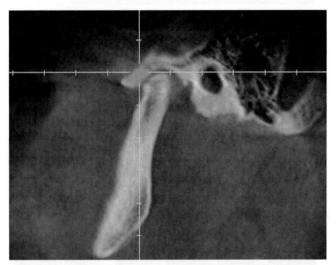

Figure 3.31 Determining the precise location of pathologies, such as bone cysts is possible with measuring tools in 3D software. Image scanned using Sirona GALILEOS and provided. (Image courtesy: http://www.dolphinimaging.com).

(Fig. 3.34). The growing understanding of the association between airway size and orthodontic treatment makes this valuable to the practitioner during treatment planning. These same software programs should also be able to locate mandibular nerves (Fig. 3.35) and their relationships to roots and other structures, making the technology invaluable for the safe execution of impaction and implant procedures. In addition, if other related medical problems are identified, the patient can be referred to the proper specialist with complete image records, aiding in communication between the orthodontist and the specialist.[30]

Endless views

A major advantage of 3D data sets over 2D is the ability to process the data using special software that by design has a very low learning curve, making it easy and practical for all staff to use. Staff can take the scan and within five minutes build an image file that includes all the images of a standard orthodontic series: from a cephalometric image to airway analysis to TMJ assessment (Fig. 3.36).[30] Once the data has been imported into the software, the user is able to isolate anatomy and segment the hard and soft tissues for closer viewing. Different colours can be assigned to different anatomy for further visual clarity (Fig. 3.37).

Further, the ability to adjust translucency and colours of the image gives an opportunity to determine the specific relationship of soft tissue to skeletal structures (Fig. 3.38). This has significant applications for orthodontic treatments, such as planning tooth movement, extractions, and other therapies that might alter facial appearance.[32] In addition, secondary reconstructions of any desired anatomical view or isolated structure can be easily generated from this single scan.[33]

Patient expectations

The sophisticated technology once exclusive to elite sectors of academia and the medical/hospital industry has permeated popular culture during the lifetime of the 21st century orthodontic patient. These new

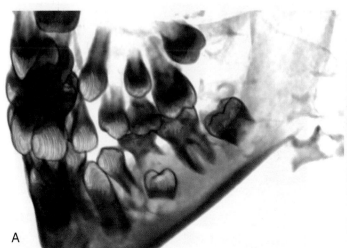

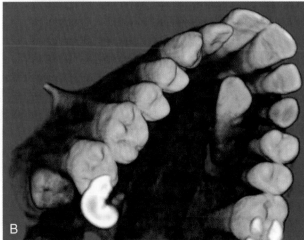

Figure 3.32 Previously hidden conditions, such as impacted teeth and supernumeraries can be clearly visualized using 3D software. (Image courtesy: (Figure A) http://www.dolphinimaging.com and (Figure B) Dr Peter Gaffey, Nowra, New South Wales, Australia).

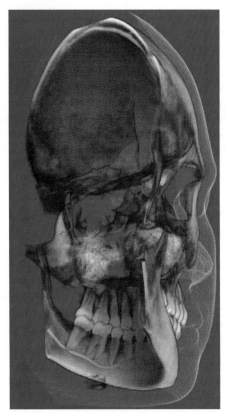

Figure 3.33 Three-dimensional software gives the clinician the ability to manipulate the image for previously impossible angles, such as viewing the occlusion from the back of the patient's head into the oral cavity. (Image courtesy: http://www.dolphinimaging.com).

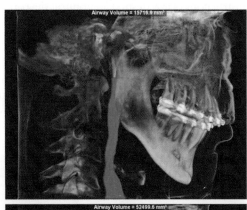

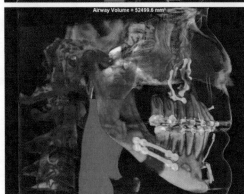

Figure 3.34 Specialized software enables the assessment and measurement of airway used in examining orthognathic surgery results. (Image courtesy: Dr Julio Cifuentes, Santiago, Chile).

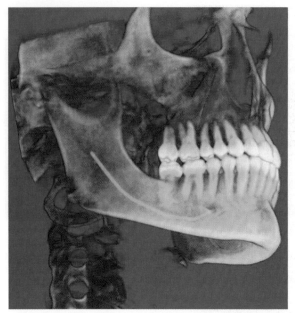

Figure 3.35 The ability to locate the mandibular nerve is especially useful when planning treatment for implants. (Image courtesy: http://www.dolphinimaging.com).

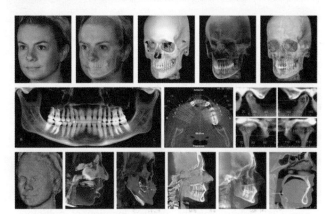

Figure 3.36 A single 20-s CBCT scan can deliver the entire series of dental diagnostic images. (Image courtesy: http://www.dolphinimaging.com).

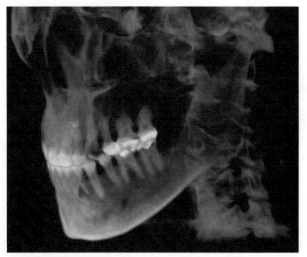

Figure 3.37 Three-dimensional software contains colour tools to better visualize anatomy. (Image courtesy: http://www.dolphinimaging.com).

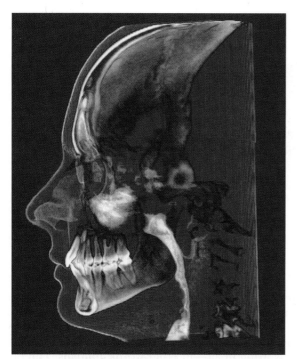

Figure 3.38 Tissue segmentation tools allow the clinician to easily visualize the relationship of soft tissue to skeletal structures. (Image courtesy: http://www.dolphinimaging.com).

patients expect the same level of sophistication for all their professional services. The ability to communicate intelligently and on the same level with this generation will promote increased case acceptance, improved outcomes, and new patient referrals (Fig. 3.39).[34]

CAVEATS OF CONE BEAM

The wealth of information delivered by cone beam CT brings with it some controversy regarding the medicolegal liability of the practitioner. For example, some practitioners have put forth that there is no responsibility for radiologic findings beyond those needed for a specific task, such as treatment planning; however, this is deemed by many to be a misconception.

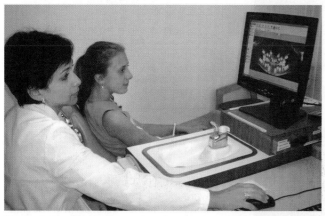

Figure 3.39 Three-dimensional records can be immediately displayed for patient consultation after the initial exam. (Image courtesy: http://www.dolphinimaging.com).

Professional organizations, such as the American Association of Maxillofacial Radiologists (AAOMR), have drafted edicts and guidelines for members to follow for the primary purpose of avoiding unpleasant legal situations.[35,36] Individual practitioners will find it wise to implement a protocol that requires each scan to be read by an outside service as a precaution. In fact, as CBCT becomes more prevalent and establishes itself as a standard of care in dental imaging, interpretation services dedicated to reading these volumetric data sets are being created to address this specific need.[37]

CBCT BASICS AND TERMINOLOGY

As with any new technology, cone beam CT is accompanied by its own nomenclature. In this section, we will review some basic terminology that clinicians and staff will need to be familiar with when utilizing CBCT.

Points of view

The third dimension brought by CBCT also brings with it perspectives that relate only to the 3D environment:

Sagittal: A vertical or longitudinal plane passing through the standing body from front to back, dividing it into left and right halves.

Coronal: A vertical plane passing through the body that divides it into front (anterior) and back (posterior) halves.

Axial: Also known as a *transverse* plane, this is horizontal and divides anatomy from top to bottom (Fig. 3. 40).

Multiplanar reconstruction (MPR): This term refers to the reconstruction of images in the coronal and sagittal planes in conjunction with the original axial data set (Fig. 3.41).

Maximum intensity projection (MIP)

This term refers to the actual computerized rendering process of the voxel data set, which allows the image to be viewed in three-dimensional object (Fig. 3. 42).

Attenuation and greyscale

As an X-ray beam passes through material, it experiences a loss of intensity that is referred to as attenuation. This loss of beam intensity will vary depending on the density of the material, and is displayed in image tissues as varying hues of grey.

Pixels and voxels

The word 'pixel' is a portmanteau of the words 'picture' and 'element.' Likewise, the word 'voxel' is formed by the words 'volume' and 'element.' A pixel represents the smallest item of information in an image, and is arranged in a two-dimensional grid. In colour systems, each pixel has typically three or four components, such as red, green and blue, or cyan, magenta, yellow and black. The intensity and hue of each pixel can vary, creating multiple combinations of data elements that make it possible to form an accurate rendering or image. In

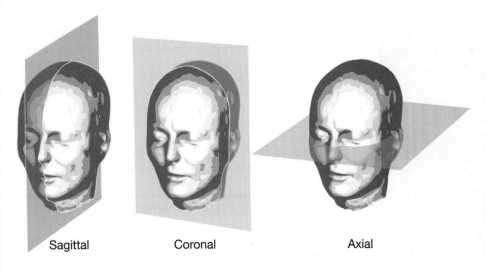

Sagittal   Coronal   Axial

Figure 3.40 Perspectives relating to 3Ds include coronal, sagittal and axial. Illustration by Ardy Ho, 2009. (Image courtesy: http://www.dolphinimaging. com).

turn, a 'voxel' is the smallest piece of information in a three-dimensional image. The voxel adds the third dimension to the pixel by adding the z-axis (depth) to the x-axis (width) and the y-axis (height). Image resolution and pixel size possess an inverse relationship: the smaller the pixel, the higher the resolution.[25]

Hounsfield units (Fig. 3.43)

The Hounsfield Unit is a measurement relating to the radiolucency of materials in a CAT scan, and is used to distinguish between the different biological structures. The Hounsfield Unit (HU) is based on the Hounsfield Scale, which determines 0 HU to be the radiodensity of distilled water at standard pressure and temperature, and −1000 HU as the radiodensity of air. These values

were chosen as universally available references, and were oriented to the key application for which CAT technology was developed: imaging the internal anatomy of living creatures based on organized water structures and mostly living in air—in other words, humans. The range of the scale goes as high as +1000 for cortical bone, +400 for cancellous bone, and as high as +3000 for metallic structures. This system was developed by Godfrey Hounsfield, the key engineer in CAT technology.[25]

Microsievert

The sievert is a unit of measurement used to measure the biological risk of radiation deposited in human tissue. Not all radiations have the same biological effect, even for the same amount of absorbed dose. Equivalent dose

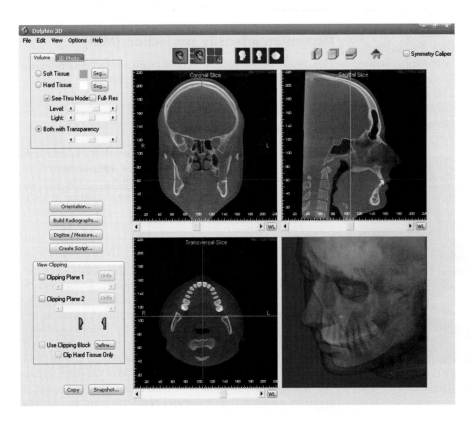

Figure 3.41 Three-dimensional software offers the ability to reconstruct images in the coronal and sagittal planes in conjunction with the original axial data set. (Image courtesy: http:// www.dolphinimaging.com).

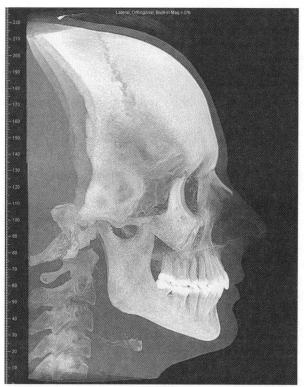

Figure 3.42 A maximum intensity projection rendered from a CBCT data set using 3D software. (Image courtesy: http://www. dolphinimaging.com).

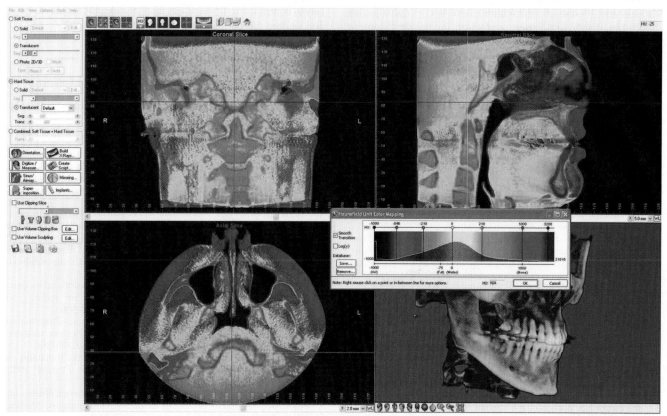

Figure 3.43 Software tools make it possible to distinguish between different biological structures via their radiolucency values in Hounsfield units. (Image courtesy: http://www.dolphinimaging.com).

is often expressed in terms of millionths of a sievert, or micro-sievert.[38]

DOSIMETRY: 2D VS 3D

Comparatively speaking, cone beam CT delivers a larger dose of radiation than a conventional 2D full mouth series.[39,40] In recent years, however, manufacturers are addressing radiation concerns with scanner technology that allows low-exposure alternative scanning options. While dose reductions are accompanied by significant reductions in image quality, these lower quality images can be suitable for interim tasks, such as recording treatment progress.[41] In addition, dose-reduction can be further achieved with protocols and techniques, such as wearing a thyroid collar and leaded glasses, and minimizing FOV exposure parameters as much as possible.[42,43]

CONCLUSION

Digital imaging technology has created a paradigm shift in the practice of orthodontics. This is a result of no single application, but rather the collective contributions of its steady—and fast-paced—course of evolution. All corners of the orthodontic practice have been impacted, from the doctor's chair to the front desk receptionist and beyond to the manner in which the patient conveys information to family and friends.

While 3D imaging represents the most recent frontier in orthodontic imaging, it is by no means the final one. To the contrary, it is paving the way for digital applications that will one day replace the need for physical diagnostic tools, such as impressions and study models, plus 4D (add time) and 5D (add function) applications in the not-so-distant future. The technologies of the future will continue to be increasingly relevant to practitioners as software developers seek guidance and direction from the clinician in a quest to answer the real-life needs of the orthodontist.

ACKNOWLEDGEMENTS

The authors would like to recognize Dr. Swann Liao and Mr. Ken Gladstone for their relentless quest to provide the orthodontic community with cutting edge software solutions. Drs Paul Thomas and Richard P. McLaughlin have been invaluable for their input, insight and expert counsel during the development of many of Dolphin's trademark software products. We would also like to thank Mr. David Fischer, Dr. David Hatcher, Ms. Jackie Hittner, Mr. Ardy Ho, Ms. Linda Homel, and Ms. Camille Mayorga, for their gracious assistance and meaningful contributions during the research and preparation of this chapter. Lastly, we would like to thank Dr. Ashok Karad for extending us this opportunity to contribute to this very special textbook, and for his guidance and wisdom throughout the process.

REFERENCES

1. Galante DL. History and current use of clinical photography in orthodontics. CDA Journal 2009; 3:173–174.
2. Sandler J, Murray A. Digital photography in orthodontics. J Orthod 2001; 28:197–201.
3. Iwamoto E. Choosing a camera. Dolphin Echoes 2007; 2: 2.
4. Wang CH. Standardized digital photography for the orthodontic practice. J Ind Orthod Soc 2005; 38:176–183.
5. Morris M. Digital photography: Your modern communication and marketing tool. DE 2009; 3:88–90.
6. McEvoy, Steven. WiFi your camera: How to save time & money taking photo records. http://blog.mmeconsulting.com/wifi-your-camera-how-to-save-time-money-takin; May 6, 2011.
7. Sawyer P. Remote shooting: Using your laptop as monitor and control for your Canon DSLR. http://photography.tutsplus.com/tutorials/remote-shooting-using-your-laptop-as-monitor-and-control-for-your-canon-dslr—photo-6583; May 19, 2011
8. Jarvis C. Wireless cameras are the future — What's in it for you? http://blog.chasejarvis.com/blog/2013/02/wireless-cameras-are-the-future-whats-in-it-for-you/; Feb 28, 2013.
9. Goode L. Sony's head-scratcher of a camera: The Lens-Style Cyber-Shot QX10 and QX100. http://allthingsd.com/20130904/sonys-head-scratcher-of-a-camera-the-lens-style-cyber-shot-qx10-and-qx100/; September 4, 2013.
10. Birnbaum NS, Aaronson HB, Stevens C, Cohen B. 3D digital scanners—a high tech approach to more accurate dental impressions. Inside Dentistry. 2009 April; 5(4).
11. Birnbaum NS, Aaronson HB. Dental impression using 3D digital scanners: virtual becomes reality. Compend Contin Educ Dent. 2008 Oct; 29(8):494, 496, 498–505.
12. Miyazaki T, Yasuhiro H, Kunii J, Kuriyama S, Tamaki Y. A review of dental CAD/CAM: current status and future perspective from 20 years of experience. Dent Mater J 2009; 28(1): 44–56.
13. Cuperus AM, Harms MC, Rangel FA, Bronkhorst EM, Schols JG, Breuning KH. Dental models made with an intraoral scanner: a validation study. Am J Orthod Dentofacial Orthop 2012 Sep; 142(3):308–13.
14. Kahn E, Malik-Kahn M. All you need to know about digital photography. DE 2002; 5:78–82.
15. Weinberger G. Optimizing practice protocols for a new century of orthodontics. Dolphin Echoes 2008; 1:4.
16. Broadbent B. A new X-ray technique and its application to orthodontia. The introduction to cephalometric radiology. Angle Orthod 1931; 1:45–66.
17. Erkan M, Gurel GH, Nur M, Demirel B. Reliability of four different computerized cephalometric analysis programs. Eur J Orthod 2012 Jun; 34(3):318–21.
18. Santoro M, Jarjoura K, Cangialosi TJ. Accuracy of digital and analogue cephalometric measurements assessed with the sandwich technique. AJO DO 2006; 3:345–351.
19. Quintero JC, Trosien A, Hatcher D, Kapila S. Craniofacial imaging in orthodontics: Historical perspective, current status, and future developments. Angle Orthod 1999; 69:491–506.
20. Roden-Johnson D, English J, Gallerano R. Comparison of hand-traced and computerized cephalograms: Landmark identification, measurement, and superimposition accuracy. AJO DO 2008; 4: 556–564.
21. Cangialosi TJ, Chung JM, Elliot DF, Meistrell ME. Reliability of computer-generated prediction tracing. Angle Orthod 1995; 4:277–284.
22. Pektas ZO, Kircelli BH, Cilasum U. The use of software systems for visualized treatment objectives in orthognathic surgery. Medical Robotics. Vienna: I-Tech Education and Publishing, 2008.
23. Jacobson A, Sadowsky PL. A visualized treatment objective. J Clin Orthod 1980; 14: 554–571.
24. Ricketts RM. The value of cephalometrics and computerized technology. Angle Orthod 1972; 42:179–199.

25. Lark MR. Cone beam technology: a brief technical overview. DE 2008; 8:70–74 & 129.

26. Khaled E, Friedland B, Scarfe WC, Ganon E. CBCT versus MDCT. www.conebeam.com.

27. Sukovic P. Cone beam computed tomography in dentomaxillofacial imaging. AADMRT Currents 2004; http://www.aadmrt.com/static.aspx?content=currents/sukovic_winter_04

28. Lagravère MO, Carey J, Toogood RW, Major PW. Three-dimensional accuracy of measurements made with software on cone-beam computed tomography images. Am J Orthod Dentofacial Orthop 2008; 134:112–116.

29. Athanasiou AE. Orthodontic cephalometry. London: Mosby-Wolfe, 1997.

30. Randazzo L. Orthodontic applications of 3D imaging. J Am Orthod Soc 2008; 4:16–19.

31. Lark M. How cone beam technology revolutionized my practice. DE 2008; 6: 62–67.

32. Valiathan A, Dhar S, Verma N. 3D CT imaging in orthodontics: Adding a new dimension to diagnosis and treatment planning. Trends Biomater Artif Organs 2008; 21(2):116–120.

33. Ziegler CM, Woertche R, Brief J, Hassfeld S. Clinical indications for digital volume tomography in oral and maxillofacial surgery. Dentomaxillofac Radiol 2002; 31:126–30.

34. Miller MK. Generation X: Are you targeting the current orthodontic market? Dolphin Echoes 2008; 1:3.

35. Farman AG, Scarfe WC. Dolphin 3D and oral and maxillofacial radiology practice. Dolphin Echoes 2009; 2:5.

36. Kincade K. Cone-beam CT raises new issues for dentists. www.drbicuspid.com; April 28, 2009.

37. Hatcher DC, Randazzo L. The dynasty that David built. Dolphin Echoes 2009; 4:1.

38. Radiation Measurement Fact Sheet. Department of Health and Human Services, Centers for Disease Control and Prevention. www.bt.cdc.gov/radiation/measurement.asp.

39. Roberts JA, Drage NA, Davies J, Thomas DW. Effective dose from cone beam CT examinations in dentistry. The British Journal of Radiology 2009; 82:35–40.

40. Grunheid T, Kolbeck Schieck JR, Pliska BT, Ahmad M, Larson BE. Dosimetry of a cone-beam computed tomography machine compared with a digital X-ray machine in orthodontic imaging. Am J Orthod Dentofacial Orthop 2012 Apr; 141(4):436–43.

41. Ludlow JB, Walker C. Assessment of phantom dosimetry and image quality of i-CAT FLX cone-beam computed tomography. Am J Orthod Dentofacial Orthop 2013 Dec; 144(6):802–17.

42. Gang L. Patient radiation dose and protection from cone-beam computed tomography. Imaging Science in Dentistry 2013; 43:63–69.

43. Qu XM, Li G, Ludlow JB, Zhang ZY, Ma XC. Effective radiation dose of ProMax 3D cone-beam computerized tomography scanner with different dental protocols. Oral Surg Oral Med Oral Pathol Oral Radiol Endod 2010 Dec; 110(6):770–76.

4 Sagittal Discrepancies

Ashok Karad

The correction of sagittal discrepancy has been considered a common goal for the patient and the orthodontist. A large proportion of clinical situations is not a single entity and is often associated with significant skeletal and dental imbalances in sagittal plane. Traditionally, orthodontic assessment and diagnosis is mainly based on Angle's sagittal classification of malocclusion.[1] Since the dentofacial abnormalities exist in sagittal, transverse and vertical planes, contemporary orthodontic assessment and interpretation must include their understanding in all three dimensions. While studying the various abnormalities in anteroposterior plane, it is also important to identify vertical discrepancies, as their presence impacts the sagittal dimension.

This chapter deals with the systematic approach to the diagnosis and treatment planning of various sagittal discrepancies based on redefined treatment goals, treatment options at various stages of development and their resolution with appropriate treatment mechanics and long-term stability.

The sagittal discrepancies essentially include Class I, Class II and Class III malocclusions; however, defining any one of these malocclusions is difficult because this arbitrary categorization consists of various abnormalities. In their original interpretation and understanding, these abnormalities represent the anteroposterior relationship between the maxillary and the mandibular first permanent molars as described by Edward H. Angle.[1] Therefore, this approach does not recognize the dysplastic skeletal sagittal relationship of the maxilla and mandible to each other and to the cranial base. It is critical to identify and assess vertical discrepancies and understand their role in anteroposterior malrelationships. Equally important has been the proper understanding of the functional adaptation to the sagittal and vertical discrepancies. This leads to a posterior and occasionally anterior condylar displacement or autorotation of the mandible due to deficient posterior or excessive anterior facial height.[2]

The traditional approach to the diagnosis of sagittal discrepancies based on the molar relationship or the habitual occlusion does not reveal the abnormalities in the vertical dimension and in the condylar position in the fossa, dictated by the occlusal guiding forces and the neuromuscular adaptation. Therefore, a contemporary approach should address all these areas in differentially diagnosing variety of sagittal discrepancies. The diagnosis, treatment planning and the orthopaedic and orthodontic management of various Class II and Class III clinical situations and their interaction with the vertical dimension form the basis for this chapter.

DEVELOPMENT OF A SAGITTAL PROBLEM

Various factors play an important role in the development of sagittal discrepancies. Identifying and understanding the involvement of specific causative factors is essential in developing an effective treatment plan. Growth disturbances, tooth size, crowding or spacing of teeth, height of palate and length and width of arch are all influenced by heredity. These, in turn, significantly contribute to the development of Class II and Class III malocclusions. An injury to the maxilla during growth can produce retardation of growth resulting in Class III relationship, while trauma during pregnancy or birth injury damaging the condyle can lead to Class II relationship. Congenital defects, like cleidocranial dysostosis leading to retruded maxilla and prognathic mandible; cerebral palsy resulting in loss of muscular coordination; Down's syndrome (Mongolism); hypothyroidism leading to underdevelopment of mandible and Pierre Robin syndrome resulting in micromandible, are all responsible for the development of Class II malocclusion. Class II relationship is also caused by certain local factors, like anomalies in number of teeth—missing teeth and supernumerary teeth; anomalies of form and position—large teeth, ectopic positions and transpositions and tooth-arch disproportion—spacing and crowding. Abnormal pressure habits, like thumb sucking and tongue thrusting, significantly contribute to the development of sagittal discrepancies. In patients with nasal obstruction, tongue is held in forward position to keep the airway patent leading to short and constricted maxilla and long and expanded mandible. Disturbances in eruption sequence and timing can often result in occlusal interferences leading to a pseudo Class III malocclusion. Certain other factors, like extracted or missing teeth and their non-replacement, result in drifting of adjacent teeth, thereby developing a dental sagittal discrepancy.

DIAGNOSIS OF SAGITTAL DISCREPANCIES

Since sagittal discrepancies consist of various components and are often associated with abnormalities in other planes of space, their accurate diagnosis is a key element in the design of any successful treatment plan. It is essential to obtain adequate information about patient's problem through the analysis of high-quality diagnostic records in order to improve diagnostic capabilities. However, increased amount of patient data requires thorough analysis and makes the process of interpretation a complex process. Therefore, a systematic approach to diagnosis is the key to redefining treatment goals and treatment planning of various sagittal discrepancies and their resolution with appropriate treatment mechanics to ensure long-term stability.

Class II malocclusion

'Class II' is a broad term designated to a set of various abnormalities that could be either simple or most complex. It is not a single clinical entity, rather it consists of various components of the craniofacial complex having variations in size, shape and position.[3] In order to plan an appropriate treatment, the clinician should localize and quantify any skeletal and dental contributions, sagittal and vertical variations and the role of abnormal function and habits to the development of Class II malocclusion. There are many different types of Class II patients with significant variations in skeletal, dental and soft tissue morphology.

Clinical examination and functional assessment

Improvement in facial profile is the most important factor considered by most patients seeking orthodontic treatment. Therefore, the focus of orthodontic treatment should be to achieve pleasing facial profile and soft tissue characteristics rather than just cephalometric norms. In the past few years, the scope of orthodontic assessment and treatment has been expanded, and the ability of the orthodontist to remarkably improve the patient's facial appearance has also been considerably enhanced.[4] During the process of clinical examination, while evaluating patient's profile, it is important to study total profile, lip projections and nasolabial angle (Fig. 4.1).

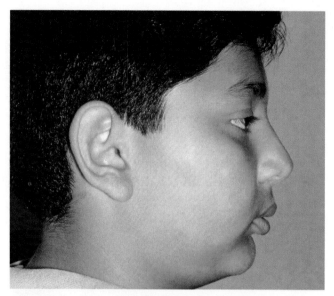

Figure 4.1   Class II facial profile.

Functional assessment

Functional assessment is performed during the clinical examination for planning treatment for Class II malocclusions, especially in growing patients.

- It is important to study the relationship between increased overjet, commonly found in Class II division 1 malocclusion, and lip function (Fig. 4.2). If the lower lip is trapped between maxillary and mandibular incisors, its posture and function in the same area along with hyperactive mentalis muscle function leads to progressive deforming activity on dentition.
- To differentiate between functionally true Class II and forced bite Class II malocclusions, it is essential to assess the relationship between rest position and occlusion.
- Tongue posture and function should be carefully assessed to find out its role in the development of malocclusion.

The above-mentioned parameters are of particular interest in establishing soft tissue or facial aesthetic goals, as the face is considered to be the determinant of orthodontic treatment.

Morphologic characteristics

As a clinician, it is critical to identify and locate the structures at fault with the help of cephalometric analysis, which are mainly contributing to the development of Class II malocclusion (Fig. 4.3). Their understanding is essential to establish treatment goals and plan a treatment to resolve them. The first simple step is to find out whether it is dental or skeletal Class II malocclusion. Dental Class II malocclusion is caused by tooth migration, which may be confined to the entire arch or a segment of the arch following a missing tooth or abnormally displaced teeth. Skeletal Class II malocclusion could be as a result of prognathic maxilla and normal mandible,

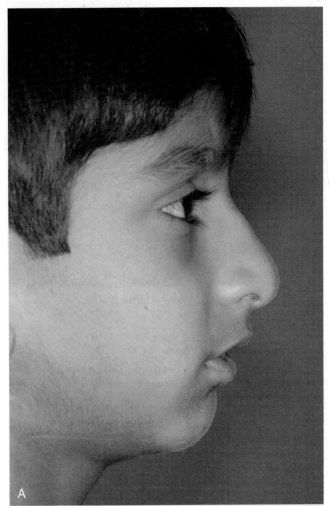

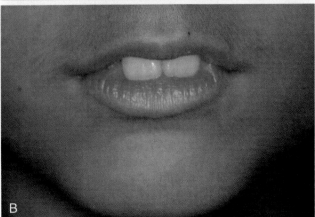

Figure 4.2 Abnormal **(A)** Lip posture and **(B)** Function.

retrognathic mandible and normal maxilla or a combination of both—prognathic maxilla and retrognathic mandible. This is just a broad understanding of Class II malocclusion, whether it is dental or skeletal, and identifying the component involved. The Class II patient should be further analyzed cephalometrically to ascertain the involvement of vertical discrepancy or whether it is purely horizontal in nature.

Björk[5] divided Class II malocclusions into forward and backward rotators and suggested that forward rotators

are more common and easier to treat than the backward rotators. Classification of Class II malocclusion to group together cases having predominantly similar features is useful for the clinician to design a common treatment. These can be broadly classified as following horizontal types.[6]

Horizontal types

There are many variations in horizontal types of Class II malocclusions ranging from those having normal skeletal features but Class II dental characteristics to distinctly different skeletal types (Fig. 4.4).

- *Type A:* It is characterized by normal sagittal position of the jaws exhibiting normal skeletal profile. The maxillary dentition is protracted with normal mandibular dentition leading to a Class II molar relationship associated with increased overjet and overbite. This type of malocclusion is also called a *dental Class II malocclusion*
- *Type B:* It exhibits a midface prominence with a mandible of normal length. The maxilla is prognathic, while the mandible is in normal anteroposterior relationship.
- *Type C:* It is characterized by retrognathic maxilla and mandible, the maxillary incisors are either upright or labially tipped and the mandibular incisors are proclined. The patient usually exhibits smaller facial dimensions than other Class II type displaying a Class II profile.
- *Type D:* It shows a retrognathic skeletal profile with maxillary and mandibular retrognathism. The maxillary incisors are typically proclined, and the mandibular incisors are either upright or lingually inclined.
- *Type E:* It displays a maxillary prognathism and a normal mandible. The maxillary and mandibular incisors are proclined. Bimaxillary protrusion Class II malocclusions are usually of horizontal type E.
- *Type F:* It is a large, heterogeneous group with mild skeletal Class II tendencies. Each type F is generally considered to be milder, non-syndromal forms of types B, C, D or E.

Functional Class II with a distally forced bite

This is a functionally created Class II malocclusion, having normal postural rest position but a forced mandibular retrusion in habitual occlusion. The path of closure of the mandible is abnormal or forced; quite often, associated with an infraocclusion of buccal segment teeth leading to an excessive overbite.

In addition to this, it is important for the clinician to predict the Class II malocclusion as forward or backward rotator. Four of the variables—mandibular inclination, shape of the lower border of the mandible, inclination of the symphysis and intermolar angle, when combined, give the best prognostic estimate of mandibular growth rotations.[7]

Class III malocclusion

Class III malocclusion generally manifests at an early age, and it is one of the difficult clinical situations to treat. The factors responsible for development of Class III malocclusion are different from those in Class II situation. As compared to Class II relationships, most Class III problems have a strong hereditary component.[8,9]

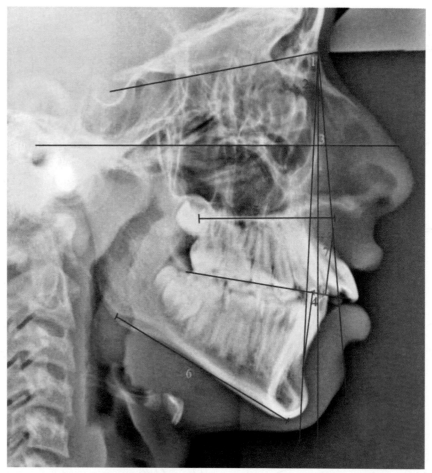

Figure 4.3 Cephalometric assessment (Class II malocclusion). 1, SNA; 2, SNB; 3, ANB; 4, Wits appraisal; 5, Maxillary length; 6, Mandibular length; and 7, Point A—nasion perpendicular. (For a detailed sagittal cephalometric assessment refer to Figures 2.21–2.25 in Chapter 2).

Environmental influences, like habits and mouth breathing, also play an important role in the development of Class III malocclusion. A growth stimulus from the constant distraction of the mandibular condyle in patients with abnormal mandibular posture can result in excessive mandibular growth.[10] Class III malrelationships are often associated with morphologic and functional consequences. Patients with Class III problems may present with an impairment of dentofacial aesthetics and occasionally with psychological issues. This clinical situation may lead to incorrect loading of the teeth; chewing and speech functions may be altered. The prosthetic rehabilitation of the case may be difficult.

Like Class II malocclusion, Class III malocclusion is not a single clinical entity, rather it consists of various components of dentofacial complex.[1] In a broader perspective, it is generally considered to be a manifestation of mandibular prognathism or midface deficiency or a functional forward shift of the mandible on closure to occlusion. Therefore, it could be skeletal Class III, dental Class III or 'pseudo' Class III, all resulting from a variety of combinations.

It is critical for the orthodontic professional to localize the disharmonious elements contributing to the Class III malocclusions. Other affected areas in the dentofacial complex of individuals having Class III malocclusions also include larger mandibular plane angles, larger gonial angles, longer mandibles and compensations of the dentition with maxillary dentoalveolar protrusion and mandibular dentoalveolar retrusion.[12] While evaluating the Class III relationships, it is important to identify whether the problem is dental, caused by the improper inclination of the maxillary and mandibular incisors; functional, caused by the occlusal interferences; or skeletal, caused by the discrepancies of the maxilla and mandible. Therefore, the evaluation of a patient with Class III morphology should have a prescribed protocol to include: (1) assessment of general facial morphology, (2) identification of abnormal components, (3) the vertical position of the mandible in posture and occlusion and (4) the position and angulation of the maxillary and mandibular incisors.

It is important to follow a well-organized and systematic approach to the diagnosis of patients with Class III malocclusion to determine the following variations in the Class III skeletal profile[13] (Fig. 4.5).

1. Normal maxilla and mandibular prognathism
2. Retruded maxilla and normal mandible
3. Maxillary retrusion and mandibular prognathism
4. Normal maxilla and mandible

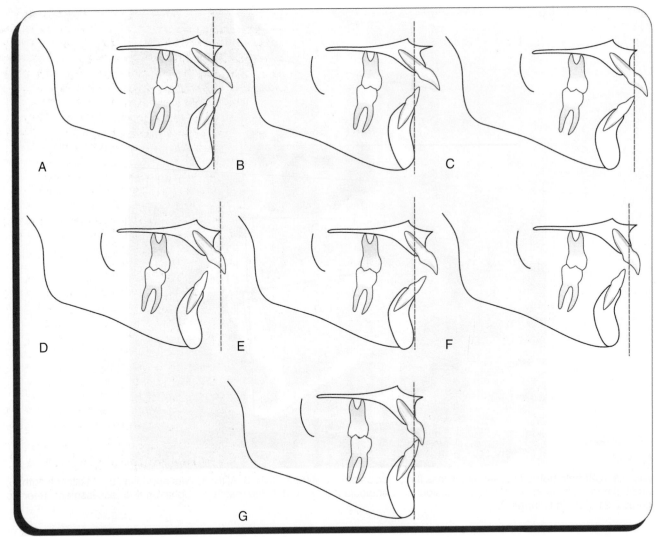

Figure 4.4 Horizontal morphologic characteristics of Class II malocclusion based upon the study by Robert Moyers. **(A)** Maxillary dental protraction. **(B)** Midface prognathism. **(C)** Maxillary retrognathism, dental protraction and mandibular retrognathism, dental protraction. **(D)** Mandibular retrognathism, maxillary retrognathism and maxillary dental protraction. **(E)** Maxillary prognathism and dental protraction. **(F)** Mandibular retrognathism. **(G)** Normal maxillary and mandibular dental and skeletal relationships.

Assessment of facial profile

An evaluation of the facial profile should include an analysis of facial proportions, midface position, chin position and vertical proportions.[14] This assessment is done to determine whether the patient's profile is straight, convex or concave (Fig. 4.6). Patients with maxillary deficiency usually exhibit a concave profile and flattening of the infraorbital rim and the area adjacent to the nose. It is essential to note that the facial convexity decreases as the patient matures.

Functional assessment

In patients with Class III malocclusion, it is critical to assess the relationship of the mandible to the maxilla to identify whether a centric relation (CR) and centric occlusion (CO) discrepancy exists. This is important because the anterior position of the mandible may be guided by abnormal tooth contacts that shift the mandible forward.

Patients having normal facial profile, Class I skeletal pattern and Class I molar relationship in CR with forward shift of the mandible on closure will exhibit concave profile, Class III skeletal and dental profile in CO. This clinical situation is called *pseudo Class III malocclusion*. However, patients with no shift of the mandible on closure are most likely to have a true Class III malocclusion. The key diagnostic feature in differentially diagnosing pseudo and skeletal Class III malocclusions is the gonial angle measurement that is usually more obtuse in skeletal Class III.[15]

Dental assessment

It is essential to assess the position and angulations of maxillary and mandibular incisors and the resultant interincisal relationship. The Class III relationship may be associated with an edge-to-edge relationship, a negative overjet or a positive overjet (Fig. 4.7). If it is associated with a negative overjet, the clinician should proceed to functional assessment to differentiate between true and pseudo Class III malocclusion. If the Class III molar relationship is associated with a positive overjet or an edge-to-edge incisal relationship, a compensated Class III malocclusion is suspected. A compensated Class III malocclusion is a clinical

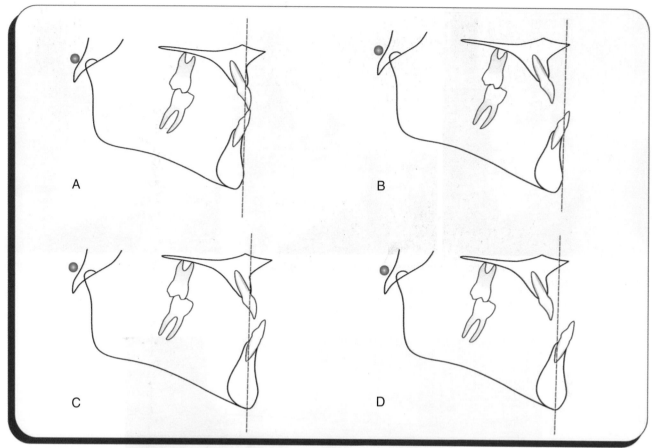

Figure 4.5 Variations in Class III skeletal profile. **(A)** Normal maxilla and mandible. **(B)** Maxillary retrusion and normal mandible. **(C)** Normal maxilla and mandibular prognathism. **(D)** Maxillary retrusion and mandibular prognathism.

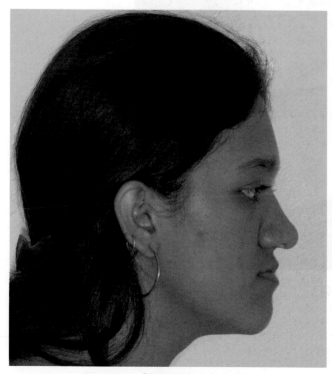

Figure 4.6 Class III facial profile.

situation where maxillary and mandibular incisors compensate for the existing skeletal Class III discrepancy.

Cephalometric assessment

Patients with Class III malocclusion may present with a variety of combinations of skeletal and dentoalveolar components often associated with vertical and transverse discrepancies. Proper understanding of these components is essential to establish appropriate treatment plan so that the underlying cause of the discrepancy can be treated effectively.

Cephalometric analysis is a valuable diagnostic tool that drives the clinician to pinpoint the components responsible for the development of Class III malocclusion. While analyzing the anteroposterior relationship of maxilla and maxillary incisors and mandible and mandibular incisors, it is important to assess the vertical and transverse discrepancies associated with Class III malocclusion. The traditional approach to analyze patients with Class III malocclusion is to use ANB discrepancy. The patients with skeletal Class III malocclusion usually exhibit negative ANB angle with a smaller SNA angle and a larger SNB angle. However, individual variations in cranial base flexure and anteroposterior displacement of nasion often alter the ANB discrepancy.[16] Therefore, alternative cephalometric measurements and analysis, like Wits appraisal, effective maxillary and mandibular length and nasion perpendicular to 'A point', can be used to assess the anteroposterior relationship of the maxilla and mandible (Fig. 4.8).

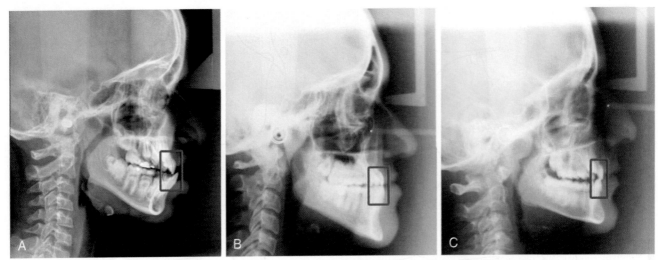

Figure 4.7 Variations in incisal relationship in Class III malocclusion. **(A)** Negative overjet. **(B)** Edge-to-edge incisor relationship. **(C)** Positive incisor overlap.

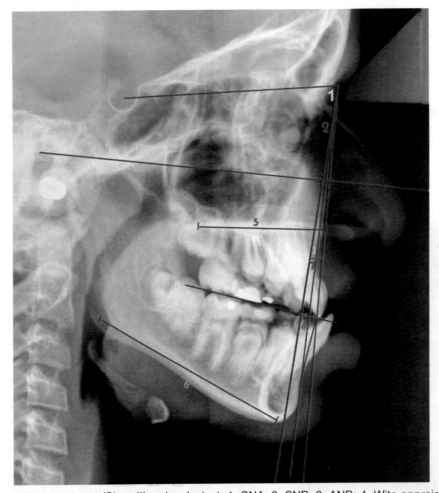

Figure 4.8 Cephalometric assessment (Class III malocclusion). 1, SNA; 2, SNB; 3, ANB; 4, Wits appraisal; 5, Maxillary length; 6, Mandibular length; and 7, Point A—nasion perpendicular. (For a detailed sagittal cephalometric assessment refer to Figures 2.21–2.25 in Chapter 2).

TREATMENT PLANNING

Establishing accurate diagnosis is the key element in formulating a successful treatment plan. The practitioner should focus on the development of an individualized treatment plan to improve the treatment results and shorten the treatment duration. The best way to approach treatment planning for a specific malocclusion is to define treatment goals as to what needs to be accomplished by treatment. These include facial, skeletal and dental goals. Making the most of available diagnostic information including the patient's chief complaint forms a basis for establishing treatment goals. This often drives the clinician to an important process of a re-exploration of the diagnostic information and consideration of some important factors.

- Determine whether the malocclusion is skeletal or dentoalveolar.
- Treatment planning for the sagittal discrepancies requires that the clinician should assess the relationship between the postural rest position of the mandible and the habitual occlusion. This will help differentiate between 'true discrepancy' with a normal path of closure from postural rest to habitual occlusion and 'functional discrepancy' with abnormal path of closure of the mandible.
- While assessing the treatment possibilities for sagittal discrepancies in a growing patient, it is essential to forecast the probable growth direction and magnitude.
- Ascertain the growth potential of the patient based upon the useful diagnostic information. The clinician should assess the growth potential and when a growth spurt can be expected to determine the treatment timing and the method. Growth increments per unit time are a prime consideration.
- Identification of aetiological factors responsible for the development of a sagittal discrepancy, the role of neuromuscular dysfunctions and differentiating hereditary malocclusions are of great value in planning a treatment.
- The dentofacial aesthetics greatly influences the treatment planning process of sagittal discrepancies since it is one of the main reasons why patients seek orthodontic treatment. The clinician must record the expectations of a patient in terms of aesthetics. The aesthetic benefits of orthodontic treatment are universally accepted by both patients and practitioners.[17,18] It has been widely recognized that attractive individuals are more likely to be successful in their academic and career accomplishments.[19,20] Orthodontic treatment affects aesthetics through three-dimensional alteration of anterior tooth position. Therefore, the impact of proposed orthodontic treatment on dentofacial aesthetics should be analyzed and required alterations, if necessary, be incorporated in the final treatment plan.
- The functional benefits of orthodontic treatment have been universally recognized by practitioners. Achievement of Class I occlusion with proper excursive guidance will lead to maximum intercuspation, optimum aesthetics and long-term stability.[21] Patients with anterior open bite or severe overjet may benefit functionally by achieving normal interincisal relationships.[22] While planning orthodontic treatment, the clinician should establish functional goals not only related to the occlusal relationships, but they should also be extended to include the relationship of the soft tissues to the teeth. Quite often, patients present with abnormal lip posture due to abnormal jaw and teeth relationships. Therefore, the treatment planning process should include selection of appropriate treatment strategy to achieve adequate lip closure at the conclusion of treatment.[23]
- One of the most important factors that influence treatment planning is the prediction of long-term stability of tooth positions. Orthodontists should plan tooth movements and determine final jaw and tooth positions that ensure stability. It has been traditionally considered that extractions are required in patients with dental crowding to achieve long-term stability; however, this treatment modality does not necessarily guarantee long-term stability.[24,25] Both extraction and non-extraction treatment approaches may result in variable amount of relapse based upon many factors, like severity of malocclusion, duration of retention and specific characteristics of individual patients. Therefore, the clinician should identify the areas of potential relapse and take appropriate measures to establish individualized retention protocol for good stability.

TREATMENT OF SAGITTAL DISCREPANCIES

There is no universal treatment approach that can address all sagittal discrepancies. As described earlier, Class II and Class III malocclusions are not a single clinical entity, rather they consist of various components. Quite often, they are associated with vertical or transverse discrepancies. Therefore, to design a treatment plan for a particular patient, the clinician should identify and locate the components involved.

There are various treatment methods and numerous appliances available to deal with different types of sagittal discrepancies depending upon the configuration of the malocclusion and the age of the patient. It should be noted that the response of the patient to a prescribed treatment plan is a major factor to be considered in achieving the desired result. Even similar malocclusions respond differently to similar treatment approach, and such differential response should be continually monitored to determine the need for necessary therapeutic alterations.

Treatment of Class II malocclusion

There are several treatment strategies available to deal with different types of Class II situations. It is essential for the practitioner to select the appropriate treatment strategy depending upon the recognition of various elements contributing to the existing clinical problems. In other words, the treatment approach should be individualized. There are many Class II cases that require one or a discretionary combination of the various available treatment strategies. These include movement of teeth and alveolar processes, guidance of eruption and alveolar development, differential restraint and control of skeletal growth, differential promotion of skeletal growth, translation of parts during growth, training of muscles and surgical translation of parts.[6]

For the purpose of discussion, various Class II malocclusions can be grouped into the following categories:

1. Dentoalveolar Class II malocclusions
2. Functional Class II with distally forced bite
3. Skeletal Class II with maxillary prognathism
4. Skeletal Class II with prognathism and anteinclination of maxilla
5. Skeletal Class II with retrognathic mandible

Treatment of dentoalveolar Class II malocclusion

Dentoalveolar Class II malocclusion patients present with normal skeletal jaw relationship and Class II molar position caused by mesial movement of maxillary molars with respect to mandibular molars during developmental stage (Fig. 4.9). The unilateral Class II situation may exist due to mesial migration of maxillary permanent first molars following missing or abnormally positioned maxillary second bicuspids or premature loss of deciduous second molar on the affected side (Fig. 4.9A and D). Patients with this abnormality are also associated with other parameters, like varying degrees of overbite, overjet, crowding, rotations, etc. Not only the severity of Class II molar relationship but parameters, like varying degrees of overbite, overjet, crowding, rotations, etc. also determine the complexity of treatment involved. After it has been established that the Class II malocclusion is dental in nature, the clinician should assess the position of all dental units in sagittal, vertical and transverse dimensions to define treatment goals and select appropriate treatment strategy. The contemporary orthodontic treatment illustrates that such patients will have numerous treatment goals and individualized treatment mechanics designed to address those goals. Specific treatment plans for individual patients fall into five major categories: growing patients, non-growing patients, sagittal discrepancies, vertical discrepancies and transverse discrepancies.

Biologic variables

The basic strategy in the management of dentoalveolar Class II malocclusion is to achieve normal molar and incisal relationships, maintaining the existing normal skeletal relationship and the vertical dimension. Efficient tooth movement is ultimately the result of optimal biologic response to the orthodontic force system. The physiologic activity of alveolar bone resorption and deposition to produce tooth movement is induced by the mechanical stimulus through the delivery of orthodontic force systems. It is important that the force levels produced by orthodontic appliances are optimal, which will promote the most efficient treatment response without any damage to the teeth and the supporting structures (Table 4.1). The clinician should avoid excessive orthodontic force levels to prevent periodontal ligament necrosis and associated pain and bring about efficient tooth movement. It is essential to update on the knowledge of the force levels delivered to teeth through the medium of the appliance to understand optimal forces.[26–28] These optimal force values depend on the type of the tooth and the size of the tooth.

Dentoalveolar problems: Early treatment

The sagittal dental discrepancies in the primary dentition, seen in children having sucking habits, are expressed in the form of anterior displacement of upper incisors and posterior displacement of lower incisors. At this stage of development, if the sucking habit stops before the eruption of permanent teeth, it is usually self-correcting and, therefore, does not require any orthodontic intervention.

The mixed dentition phase is a very critical developmental stage. During this phase, children should be carefully examined and assessed for existing and potential or developing discrepancies. There are many treatment options available, depending upon the severity of the problem. The discrepancies in their severe form are best treated with two phases of treatment: phase 1 in the mixed dentition and phase 2 during the early permanent dentition period. It has been universally recognized that prevention is better than cure. The development of a space discrepancy when primary first or second molars are missing is best prevented by space maintenance protocol. This is indicated when there is adequate available space, and the premolar eruption will take more than 6 months. If the patient presents with bilateral problem, it is better to use lingual arch rather than two isolated appliances in the posterior segments. However, if the available space is not adequate for the permanent tooth or if there is significant amount of space loss due to the drifting of adjacent teeth, the lost space should be regained by repositioning the drifted dental units.

One of the basic tenets of any mixed dentition treatment protocol is to monitor the transition from the mixed to the permanent dentition. The simple procedure of maintaining the available arch length during the mixed dentition period helps to resolve minor to moderate tooth-size and arch-size discrepancies[29] along with the other methods of space gaining.

In the mandibular arch, the combined average width of the deciduous cuspid, the first deciduous molar and the second deciduous molar is approximately 1.7 mm greater than the combined width of the canine, the first premolar and the second premolar teeth (Fig. 4.10A). In the maxillary arch, this combined width difference is approximately 0.9 mm.[30] The practitioner should assess each patient radiographically to determine the size differential between the second deciduous molars and their successors, as the tooth size varies significantly among individuals[31] (Fig. 4.10B).

Patients with thumb sucking habit present with flared maxillary incisors and loss of vertical contact with the mandibular incisors and are frequently associated with variable degree of narrowing of the maxillary arch. Prolonged thumb sucking habit increases the severity of symptoms, leading to the development of anterior open bite. In an effort to improve swallowing and speech, the child often positions the tongue anteriorly between the maxillary and mandibular incisors to seal off the anterior open bite with the consequent development of 'tongue thrust'. In patients with such problems in mixed dentition stage, the treatment goal should be to establish proper lip seal by retraction of maxillary incisors. It is interesting to note that the tongue thrust habit usually disappears following the retraction of maxillary incisors, since it is considered to be due to 'physiologic adaption'.

Maxillary molar distalization

Contemporary orthodontic treatment ideologies focus on soft tissue assessment and management. There is a

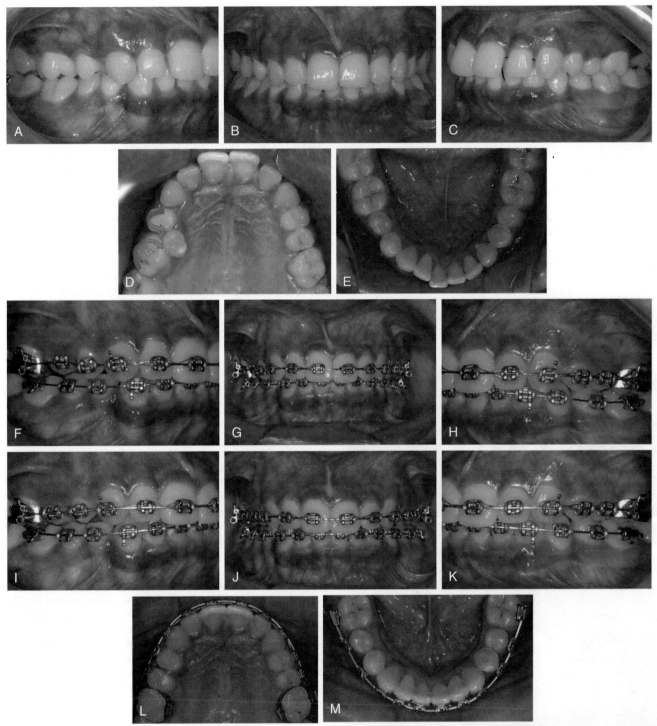

Figure 4.9 **(A–E)** Pretreatment intraoral photographs showing Class II molar relationship on right side, Class I molars on the left side and deep overbite. The Class II relationship on right side is due to mesiopalatal rotation of the first molar and distopalatal rotation of the first premolar as a result of palatal displacement of the second bicuspid. **(F–H)** After mesiobuccal rotation and distalization of the first molar to correct molar relationship and gain adequate space for the palatally placed second bicuspid, the second bicuspid is being moved into proper occlusion. **(I)** Establishing proper torque and fine-tuning the position of the maxillary right second bicuspid with finishing wires. **(J–M)** Midlines are corrected and proper occlusal relationship and coordinated upper and lower archforms are achieved.

Table 4.1   Optimal force levels for orthodontic tooth movement

Type of Tooth Movement	Force (g)
Tipping	45–70
Bodily movement (translation)	90–140
Root uprighting	70–115
Rotation	45–90
Extrusion	45–90
Intrusion	15–20

Force values vary according to the size of the tooth and periodontal condition; smaller values for incisors and higher values for posterior teeth.

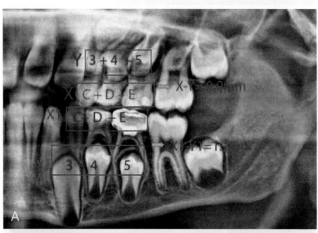

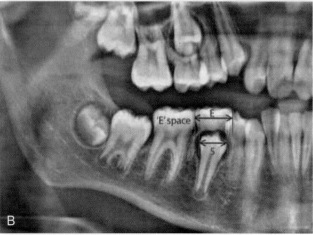

Figure 4.10 (A) Leeway space. On the average, the combined width of the deciduous canine and first and second deciduous molars is 1.7 mm greater than the permanent successors in the mandibular arch and 0.9 mm in the maxillary arch. **(B)** E-space.

general shift from hard tissue goals, where the face is the determinant of orthodontic treatment. Advances in mechanotherapy and changes in treatment concepts and philosophies now minimize the need for extractions, even in severe discrepancies. One non-extraction treatment

approach is the distal movement of maxillary molars to establish Class I molar relationship.

Precise distalization of maxillary molars is of significant value for non-extraction treatment of dentoalveolar Class II malocclusion with a normal mandible. Over the past few years, the focus of the maxillary molar distalization treatment modality has been on the introduction of fixed intra-arch appliances to eliminate the need for patient compliance, following the findings of rapid Class II corrections with non-removable appliances.[32,33]

Essentially, this approach is very useful in cases with midline discrepancies, to regain the space lost due to mesial drifting of first molars following premature loss of deciduous teeth, and in cases with Class II molar relationship due to ectopic eruption of first or second bicuspids and impacted or high labially placed cuspids. Based on the author's extensive experience in this field, spanning over last many years, there are basically three elements that determine the efficiency and effectiveness of distal driving of maxillary molars. They are:

1. Three-dimensional control of molars while they are being moved distally.
2. Maximum anchorage preservation during the distalization phase
3. Stabilization of molars in their new positions post-distalization during the subsequent phase of space consolidation.

Several appliances have been introduced to accomplish distal molar movement with or without the need for patient cooperation.[34–42] Most produce tipping, rotation and extrusion of the molars during distalization therapy; some produce a significant amount of incisor flaring due to anchorage loss, which is seen clinically as increased overjet.[39] After distalization of the molars, the distalizing modules and existing palatal anchorage appliances are removed and a Nance palatal button is delivered to maintain the first molars in their new positions.

Case selection criteria. The degree of space discrepancy and the facial profile characteristics of the patient are the two main important factors that should be considered in case selection criteria. Patients with mild to moderate space discrepancy are good candidates for maxillary molar distalization therapy. A maximum of 8 mm space has been achieved by certain appliances.[43] Even up to 10.5 mm of space gain has been achieved by some clinicians.[44]

Ideally, the patient should have orthognathic profile; and it is not the modality of choice when there is significant dental protrusion and/or convexity of profile as intraoral distalizing appliances do not cause significant soft tissue changes.[45] On the contrary, certain appliances may cause mild increase in profile convexity.[46] Therefore, the maxillary molar distalization therapy should be employed when the maxilla and mandible are skeletally normal with mild to moderate maxillary dental proclination or crowding. The patient should exhibit normal lower facial height as most distalizing appliances have an extrusive effect on the molars when they are distalized, leading to an increase in lower facial height.

Also, the patient should not have posterior arch crowding. According to Ricketts,[47] the distance between the pterygoid vertical (PTV) plane and the distal aspect of the

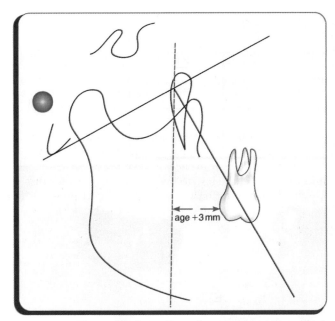

Figure 4.11 The sagittal maxillary first molar relationship is given by its distance to the PTV plane, the norm being 'age +3 mm'. Under normal circumstances, the facial axis passes through the mesiobuccal cusp of the first molar.[46]

maxillary first molar should be 'age + 3 mm' (Fig. 4.11). In normal skeletal and dental relationship, the facial axis passes through the mesiobuccal cusp of the first molar. If the distance M1-PTV is shorter than the normal, the possibility for molar distalization is less and extractions may be required depending upon the growth potential and the presence of third molars.[47]

In distalization therapy, the position of the second molar determines the type of the first molar movement.[48] If second molar is developing, one should expect more tipping of first molar as compared to fully erupted second molar, as the developing second molar tooth bud acts as a fulcrum for the distal movement of first molar. In the absence of third molars, if second molars are fully erupted, molars will be distalized bodily, requiring greater force levels that result in more anchorage loss.

Appliance selection. An ideal distalizing appliance should be rigid and compliance free. It should distalize molars bodily with minimal anchorage loss. Also, it should allow passive free floating of teeth immediately anterior to the distalized teeth. The design of the appliance should be such that it should readily be convertible into a holding appliance after the distalization.

Anchorage. The anchorage for intraoral distalizing appliances should ideally be derived from non-dental sources, like palatal vault and mid-palatal screws. However, in most appliances, it is partially obtained from bicuspids. In planning the anchorage system, it is important to consider that rigidity is essential for good anchorage, and the reactive anterior forces generated by the active components are distributed over a large area of the palate. A large acrylic button is made in the region of the vertical portion of the palatal vault.

It extends to approximately 5 mm from the teeth, relieving the incisive papilla anteriorly. The precise fabrication of the palatal button is the key to anchorage preservation, as any space between the palatal tissues and the inner surface of the button would lead to anchorage loss. There is little anchorage value to mobilized teeth. Simultaneous levelling and aligning the rest of the dentition taxes the anchorage, resulting in lesser amount of net distal molar movement. Therefore, it is advisable to distalize maxillary molars without full arch fixed appliance.[49]

Expansion. Some maxillary expansion is often a prerequisite for Class II molar correction. It should either precede or be concomitant with the distalization, which can be made possible by incorporating an expansion device in the distalizing appliance.[40]

Force levels. For efficient and effective distal molar movement, force levels in the range of 100–120 g are considered to be ideal. Continuous forces are preferred than intermittent or interrupted forces. The direction of force should be along the line of arch and should be as close to the centre of resistance of the molar as possible. A good control over the direction and the magnitude of distalizing forces is essential to avoid tipping, rotations and intrusion or extrusion of molars. It is advisable to distal drive maxillary first molars into super Class I relationship to compensate for some anchorage loss during the postdistalization phase of orthodontic treatment.

Stabilization of molars. There are various options available to stabilize molars in their new positions, postdistalization. These include utility arch, continuous archwire with molar stops, headgears, Nance holding arch, etc. A secure molar stabilization system should be stable and rigid enough to hold molars and should serve as good anchorage units during the subsequent phase of treatment mechanics.

Postdistalization mechanics. Postdistalization stabilization of molars is difficult and highly critical. It should be immediate and as rigid and precise as possible. A lag phase of 3–6 months is desirable before commencing further mechanics to allow passive free floating of bicuspids. It is highly recommended to monitor new molar position and use minimal force levels in postdistalization treatment mechanics.

The Karad's Integrated Distalizing System (KIDS) was developed to address the disadvantages of other distalizing appliances (Figs 4.12– 4.16).[42] This appliance system is designed on the following principles:

- Light, continuous force system to achieve efficient and predictable molar movement
- Desired moment-to-force ratio for bodily movement of first molars
- Three-dimensional molar control throughout distalization therapy
- Maximum anchorage preservation throughout treatment
- Elimination of need for new Nance palatal button to hold the molars in their new positions after distalization
- Economically viable

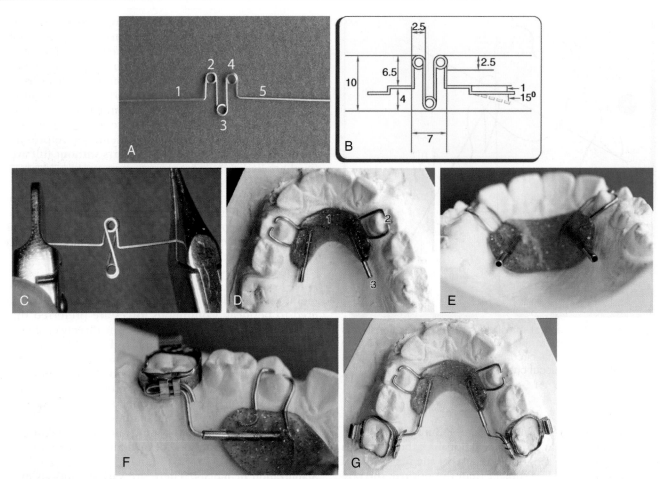

Figure 4.12   (A) Triple helical distalizing spring made from 0.017 × 0.025 TMA wire. 1, Mesial leg; 2, Mesial helical loop; 3, Occlusal helical loop; 4, Distal helical loop; 5, Distal leg. **(B)** Dimensions of average-sized distalizing spring in mm. **(C)** Compressed spring when activated. **(D)** Modified Nance palatal button. 1, Acrylic part; 2, Occlusal rests; and 3, Guiding tubes. **(E)** Location of the guiding tubes on the lateral curvatures of the palate. **(F)** Position of sliding tubes into the guiding tubes (palatal button). **(G)** Components of Karad's Integrated Distalizing System (except for the triple helical distalizing spring). (Source: Karad A. World J Orthod 2008; 9:244–254 (Figs 4.12–4.16, Reproduced with permission from Quintessence Publishing Co Inc).

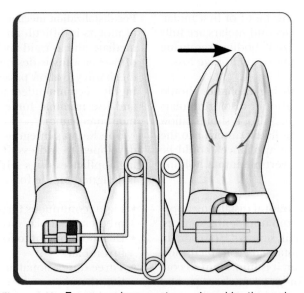

Figure 4.13   Forces and moments produced by the spring.

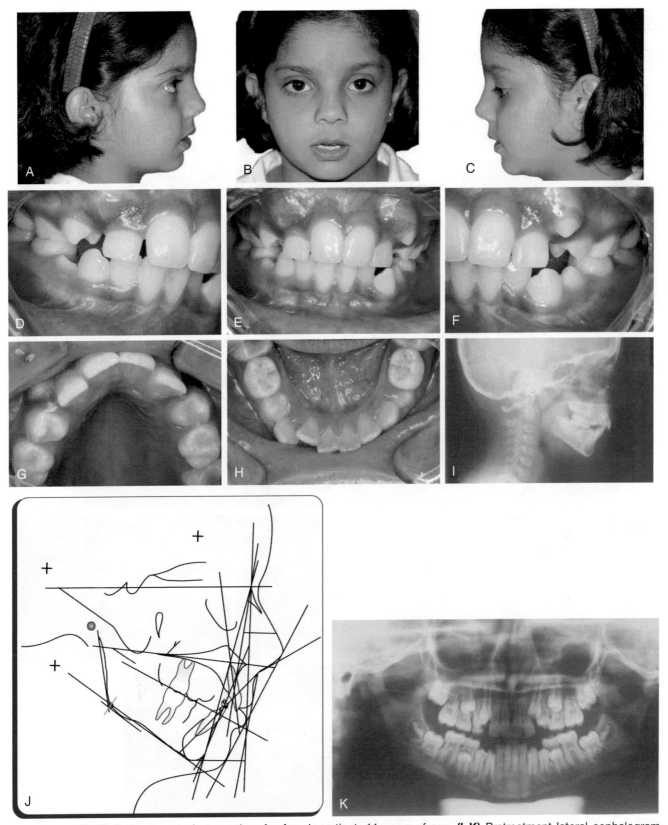

Figure 4.14   **(A–H)** Pretreatment photographs of a female patient, 11 years of age. **(I–K)** Pretreatment lateral cephalogram, cephalometric tracing and orthopantomogram.

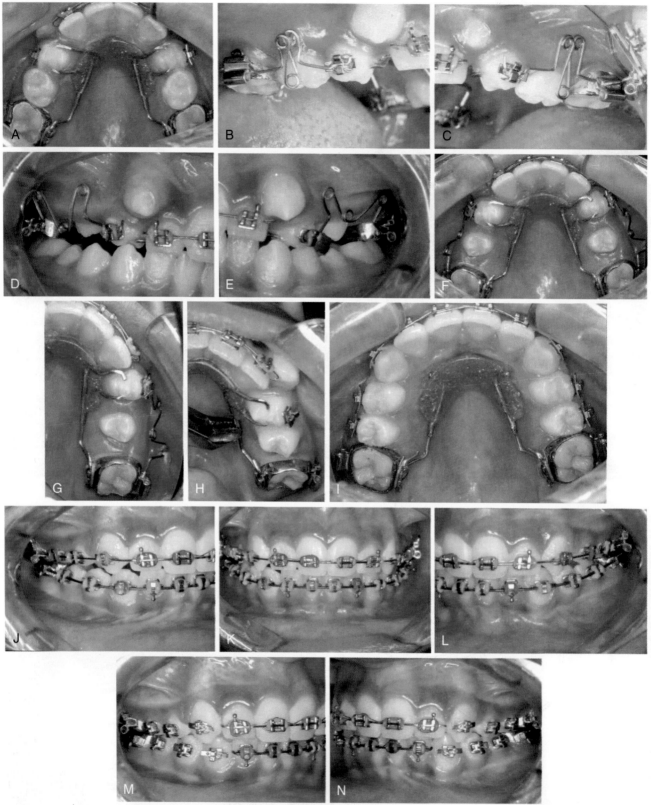

Figure 4.15 **(A)** Palatal and molar assemblies are bonded and cemented, respectively. **(B and C)** Initial activation and placement of the distalizing springs. **(D–G)** Maxillary molars are distalized into super Class I relationship. **(H)** After the desired amount of distalization, the guiding tubes are crimped with the utility pliers to stabilize the molars in their new positions. **(I)** Occlusal rests are cut at the palatal button to convert the whole assembly into a holding appliance. **(J–N)** Finishing and detailing procedures.

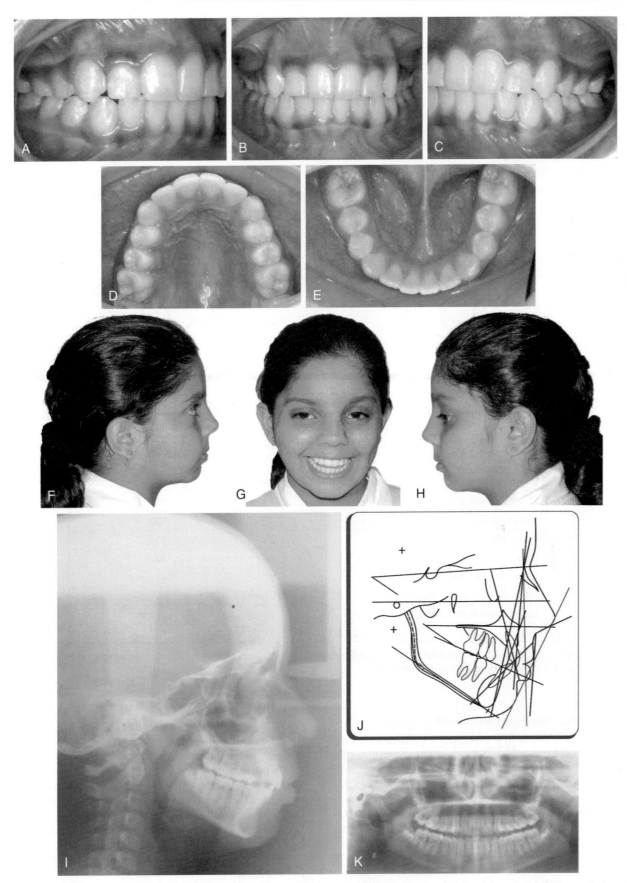

Figure 4.16 **(A–H)** Post-treatment intraoral and extraoral photographs. **(I–K)** Post-treatment lateral cephalogram, cephalometric tracing and panoramic radiograph.

Continued

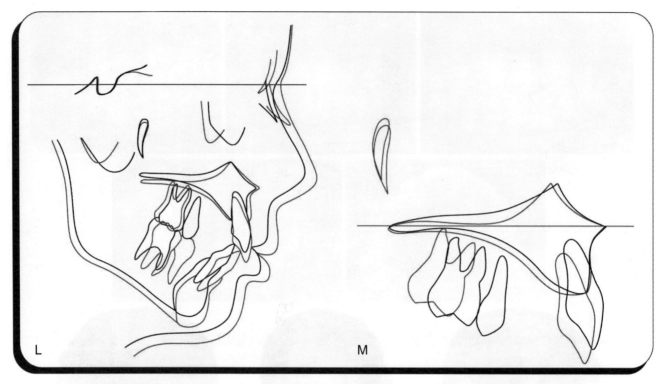

Measurement	Norm	Pretreatment	Post-treatment
SNA	82 ± 3	80	80
SNB	79 ± 3	76	76
ANB	3 ± 1	4	4
U1 – maxillary plane	108 ± 5	104	107
L1 – mandibular plane	92 ± 5	100	101
Interincisal angle	133 ± 10	126	120
MM angle	27 ± 5	28	30
FMA	25 ± 5	20	20
Upper anterior face height		42 mm	43 mm
Lower anterior face height		53 mm	55 mm
Lower incisor to APO line	0–2 mm	+1 mm	+1 mm
U1 – SN	102 ± 2	97	102

Figure 4.16, cont'd (L and M) Pretreatment and post-treatment overall and maxillary superimpositions. **(N)** Table showing pretreatment and post-treatment cephalometric data.

Non-extraction headgear treatment

The use of headgears in contemporary management of Class II malocclusions is mainly aimed at controlling the anchorage and the cant of the occlusal plane, tooth movement and orthopaedic correction (Figs 4.17–4.22).

With the introduction of fixed intraoral appliances to distalize maxillary molars or other tooth movements in noncompliant patient, the use of headgear has been considerably reduced. However, there are certain clinical situations that require headgear forces to be used in association with contemporary mechanotherapy to prevent adverse effects of intraoral forces from the archwire in order to achieve high quality and stable correction of Class II malocclusions.

For successful use of headgears in clinical practice, sound knowledge of force systems produced by various designs of headgears is essential. In tipping orthodontic tooth movement, even if the forces are light, the stress levels at the periodontal-tooth and bone interfaces are beyond acceptable physiologic limits.[50] Therefore, the practitioner should avoid distal tipping headgear forces to prevent any untoward tissue reactions due to high localized stress levels at the marginal ridge and at the root apices. However, the bodily movement of teeth produced by headgears takes considerable amount of time. In patients with Class II dentoalveolar malocclusion, the use of headgear for 14 hours each night, consistently with a force direction passing through the centre of resistance of the

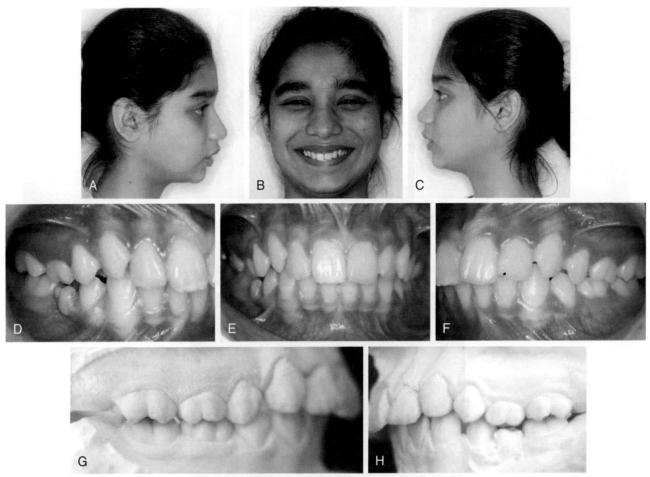

Figure 4.17 **(A–C)** Pretreatment extraoral photographs of a female patient (age 12 years) showing convex profile, acute nasolabial angle and incompetent lips. **(D–F)** Pretreatment intraoral features include proclination of maxillary incisors with crowding. **(G–H)** Pretreatment models show Class II molar and canine relationship.

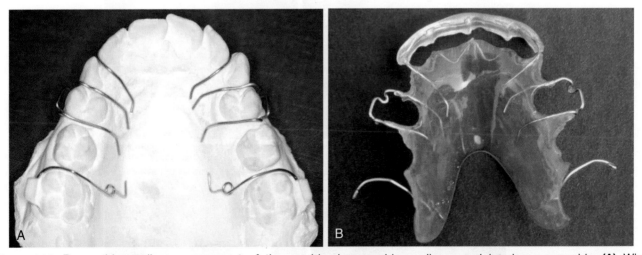

Figure 4.18 Removable appliance component of the combined removable appliance and headgear assembly. **(A)** Wire components on the model. **(B)** An appliance with molar distalizing springs, acrylic shield on incisors and Adams clasps on first bicuspids.

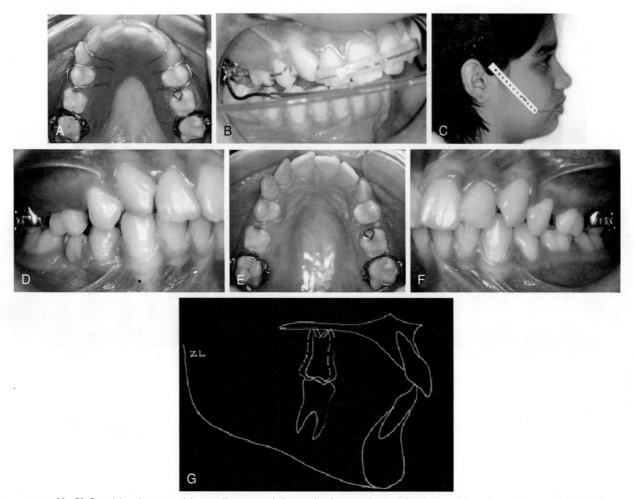

Figure 4.19 **(A–C)** Combined removable appliance and the molar-inserted combination-pull headgear therapy to distalize maxillary first molars. **(D–F)** The molars are driven distally into Class I relationship. **(G)** Pretreatment and postdistalization cephalometric superimposition shows bodily movement of maxillary molars.

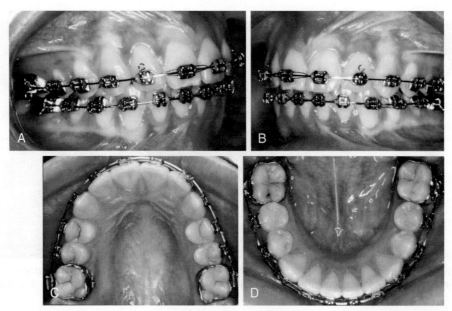

Figure 4.20 **(A and B)** Postdistalization fixed appliance therapy to resolve anterior discrepancy. **(C and D)** Coordinated and compatible upper and lower archforms.

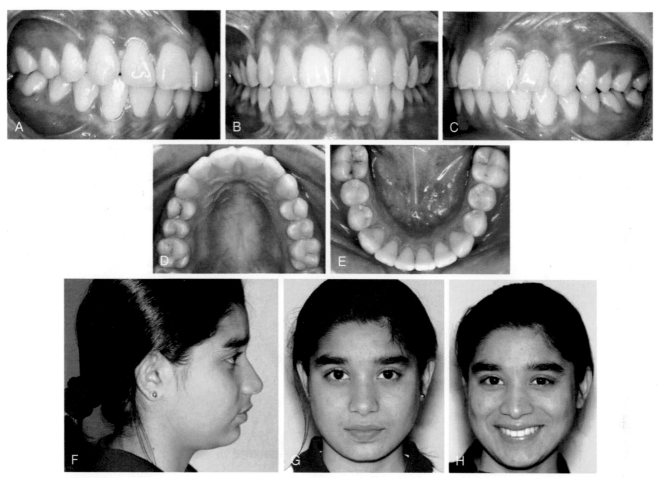

Figure 4.21 **(A-H)** Post-treatment records show good occlusion, archforms, improvement in facial profile, competent lips and pleasing smile.

maxillary first molar, will move the teeth distally by 2 mm in 2–4 months without tipping.[51] In a treatment approach that uses a combination of removable appliance and headgear to gain maxillary arch length, the removable appliance tips the maxillary first molar crown distally and the molar-inserted headgear moves the root distally, resulting in a net bodily distal movement of the tooth.[35]

The combined removable appliance and headgear essentially consists of three components.

1. Removable appliance consists of molar distalizing springs, modified Adams clasps, acrylic shield on incisors and acrylic plate covering the palate (Fig. 4.18).
2. Headgear (Fig. 4.19C).
3. Maxillary first molar bands with headgear tubes and lingual sheaths (Fig. 4.19B).

The active components of the removable appliance are distalizing springs made from 0.028 inch stainless steel wires, which are activated by 1–1.5 mm exerting a force of approximately 30 g per side. This appliance is worn by the patient for 24 hours a day except for meals and hygiene. The headgear, either cervical pull or combination pull, is worn by the patient for 12–14 hours per day, exerting a force of approximately 150 g per side. Postdistalization, molars are held in their new positions during the subsequent phase of space consolidation.

For any orthodontic application, the following sequential steps may guide a clinician to design the headgear force system.[51,52]

1. Select the appropriate size of the inner bow of the facebow. It should be adjusted by placing it against the maxillary plaster model so that it is approximately 3–4 mm away from all teeth except the first molars. At the molar region, it can be adjusted to rest passively in the molar tubes or can be expanded by 1–1.5 mm. The inner bow should rest comfortably between the lips.
2. Determine the centre of resistance of the body to which the headgear force is being applied (tooth or segment or arch or maxilla; Fig. 4.22).
3. Mentally, mark the centre of resistance on the patient's cheek.
4. Choose the type of headgear pull—cervical, occipital or combination pull—depending on the vertical relationships observed in the patient.
5. Determine the force system (force and moment at the centre of resistance) through the centre of resistance that will produce the desired changes.
6. Allow the outer bow to rest away from the cheeks and adjust its length and vertical position with respect to the centre of resistance to achieve proper line of force.

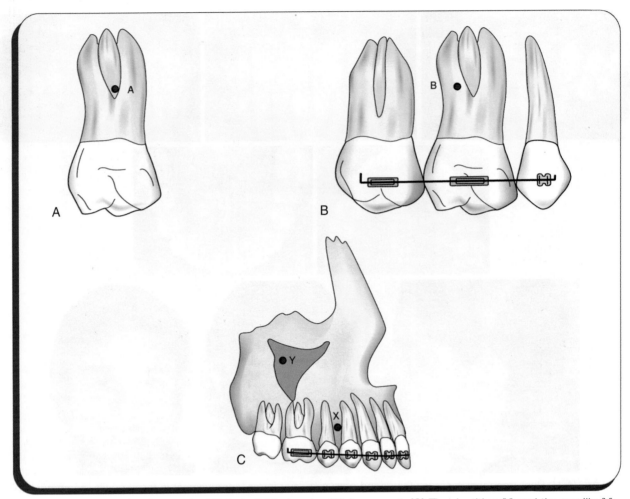

Figure 4.22 Centre of resistance for **(A)** An individual molar, **(B)** A segment, **(C)** The dentition (X) and the maxilla (Y).

7. Choose the headgear force magnitude.
   a. In rotating the unit (use a large moment in comparison to the applied force through the centre of resistance), use low-strap forces to avoid high local stress in the periodontal ligament (approximately 150 g per side).
   b. If the line of action of the headgear force passes close to or through the unit's centre of resistance, 350–450 g per side can be used.
8. Monitor for changes as treatment proceeds. Adjust the force line of action and force magnitude as necessary.

Extraction treatment approach

Over the last few years, it is certainly true that the advances in orthodontic treatment mechanics, philosophies and material science have curtailed the need for extractions in severe discrepancies. However, on many occasions, it has always been a difficult task for the clinician to make the extraction or non-extraction treatment decision to resolve a specific malocclusion. There are several factors that influence this decision. The severity of malocclusion, like the amount of intra-arch crowding, requires extraction of some dental units; however, its impact on the soft tissue profile of the face should be considered in the treatment planning process.

Management of extraction space. One of the most important factors in extraction treatment approach is effective utilization of extraction space to resolve the existing discrepancy (Fig. 4.23). There are several techniques that may be employed for orthodontic space closure; however, the clinician should select the technique that efficiently brings about the desired tooth movement. Also, the orthodontic space closure planning should be individualized and should address the individual patient problems and the patient's chief complaint. One can use either a two-step space closure mechanics in which individual retraction of cuspids is followed by incisor retraction, or an en masse retraction of all six anterior teeth in a single stage (Fig. 4.23E and F). However, it is the author's experience that the two-step space closure method, which is believed to be less detrimental to the anchorage, temporarily impairs the anterior aesthetics due to shifting of the extraction space from the distal of canine to the mesial of canine and prolongs the treatment duration. However, independent cuspid retraction can be the method of choice in certain cases, which requires space for decrowding of anterior teeth.

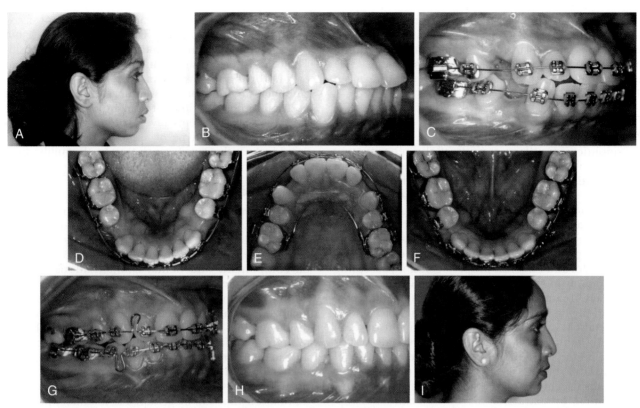

Figure 4.23 Extraction treatment approach. **(A)** Pretreatment facial profile of an adult female patient exhibiting acute nasolabial angle and protrusive lips. **(B)** Class I molar relationship and severe maxillary and mandibular incisor proclination. **(C)** Alignment and levelling of maxillary and mandibular arches before the initiation of retraction mechanics. **(D)** The management of extraction space is based upon the concept of differential extraction space closure (anterior retraction versus posterior protraction). **(E)** A two-step space closure mechanics (retraction of cuspids followed by incisor retraction) in the maxillary arch. **(F)** En masse retraction of six anterior teeth in a single stage in the mandibular arch. **(G)** Closure of extraction spaces with loop mechanics. **(H–I)** Post-treatment occlusal relationships and post-treatment balanced facial profile.

The following factors influence extraction space closure.[53]

1. *Severity of discrepancy:* The severity of the problems, like the degree of proclination, crowding, etc., plays an important role in determining the extent of extraction space required to resolve the discrepancy. The practitioner should plan the mechanism of space closure by determining the amount of extraction space to be utilized by anterior retraction as against the residual space closure by protraction of posterior teeth. This differential space closure mechanics demands a good control over the anterior and posterior dental units.

2. *Midline discrepancies:* Patients with transverse dental problems present with or without asymmetric left- and right-side occlusal relationships. Application of asymmetric forces in an effort to correct midline discrepancies can produce untoward effects, like asymmetric anchorage loss, unilateral vertical forces, etc. An efficient and effective approach to the resolution of midline discrepancies is to correct the asymmetries in the early part of treatment followed by symmetric mechanics for the residual discrepancies.

3. *Anchorage:* Control of anchorage units is one of the important elements in space closure mechanics.

While planning space closure, the clinician should assess the anchorage units, understand the concept of differential anchorage and determine whether entire extraction space will be closed by retraction or decrowding and alignment of anterior teeth or if some degree of sagittal movement of molars is desired to close the space and then plan the mechanics accordingly. Using the same universal mechanics for different anchorage requirements limits the ability of the practitioner to achieve desired results.

4. *Axial inclination of canines and incisors:* Patients with Class II malocclusions present with variable axial inclinations of cuspids and incisors—mesially inclined, upright or distally inclined. The same degree of force or moment applied to these teeth during the space closure mechanics will result in different types of tooth movements. Therefore, the clinician should assess the axial inclinations of cuspids and incisors and design the force system accordingly to achieve desired tooth movement.

Management of vertical dentoalveolar problems

As mentioned earlier, the sagittal discrepancies are not a single entity and are often associated with vertical problems. Class II malocclusions are also associated with vertical discrepancies, like deep overbite or open bite. For the successful and stable correction of Class II malocclusion, the treatment plan must include the identification and the correction of these vertical components. The management of these problems is explained in detail in Chapter 5.

Orthodontic camouflage: A treatment alternative for skeletal discrepancy

Orthodontic camouflage consists of the repositioning of the dentition in order to obtain proper molar and incisor relationships in patients with underlying skeletal discrepancies with a favourable effect on facial aesthetics. For some reason, if the patient does not accept the orthosurgical treatment approach for the correction of a dentofacial deformity, camouflage proves to be quite useful. The goal is to achieve certain degree of dentofacial aesthetics and establish proper occlusion, accepting the limitations in skeletal relationships. The success of camouflage treatment approach depends on the severity of underlying sagittal discrepancy. In mild to moderate skeletal Class II malocclusions, movement of teeth to achieve dentoalveolar changes and aesthetic results is much better than those in severe skeletal Class II problems. In severe Class II patients, the need for greater displacement of teeth relative to their bony bases, either by extraction or by non-extraction approach is possible due to improvements in orthodontic treatment mechanics but only at considerable expense to facial aesthetics. Therefore, the clinician should assess the case carefully for camouflage approach for the underlying skeletal discrepancy to plan treatment mechanics and strike a balance between occlusal and facial aesthetic goals.

Management of functional Class II malocclusion

There are many systematic, definitive treatment methods available and possible in typical Class II malocclusions, and there are some cases that require a specific diagnostic protocol to identify the problem and design a treatment plan. One such type of discrepancy is a functional Class II malocclusion (Figs 4.24–4.26).

Functional criteria as the determinant of treatment method

In functional retrusion cases, it is essential to perform a functional analysis as a part of the clinical examination before selecting a specific appliance therapy. The practitioner should determine the path of closure of the mandible and analyze the relationship between the postural rest and habitual occlusal position. The mandible moves upward and backward from rest position into a forced retrusive habitual occlusion. There is a rotary action of the condyle in the glenoid fossa from postural rest to initial contact of teeth. From the initial contact to habitual occlusion, the action of the condyle is rotary and translatory—upward and backward. This is also called a *distally forced bite* or *posterior shift*. This type of condylar movement is commonly seen in patients with excessive overbite. The Class II malocclusion with functional disturbances appears more severe than it actually is sagittally.

Usually, the base of the mandible is of normal size with no growth deficiency. The SNB angle is smaller in habitual occlusion, but it improves in the postural resting position. The Class II relationship is mainly of dental nature caused by improper intercuspation. The treatment goal is to eliminate the functional disturbance and not to alter the postural resting position of the mandible. The early treatment of such problems involves interceptive functional therapy—screening type of appliances or activators and twin-blocks with or without the occlusal equilibration in the later stages of therapy.

Treatment of skeletal Class II malocclusion

The treatment of skeletal Class II malocclusion is based on careful and accurate diagnosis. In skeletal Class II malocclusions, it is not just that the skeletal bases are at fault; there are many variations involving various skeletal components and dental compensations in anteroposterior plane, often associated with vertical problems. Before planning the treatment, the orthodontist should localize and quantify skeletal contributions and dental displacements associated with the problem. There are numerous variations of skeletal Class II discrepancies, and it is beyond the scope of this chapter to identify each type and discuss its treatment; however, for the purpose of description, the commonly observed skeletal relationships can be grouped as maxillary protrusion with normal mandible, normal maxilla and retrognathic mandible, a combination of maxillary protrusion and mandibular retrusion and a vertical problem. There is no universal treatment approach to deal with skeletal Class II problems; therefore, the treatment should be directed at the individual patient's specific problem area.

Maxillary prognathism

It is characterized by a large maxillary base or a normal maxilla, which is positioned anteriorly with respect to the cranial base associated with a normal mandible (Fig. 4.27). In the management of patients with skeletal problems, the growth direction plays an important role in the selection of a treatment strategy. In a Class II relationship, with a fault in the maxilla during mixed dentition, the treatment goal is to inhibit growth in the mid-face region and allow the normal growth of the mandible. This produces orthopaedic mid-face changes to alter the maxillary position in relation to the mandible and the anterior cranial base.

Extraoral heavy forces, with the help of a headgear assembly, applied to the maxillary first molars, are used for growth inhibition in the mid-face region. This treatment approach used in growing patients produces a desired maxillary skeletal change.[54] A headgear used for this purpose should be designed to deliver an optimal extraoral orthopaedic force to compress the maxillary sutures, modifying the pattern of bone apposition at these sites. To be effective for this purpose, the extraoral force should be of much greater magnitude, in the range of 400–600 g per side, worn at least 12–14 hours per day to produce a skeletal change and to minimize dental effects.[52]

Apart from the force magnitude and duration, the direction of the extraoral force should be determined

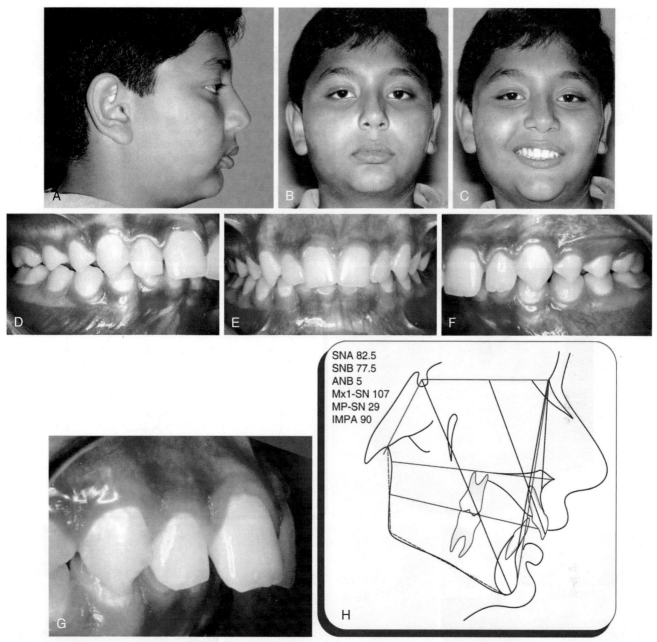

SNA 82.5
SNB 77.5
ANB 5
Mx1-SN 107
MP-SN 29
IMPA 90

Figure 4.24 Pretreatment records of a growing patient. **(A–C)** Convex profile and deep mentolabial groove. **(D–G)** Class II division 1 malocclusion with severe overjet and overbite. The functional examination demonstrated a distally-forced-bite. **(H)** Pretreatment lateral cephalometric tracing.

based on the vertical relationships observed in the patient or the growth pattern. The extraoral attachment can be cervical or occipital to establish a low or a high angle of force vector. To achieve the maximum skeletal improvement by affecting the maxillary sutures, a superior and posterior force vector through the centre of resistance of the maxilla appears to be the most appropriate direction. The extraoral force vector also depends on the height and length of outer bow. Raising or shortening the outer bow moves the force vector superiorly, and lowering or lengthening the outer bow moves the force vector inferiorly. Often,

the mandibular arch is normal and the occlusal plane is flat; however, if the maxillary incisors are flared and tipped labially, they should be retracted first. If the maxillary arch is constricted, an extraoral traction should be preceded by an initial phase of maxillary expansion.

The goal of orthopaedic treatment with the head-gear is to restrict normal downward and forward maxillary growth by compressing the maxillary sutures and altering the growth and apposition of bone at these sutures, while allowing the mandible to grow normally.

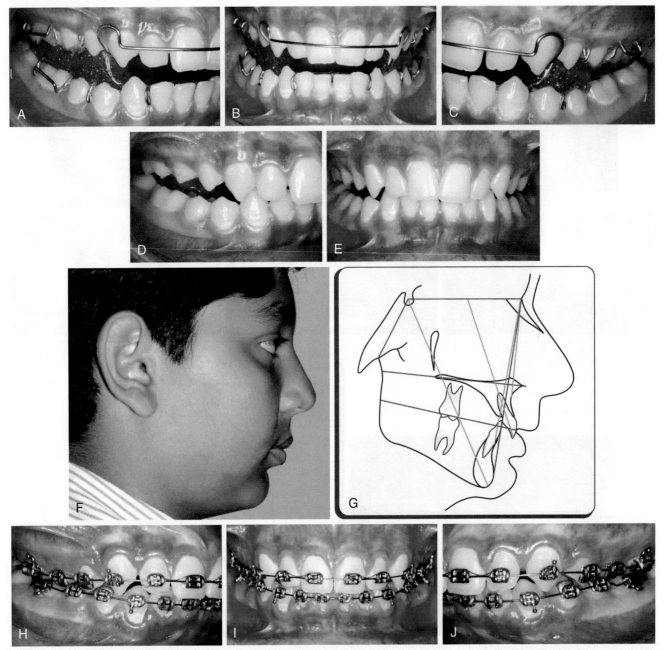

Figure 4.25   The treatment strategy included 8-month use of a twin-block appliance to improve abnormal skeletal relationships, followed by fixed appliance therapy to fine-tune the dentition. **(A–C)** Use of a twin-block appliance. **(D–G)** Post-twin-block therapy occlusion, facial profile and lateral cephalometric tracing. **(H–J)** Fixed appliance therapy.

Mandibular retrusion

The Class II malocclusion, characterized by mandibular deficiency and orthognathic maxilla, is often associated with some degree of dental compensations. The treatment strategies in such cases are directed to establish orthognathic profile and lip seal and to improve facial muscle function by promoting optimal mandibular growth in the first phase of treatment, followed by detailing of dentition using the contemporary fixed appliances in the second phase (Figs 4.28–4.30). This desired sagittal change can be achieved by posturing the mandible

forward using one of the functional jaw orthopaedic appliances.

This sagittal change is dependant on growth guidance and adaptive processes for the desired skeletal modification. One of the treatment methods in patients with deficient mandible is to hold the normally positioned maxilla and allow the mandible to express its normal growth. The literature shows that the patients wearing headgear that is attached to the maxilla exhibit more mandibular growth than untreated Class II patients.[55] It remains to be seen whether this statistically significant

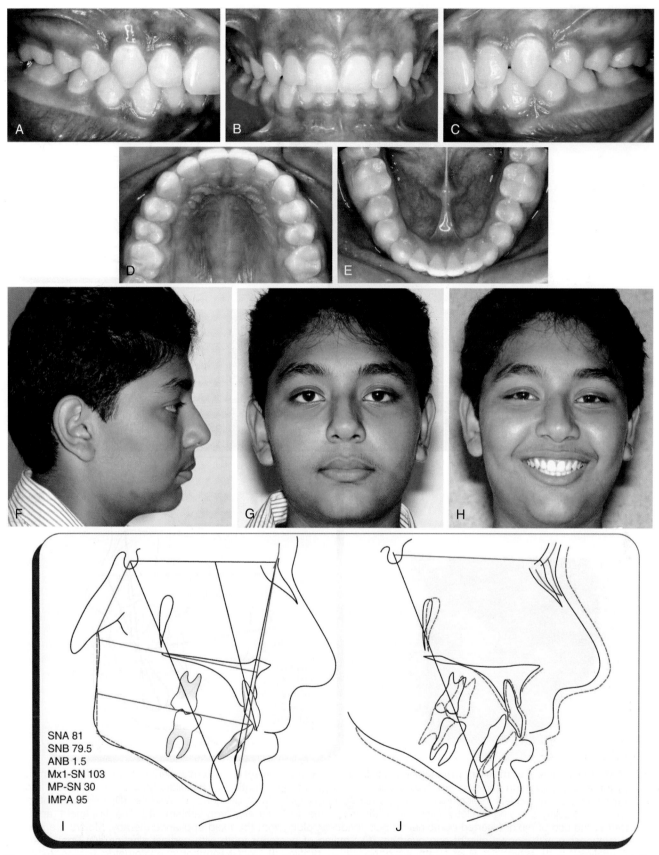

SNA 81
SNB 79.5
ANB 1.5
Mx1-SN 103
MP-SN 30
IMPA 95

Figure 4.26 Post-treatment records. **(A–E)** Normal occlusal relationships and archforms. **(F–H)** Orthognathic profile. **(I)** Post-treatment lateral cephalometric tracing. **(J)** Pretreatment and post-treatment lateral cephalometric superimposition.

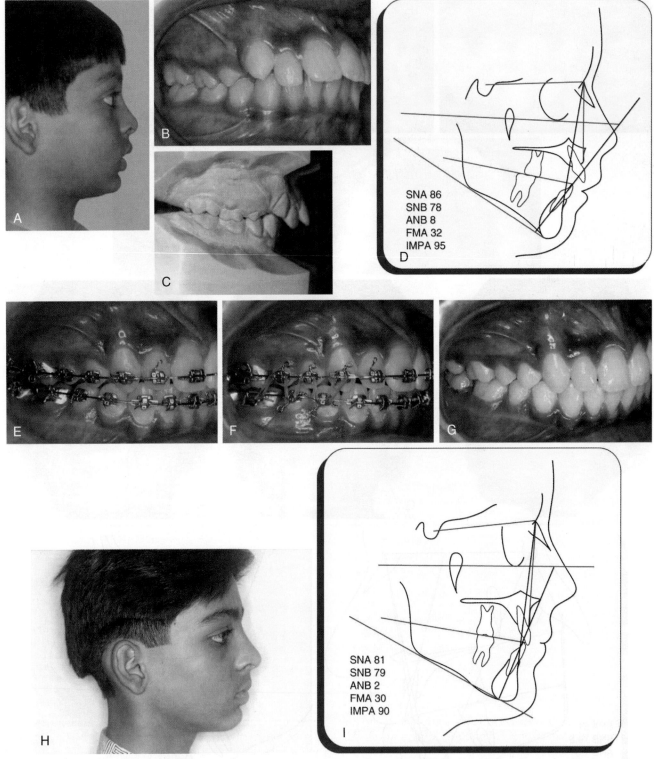

Figure 4.27 Management of maxillary prognathism in a 12-year-old male patient. **(A)** Pretreatment convex profile, incompetent lips. **(B)** Intraoral photograph showing late mixed dentition stage and proclination of maxillary incisors and Class II molars. **(C)** Pretreatment study models in occlusion to demonstrate the magnitude of overjet and overbite. **(D)** Pretreatment lateral cephalometric tracing showing skeletal Class II relationship due to maxillary prognathism. **(E)** The treatment approach consisted of the use of molar-inserted combination pull headgear, along with the fixed appliance therapy. Molars are in super Class I relationship with normal overjet and overbite. **(F)** Settling of posterior teeth with vertical elastics. **(G)** Post-treatment normal occlusal relationship. **(H)** Post-treatment orthognathic profile. **(I)** Post-treatment cephalometric tracing exhibiting normal skeletal and dental relationships.

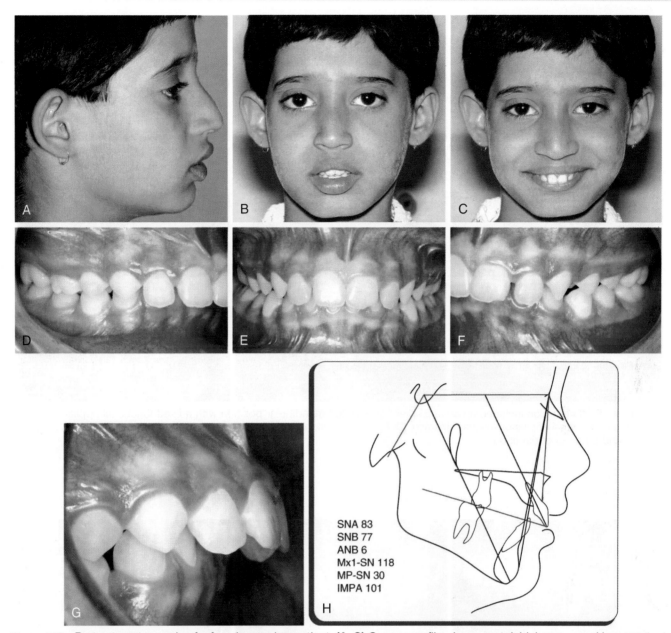

SNA 83
SNB 77
ANB 6
Mx1-SN 118
MP-SN 30
IMPA 101

Figure 4.28 Pretreatment records of a female growing patient. **(A–C)** Convex profile, deep mentolabial groove and incompetent lips. **(D–G)** Class II division 1 malocclusion with severe overjet and overbite. It is characterized by mandibular skeletal retrusion. **(H)** Pretreatment lateral cephalometric tracing.

extra-mandibular growth is clinically significant. The author's treatment of choice in patients with mandibular deficiency is to enhance the mandibular growth using a variety of functional appliances. It is believed that mere unloading of the condyle by forward mandible posturing contributes to a significant condylar growth.[56,57] It should be recognized that it is not only the apparent condylar position in glenoid fossa but the more retruded fossa itself to be used as a criterion in Class II malocclusion.[58,59] More condylar growth increments and a change in the direction of growth to a more upward and backward vector are associated with the use of functional appliances.[60,61] The research has also shown significant change in the position of the glenoid fossa with respect to the

anterior cranial base.[62] Unloading of the condyle associated with downward and forward posturing of the mandible also enhances metabolic action in the temporomandibular joint (Fig. 4.31).[63] It is not just a mere forward posturing of the mandible but an increased anabolic and catabolic exchange that may contribute to enhanced growth of the condyle and posterior wall proliferation.[64,65]

Treatment of Class III malocclusion

The treatment options for the management of Class III malocclusion are dependant on the age of the patient and the components involved. There are various types of

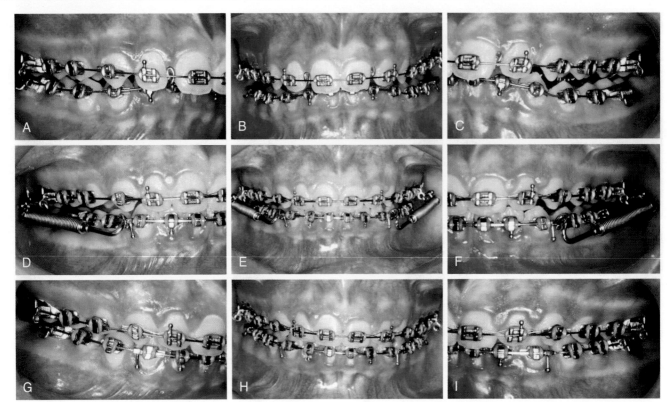

Figure 4.29 Treatment plan included an advancement of retruded mandibular position with a fixed functional appliance. **(A–C)** Prior to fixed functional appliance mechanotherapy. **(D–F)** Fixed functional appliance therapy. **(G–I)** After fixed functional appliance finishing and detailing of dentition.

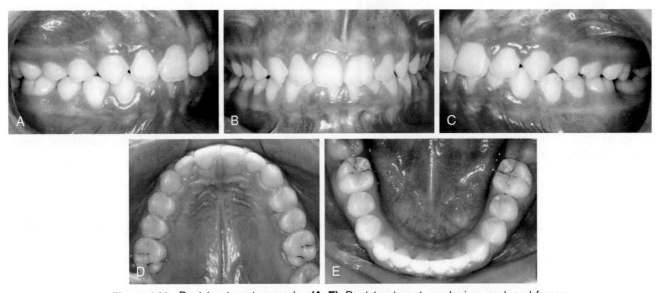

Figure 4.30 Post-treatment records. **(A–E)** Post-treatment occlusion and archforms.

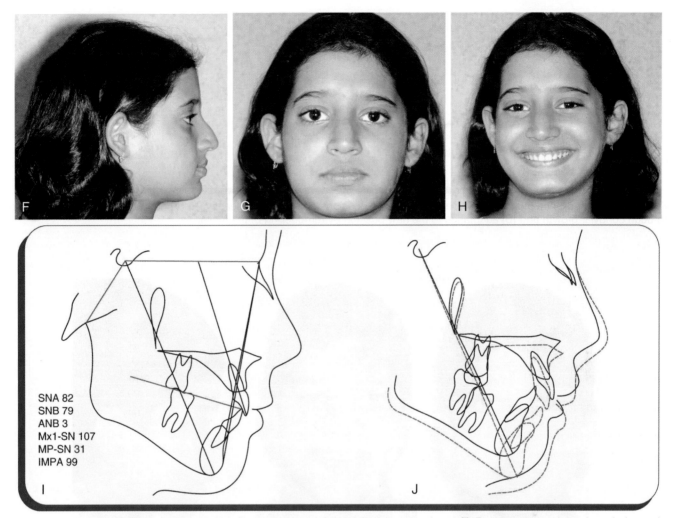

SNA 82
SNB 79
ANB 3
Mx1-SN 107
MP-SN 31
IMPA 99

Figure 4.30, cont'd **(F–H)** Orthognathic profile and normal frontal facial proportions. **(I)** Post-treatment lateral cephalometric tracing. **(J)** Pretreatment and post-treatment lateral cephalometric superimposition.

Class III malocclusions; however, for the purpose of discussion, these can be categorized into following groups:

1. Dentoalveolar Class III
2. Functional Class III malocclusion (with pseudo-forced bite or anterior displacement)
3. Class III malocclusion with retruded maxilla
4. Class III malocclusion with mandibular prognathism
5. Class III malocclusion with a combination of maxillary retrognathism and mandibular prognathism

The treatment approach to the correction of Class III malocclusion should be individualized, and it should be designed to address the specific nature of the dental, skeletal or functional imbalances. It has been generally recognized that Class III malocclusions are one of the most difficult problems to treat. It has been observed that before adolescence, some of the features of vertical discrepancy, like increased lower anterior face height, steep mandibular plane angle, excessive eruption of posterior teeth, anterior open bite, etc., are located below the palatal plane.[66] The goal of early Class III treatment is to create an environment that promotes favourable dentofacial growth.[67]

Dentoalveolar Class III malocclusion

The dentoalveolar Class III malocclusion is characterized by abnormal sagittal incisor position; the ANB angle within normal limits is suggestive of normal basal relationship. In such cases, the maxillary incisors are tipped lingually and the mandibular incisors are tipped labially. Most Class III malocclusions exhibit these characteristics during the initial stages of development; however, after the eruption of the permanent teeth, these problems become more severe. It has been reported that Class III skeletal discrepancies tend to worsen with age.[68] If anterior crossbite exists for prolonged duration, it may enhance the mandibular prognathism and retard the maxillary sagittal development. This demands early institution of appropriate treatment, the goal being the establishment of a normal functional engram and stimulus in the developing face. The treatment is aimed at uprighting lingually tipped maxillary incisors and labially tipped lower incisors (Figs 4.32–4.34). Quite often, maxillary arch expansion is required to unravel the transverse component. Several researchers have attempted to predict the growth of Class III malocclusion.[69,70] It is in fact difficult to predict as to which case will primarily remain as dentoalveolar in nature and which one will become more severe,

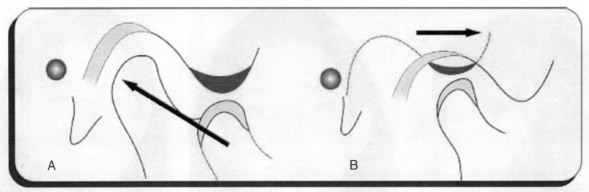

Figure 4.31 An appliance-induced downward and forward positions of the condyle leading to **(A)** adaptation to the new position through condylar growth and **(B)** adaptation to the new position by remodelling of the fossa.

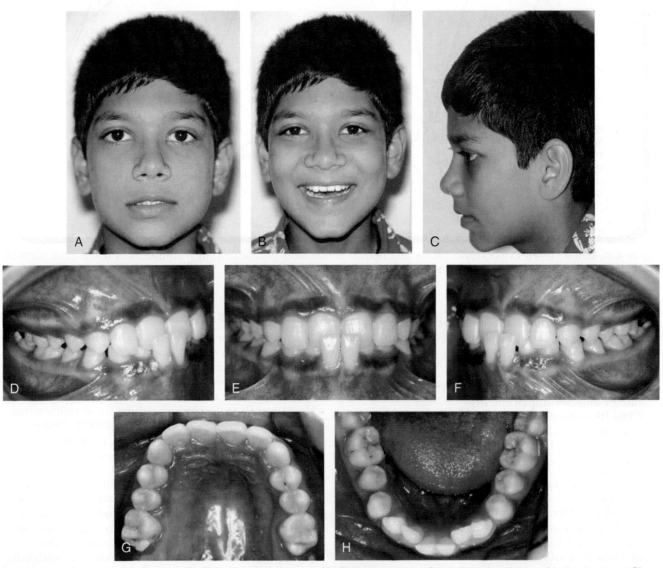

Figure 4.32 Pretreatment records. **(A–C)** Facial photographs. **(D–F)** Dentoalveolar Class III malocclusion. Molars in super Class I relationship and canines in Class III relationship; incisors are in crossbite. **(G and H)** Square maxillary archform and mild mandibular anterior crowding.

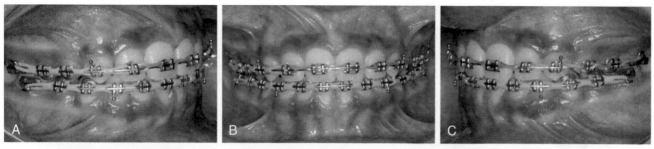

Figure 4.33   Transitional orthodontic treatment mechanics.

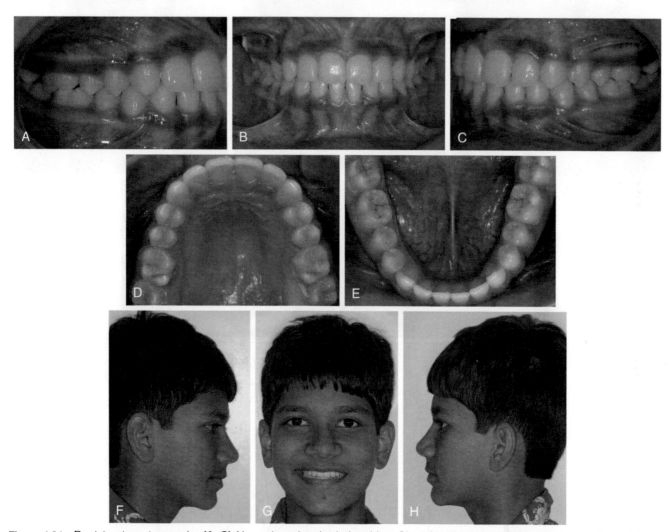

Figure 4.34   Post-treatment records. **(A–C)** Normal occlusal relationship—Class I molars and canines and normal overjet and overbite. **(D and E)** Coordinated and compatible archforms. **(F–H)** Normal facial features.

involving the skeletal components. However, hereditary pattern plays an important role in early prediction.

In some patients, early diagnosis of the problem is sometimes possible with the help of the lateral cephalogram. A long mandibular base with spaces between the developing unerupted teeth may be an indication of future prognathism.

Dentoalveolar movements to camouflage skeletal Class III discrepancy

For patients with Class III malocclusions diagnosed during the permanent dentition period, treatment options are very limited. Such problems that are not resolved during the

mixed dentition by orthopaedic treatment usually require comprehensive fixed appliance therapy or surgical intervention. For some reasons, if surgical correction is not considered in the final treatment plan to resolve the underlying skeletal discrepancy, camouflage by dentoalveolar movements is the only treatment option (Figs 4.35–4.37). In mild discrepancy cases, camouflage involves the use of mid-Class III elastics with or without extraction of teeth to produce acceptance facial profile change.

Though this approach improves interincisal relationship and overall occlusion, retraction of mandibular incisors makes the chin more prominent and often magnifies the facial aesthetic problems. Therefore, camouflage

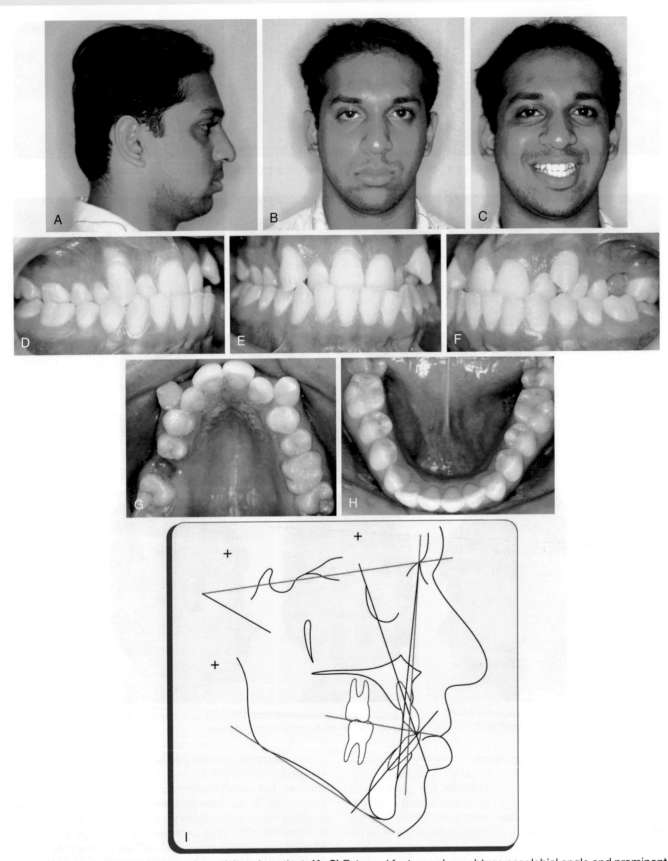

Figure 4.35 Pretreatment records of an adult male patient. **(A–C)** Extraoral features show obtuse nasolabial angle and prominent lower lip. **(D–F)** Bilateral posterior crossbite, anterior crossbite and high labially placed maxillary canines. **(G)** Severe maxillary anterior crowding and contracted arch. **(H)** Normal mandibular arch. **(I)** Pretreatment lateral cephalometric tracing.

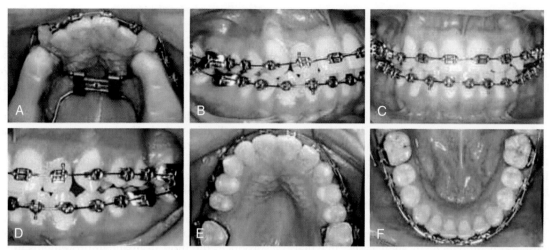

Figure 4.36 Treatment plan involved dentoalveolar movements to camouflage skeletal Class III discrepancy. **(A)** Optimal maxillary arch expansion to correct posterior crossbite and gain adequate space for the cuspids. **(B–D)** Orthodontic treatment mechanics to improve occlusal relationship. **(E and F)** Normal maxillary and mandibular archforms.

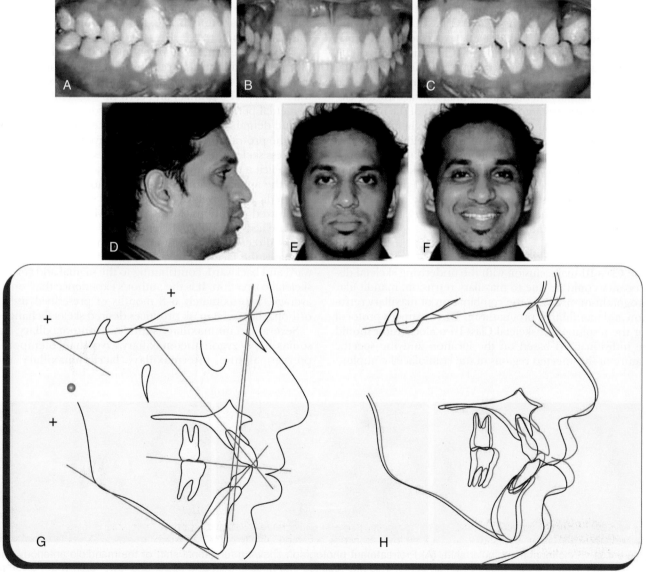

Figure 4.37 **(A–F)** Post-treatment records demonstrate improved dentition and soft tissue facial features. **(G)** Post-treatment lateral cephalometric tracing. **(H)** Pretreatment and post-treatment lateral cephalometric superimposition.

treatment in Class III malocclusions is generally considered less successful than in Class II problems.

Functional Class III malocclusion

Functional Class III malocclusion is characterized by an edge-to-edge incisor relationship or by an anterior crossbite caused by a premature tooth contact or by an abnormal positioning of the maxillary and mandibular incisors. At an early stage, patients with functional Class III do not show abnormal skeletal relationships. Usually, the mandible slides anteriorly due to tooth guidance in the canine region (Fig. 4.38). The early correction of this clinical situation involves a careful equilibration of canines to eliminate the prematurity. Some patients having chronic nasorespiratory problems often present with contracted maxillary arch leading to decreased intercanine width with resultant tooth guidance. In such cases, maxillary arch expansion without equilibration of canines is just what is required to eliminate the tooth guidance and settle the occlusion. Such discrepancies should be resolved at an early stage as they are generally considered the beginning signs of true Class III malocclusions.

In some instances, anterior displacement of the mandible is also associated with skeletal Class III malocclusion. The natural compensation of teeth, expressed as the labial tipping of the maxillary incisors and lingual tipping of the mandibular incisors, makes the patient slide the lingual surfaces of the mandibular incisors against the incisal edges of maxillary incisors after initial contact during closure. This produces anterior displacement of the mandible on the path of closure from postural rest to habitual occlusion. In habitual occlusal position, the mandible appears to be even further anteriorly positioned. This abnormal position of the mandible, coupled with sagittal skeletal discrepancy and unfavourable axial inclinations of maxillary and mandibular incisors makes the orthodontic treatment extremely difficult. The treatment usually consists of surgical orthodontic intervention in adults.

Skeletal Class III malocclusion

The Class III malocclusion with the underlying skeletal discrepancy could be due to maxillary retrusion, mandibular prognathism or due to the combination of maxillary retrusion and mandibular prognathism. The treatment protocol for the resolution of skeletal Class III malocclusion should be individualized based on the location and the specific nature of the affected regions of the craniofacial complex.

Maxillary skeletal retrusion

The skeletal Class III malocclusion due to maxillary skeletal retrusion is characterized by small and retrognathic maxillary base with small SNA and normal SNB angles. Early treatment of such patients involves growth guidance during the eruption of the maxillary incisors.

The orthopaedic facial mask. The orthopaedic facial mask is the appliance of choice in the management of patients with mild to moderate Class III malocclusions having a retruded maxilla and a hyperdivergent growth pattern in the early mixed or late deciduous dentition (Figs 4.39–4.41). For patients exhibiting vertical or hyperdivergent growth pattern, the use of bonded acrylic maxillary expansion appliance controls the vertical eruption of molars. The orthopaedic facial mask is a very versatile appliance and produces the most dramatic improvements in the shortest period of time. It affects almost all areas contributing to the development of Class III malocclusion, like maxillary basal retrusion, retrusion of maxillary dentoalveolar region, prognathic mandible and decreased lower facial height.

The orthopaedic facial mask system has various components: an acrylic bonded maxillary splint that provides a rigid maxillary anchorage, the facial mask and elastics (Fig. 4.40C and D).

The optimal time to resolve skeletal Class III malocclusion with maxillary basal retrusion and orthopaedic facial mask is at the time of initial eruption of the maxillary central incisors. The primary and early mixed dentition developmental periods are considered to promote better skeletal and dental response.[71] However, recent evidence shows that the protraction of maxilla is effective through puberty with less skeletal response as the sutures mature.[72,73]

To elicit a maximum skeletal change, the patient should wear the appliance for at least 12–14 hours a day, with orthopaedic force levels of 300–400 g per side in the primary and mixed dentitions. Most patients with maxillary retrusion are also vertically deficient. Therefore, the elastic pull can be directed little downward to lower the maxilla, which increases the face height and rotates the mandible downward and backward, contributing to the sagittal and vertical skeletal correction. It is the author's experience that, on an average, approximately 6–8 months of prescribed use of orthopaedic facial mask produces desired skeletal changes.

Several circummaxillary sutures—frontomaxillary, nasomaxillary, zygomaticomaxillary, zygomaticotemporal, pterygopalatine, intermaxillary, lacrimomaxillary and

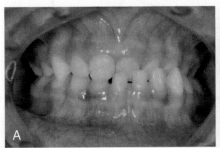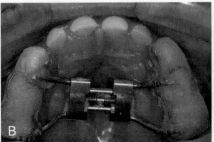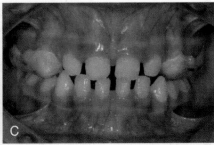

Figure 4.38 Functional mandibular shift. **(A)** Pretreatment photograph showing functional shift of the mandible anteriorly and laterally (left side) in a deciduous dentition stage. This has resulted into midline shift and upper and lower arch width discrepancy. **(B)** Expansion appliance with posterior occlusal coverage. **(C)** Before the appliance removal, the mandible is in normal position in both sagittal and transverse planes.

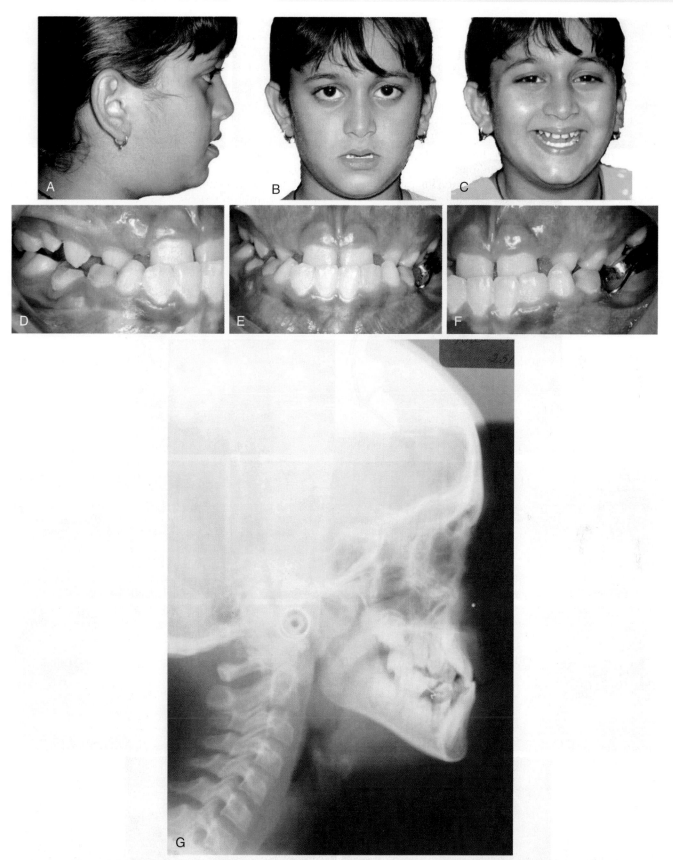

Figure 4.39 Pretreatment records of a female patient in the early mixed dentition stage. **(A–C)** Extraoral photographs demonstrate premaxillary deficiency. **(D–F)** Intraoral pictures show anterior and bilateral posterior crossbite. **(G)** Pretreatment lateral cephalogram.

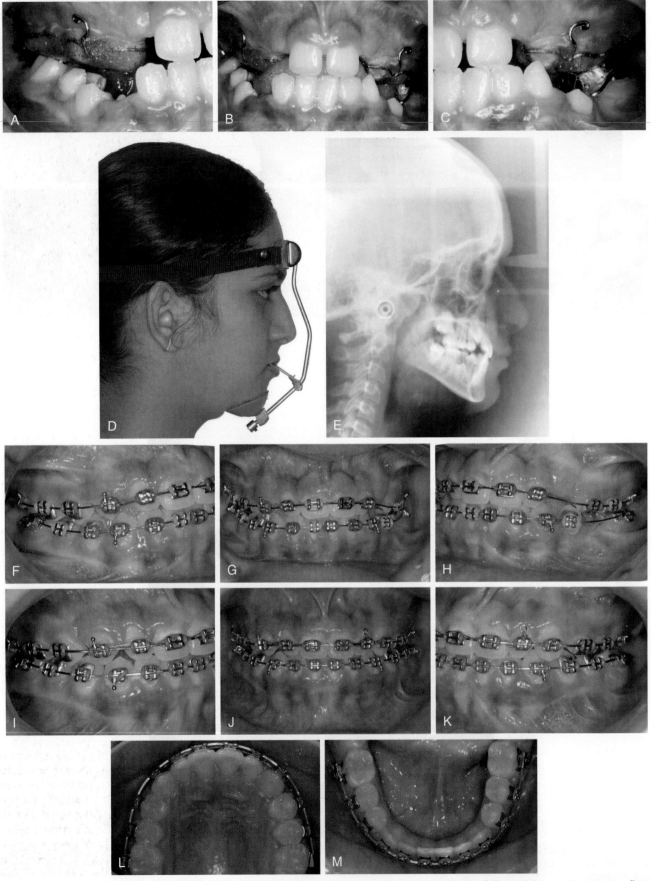

Figure 4.40 Treatment plan consisted of maxillary protraction with reverse pull headgear followed by contemporary fixed appliance therapy for detailing of the dentition. **(A–C)** Cemented maxillary splint with occlusal coverage and expansion device. **(D)** Orthopaedic facial mask. **(E)** Postmaxillary protraction lateral cephalogram. **(F–H)** Initial alignment and levelling of teeth. **(I–K)** Finishing and detailing. **(L and M)** Normal maxillary and mandibular archforms.

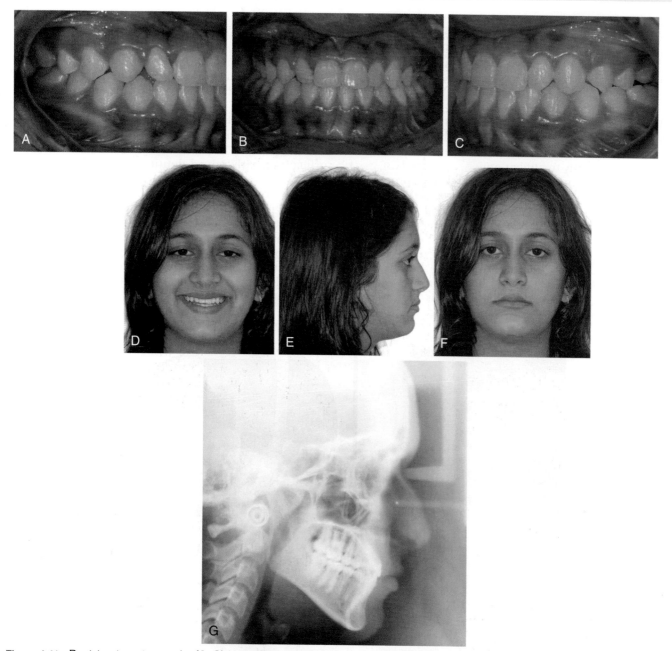

Figure 4.41 Post-treatment records. **(A–C)** Normal occlusal relationships. **(D–F)** Balanced facial profile. **(G)** Lateral cephalogram exhibiting normal skeletal, dental and soft tissue relationships.

ethmomaxillary sutures—contribute to the development of the nasomaxillary complex. To bring about rapid and significant maxillary protraction, it is essential to disarticulate the maxilla and initiate cellular response in the circummaxillary sutures. It has been found that the forward displacement of the maxilla is significantly greater when face mask is used in association with rapid maxillary expansion when compared with the protraction without rapid maxillary expansion.[74] The timing of the protraction pull on the retruded maxilla is critical. The protraction of the maxilla appears to be greater when it is carried out during maxillary expansion when compared with protraction after expansion.[74]

In pseudo-Class III patients, it is common to observe a rapid shift in the occlusal relationship and a correction of a CO-CR discrepancy. Along with skeletal improvements,

the face mask produces forward movement of maxillary dentition and lingual tipping of mandibular incisors.

In patients who do not require increase in transverse dimension, it is still advisable to activate the expansion appliance for a week to disrupt the maxillary sutural system to generate more positive reaction to protraction forces.[75]

The key to prevent post-treatment relapse is to maintain a positive overjet and overbite during the retention period. As some degree of regression of the overjet is expected during the early post-treatment period, it is important to achieve a positive overjet of approximately 4 mm before the facial mask therapy is discontinued.

Mandibular skeletal protrusion

Skeletal Class III malocclusion with a mandibular prognathism and normal maxilla is characterized by larger

SNB angle and normal SNA angle, producing a negative ANB difference. The mandible is longer with frequent findings of large gonial angle and small articular angle. Quite often, it is also anteriorly positioned. Patients with this malocclusion exhibit dentoalveolar compensation—maxillary incisors are tipped labially and the mandibular incisors are lingually inclined. A wider part of the mandible occludes with a narrower part of the maxilla, leading to a posterior crossbite. These malocclusions are extremely difficult to correct, and in severe problems, surgery is the only treatment option.

The early treatment of mandibular skeletal protrusion involves the use of functional appliances and orthopaedic chin cups. Functional appliances have very limited role in the management of mandibular prognathism and usually work by rotating the mandible downward and backward, allowing the maxillary posterior teeth to erupt downward and forward while inhibiting the eruption of mandibular teeth and promoting proper occlusal relationships. This treatment approach is indicated in patients with normal or decreased lower anterior facial height and mild mandibular skeletal problem.

Another approach to deal with mandibular prognathism is the use of orthopaedic chin cups of two different types; the occipital-pull chin cup that is indicated in case of mandibular prognathism and vertical-pull chin cup that is advocated in patients with increased lower facial height and steep mandibular plane angle. The treatment with chin cup to influence mandibular skeletal protrusion is effective in patients during the primary or early mixed dentition period[76] (Fig. 4.42A and B).

There are two ways in which the direction of the chin cup pull is applied. If the orthopaedic force is directed below the condyle, the downward and backward rotation of the mandible is expected. This is helpful in patients with short lower anterior facial height; however, in patients in whom the vertical dimension needs to be maintained, the force should be applied through the condyle to help restrict mandibular growth (Fig. 4.42C).

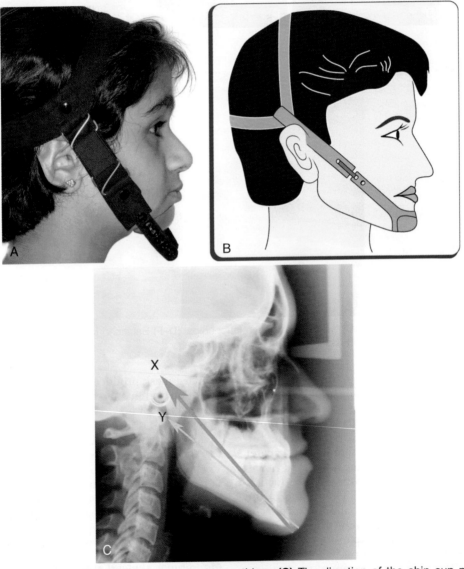

Figure 4.42 **(A and B)** Chin cup therapy for mandibular prognathism. **(C)** The direction of the chin cup pull can be applied through the mandibular condyle, if the objective is to impede mandibular growth (X), and the line of chin cup force can be below the mandibular condyle to deliberately rotate the chin downward and backward (Y).

It is recommended that the patient should use the chin cup for 12–14 hours per day with orthopaedic force levels of 300–400 g per side. It has been shown that the early correction of an anterior crossbite with a chin cup appliance prevents impaired sagittal growth of the maxilla.[76] There has been some concern among clinicians about chin cups creating pressure on the TMJ, since several patients were reported of having temporary soreness of TMJ.[77] It is recommended that patients undergoing chin cup therapy should be monitored for TMD signs and if noted, the treatment should be discontinued immediately.

CONCLUSION

A large portion of sagittal discrepancies are not just a single entity and are often associated with a variety of combinations of significant skeletal, dental and functional imbalances not just in anteroposterior plane but in vertical plane as well. In dealing with these malocclusions, contemporary orthodontic assessment and interpretation must include their proper understanding with respect to the recognition of various components involved and their interaction with the sagittal dimension. However, it should be recognized that the reliable identification of such cases requires the development of extensive diagnostic skills.

In the existing scenario, there appears to be a controversy regarding the facial growth modification, its optimal timing and the efficacy of the various appliances used. The current methods of management of these problems also reveal a great deal of variability in the clinical response of different patients to similar treatment modality. The key to successful resolution of various sagittal discrepancies is that the treatment protocol for each patient be individualized, based on the recognition, location and the specific nature of the affected regions of the craniofacial complex.

A wide spectrum of treatment modalities exist for the sagittal discrepancies at different developmental stages—acceleration or inhibition of the craniofacial growth, and the correction of abnormal dental relationships. This chapter has provided the systematic approach to the diagnosis and treatment planning of various sagittal discrepancies based on refined treatment goals, treatment options for various stages of development and their resolution with appropriate treatment mechanics and long-term stability.

REFERENCES

1. Angle EH. Treatment of malocclusion of the teeth and fractures of the maxillae: angle's systems. 6th edn. Philadelphia: SS White Dental Manufacturing; 1900.
2. Graber TM, Rakosi T, Petrovic AG. Treatment of Class II malocclusions. In: Dentofacial orthopedics with functional appliances. St Louis, Missouri: The C.V. Mosby company; 1985. 346–380.
3. Moyers RE, Guire KE, Riolo M. Differential diagnosis of Class II malocclusion. Am J Orthod 1980; 78:477–494.
4. Sarver DM. The esthetic impact of orthodontics: planning treatment to meet patient's needs. J Am Dent Assoc 1993; 124:99–102.
5. Björk A. Prediction of mandibular growth rotation. Am J Orthod 1969; 55:585–599.
6. Moyers RE. Analysis of craniofacial skeleton: cephalometrics. In: Handbook of orthodontics. Year Book Medical publishers; 1988. 270.
7. Skieller V, Björk A, Linde-Hansen T. Prediction of mandibular growth rotation evaluated from a longitudinal implant sample. Am J Orthod 1984; 86:359–370.
8. Litton SF, Ackermann LV, Isaacson RJ, et al. A genetic study of Class III malocclusion. Am J Orthod 1970; 58:565–577.
9. Harris JE, Kowalski CJ, Watnick SS. Genetic factors in the shape of the craniofacial complex. Angle Orthod 1973; 43:109–111.
10. Rakosi T, Schilli W. Class III anomalies: a coordinated approach to skeletal, dental and soft tissue problems. J Oral Surg 1981; 39:860–870.
11. Ellis EE, McNamara Jr JA. Components of adult Class III malocclusion. J Oral Maxillofac Surg 1984; 42:295–305.
12. Guyer EC, Ellis E, McNamara Jr JA, Behrents RG. Components of Class III malocclusion in juveniles and adolescents. Angle Orthod 1986; 56:7–31.
13. Ngan P, Hägg U, Yiu C, et al. Soft tissue and dentoskeletal profile changes associated with maxillary expansion and protraction headgear treatment. Am J Orthod Dentofacial Orthop 1996; 109:38–49.
14. Turley P. Orthopaedic correction of Class III malocclusion with palatal expansion and custom protraction headgear. J Clin Orthod 1988; 22:314–25.
15. Kwong WL, Lin JJ. Comparison between pseudo and true Class III malocclusion by Veterans' General Hospital cephalometric analysis. Clin Dent 1987; 7(2):69–78.
16. Latham RA. The sella point and postnatal growth of the human cranial base. Am J Orthod 1972; 61:156–162.
17. Breece GL, Nieberg LG. Motivations for adult orthodontic treatment. J Clin Orthod 1986; 20:166–171.
18. Shaw WC, Rees G, Dawe M, Charles CR. The influence of dentofacial appearance on the social attractiveness of young adults. Am J Orthod 1985; 87:21–26.
19. Shaw WC. The influence of children's dentofacial appearance on their social attractiveness as judged by peers and lay adults. Am J Orthod 1981; 79:399–415.
20. Adams GR. Physical attractiveness research: toward a developmental social psychology of beauty. Hum Dev 1977; 20:217–239.
21. Harris EF, Behrents RG. Intrinsic stability of Class I molar relationship: a longitudinal study of untreated cases. Am J Orthod Dentofacial Orthop 1988; 94:63–67.
22. Laine T. Malocclusion traits and articulatory components of speech. Eur J Orthod 1992; 14:302–309.
23. Burstone CJ. Lip posture and its significance in treatment planning. Am J Orthod 1967; 53:262–284.
24. Little RM, Wallen TR, Riedel RA. Stability and relapse of mandibular anterior alignment. First premolar extraction cases treated by traditional edgewise orthodontics. Am J Orthod 1981; 80:349–365.
25. Sadowsky C, Sakols EI. Long-term assessment of orthodontic relapse. Am J Orthod 1982; 82:456–463.
26. Nikolai RJ. On optimum orthodontic force theory as applied to canine retraction. Am J Orthod 1975; 68:290–302.
27. Tanne K, Koenig HA, Burstone CJ. Moment to force ratios and the centre of rotation. Am J Orthod 1988; 94:426–431.
28. Hixon EH, Aasen TO, Arango J, et al. On force and tooth movement. Am J Orthod 1970; 57:476–488.
29. Gianelly AA. Crowding: timing of treatment. Angle Orthod 1994; 64:415–418.
30. Nance HN. The limitations of orthodontic treatment. Part 1. Am J Orthod 1947; 33:177–223.
31. Leighten BC. The early signs of malocclusion. Trans Eur Orthod Soc 1969; 45:353–368.
32. Armstrong M. Controlling – the magnitude, direction and duration of extraoral force. Am J Orthod 1971; 59:217–243.
33. Pancherz H. Treatment of Class II malocclusions by jumping the bite with Herbst appliance. A cephalometric investigation. Am J Orthod 1979; 76:423–442.
34. Poulton DR. The influence of extraoral traction. Am J Orthod 1967; 53:8–18.
35. Cetlin NM, Ten Hoeve A. Non-extraction treatment. J Clin Orthod 1983; 17:396–413.
36. Gianelly AA, Vaitas AS, Thomas WM. The use of magnets to move molars distally. Am J Orthod 1989; 96:161–167.

37. Locatelli R, Bednar J, Dietz VS, et al. Molar distalization with super elastic NiTi Wire. J Clin Orthod 1992; 26:277–279.

38. Carano A, Tests M. The distal jet for upper molar distalization. J Clin Orthod 1996; 30:374–380.

39. Jones RD, White JM. Rapid Class II molar correction with an open coil jig. J Clin Orthod 1992; 26:661–664.

40. Hilgers JJ. The pendulum appliance for Class II non-compliance therapy. J Clin Orthod 1992; 26:706–714.

41. Kalra V. The K-loop molar distalizing appliance. J Clin Orthod 1995; 29:298–301.

42. Karad A. KIDS: a new approach to distalize maxillary molars. World J Orthod 2008; 9:244–254.

43. Fortini A, Lupoli M, Pari M. The first class appliance for rapid molar distalization. J Clin Orthod 1999; 33(6):322–328.

44. Pieringer M, Droschl H, Permann R. Distalization with a Nance appliance and coil springs. J Clin Orthod 1997; 31(5): 321–326.

45. Polat-Ozsoya O, Gokcelikb A, Güngör-Acarc A, et al. Soft-tissue profile after distal molar movement with a pendulum. K-loop appliance versus cervical headgear. Angle Orthod 2008; 78(2): 317–323.

46. Sayinsu K, Isik F, Nur Ülgen A. A comparative study of profile changes with three different distalization mechanics. World J Orthod 2007; 8(1):65–71.

47. Ricketts RM, Bench RW, Gugino CF, et al. Bioprogressive therapy. Denver, CO: Rockey Mountain Orthodontics; 1979.

48. Kinzinger GSM, Fritz UB, Sander FG, et al. Efficiency of a pendulum appliance for molar distalization related to second and third molar eruption stage. Am J Orthod Dentofacial Orthop 2004; 125(1):8–23.

49. Gutierrez VME. Treatment effects of the distal jet appliance with and without edgewise therapy. St Louis: Department of Orthodontics, St. Louis University; 2001.

50. Tanne K, Sakuda M, Burstone CJ. Three dimensional finite element analysis for stress in the periodontal tissue by orthodontic forces. Am J Orthod 1987; 92:499–505.

51. Siatkowski R. The role of headgear in Class II dental and skeletal corrections. In: Nanda R, Kuhlberg A, eds. Biomechanics in clinical orthodontics. Philadelphia: WB Saunders; 1996. 109–142.

52. Proffit WR, et al. Contemporary orthodontics. 2nd edn. St Louis: Mosby; 1993.

53. Nanda R, Kuhlberg A. Biomechanical basis of extraction space closure. In: Nanda R, Kuhlberg A, eds. Biomechanics in clinical orthodontics. Philadelphia: WB Saunders; 1996. 156–187.

54. Wieslander L. The effect of force on craniofacial development. Am J Orthod 1974; 65:531–538.

55. Baumrind S, Korn EL, Molthen R, et al. Changes in facial dimensions associated with the use of forces to retract the maxilla. Am J Orthod 1981; 80:17–30.

56. Melanson E, Van Dyken C. Studies in condylar growth, master's thesis. Ann Arbor: University of Michigan; 1972.

57. Mills CM, Mc Culloch KJ. Treatment effects of the twin block appliance. Am J Orthod Dentofacial Orthop 1998; 114:15–24.

58. Droel R, Isaacson RJ. Some relationship between glenoid fossa position and various skeletal discrepancies. Am J Orthod 1972; 61:64–78.

59. Liselot B, Melsen B, Terp S. A laminographic study of the alterations of the temporomandibular joint following activator treatment. Eur J Orthod 1984; 6:157.

60. Woodside DG, Metaxas A, Altuna G. The influence of functional appliance therapy on glenoid fossa remodeling. Am J Orthod Dentofacial Orthop 1987; 92:181–198.

61. Woodside DG. Do functional appliances have an orthopaedic effect? Am J Orthod Dentofacial Orthop 1998; 113:11–14.

62. Buschang PH, Santos-Pinto A. Condylar growth and glenoid fossa displacement during childhood and adolescence. Am J Orthod Dentofacial Orthop 1998; 113:437–442.

63. Ward DM, Behrents RG, Goldberg JS. Temporomandibular joint fluid pressure response to altered mandibular position. Am J Orthod Dentofacial Orthop 1990; 98:22–28.

64. Graber TM. The unique nature of temporomandibular joint metabolism: the clinical implications. In: Rabie AM, Urist MRB, eds. Bone formation and repair. Amsterdam: Elsevier; 1997; 143–153.

65. Ikai A, Sugisaki M, Young-Sung K, et al. Morphologic study of the mandibular fossa and the eminence of the temporomandibular joint in relation to facial structures. Am J Orthod Dentofacial Orthop 1997; 112:634–638.

66. Fields HW, Proffit WR, Nixon WL, et al. Facial pattern difference in long-faced children and adults. Am J Orthod 1984; 85:217–223.

67. Joondeph DR. Early orthodontic treatment. Am J Orthod 1993; 104:199–200.

68. Dietrich UC. Morphological variability of skeletal Class III relationships as revealed by cephalometric analysis. Rep Congr Eur Orthod Soc 1970; 131–143.

69. Aki T, Nanda RS, Currier GF, et al. Assessment of symphysis morphology as a predictor of the direction of mandibular growth. Am J Orthod Dentofacial Orthop 1994; 106:60–69.

70. Schulof RJ, Nakamura S, Williamson WV. Prediction of abnormal growth in Class III malocclusions. Am J Orthod 1977; 71:421–430.

71. Baccetti T, McGill JS, Franchi L, et al. Skeletal effects of early treatment of Class III malocclusion with maxillary expansion and face-mask therapy. Am J Orthod Dentofacial Orthop 1998; 113:333–343.

72. Merwin D, Ngan P, Hagg U, et al. Timing of effective application of anteriorly directed orthopaedic force to the maxilla. Am J Orthod Dentofacial Orthop 1997; 112:292–299.

73. Kapust AJ, Sinclair PM, Turley PK. Cephalometric effects of face mask/expansion therapy in Class III children: a comparison of three age groups. Am J Orthod Dentofacial Orthop 1998; 113:204–212.

74. Baik HS. Clinical results of the maxillary protraction in Korean children. Am J Orthod Dentofacial Orthop 1995; 108:583–592.

75. Haas AJ. The treatment of maxillary deficiency by opening the mid-palatal suture. Angle Orthod 1965; 35:200–217.

76. Üner O, Yüksel S, Üçüncü N. Long-term evaluation after chin cup treatment. Eur J Orthod 1995; 17:135–141.

77. Deguchi T, Kitsugi A. Stability of changes associated with chin cup treatment. Angle Orthod 1996; 66:139–146.

Vertical Discrepancies 5

Ashok Karad

The vertical dimension of face is often altered, either intentionally or non-intentionally, during orthodontic treatment of various dentofacial problems by the extrusion or intrusion of teeth and by growth modification and orthognathic surgery. These changes have a great impact on the way the mandible rotates, either open or closed, with corresponding alterations in maxillomandibular dental relationships, lip and tongue function and, importantly, the facial aesthetics. Therefore, before the initiation of orthodontic therapy, it is vital for the clinician to clearly define the treatment goals related to the vertical dimension of face and design a detailed individualized treatment strategy and mechanics plan based on sound biomechanical principles.

The orthodontic literature related to the management of sagittal discrepancies and to certain extent transverse discrepancies is replete with research, case studies and publications. However, for the most part in the past and still to a large extent in the present, there has been much less research and discussion on the treatment of vertical problems. A large variation in craniofacial growth in the vertical dimension should play a prominent role in orthodontist's approach to the diagnosis and treatment of malocclusion. The relevance of assessing the vertical dimension to clinical practice is to determine, if there is a vertical component contributing to the development of a problem. In a clinical practice, vertical discrepancies are often considered to be the most difficult dentofacial problems to treat. To successfully treat vertical discrepancies, it is important for the clinician to have good understanding of the factors having the greatest influence on the vertical dimension problem. The author believes that in dealing with malocclusions with abnormal vertical component, the simplicity or complexity of the force system is not the deciding factor in producing the best treatment results. Rather, clinicians should have sound knowledge of facial growth and development, interplay between the horizontal and vertical growth, function of the lips and tongue, etc.

DEVELOPMENT OF A VERTICAL PROBLEM

Facial growth in relation to the cranial base proceeds along a vector with variable amounts of horizontal and vertical growth. It is important to consider, understand and appreciate the value of vertical growth, as it relates to anteroposterior growth. Vertical growth carries the chin downward, while anteroposterior growth carries it forward (Fig. 5.1). The major sites of bony additions contributing to the facial growth include the facial sutures, maxillary alveolar processes, mandibular condyle and mandibular alveolar processes.[1] If vertical growth increments at the facial sutures and the maxillary and mandibular alveolar processes exceed the condylar growth, the mandible would rotate backward. However, if growth at the condyle exceeds the total vertical growth at the facial sutures and alveolar processes, the mandible would rotate forward.[2] These growth changes significantly alter the lower facial height and the position of chin horizontally and vertically.

Growth

For the facial proportions and the occlusal relationships to be normal, the components of the craniofacial complex consisting essentially of the cranial base, nasomaxillary complex and the mandible should exhibit harmonious growth and should maintain a reasonable proportion in size and form. It is well recognized that the spatial position of the maxillary dentition is influenced by the eruption pattern of the teeth and the growth of the maxilla and its contiguous bones. It is also affected by the

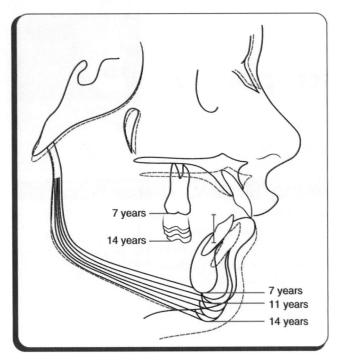

Figure 5.1 Cephalometric superimpositions showing the chin position as a result of growth changes in a patient between 7 and 14 years of age. It was observed that the chin moved downward and forward till the age of 11 years; thereafter, it was displaced downward and backward as a result of less condylar growth and more vertical growth in the molar area.

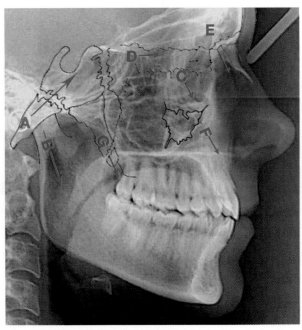

Figure 5.2 Growth at the spheno-occipital synchondrosis during the first decade displaces the maxillary complex anterosuperiorly, while the mandibular condylar growth displaces the mandible anteroinferiorly producing diverging growth vectors to create a space for vertical facial growth, alveolar growth and tooth eruption. Cartilaginous growth: **A,** spheno-occipital synchondrosis; **B,** reflection of mandibular condylar growth; **C,** nasal septum; **D,** sphenoethmoidal; **E,** frontomaxillary; **F,** zygomaticomaxillary; **G,** pterygopalatine.

growth of the anterior cranial base, the area between the pituitary fossa and the internal plate of the frontal bone, to which the maxillary complex is attached. The growth at the sphenoethmoidal suture significantly contributes to the increase in depth of the anterior cranial base and upper face until the suture closes by the age of 7 years.[3] After the age of 7 years, further growth in this area until adulthood takes place by surface remodelling of bone on the frontonasal surface, with the sella to the internal plate of the frontal bone dimension unchanged.[4]

After the cessation of anterior cranial base growth at an early age, the anterior half of the craniomaxillary complex is displaced in an anterosuperior direction by the growth at the spheno-occipital suture until the suture closes after puberty.[5] This expression of growth shows a great degree of variation in the direction and rate among individuals. The spatial position of the mandibular dentition is determined by the growth of the mandible and its relationship to the temporal bone. It has been shown that the relationship of the mandible to the anterior border of the foramen magnum (Ba-Ar) does not vary.[6] Condylar head, being the primary growth centre of the mandible, grows in upward and backward directions with the resultant downward and forward displacements of the mandible and carries the mandibular dentition away from the vertebral column and cranial base. Therefore, the growth at the spheno-occipital synchondrosis displaces the maxillary complex anterosuperiorly, while the growth at the mandibular condyle displaces the mandible downward and forward (Fig. 5.2). These two diverging growth vectors create a space for vertical facial growth, alveolar

growth and tooth eruption. Annual incremental growth of various craniofacial components is shown in Figure 5.3.

The mandible demonstrates a great degree of variation in the direction of its growth in the normal population as shown in studies on facial growth by Björk and Skieller using metallic implants.[7–13] The most common direction of condylar growth is vertical with some anterior component; however, the posterior growth is less frequently observed. Patients with upward and forward growth of the condyle are usually characterized by reduced anterior face height and deep overbite, as seen in Class II division 1 malocclusion. Patients with extreme cases of upward and forward growth of the condyle exhibit a skeletal deep bite, as observed in Class II division 2 malocclusion. Typically, the maxillary and mandibular dentitions are characterized by considerable degree of mesial migration of teeth with some amount of mandibular incisor proclination. Patients with a more posteriorly directed mandibular condylar growth demonstrate a pronounced increase in lower face height and an anterior open bite. The erupting posterior dentition is generally vertical, and quite often, the anterior teeth may even become more proclined with time.

It is important for the clinician to consider, understand and recognize the importance of mandibular growth rotation, as it relates to anterior facial height (AFH) and overbite relationship. Björk[11] suggested that under normal situations, the fulcruming point for anterior mandibular growth rotation is located at the

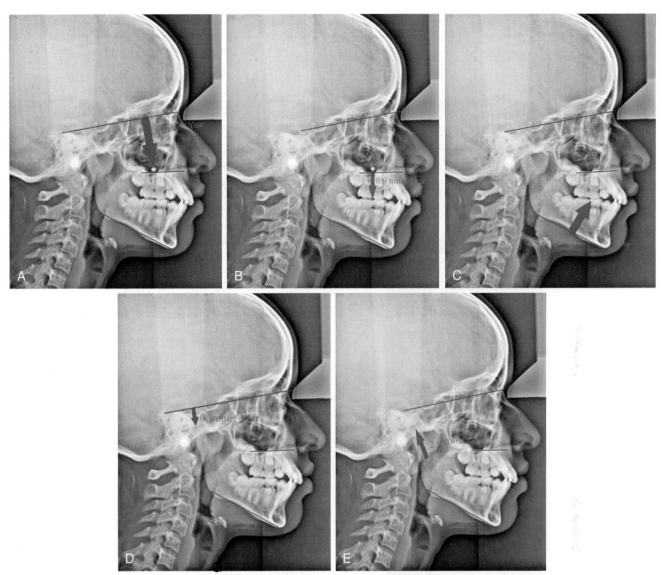

Figure 5.3 Annual incremental growth of various craniofacial components. **(A)** Average basal maxillary vertical displacement. **(B)** Vertical maxillary dentoalveolar growth. **(C)** Mandibular vertical dentoalveolar growth. **(D)** Vertical displacement of the articular fossa. **(E)** Condylar growth.

incisors (Fig. 5.4). In the absence of proper incisal contact due to lip dysfunction, finger sucking habit or severe sagittal jaw discrepancy, the fulcruming point moves posteriorly along the occlusal plane leading to the development of skeletal deep bite. In patients with posterior condylar growth rotation, the fulcruming point is located near the mandibular condyles, with the development of anterior open bite and increased anterior face height.

In addition to the condylar growth direction, differences in AFH and posterior facial height (PFH) development do play an important role in the development of vertical skeletal discrepancies (Figs 5.5 and 5.6). These differences significantly contribute to rotational growth or to changes in mandibular position, influencing the position of the chin.[14] The research findings show that the dentoalveolar heights are significantly greater in long AFH patients and smaller in short lower AFH group.[15,16] The excessive maxillary posterior dentoalveolar development may be associated with weaker masticatory musculature in high-angle patients compared with stronger musculature associated with low-angle patients.

Environmental factors

The role of certain environmental factors, like swallowing, breathing and tongue posture in altered vertical dimension, still continues to be the subject of debate. However, breathing problems due to large adenoids, tonsils, deviated nasal septa, etc. are frequently associated with high-angle patients, which alter mandibular posture, creating more room for posterior teeth eruption. It has been shown that the removal of adenoids and tonsillectomy have resulted in closing of the mandibular plane (MP) angle and reduction in the anterior face height.[17,18] The significance of tongue posture and tongue thrust has been evaluated by many with regard to its role as a causative factor in the development of malocclusion.

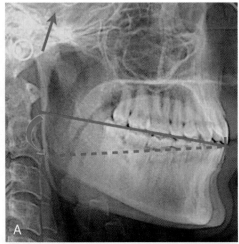

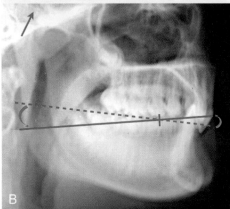

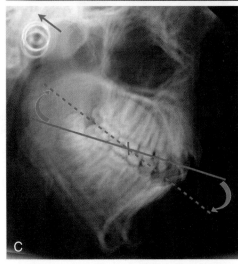

Figure 5.4 Photos showing mandibular growth rotations. **(A)** Patients with a stable occlusion demonstrate anterior rotation of the mandible with the fulcrum point located at the incisors. **(B)** Patients with lack of anterior occlusion tend to have the fulcruming point located posteriorly along the occlusal plane. **(C)** In patients with posterior mandibular rotation, the fulcruming point is located near the mandibular condyles.

DIAGNOSIS OF VERTICAL DISCREPANCIES

Vertical discrepancies consist of various components of the craniofacial complex and are often associated with abnormalities in other planes of space. Their accurate diagnosis is a key element in the design of any successful treatment plan. In order to plan an appropriate treatment strategy, the clinician should localize and quantify any skeletal and dental contributions, vertical and sagittal variations and the role of abnormal function to the development of vertical problems.

Facial evaluation

Facial evaluation should begin with a systematic, three-dimensional assessment of the frontal and profile views in the vertical, sagittal and transverse planes. The goal of this assessment is to establish an accurate description of the aesthetic, skeletal and occlusal abnormalities, as well as functional disorders. Based on the extraoral features, patients with vertical discrepancies may be broadly classified as long-face and short-face patients.

Long-face patients are usually characterized by leptoprosopic facial form and dolichocephalic head form, increased lower facial height, narrow alar bases, prominent nasal dorsum, retrognathic mandible, orthognathic or prognathic maxilla, incompetent lips with mentalis strain, shallow mentolabial sulcus and flattened or recessive chin. Such patients usually exhibit Class II malocclusion with the appearance of mandibular deficiency and are often associated with excessive gingival display upon smile.

Short-face patients can be found in Angle's Class II and Class III malocclusions. Short-face patients with the most common Class II malocclusion present with decreased lower anterior face height, normal upper lip length, obtuse nasolabial angle, acute mentolabial sulcus, retruded mandible and adequate or excessive soft tissue chin. Short-face patients having Class III malocclusion exhibit many opposite facial characteristics with decreased lower anterior face height, short upper lip, acute nasolabial angle, prognathic appearing mandible and obtuse mentolabial sulcus.

Intraoral examination of the long-face patients reveals maxillary–mandibular dentoalveolar protrusion, upright and supraerupted maxillary and mandibular incisors, excessive eruption of posterior teeth, anterior open bite, high and narrow palate with posterior crossbite, etc. Intraoral features common to short-face patients of both Angle's Class II and Class III groups include excessive deep overbite and deep curve of Spee. The maxillary and mandibular incisors are often upright exhibiting a bidentoalveolar retrusion.[19] A short face in these patients is often caused by overclosure of the mandible either due to vertical maxillary deficiency or due to deficient teeth eruption in either the maxilla or the mandible.

Functional assessment

An assessment of function is a very important part of the clinical examination for planning treatment of vertical discrepancies. Associated disorders involving airway, speech and tongue function should be carefully evaluated. It has been generally recognized that environmental factors that are responsible for keeping the maxillary and mandibular teeth apart promote elongation of the posterior teeth, leading to an increase in lower face height. Excessive posterior dentoalveolar development in the maxilla is considered to be associated with weaker

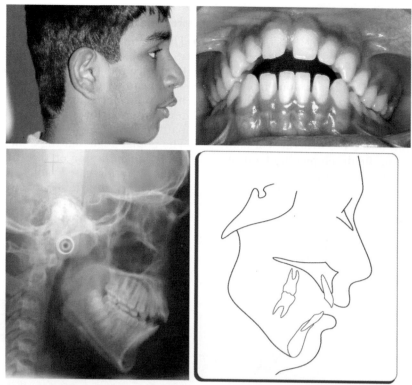

Figure 5.5 Facial profile photograph, intraoral photograph and lateral cephalogram of a 15-year-old male patient having convex profile, open bite and increased lower facial height.

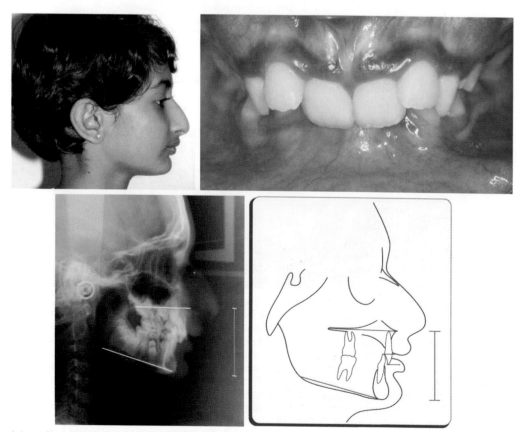

Figure 5.6 Facial profile photograph, intraoral photograph and lateral cephalogram of a 12-year-old female patient exhibiting extreme skeletal deep bite, decreased anterior face height and insufficient dentoalveolar compensation.

musculature in high-angle patients compared with stronger musculature in low-angle patients.[20]

Morphologic characteristics

Classifying patients into high-angle or long-face patients and low-angle or short-face patients is just a broad understanding of vertical discrepancies. Patients with vertical problems should be further analyzed cephalometrically to identify and locate the structures at fault, which mainly contribute to the development of a problem (Fig. 5.7). Their understanding is essential to define the treatment goals and plan a treatment strategy to resolve them. Vertical discrepancies can be divided into those that are dentoalveolar in nature and into those that are predominantly skeletal as a result of the growth patterns of the jaws.

Cephalometric assessment

- The cranial flexure angle (N-S-Ar), articular angle (S-Ar-Go) and gonial angle (Ar-Go-Me) are often used to determine the growth pattern of an individual. The mean value of sum of these angles is $396° \pm 4°$; high values are suggestive of a vertical growth pattern, whereas low values indicate horizontal growth pattern.[21,22]
- The gonial angle, having a mean value of $130° \pm 7°$, is a good indicator of vertical or horizontal growth pattern. An increased value shows that the individual is backward growth rotator, while a decreased value indicates a forward rotator.[21,23] To be more precise, if the ratio of the upper gonial angle (Ar-Go-Na) to the lower gonial angle (Na-Go-Me) is more than 75%, it is considered a horizontal growth rotation; however,

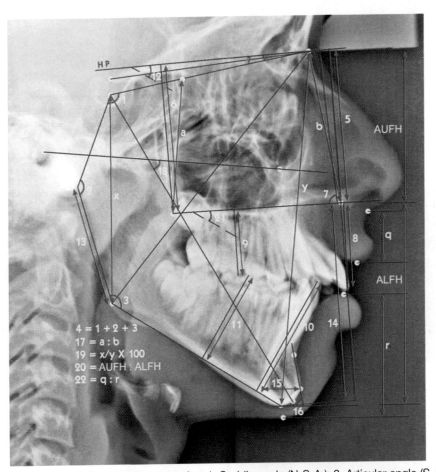

Figure 5.7 Cephalometric assessment of vertical discrepancies. 1. Saddle angle (N-S-Ar); 2. Articular angle (S-Ar-Go); 3. Gonial angle (Ar-Go-Me), upper gonial angle (Ar-Go-N) and lower gonial angle (N-Go-Me); 4. Björk's sum = saddle angle (N-S-Ar) + articular angle (S-Ar-Go) + gonial angle (Ar-Go-N); 5. Distance between N and ANS (perpendicular to HP); 6. Distance between N and PNS (perpendicular to HP); 7. J angle—angle between palatal plane and perpendicular to N-Se passing through N'; 8. Upper incisor edge to nasal floor (NF) (perpendicular distance to NF); 9. Upper first molar mesiobuccal cusp tip to NF (perpendicular distance to NF); 10. Lower incisor edge to mandibular plane (MP) (perpendicular distance to MP); 11. Lower first molar mesiobuccal cusp tip to MP (perpendicular distance to MP); 12. MP-HP (angle); 13. Length of mandibular ramus (Ar-Go); 14. Distance between ANS and Gn (perpendicular to HP); 15. Width of symphysis measured at Pg, parallel to true horizontal; 16. Symphysis angle—angle between line passing through point B and Pog and true horizontal; 17. Ratio of posterior maxillary height (E-PNS) to anterior maxillary heights (N-ANS); 18. Angle between FH plane and y-axis (S-Gn); 19. Jarabak's ratio posterior facial height (S-Go)/anterior facial height (N-Me) × 100; 20. Anterior upper facial height (vertical distance from N to ANS): anterior lower facial height (vertical distance from ANS to Me); 21. Angle between palatal plane (ANS-PNS) and mandibular plane; 22. Upper lip length (subnasale to stomion superior): lower lip length (stomion inferior to soft tissue menton).

higher lower gonial angle indicates a vertical growth pattern.[21]

- The MP angle (Go-Me—true horizontal) having a mean value of $27° \pm 5°$ is one of the most commonly used parameters. It is increased in patients with a vertical growth pattern, while horizontally growing patients exhibit low angle.

- An assessment of symphysis morphology is useful in determining the growth pattern of an individual. The width of symphysis, measured at pogonion (Pg) parallel to the true horizontal, has a mean value of 16.5 ± 3 mm, with greater values in horizontally growing patients and smaller values in vertically growing patients.[23] The symphysis angle, formed by the line passing through point B, Pg and the true horizontal, having a mean value of $75° \pm 5°$, is acute in a forward growth rotational pattern and obtuse in a backward rotation.[23,24]

- In an individual with average facial growth, the ratio of posterior face height (S-Go) to anterior face height (Na-Me) is 65%, with higher values in a forward growth pattern and smaller values in a backward growth pattern.

- The vertically growing patients tend to have a ratio of posterior to anterior maxillary height higher than 90%, while in horizontally growing patients, this ratio is lower than 90%.

High-angle patients are usually characterized by the following:

- Steep MP angle
- Rotation of palatal plane down posteriorly
- Large gonial angle
- Short ramus height or decreased posterior face height
- Increased maxillary and mandibular dentoalveolar height
- Antegonial notching

Low-angle patients are usually characterized by the following:

- Decreased MP angle
- Decreased lower face height
- Normal or long posterior face height
- Reduced maxillary molar height is the strongest measure of vertical maxillary deficiency
- Reduced incisor height may be associated with deficient incisor display

Vertical Class II types

While assessing various problems in vertical dimension, it is essential for the clinician to understand their impact on the sagittal dimension. Björk[11] described morphologic method of predicting growth rotation from a single cephalogram and found seven structural signs for predicting forward or backward growth rotation.

1. Inclination of the condylar head: The condylar head curves forward in forward rotator, while it is straight or slopes up and back in backward rotator.
2. Curvature of the mandibular canal: The mandibular canal is curved in forward rotator and straight in backward rotator.
3. Shape of the mandibular lower border: In forward rotator, it is curved downward, whereas in backward rotator, it is notched.

4. Inclination of the symphysis (anterior aspect just below point 'B'): This slopes backward in forward rotator and forward in backward rotator.
5. Interincisal angle: This angle is vertical or obtuse in forward rotator and acute in backward rotator.
6. Interpremolar or intermolar angles: These angles are vertical or obtuse in forward rotator and acute in backward rotator.
7. Anterior lower face height: This height is short in forward rotator and long in backward rotator.

Of these seven original signs, four of the variables when combined give the best prognostic estimate of mandibular growth rotations.[24]

These parameters are as follows:

1. Mandibular inclination: This can be assessed by the gonial angle measurement, the inclination of the lower border or a proportion between posterior and AFH.
2. Shape of the lower border: The backward rotator has convex or notched lower border as against the concave lower border of the forward rotator.
3. Inclination of the symphysis: If the symphysis points behind nasion or posterior to nasion, a forward rotational pattern is likely present. If it points forward or anterior to nasion, it is an indication of backward rotation.
4. Intermolar angle: In backward growth rotation, the premolars and molars are more inclined, while in the forward growth rotation, these teeth are more upright to one another.

Class II malocclusions with vertical discrepancies have been identified as having five vertical types[25] (Fig. 5.8).

Type 1: It is characterized by the disproportionately increased anterior face height than by the posterior face height. The palate may be tipped downward, and the anterior cranial base tends to be upward. The mandibular and functional occlusal lines are steeper than normal. This vertical type of Class II malocclusion is also called *high-angle case* or *long-face syndrome*.

Type 2: It displays more horizontal or nearly parallel mandibular, functional occlusal and palatal planes. The gonial angle is small, and the anterior cranial base is horizontal. The patient displays a 'square face' with more vertical incisor position and skeletal deep bite.

Type 3: Patients having type 3 vertical pattern exhibit a palatal plane that is tipped upward anteriorly resulting in a decreased anterior upper face height and an open bite. When it is associated with steep MP angle, a severe skeletal open bite is developed.

Type 4: It is a rare type of Class II malocclusion having palatal and functional occlusal planes that are tipped downward, and the mandible plane is almost normal. The gonial angle is relatively obtuse. The maxillary incisors are tipped labially, and the mandibular incisors are lingually inclined. Patients usually exhibit high lip line on the maxillary alveolar process.

Type 5: The features of this type include the palatal plane that is tipped downward with normal mandibular and functional occlusal planes. The gonial angle is smaller than normal. This leads to skeletal deep bite.

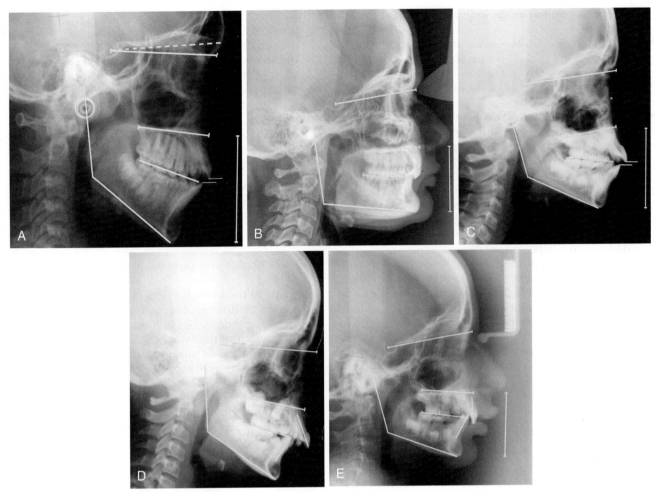

Figure 5.8 Differential diagnosis of vertical discrepancies. Class II malocclusions having five vertical types based on the research by Moyers et al[25]: **(A)** Type 1, **(B)** Type 2, **(C)** Type 3, **(D)** Type 4 and **(E)** Type 5.

The maxillary incisors are almost vertical, and the mandibular incisors are severely labially placed.

TREATMENT PLANNING

Establishing accurate diagnosis is an integral part of designing a successful treatment strategy. An ideal treatment plan maximizes treatment results and shortens the treatment duration. Defining treatment goals—facial, skeletal and dental—is the best way to approach treatment planning for the vertical discrepancies. At the treatment planning stage, as the clinician gets involved into an important process of reexploration of the available relevant diagnostic information, several critical factors must be considered.

• A careful evaluation of the vertical proportions of the face to determine long lower face height (high angle) or short lower face height (low angle) is the first step in the treatment planning process. Control of the vertical dimension is considered the most important factor in successfully treating high-angle patients. These patients usually have a tendency to further bite opening during

treatment as a result of significantly less bite force than low-angle patients.[26] The treatment of such patients should result in:

• Preventing further development of upper and lower posterior dentoalveolar segments of maxilla
• An increased posterior-to-anterior face height ratio
• A forward autorotation of the mandible
• An enhanced vertical growth of the condyle and ramus

Conversely, a vertical discrepancy patient involving a disproportionately short lower facial height would have different and opposite treatment goals and approach.

• Determine whether the malocclusion is dentoalveolar or skeletal. It is possible to have abnormalities of teeth in vertical dimension without affecting the lower anterior face height. It is also important to identify the dentoalveolar compensation masking the underlying severe vertical skeletal discrepancy. In the maxilla, the angle between the palatal plane and the maxillary occlusal plane (mean $10° \pm 3°$) describes the extent of compensatory or dysplastic development, while in the mandible, it is described by the measurement between the MP and the mandibular occlusal plane (mean $20° \pm 4°$).[27]

- Vertical discrepancy is not a single entity and involves many components. Identification of their involvement is essential to formulate an effective treatment strategy.
- Age of the patient and the severity of malocclusion significantly influence the treatment planning process. It is recommended to ascertain the growth potential of the patient based on the useful diagnostic information. It is not only the differences in condylar growth direction but also the result of differences in AFH and PFH development that significantly contribute to two extreme growth patterns—long face and short face.
- Identification of aetiological factors responsible for the development of a vertical discrepancy and the role of neuromuscular dysfunctions are of great value in planning a treatment. Though the role of environmental factors, like abnormal tongue posture, swallowing and mouth breathing, is still a subject of debate, it needs serious consideration.
- The dentofacial aesthetics is considered one of the main reasons for patients to undergo orthodontic treatment. The vertical discrepancies, especially the skeletal involvement, expressed clinically either as a long-face problem or as a short-face problem, significantly contribute to the impairment of facial aesthetics. Therefore, aesthetic benefits of proposed treatment plan should be analyzed, and if required, necessary alterations should be incorporated to maximize facial aesthetics.
- Clinicians are quite often faced with the difficult task of treating patients with anterior open bite or deep bite with subsequent challenge to retention. Various treatment modalities have been used to address these problems; however, the success of any therapy is ultimately measured by long-term stability. The best way to approach any vertical discrepancy is to identify the areas of potential relapse and take appropriate measures to enhance stability.

TREATMENT OF VERTICAL DISCREPANCIES

While dealing with the patients with vertical problems, it must be recognized that all cases cannot be treated in a similar manner due to extreme variation in facial pattern and morphological characteristics. The facial pattern is not constant since it is changed by growth and by orthodontic treatment. Also, the effects of vertical growth increments on different facial types are different. Therefore, in patients with compromised AFHs, the relative methods of mandibular rotation (opening versus closure) as a part of orthodontic treatment should be recognized as either desirable or undesirable.

For the purpose of discussion, treatment of vertical discrepancies can be grouped and explained under following categories (Fig. 5.9):

1. Vertical discrepancies with increased lower anterior face height or long-face patient
2. Vertical discrepancies with normal vertical dimension of face
3. Vertical problems with decreased lower AFH or low-angle patient

Management of long-face patients

Treatment of excessive lower facial height or long-face patients depends on an accurate diagnosis that requires precise identification of various components. As opposed to simple open bite malocclusions that do not include skeletal components, high-angle patients have underlying skeletal problems that have proven to be extremely challenging for orthodontists. The clinician should expect a great degree of variation of traits among individuals; some show severe anterior open bite, while others, despite the underlying severe skeletal discrepancy, exhibit less severe open bite due to dentoalveolar compensation (Fig. 5.10). Dentoalveolar compensation that masks discrepancies in all three planes of space should be measured cephalometrically to design an appropriate treatment strategy.

The most consistent morphologic characteristics in the maxillary zone include excessive anterior and posterior dentoalveolar heights;[28] the palatal plane angles tend to be flatter due to decreased upper AFHs;[29] however, upper PFHs appear to be unchanged. The maxillary length is usually shorter,[29] and the width is reduced with a tendency for posterior crossbites.[14] The most constant morphologic features in the mandibular region include steeper MP angle, increased lower anterior heights and larger gonial angle.[28,29] Most patients exhibit shorter

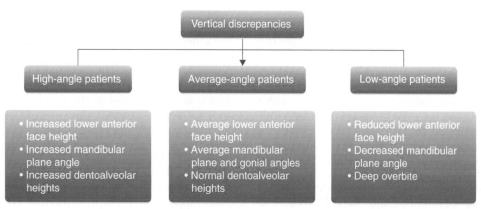

Figure 5.9 Three broad groups of vertical discrepancies.

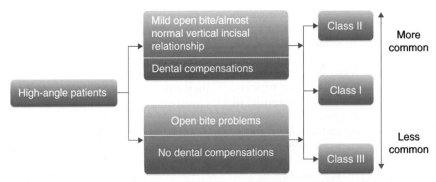

Figure 5.10   High-angle patient types.

ramus heights leading to decreased PFHs. Mandibular dentoalveolar heights generally tend to be excessive. The glenoid fossa is often positioned more superior relative to sella turcica. All these features combine to produce overall proportional increase in lower facial height to upper and total AFHs.

It is clear from these findings that the vertical discrepancies are often associated with problems in sagittal and transverse dimension. Therefore, a well-designed treatment strategy must address the three-dimensional problems pertaining to the dental, alveolar and skeletal structures of both the jaws. Hyperdivergent Class III open bite cases are less frequently observed and are more difficult to treat non-surgically than hyperdivergent Class II patients. Control of vertical dimension is considered to be the most important factor in successfully treating patients with hyperdivergency.

Treatment goals for hyperdivergent Class II patients are as follows:

1. Reductions in maxillary and mandibular dentoalveolar heights
2. Reduction in gonial angle
3. Increase in palatal plane angulations
4. Maxillary expansion
5. Mandibular autorotation to decrease lower facial height and reposition the chin forward

Orthopaedic and orthodontic treatment options to manage hyperdivergent patients include the use of high-pull headgear, posterior bite-blocks, vertical-pull chin cup, extractions, etc.

Mixed dentition treatment

Overall growth potential of an individual and the ability of certain morphological features to change are greater during childhood than adolescence. This potential combined with psychosocial benefits best justifies early intervention of skeletal open bite problems. Early treatment holds the key to nonsurgical correction of these complex malocclusions. It is based on the premises that this condition can be diagnosed at an early stage of development; potential for mandibular autorotation is maximum during childhood, and certain components of these discrepancies require long periods of growth for maximum correction. These problems do not self-correct; psychosocial benefits of correction and various treatment

options are available to address associated discrepancies in transverse and sagittal dimensions.

Therefore, early diagnosis and interceptive treatment are of utmost importance since the prognosis becomes progressively poor longer the open bite persists. Certain early signs of subtle structural changes in the craniofacial complex should be carefully observed by the clinician. Elimination of all possible aetiological factors as soon as the case is diagnosed is important. Since these patients are difficult to treat and often challenge the experience and skills of the best orthodontist, early mistakes in the treatment may compound the existing problem.

High-pull headgear has been the appliance of choice in the management of hyperdivergent open bite patients (Figs 5.11–5.14). This appliance system has good control over maxillary sutural growth and vertical dentoalveolar development.[30,31] Author prefers high-pull or occipital-pull headgear attached to the maxillary acrylic splint to prevent unfavourable tipping of molars. This appliance has good vertical control over the maxillary molars and produces superior and distal displacement of the maxilla, clockwise rotation of the palatal plane, reductions in SNA angle and relative intrusion of the maxillary molars.[32] As the maxillary molars are intruded, the mandible hinges upward, closes the open bite, displaces the chin forward and reduces the lower AFH (Figs 5.13 and 5.14). It is critical to be aware of the associated molar extrusion in this type of situation unless appropriate mechanics has been designed to control their eruption. The addition of a vertical-pull chin cup to this appliance system helps to prevent the eruption of mandibular molars.[33]

As stated earlier, vertical discrepancies are often associated with abnormalities in other two planes of space. Skeletal open bite malocclusions, occasionally, exhibit constricted maxillary arch leading to unilateral or bilateral posterior crossbites. The best way to approach maxillary transverse discrepancy is to use rapid palatal expansion device along with full posterior occlusal coverage appliance for better vertical molar control (Figs 5.15–5.18).

This also prevents undesirable buccal tipping of the posterior teeth and concomitant overhanging of palatal cusps that further accentuates mandibular backward rotation. After the desired amount of maxillary orthopaedic expansion, the appliance is removed prior to fixed appliance therapy; however, continued vertical

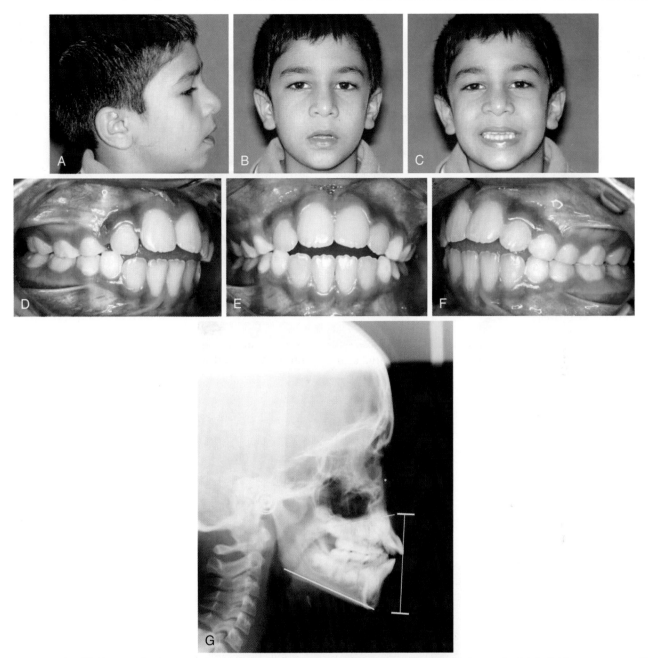

Figure 5.11 **(A–C)** Extraoral photographs of a growing male patient having increased lower facial height, convex profile and incompetent lips. **(D–F)** Intraoral photographs show mixed dentition stage, anterior open bite and tongue-thrusting habit. **(G)** Pretreatment lateral cephalogram shows high mandibular plane angle, increased lower anterior facial height and superiorly tipped palatal plane in the anterior region.

control of the posterior teeth is maintained by giving mandibular posterior bite blocks. This is frequently combined with vertical-pull chin cup to maximize the result, along with the prevention of mandibular molar eruption.

The significance of the role of certain environmental factors, like tongue posture and tongue thrust, has been evaluated by many with regard to their contribution as a causative factor in the development of a vertical problem. The management of patients with such problems is illustrated in Figures 5.19–5.22.

Extraction treatment approach

Extractions of teeth in the management of high-angle patients is considered to be useful; it is based on the belief that molars tend to move mesially out of the occlusal wedge promoting mandibular autorotation, decrease in lower anterior face height and closure of open bite relationship (Figs 5.23–5.26). Following extractions, Class II patients demonstrate decrease in ANB angle, supraeruption of the mandibular molars and increase in MP angle.[44] Patients with steep MP angles and treated with extractions and occipital headgears have

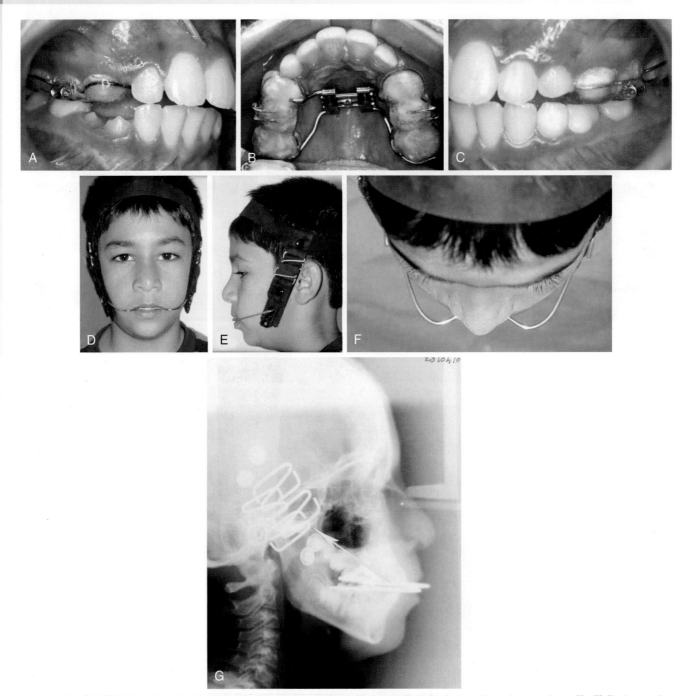

Figure 5.12 **(A–C)** Full occlusal coverage maxillary splint with rapid expansion device and headgear tubes. **(D–F)** Patient using high-pull headgear. **(G)** Extraoral orthopaedic force passing through the centre of resistance of the maxilla.

also demonstrated significant amount of vertical movement of mandibular molars.[35] Following extractions in a patient with an increased vertical dimension, the treatment mechanics of extraction space closure must be carefully planned to prevent eruption of posterior teeth. A common mistake by most clinicians in dealing with the closure of extraction space is to use heavy forces with either horizontal chains or coil springs while the teeth are engaged on a relatively light archwire. This approach typically promotes tipping of both the anterior and posterior teeth into the extraction space.

After the resolution of anterior discrepancy in a high-angle patient, the residual extraction space to a large extent is closed by controlled protraction of the posterior teeth into the extraction sites. Extraction treatment approach when compared with non-extraction treatment has shown no significant differences in changes of MP angle, AFH or vertical position of maxillary and mandibular molars.[36] Vertical movement of upper molars is better controlled with a combination of high-pull headgear and extraction treatment; however, mandibular molars show even greater compensatory vertical

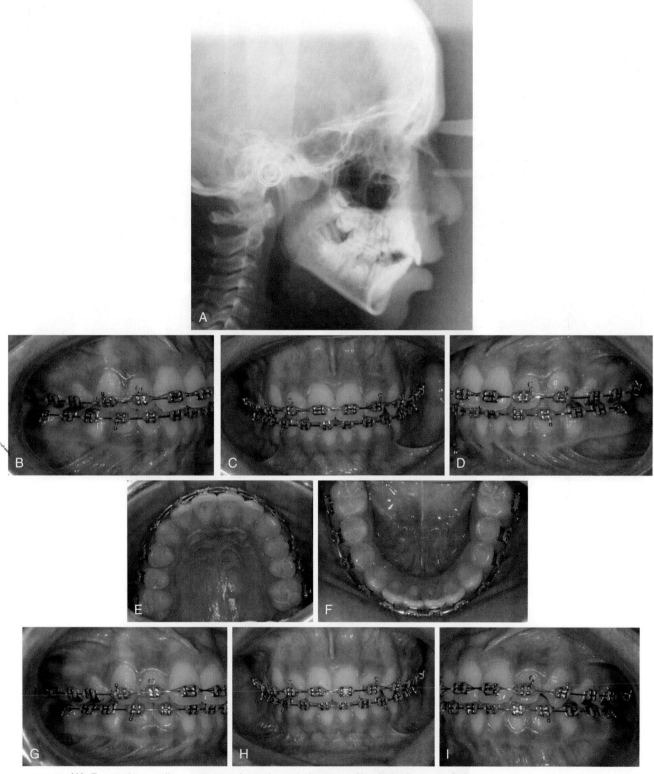

Figure 5.13 **(A)** Postorthopaedic treatment lateral cephalogram showing closure of the mandibular plane angle, positive incisor overlap and favourable orientation of the palatal plane. **(B–I)** Postorthopaedic treatment fixed appliance therapy to establish a well-coordinated maxillary and mandibular archforms, alignment, levelling and torque control of anterior and posterior teeth.

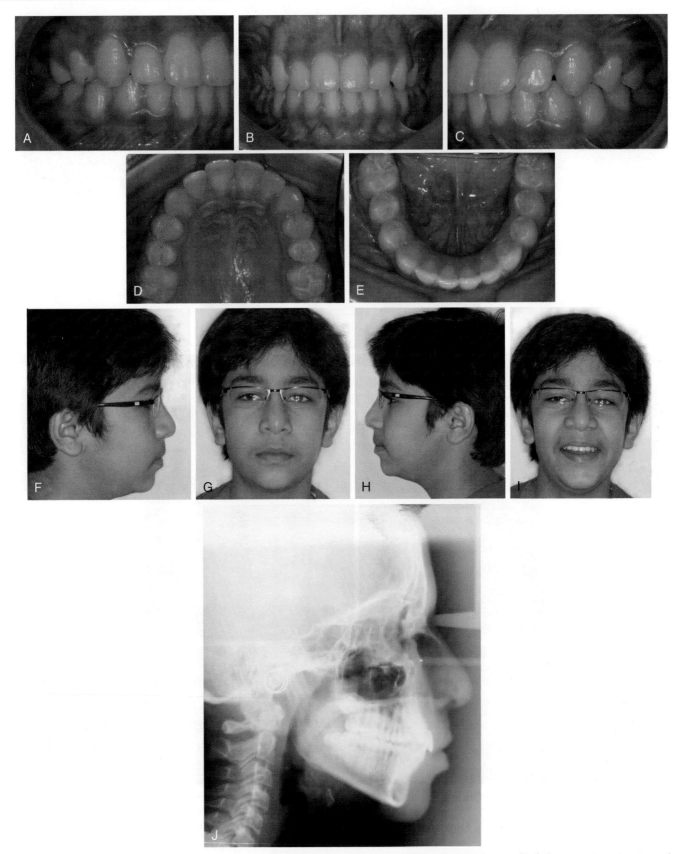

Figure 5.14 **(A–E)** Post-treatment intraoral photographs showing good occlusion and archforms. **(F–I)** Post-treatment extraoral photographs show normal facial features and a pleasing smile. **(J)** Post-treatment lateral cephalogram showing normal orientation of the palatal plane, good interincisal relationship and reduction in the lower anterior face height.

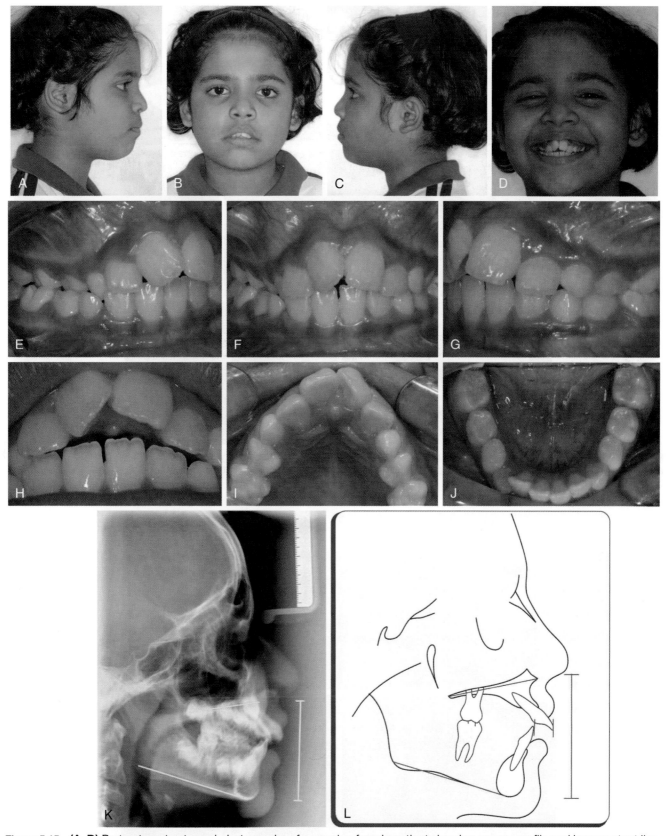

Figure 5.15 **(A–D)** Pretreatment extraoral photographs of a growing female patient showing convex profile and incompetent lips. **(E–J)** Intraoral photographs show mixed dentition stage with unilateral crossbite on the right side, anterior open bite, constricted maxillary arch and upper and lower arch anterior crowding. **(K and L)** Pretreatment lateral cephalogram shows tipped-up palatal plane in the anterior region, anterior open bite, increased lower anterior face height, incompetent lips and upper lip line high on the maxillary alveolar process.

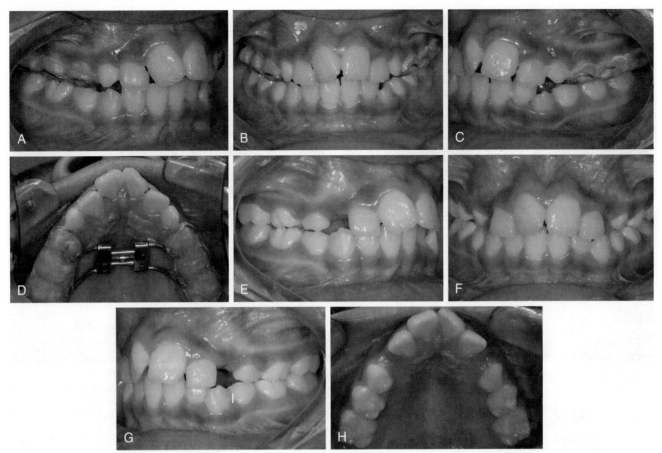

Figure 5.16 **(A–D)** Bonded rapid palatal expansion device given to split the maxillary suture and achieve desired orthopaedic expansion. **(E–H)** Postorthopaedic expansion intraoral photographs show the correction of posterior crossbite and the closure of anterior open bite.

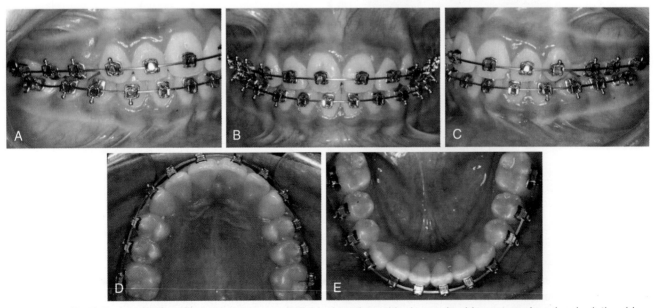

Figure 5.17 **(A-E)** Fixed appliance therapy to improve individual tooth positioning and achieve normal occlusal relationships.

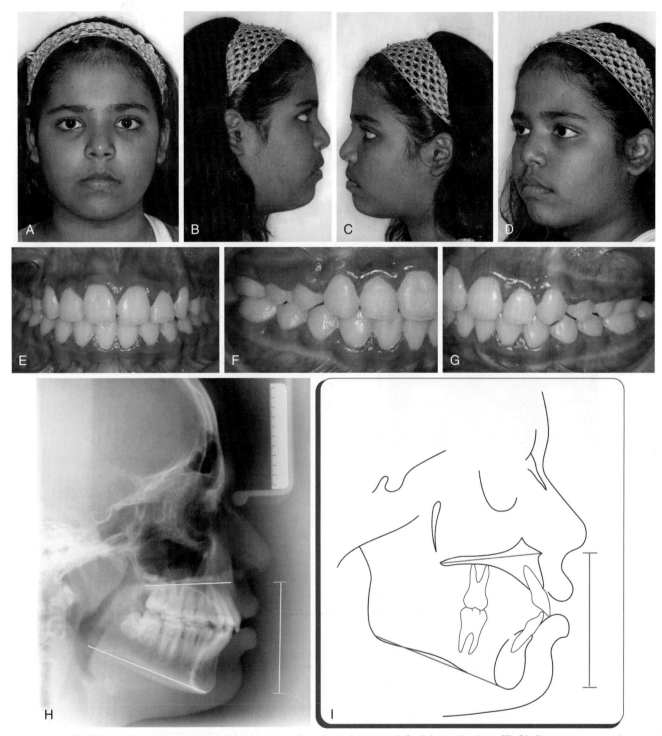

Figure 5.18 (A–D) Post-treatment extraoral photographs show improved facial aesthetics. **(E–G)** Post-treatment intraoral photographs show good individual teeth position and interarch relationship. **(H and I)** Post-treatment lateral cephalogram and tracing demonstrate normal orientation of palatal plane, reduction in lower anterior facial height, closure of mandibular plane angle and normal interincisal relationship.

movement.[34,35] It has been shown that the combined treatment of extractions and vertical-pull chin cup produces significant decrease in AFH and gonial angle.[37]

Mandibular bite blocks and vertical-pull chin cup

Another method used in the management of high-angle cases is the use of mandibular bite blocks combined with vertical-pull chin cup.[38] Mandibular bite block along with vertical chin cup therapy intrudes posterior teeth, brings about counterclockwise rotation of the mandible, promotes favourable vertical height control throughout the growth period and facilitates closure of anterior open bite.[39] However, the positive effects of extraction treatment combined with the use of a

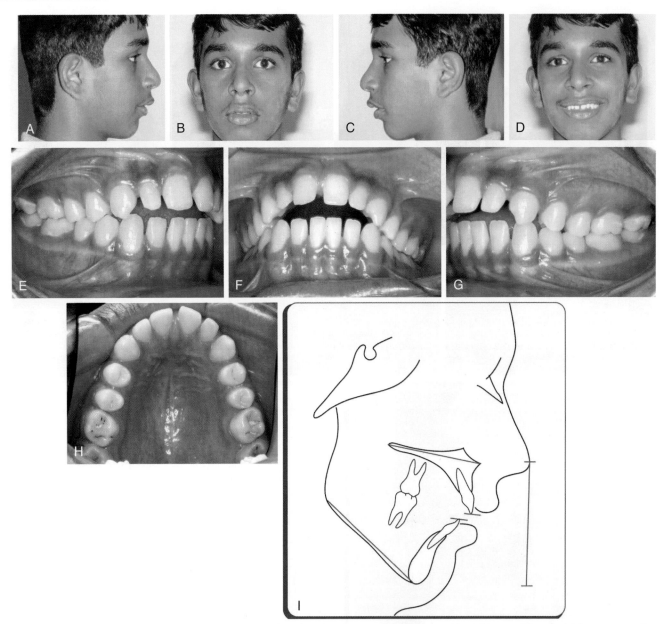

Figure 5.19 (A–D) Pretreatment extraoral photographs showing convex profile, posterior chin position and incompetent lips. **(E–H)** Intraoral photographs showing early permanent dentition with anterior open bite, interproximal spacing and Class I molar and Class II canine relationships. **(I)** Pretreatment lateral cephalometric tracing showing downward and backward rotation of the mandible, anterior open bite and increased lower anterior facial height.

high-pull headgear are confined mainly to the maxillary dentoalveolar region.

Vertical-pull chin cup, used in association with a Kloehn cervical headgear, produces significant favourable skeletal and dental alterations by inhibiting maxillary molar eruption and descent of the maxilla and redirecting mandibular growth in a more horizontal direction.[40] An increase in PFH has been the main contributing factor in the success of this approach. It is evident from the above discussion that the vertical-pull chin cup is the only appliance that effectively alters mandibular shape by decreasing gonial angle, redirecting condylar growth and increasing posterior heights. This modality seems to be favourable in achieving the main goal of hyperdivergent skeletal open

bite treatment to improve the orientation, position and shape of the mandible.

Management of vertical problems in average-angle patients

Vertical dentoalveolar discrepancies, like open bite, deep bite, etc., are often associated with individuals with normal vertical dimension (Fig. 5.27). Vertical problems in patients having average or normal MP angle are mainly dentoalveolar in nature involving single or group of teeth. Treatment of such patients is aimed at improving vertical abnormalities of teeth while simultaneously maintaining the vertical dimension.

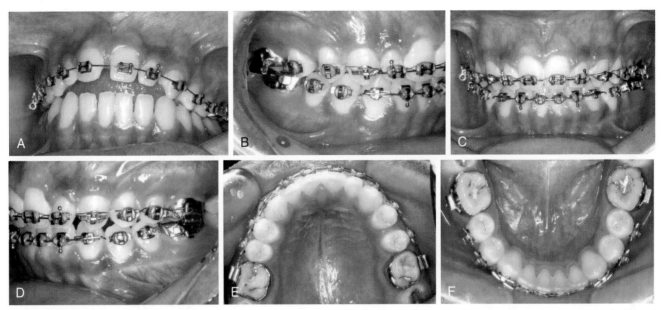

Figure 5.20   (A–F) Fixed appliance therapy was initiated along with the use of a molar-inserted high-pull headgear to intrude maxillary posterior teeth to achieve closure of interproximal spaces and open bite, normal interincisal relationship and well-coordinated and compatible maxillary and mandibular archforms.

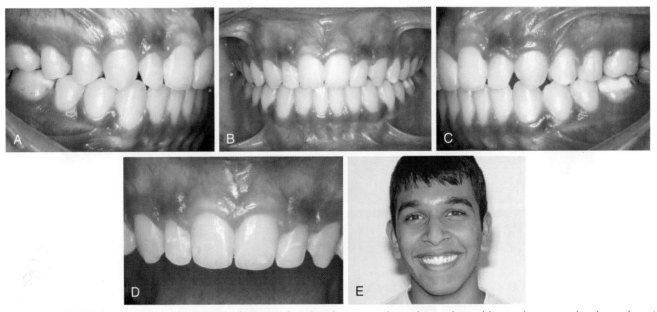

Figure 5.21   (A–D) Post-treatment intraoral photographs showing normal overjet and overbite and progressive buccal root torque of the posterior teeth. Note: The maxillary and mandibular midlines are not coinciding with each other due to disproportionate widths of maxillary lateral incisors. **(E)** Post-treatment pleasing smile.

Dentoalveolar open bite

Patients with anterior open bite due to displacement of the teeth should be carefully analyzed to design a treatment plan. Tongue posture, tongue function and eruption problems should be primarily considered in such cases. It is important to correlate the findings of the functional assessment and cephalometric analysis to establish an accurate diagnosis. In dentoalveolar open bite, the severity of the condition depends on the extent of the eruption of the teeth—infraocclusion of the incisors or

supraocclusion of the molars. The dentoalveolar profile of a patient with a vertical growth pattern consists of upper anterior protrusion combined with lingual inclination of the lower incisors. The proclination of both upper and lower incisors due to tongue posture and thrust is usually present in patients with horizontal growth pattern.

The proper treatment time and type depend on the aetiology and the localization of the problem. There are various treatment modalities possible during the various

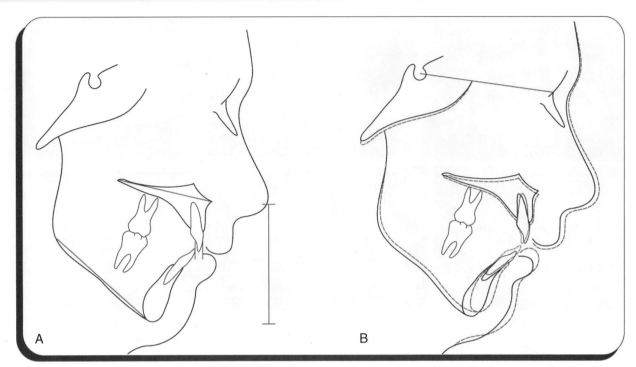

Figure 5.22 **(A)** Post-treatment lateral cephalometric tracing shows significant reduction in the lower anterior face height and improved vertical incisor and lip relationship. **(B)** Pretreatment and post-treatment cephalometric tracing superimpositions showing favourable dental, skeletal and soft tissue changes.

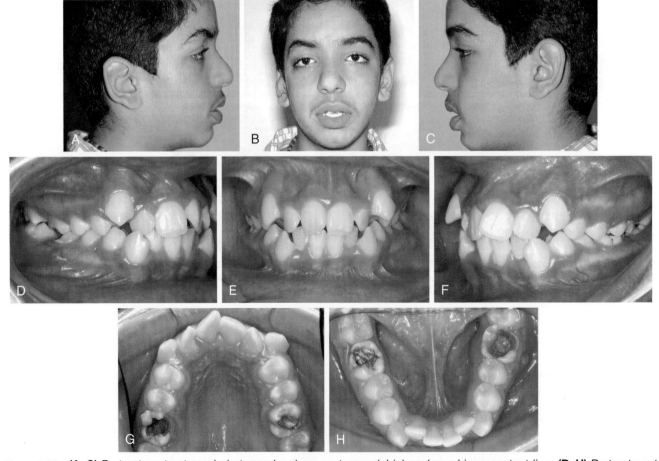

Figure 5.23 **(A–C)** Pretreatment extraoral photographs show acute nasolabial angle and incompetent lips. **(D–H)** Pretreatment intraoral photographs show severe maxillary and mandibular crowding, labially placed maxillary and mandibular cuspids and badly decayed and filled maxillary and mandibular permanent first molars.

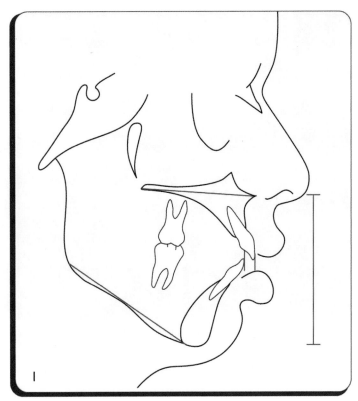

Figure 5.23, cont'd   **(I)** Pretreatment lateral cephalometric tracing shows increased mandibular plane angle, incompetent lips, acute nasolabial angle and significantly increased lower anterior facial height.

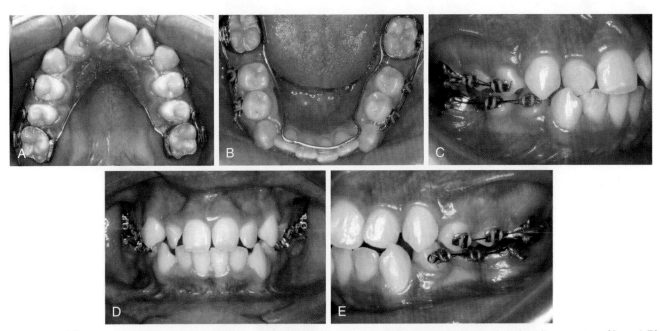

Figure 5.24   The treatment plan included the extraction of all permanent first molars to resolve the discrepancy. **(A** and **B)** Modified Nance palatal button cemented on the maxillary second molars, and the lingual arch cemented on the mandibular second molars. **(C–E)** Posterior segmental arch mechanics to retract the bicuspids to create space anteriorly to allow decrowding of the anterior teeth.

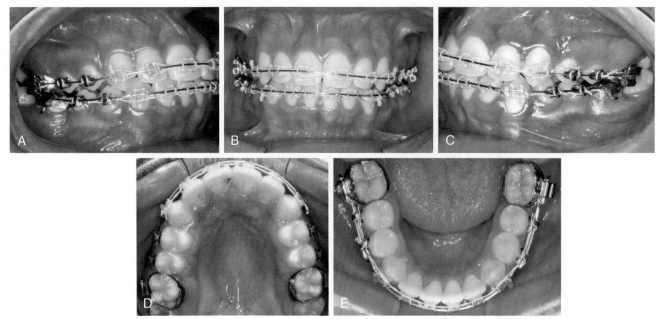

Figure 5.25   (A-E) Fixed appliance treatment protocol to achieve occlusal objectives.

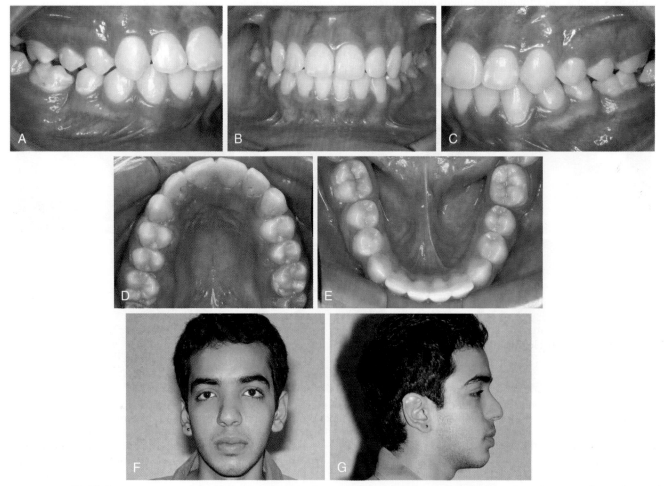

Figure 5.26   (A–E) Post-treatment intraoral photographs show good alignment and levelling of teeth, normal overjet and overbite relationships and good archforms. **(F** and **G)** Post-treatment extraoral photographs showing a good facial balance exhibiting normal nasolabial angle, lip competency and chin position.

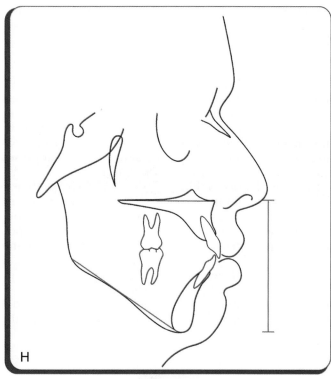

Figure 5.26, cont'd **(H)** Post-treatment lateral cephalometric tracing showing significantly improved dental, skeletal and soft tissue relationships.

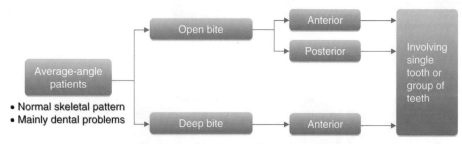

Figure 5.27 Average-angle patient types.

developmental periods of the dentition. The resolution of anterior open bite in the deciduous dentition should involve the control of the abnormal habits and the elimination of dysfunctions. If the anterior open bite is not associated with crowding of the maxillary anterior teeth or crossbite, one can expect spontaneous improvement once the deforming muscle activity is eliminated. In the early mixed dentition stage, screening therapy to eliminate abnormal muscle forces on the dentition is effective. This approach may not be useful in the late mixed dentition stage, wherein fixed appliance therapy along with swallowing exercises is the treatment modality of choice. Following the fixed appliance therapy, patient usually requires a long-term post-treatment retention until the abnormal muscle function is eliminated. Swallowing exercises, like asking the patient to put the tip of the tongue behind the upper and lower incisors, promote the transition from the infantile to a mature deglutitional and functional pattern of the tongue.

If the dentoalveolar anterior open bite is because of supraeruption of posterior teeth, it is advisable either to intrude posterior teeth or to prevent further eruption of these by using posterior bite blocks with or without the headgear.

Dentoalveolar deep overbite

The deep overbite is the amount and percentage of vertical overlap of the lower incisors by the upper incisors. The overbite varies from childhood to adulthood; between 9 and 12 years of age, it increases, whereas between the age 12 and adulthood, it decreases.[41] In the management of the deep overbite, it is important to consider the sagittal relationship and the direction and amount of growth to be expected for a particular patient. The dentoalveolar deep overbite could be either due to infraocclusion of posterior teeth or due to supraeruption of incisors. An accurate diagnosis should be established before planning the treatment. The dentoalveolar deep bite due to infraocclusion of molars is characterized by partially erupted molars, large interocclusal space and short distances between the maxillary basal plane, occlusal plane and mandibular basal plane. The deep overbite caused by supraeruption of incisors is characterized by fully erupted molars, normal interocclusal space, excessive curve of Spee and incisal edges of incisors extending beyond the functional occlusal plane (Figs 5.28–5.31). Therefore, the correction of dental deep overbite can be achieved by intrusion of incisors, extrusion of molars or combination of incisor intrusion and molar extrusion.

In patients with deep overbite caused by the supraeruption of maxillary incisors, intrusion of incisors is the treatment of choice. Before implementing the intrusion mechanics, it is essential to assess the inclination of incisors and the position of the incisor root apex with respect to the nasal floor (NF). The vertical space within the alveolar process, between the root apex and the NF, should permit the desired amount of incisor intrusion.

Burstone[42] has outlined six principles that must be considered in incisor or canine intrusion mechanics.

1. Force levels—optimal magnitude, constant delivery and low-load deflections
2. Selection of the point of force application with respect to the centre of resistance of the teeth to be intruded

3. Use of the single-point contact in the anterior region
4. Selective intrusion based on anterior tooth geometry
5. Posterior anchorage to control over the reactive unit
6. Control over the undesirable extrusive effects on the posterior teeth

One of the primary goals of deep overbite correction in Class II malocclusion, especially in Class II division 2 cases, is to achieve long-term stability of the corrected overbite. The proclination of the incisors during orthodontic therapy may cause relapse of the corrected deep overbite in the post-retention period.[43] The relapse of corrected deep overbite is mainly due to continued lower incisor eruption, retroclination of incisors and forward rotation of the mandible with continued growth.[44] The relapse potential of treated overbite is also associated with the interincisal angle and the lower AFH.[45]

The correction of deep overbite is considered to be stable in patients with a post-treatment interincisal angle between 125° and 135°, showing more relapse potential in brachycephalic patients than others. Therefore, the primary goal of deep overbite correction is to

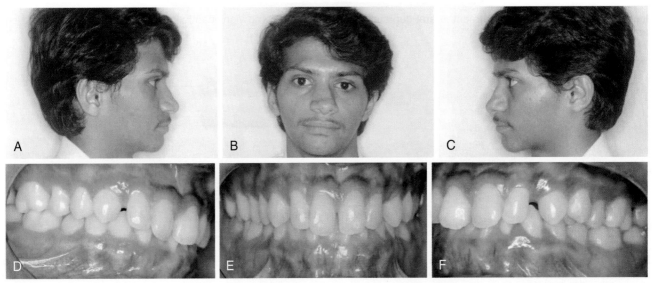

Figure 5.28 **(A–C)** Pretreatment extraoral photographs of a patient with normal vertical facial relationships. **(D–F)** Pretreatment intraoral photographs showing Class I molar relationship, rotated maxillary central incisors with median diastema and deep overbite.

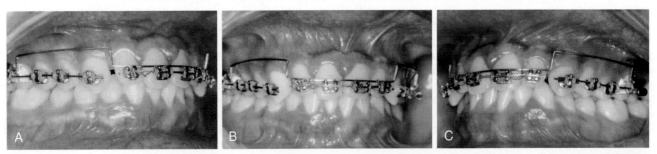

Figure 5.29 Since vertical skeletal relationships are normal, the treatment plan included the alignment and intrusion of maxillary incisors while simultaneously maintaining the lower anterior facial height. **(A–C)** The initial treatment mechanics involved the use of maxillary intrusion arch tied to the segmental archwire on the incisors between central and lateral incisors, along with rigid posterior segmental archwires to reinforce the anchorage.

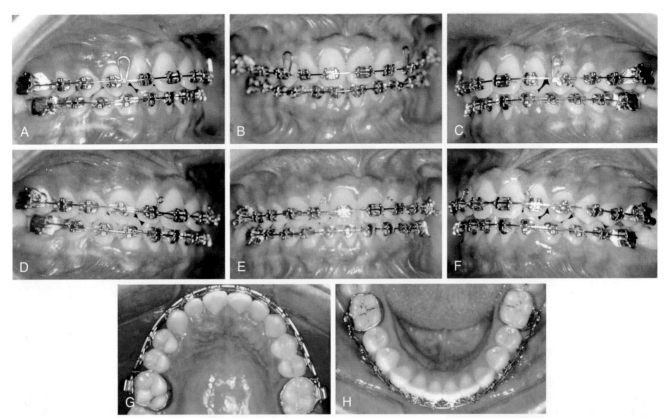

Figure 5.30 **(A–C)** Post-intrusion treatment mechanics involved the use of teardrop-looped archwire in the maxillary arch to close the residual space distal to the lateral incisors and the alignment, levelling and torque control in the mandibular arch. **(D–F)** Continuous finishing archwires in the maxillary and mandibular arches. **(G and H)** Well-coordinated and compatible maxillary and mandibular archforms.

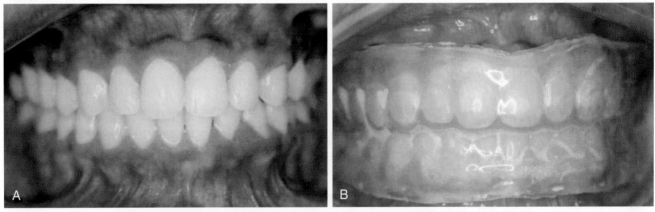

Figure 5.31 **(A)** Post-treatment intraoral photographs showing normal overbite and overjet relationships, levelling, alignment and interproximal space closure. **(B)** Post-treatment use of a gnathological tooth positioner.

achieve proper torque of incisors and proper interincisal angle to prevent their continued eruption, with a special attention to the lower anterior face height and forward rotation of the mandible with continued growth (Figs 5.32–5.35).

Intrusion of incisors

It is challenging for the orthodontists to correct deep overbite in patients with flared incisors by using conventional continuous archwires without producing any

untoward movements. In such patients, uprighting flared incisors to their better axial inclinations is often associated with lengthening their crowns, leading to the deepening of the overbite. In order to prevent further flaring of incisors during treatment, the simultaneous overbite correction and space closure is the treatment mechanics of choice in dealing with such cases. It has been observed that the possibility of flaring out of the maxillary incisors is more in Class II division 1 than in Class II division 2 malocclusions.[46,47] When using a utility arch to intrude

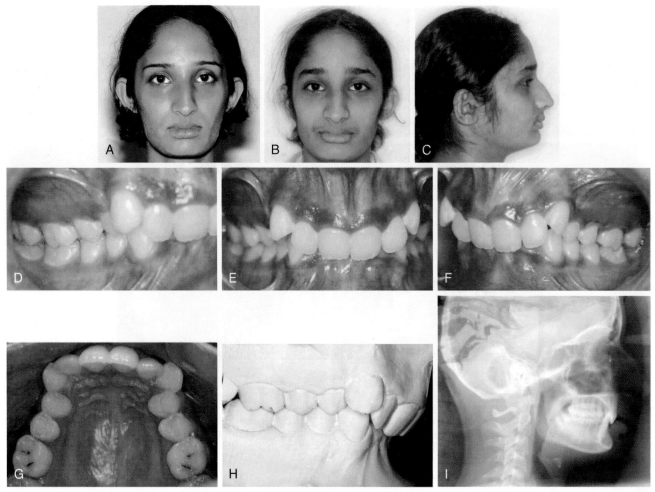

Figure 5.32 **(A–C)** Pretreatment extraoral photographs exhibiting severe decrease in lower facial height and deep mentolabial groove. **(D–G)** Pretreatment intraoral photographs demonstrate severe deep bite, retroclined maxillary incisors, high labially placed upper cuspids, square maxillary archform and Class II molar relationship. **(H)** Pretreatment study model demonstrates severe discrepancy between the posterior and anterior occlusal planes. **(I)** Pretreatment lateral cephalogram exhibits decreased lower anterior facial height, nearly parallel mandibular and palatal planes and retroclined and supraerupted maxillary incisors.

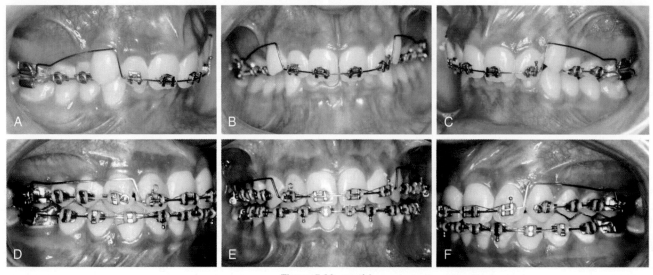

Figure 5.33, cont'd

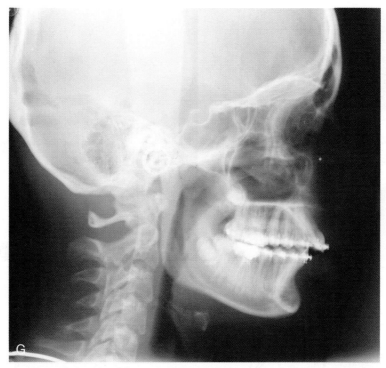

Figure 5.33, cont'd Since severely compromised lower anterior facial height and severe deep bite are the main components contributing to the development of a problem, the primary treatment goal is to intrude maxillary incisors and encourage vertical movement of posterior dentoalveolar segments to increase the lower anterior facial height. **(A–G)** Maxillary intrusion arch is in place to intrude and establish proper incisor torque.

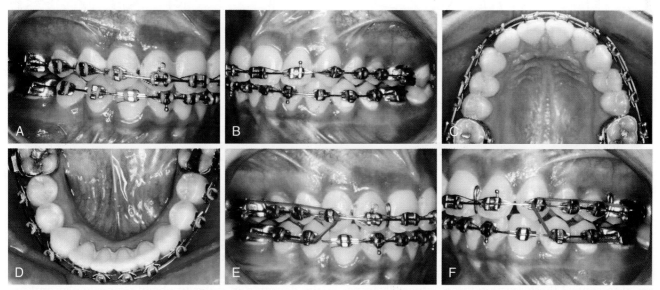

Figure 5.34 **(A–D)** Post-intrusion treatment mechanics to resolve upper and lower anterior arch discrepancy, establish proper archforms and detailing of dentition. **(E and F)** Patient wearing anterior bite plate and posterior box elastics to encourage vertical eruption of posterior dentoalveolar units.

incisors, the mechanics should be based on sound biomechanical principles for efficient tooth movement. An application of force should be directed through the centre of resistance of a tooth to be intruded to ensure translation without any tipping. It is, therefore, important to determine the centre of resistance of a particular tooth to design biomechanically sound force system. The intrusion arch should be attached to a sectional

archwire in the four upper incisors distal to the lateral incisors as the centre of resistance of the upper front teeth is supposed to be situated at this point anteroposteriorly.[46,48]

The reaction forces exerted by the intrusion arches during the intrusion mechanics should be controlled and neutralized by the posterior units. When the posterior units consist of only the first molars on either side,

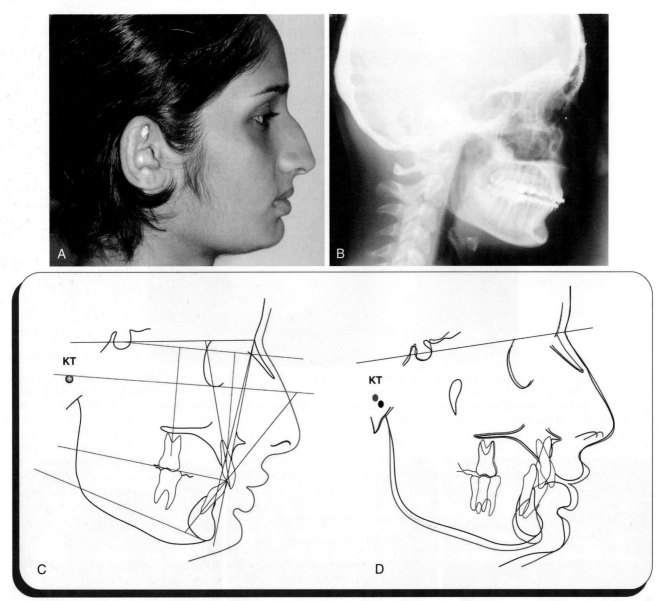

Figure 5.35 **(A)** Post-treatment extraoral photograph exhibiting improved facial features and vertical facial relationships. **(B)** Post-treatment lateral cephalogram. **(C)** Post-treatment cephalometric tracing. **(D)** Pretreatment and post-treatment cephalometric superimpositions.

the reaction forces will cause extrusion, distal tipping and, occasionally, the palatal tipping of these teeth. Therefore, the posterior anchorage units must be reinforced to control these reaction forces, especially in patients with increased lower facial height, to prevent clockwise rotation of the mandible and further lengthening of the face. The use of a transpalatal arch along with the rigid rectangular posterior sectional archwires, headgear and bite plate covering the occlusal surfaces of premolars and molars are some of the methods to stabilize the posterior units. Also, apical root resorption is found in patients with isolated incisor intrusion; however, there was no correlation between the amount of root resorption and the tooth type—central or lateral incisor[49]—and between the position of the apex in relation to the NF[50] and the amount of intrusion.[51]

Orthodontic camouflage: A treatment alternative for skeletal discrepancy

Orthodontic camouflage consists of the repositioning of the dentition in order to obtain proper molar and incisor relationships in patients with underlying skeletal discrepancies with a favourable effect on facial aesthetics. For some reason, if the patient does not accept the orthosurgical treatment approach for the correction of a dentofacial deformity, camouflage proves to be quite useful. The goal is to achieve certain degree of dentofacial aesthetics and is to establish proper occlusion, accepting the limitations in skeletal relationships. The success of camouflage treatment approach depends on the severity of underlying skeletal discrepancy. In mild to moderate skeletal malocclusions, movements of teeth to achieve dentoalveolar changes and aesthetic results are much better than those in severe skeletal problems. In severe Class II patients, the need for greater displacement of teeth relative to their bony bases, either by extraction or by non-extraction approach, is possible due to improvements in orthodontic treatment mechanics but only at considerable expense to facial aesthetics. Therefore, the clinician should assess the case carefully for the underlying skeletal discrepancy to plan treatment mechanics and strike a balance between occlusal and facial aesthetic goals using camouflage approach.

Management of short-face patients

As there is a strong correlation between the vertical and sagittal dimensions, any discrepancy in the vertical dimension contributing to the development of a problem can influence the anteroposterior dental and skeletal relationships (Fig. 5.36). An increased overbite relationship may be associated with average lower facial height; however, when it is related to the overclosure of the mandible through an excessive freeway space, it results in a decreased lower anterior face height. It has been observed that the mandibular rest position remains unchanged as growth progresses, and neither the presence nor the absence of teeth affects this position.[52] The excess interocclusal clearance or the freeway space as seen in the patients with mandibular overclosure may be due to a lack of vertical development in the buccal alveolar segments.[53] This could be the result of defects in tooth eruption or interference with normal tooth eruption.

The primary goal of treatment in the management of patients with diminished lower face height should be to improve vertical facial proportions. This can be accomplished in growing patients by encouraging vertical growth of the maxillary complex with headgears and by growth of the posterior alveolar processes along with the use of functional appliances, in adolescent patients by allowing posterior teeth eruption, and in adult population by surgical correction.

In growing patients with decreased lower AFH, orthopaedic repositioning of the maxilla and the mandible should be considered. Most patients can benefit from maxillary expansion due to desired downward movement associated with this procedure.[54,55] The use of cervical-pull headgear plays an important role in increasing the lower facial height through encouragement of vertical growth of maxillary complex and dental eruption. This vertical movement promotes downward and backward rotation of the mandible with a resultant increase in lower facial height and a change in the interarch relationship in a Class II direction. This unfavourable Class II relationship should be minimized by the distal component of the cervical-pull headgear force and mandibular growth. Treatment mechanics to achieve desired tooth movements depends on the age of the patient and whether the Class II correction is being carried out with the functional appliance (Figs 5.37–5.39). In the early correction of dental deep overbite, if the patient is undergoing sagittal correction with the functional appliances, like activator and twin-block appliance, the desired posterior teeth extrusion can be achieved by prescribed occlusal relieving of molars and premolars to encourage orthodontic tooth guidance while simultaneously exerting an intrusive force on the anterior teeth. This also promotes the levelling of curve of Spee. In growing patients with lateral tongue thrust and posture, the abnormal tongue function prevents the full eruption of posterior teeth. This can be controlled by a removable plate-type appliance with lateral tongue crips and buccinator loop extensions of the labial bow to permit extrusion and elongation of bicuspids and molars. Therefore, functional appliance therapy may be the treatment modality of choice to correct the sagittal relationships and to allow for vertical development of the lower face in growing patients exhibiting Class II dental relationships.

The orthopaedic face mask commonly used in the treatment of Class III malocclusions in growing patients consists of bilateral forces emanating from a face mask and applied to the intraoral appliance to the first molar or canine regions (Figs 5.40–5.42). The line of the protraction forces as determined sagittally by the commissure of the lips and the intraoral points of attachment influences the type of dentomaxillary complex movement. For true protraction to occur, the direction of protraction forces must pass through the centres of resistance of the dentomaxillary complex and parallel to the occlusal plane. It is, therefore, essential to locate the centres of resistance of the dentomaxillary complex. The centre of resistance of the dentomaxillary complex, as seen on a lateral cephalogram, is located on a line drawn perpendicular to the functional occlusal plane through the distal aspect of the maxillary first molar.[56] It is identified on this perpendicular line at one-half the distance from the functional occlusal plane to a line through the inferior border of the orbit (parallel to the functional

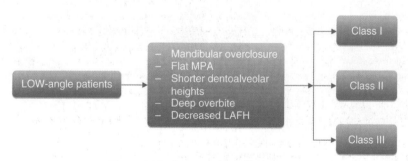

Figure 5.36 Low-angle patient types.

occlusal plane). It is recognized that the protraction forces of the face mask cause dentomaxillary rotation (counterclockwise) that results in an increase in the lower facial height and a decrease in the upper facial height.[57]

In a growing patient undergoing fixed appliance therapy where a clockwise rotation of the mandible is desirable, extrusion of molars may prove to be useful. There are many methods to bring about this change, e.g. anterior bite plate, leaving molars free to erupt, cervical-pull headgear, Class II elastics and anchorage bends or tip-back bends in the upper and lower arches. It is the author's experience that to achieve this result, the use of anterior bite plate, leaving the molars free to erupt, along with the use of posterior box elastics works very well. In a growing individual, the use of reverse curve of Spee mechanics produces supraeruption of the mandibular posterior teeth leading to downward and backward rotation of the mandible. This results in a reduction of a deep overbite and in an increase in the MP angle, the AFH and facial convexity. The use of intermaxillary elastics over a period of time in a Class II clinical situation

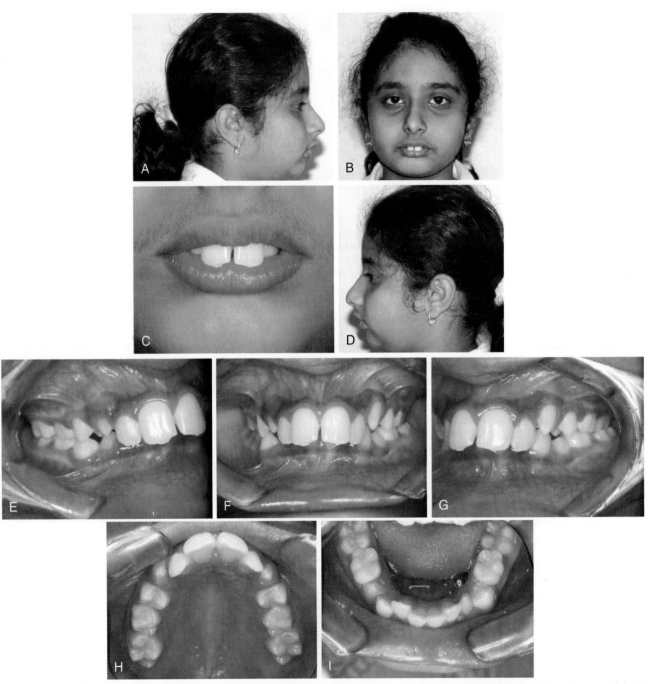

Figure 5.37 (A–D) Pretreatment extraoral photographs of a growing female patient showing convex profile, decreased lower facial height, incompetent lips, deep mentolabial groove, receding chin and lower lip trap. **(E–I)** Pretreatment intraoral photographs showing typical features of a severe Class II division 1 malocclusion in a late mixed dentition stage. Patient also exhibits moderate crowding in the upper and lower arches.

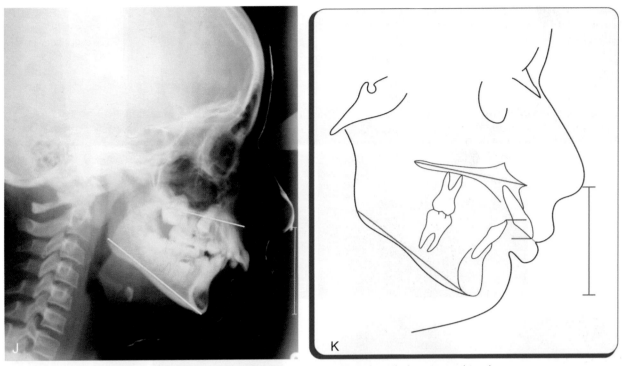

Figure 5.37, cont'd   (J and K) Pretreatment lateral cephalogram and tracing.

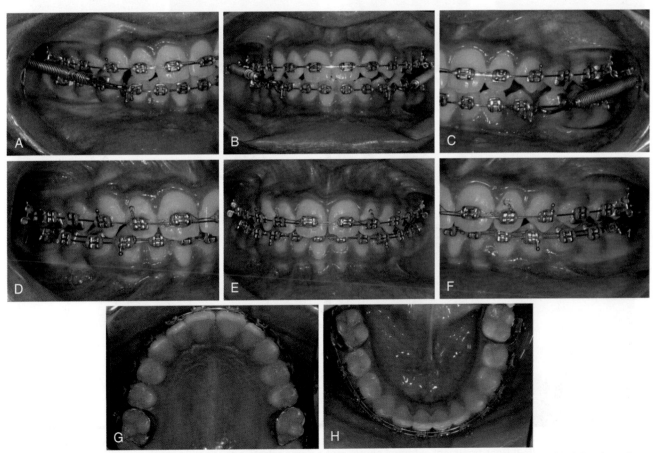

Figure 5.38   Since the patient's problem is characterized by receding chin and decreased lower anterior facial height, the primary focus of treatment is on advancing the mandible downward and forward and promoting posterior vertical dentoalveolar growth. **(A–C)** Fixed functional appliance in place to advance the mandible. **(D–H)** Settling of occlusion and coordination of upper and lower archforms during the postfixed functional therapy.

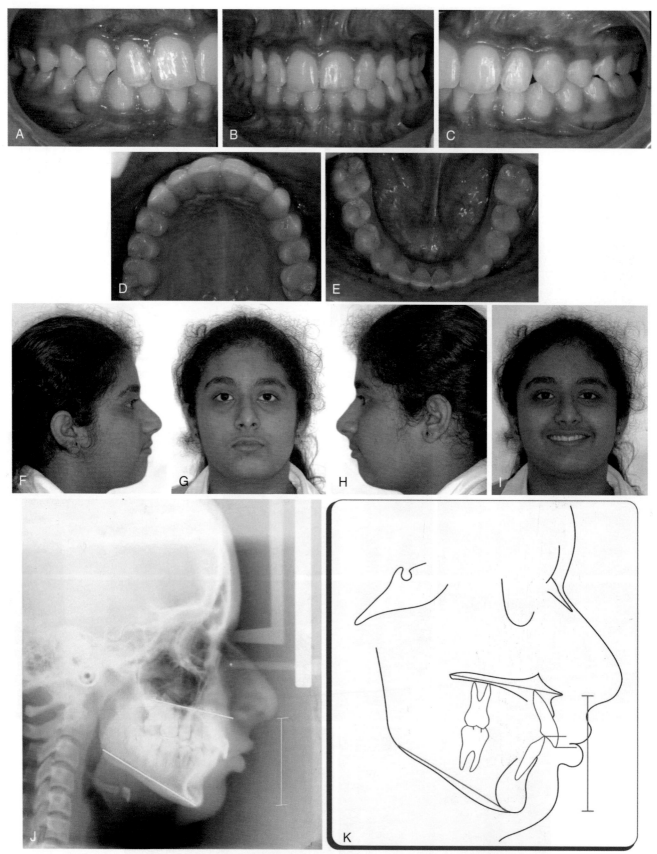

Figure 5.39 **(A–E)** Post-treatment Class I molar and cuspid relationships, normal overjet and overbite and well-coordinated and compatible archforms. **(F–I)** Post-treatment extraoral photographs demonstrate orthognathic profile exhibiting improved vertical dimension of lower face. **(J and K)** Post-treatment lateral cephalogram and tracing.

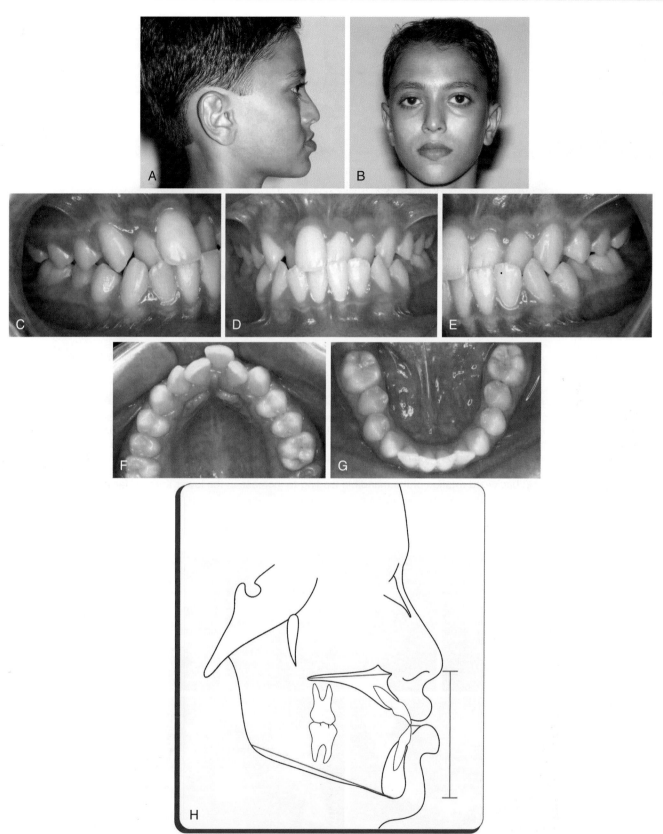

Figure 5.40 **(A** and **B)** Pretreatment extraoral photographs demonstrating decreased lower facial height, concave profile, malar insufficiency and prominence of the lower lip and chin. **(C–G)** Pretreatment intraoral photographs show a Class III molar relationship, anterior crossbite and crowding in the upper and lower anterior segments. **(H)** Pretreatment lateral cephalometric tracing exhibits the typical features of Class III malocclusion characterized by a combination of maxillary deficiency and mandibular prognathism.

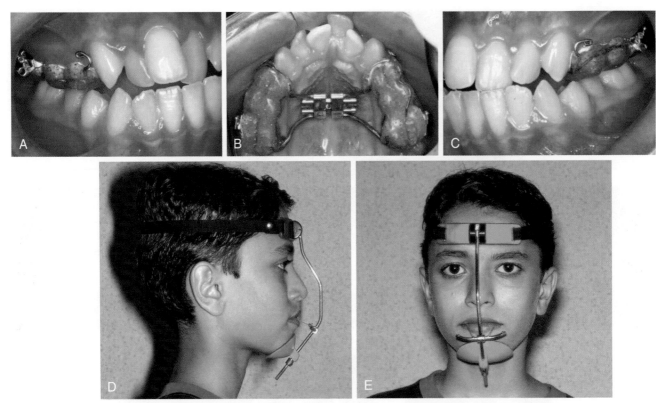

Figure 5.41   Since decreased lower facial height, deficient premaxilla and prognathic mandible are the main components contributing to the development of patient's problem, the treatment goal is to protract the maxilla and increase the lower anterior facial height. It was, therefore, decided to initiate the treatment with the orthopaedic facial mask followed by a fixed appliance therapy. **(A–C)** Maxillary bonded splint with a rapid palatal expansion device in place. **(D and E)** The use of orthopaedic facial mask. Note: The force exerted on the maxilla is downward and forward that will displace the maxilla anteriorly and inferiorly with a resultant downward and backward rotation of the mandible leading to increase in the lower anterior facial height.

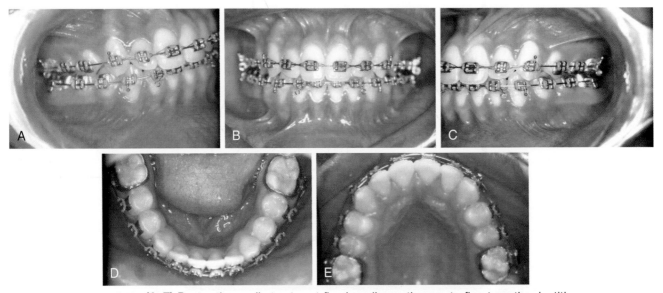

Figure 5.42   **(A–E)** Post-orthopaedic treatment fixed appliance therapy to fine-tune the dentition.

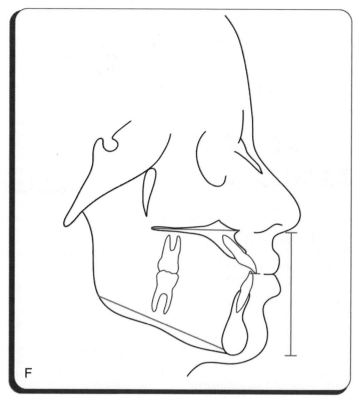

Figure 5.42, cont'd **(F)** Post-treatment lateral cephalometric tracing exhibiting an improvement in dental, skeletal and soft tissue relationships with an emphasis on improved vertical dimension of lower face.

leads to the eruption of mandibular molars and in Class III traction leads to the eruption of the maxillary posterior teeth. These changes are often associated with the rotation of the occlusal plane.

The use of a reverse curve of Spee in archwire in the edgewise brackets produces undesirable changes in the axial inclinations of the posterior teeth and flaring of the incisors.[48]

CONCLUSION

Vertical discrepancies consist of various components of the craniofacial complex. The clinician must establish differential diagnosis of vertical problem as it forms an integral part of designing a successful treatment strategy. While dealing with the patients with vertical problems, it must be recognized that all cases cannot be treated in a similar manner due to extreme variation in facial pattern and morphological characteristics. Therefore, in patients with compromised AFHs, various treatment methods of mandibular rotation—opening versus closure—as a part of orthodontic treatment should be recognized as either desirable or undesirable.

Control of vertical dimension is considered to be the most important factor in successfully treating patients with vertical discrepancies. The primary treatment goal in patients with hyperdivergent malocclusions is to autorotate the mandible to decrease the lower facial height; in patients with average facial height, the goal is to correct vertical dental problems while simultaneously maintaining the vertical dimension; and in low-angle patients, various treatment procedures should contribute to the downward and backward rotation of the mandible resulting into an increased lower facial height.

REFERENCES

1. Brodie AG. On the growth pattern of the human head from the third month to the eighth year of life. Am J Anat 1941; 68:209–262.
2. Schudy FF. Vertical growth versus anteroposterior growth as related to function and treatment. Angle Orthod 1964; 34(2):75–93.
3. Coben SE. Growth and Class II treatment. Am J Orthod 1966; 52(1):5–26.
4. Pederson RA. Cranial base growth. Individual variation studied roentgenographically, MS Thesis. Philadelphia, USA: Temple University; 1962.
5. Powell TV, Brodie AG. Closure of the spheno-occipital synchondrosis. Anat Rec 1963; 147:15–23.
6. Coben SE. The integration of facial skeletal variants. Am J Orthod 1955; 41:407–434.
7. Björk A. Facial growth in man, studied with the aid of metallic implants. Acta Odontol Scand 1955; 13:9–34.
8. Björk A. Variations in the growth pattern of the human mandible: longitudinal cephalometric study by the implant method. J Dent Res 1963; 42(1):400–411.
9. Björk A. Sutural growth of the upper face studied by the implant method. Acta Odontol Scand 1966; 24:109–129.
10. Björk A. The use of metallic implants in the study of facial growth in children: method and application. Am J Phys Anthropol 1968; 29:243–254.

11. Björk A. Prediction of mandibular growth rotation. Am J Orthod 1969; 55:585–599.

12. Björk A, Skieller V. Facial growth and development. An implant study at the age of puberty. Am J Orthod 1972; 48:61–74.

13. Björk A, Skieller V. Normal and abnormal growth of the mandible. A synthesis of longitudinal cephalometric implant studies over a period of 25 years. Eur J Orthod 1983; 5:1–46.

14. Isaacson RJ, Zapfel RJ, Worms FW, et al. Effects of rotational jaw growth on the occlusion and profile. Am J Orthod 1977; 72(3):276–286.

15. Issacson JR, Issacson RJ, Speidel TM, et al. Extreme variation in vertical facial growth and associated variation in skeletal and dental relationships. Angle Orthod 1971; 41:219–228.

16. Janson G, Metaxas A, Woodside D. Variation in maxillary and mandibular molar and incisor vertical dimension in 12 years old subjects with excess, normal, and short lower anterior face height. Am J Orthod Dentofacial Orthop 1994; 106:409–418.

17. Linder-Aronson S. Effects of adenoidectomy on the dentition and facial skeleton over a period of five years. In: Cook JT, ed. Transactions of the third International orthodontic congress. St. Louis: Mosby; 1975. 85–100.

18. Woodside DG, Linder-Aronson S, Lundstrom A, et al. Mandibular and maxillary growth after changed mode of breathing. Am J Orthod Dentofacial Orthop 1991; 100:1–18.

19. Sassouni V, Nanda S. Analysis of dentofacial vertical proportions. Am J Orthod 1964; 50:801–823.

20. Ingervall B, Thilander B. Relationship between facial morphology and activity of the masticatory muscles. J Oral Rehabil 1974; 1: 131–147.

21. Jarabak JR, Fizzell JA. Technique and treatment with light wire edgewise appliances. 2nd ed. St. Louis: CV Mosby; 1972.

22. Björk A. The face in profile: an anthropological X-ray investigation on Swedish children and conscripts. Sven Tandlak Tidskr 1947; 40(suppl).

23. Björk A. Prediction of mandibular growth rotation. Am J Orthod 1969; 55:585–599.

24. Skieller V, Björk A, Linde-Hansen T. Prediction of mandibular growth rotation evaluated from a longitudinal implant sample. Am J Orthod 1984; 86:359–370.

25. Moyers RE, Guire KE, Riolo M. Differential diagnosis of Class II malocclusion. Am J Orthod 1980; 78:477–494.

26. Proffit WR, Fields HW, Nixon NL. Occlusal forces in normal and long-face adults. J Dent Res 1983; 62:566–570.

27. Björk A. The relationship of the jaws to the cranium. In: Lundstrom A, ed. Introduction to orthodontics. London: McGraw-Hill; 1961. 104–140.

28. Subtelny JD, Sakuda M. Open-bite: diagnosis and treatment. Am J Orthod 1964; 50:337–358.

29. Nahoum HI, Horowitz SL, Benedicto EA. Varieties of anterior open-bite. Am J Orthod 1972; 61:486–492.

30. Armstrong MM. Controlling the magnitude, direction and duration of extraoral force. Am J Orthod 1971; 59:217–243.

31. Firouz M, Zernik J, Nanda R. Dental and orthopaedic effects of high-pull headgear in treatment of Class II division 1 malocclusion. Am J Orthod 1992; 102:197–205.

32. Caldwell SF, Hymas TA, Timm TA. Maxillary traction splint: a cephalometric evaluation. Am J Orthod 1984; 85:376–384.

33. Pearson LE. Vertical control in treatment of patients having backward rotational growth tendencies. Angle Orthod 1978; 48(2): 132–140.

34. Dougherty HL. The effect of mechanical forces upon the mandibular buccal segments during orthodontic treatment. Am J Orthod 1968; 54:29–49.

35. Pearson LE. Vertical control through use of mandibular posterior intrusive forces. Angle Orthod 1973; 43:194–200.

36. Staggers JA. Vertical changes following first premolar extractions. Am J Orthod Dentofacial Orthop 1994; 105:19–24.

37. DiPalma D. A morphometric study of orthopaedic and functional therapy for the hyperdivergent skeletal pattern, Master's thesis. Celveland, Ohio: Case Western Reserve University; May 1982.

38. Woodside D, Linder-Aronson S, Graber LW, eds. Progressive increase in lower anterior face height and the use of posterior occlusal bite-block in its management. In: Orthodontics: state of the art, essence of the science. St. Louis: Mosby; 1986;200–221.

39. Pearson LE. Case report KP. Treatment of a severe open-bite excessive vertical pattern with an eclectic nonsurgical approach. Angle Orthod 1991; 61:71–76.

40. Haas AJ. A biological approach to diagnosis, mechanics and treatment of vertical dysplasia. Angle Orthod 1980; 50:279–300.

41. Flemming HB. Investigation of the vertical overbite during the eruption of the permanent dentition. Angle Orthod 1961; 31:53–62.

42. Burstone CR. Deep overbite correction by intrusion. Am J Orthod 1977; 72(1):1–22.

43. Simons ME, Joondeph DR. Change in overbite: a ten year postretention study. Am J Orthod 1973; 64(4):349–367.

44. Ball JV, Hunt NP. The effect of Andresen, Harvold and Begg treatment on overbite and molar eruption. Eur J Orthod 1991; 13:53–58.

45. McAlpine JE. A comparison of overbite relapse to age, interincisal angle and lower face height in Class II deep bite cases, Master's thesis. USA: Loma Linda University; 1976.

46. Melsen B, Agerbaek N, Eriksen J, et al. New attachment through periodontal treatment and orthodontic intrusion. Am J Orthod 1988; 94(2):104–116.

47. Demange C. Equilibrium situations in bend force systems. Am J Orthod 1990; 98:333–339.

48. Nanda R. The differential diagnosis and treatment of excessive overbite. Dent Clin North Am 1981; 25(1):69–84.

49. Dermaut LR, DeMunck A. Apical root resorption of upper incisors caused by intrusive tooth movement: a radiographic study. Am J Orthod 1986; 90(4):321–326.

50. Linge BO, Ling J. Apical root resorption in upper anterior teeth. Eur J Orthod 1983; 5:173–183.

51. Costopoulous G, Nanda R. An evaluation of root resorption incident to orthodontic intrusion. Am J Orthod 1996; 109(5):543–548.

52. Thompson JR, Brodie AG. Factors in the position of the mandible. J Am Dent Assoc 1942; 29:925–942.

53. Linder-Aronson S, Woodside DG. Some craniofacial variables related to small or diminishing lower anterior face height. Swed Dent J Suppl 1982; 15:131–146.

54. Da Silva OG, Boas MCV, Capelozza L. Rapid maxillary expansion in the primary and mixed dentitions: a cepahlometric evaluation. Am J Orthod Dentofacial Orthop 1991; 100:171–181.

55. Davis WM, Kronman JH. Anatomical changes induced by splitting of the midpalatal suture. Angle Orthod 1969; 39:126–132.

56. Lee K, Young KR, Young CP, et al. A study of holographic interferometry on the initial reaction of the maxillofacial complex during protraction. Am J Orthod Dentofacial Orthop 1997; 111:623–632.

57. Nanda R, Bruce G. Biomechanical approaches to the study of alterations of facial morphology. Am J Orthod 1980; 78:213–226.

Transverse Discrepancies

6

Ashok Karad

Transverse discrepancies warrant special consideration in orthodontic diagnosis and treatment planning. Determination of the underlying cause of the asymmetric or symmetric transverse problem must be an important ingredient in the process of formulation of an appropriate treatment plan. Depending upon the structures involved, these problems may be primarily dental, skeletal, functional in origin or may even have combination of these factors present. It is equally important to determine the relationship of the transverse discrepancy with the sagittal and vertical problems, which often have a significant impact on designing a treatment strategy. The management of transverse discrepancies has been universally recognized as one of the most challenging aspects of orthodontic therapy, and this chapter comprehensively deals with the development, differential diagnosis and treatment of such problems.

Asymmetry in craniofacial morphology can be recognized as differences in the size or relationship of the right and left sides. This may be the result of imbalances in the individual position and form of teeth, variation in the position of bones of the craniofacial complex, and it may also be limited to the overlying soft tissues. It is recognized that the human face displays bilateral symmetry exhibiting mirror image characteristics between right and left halves. Is this perfect bilateral dentofacial or craniofacial symmetry predominantly a theoretical concept that seldom exists? Due to large biological variations, either inherent in the developmental process or caused by environmental disturbances, such symmetry is rarely encountered. Certain degree of asymmetry goes unnoticed and is often considered normal; however, the point at which this mild transverse discrepancy becomes abnormal cannot be easily defined, as it is influenced by the clinician's understanding of asymmetry and the patients' perception of imbalance.

As patients view themselves from the frontal perspective enabling them to compare right and left sides of the face, contemporary orthodontic diagnosis and treatment planning should incorporate identification of transverse problems and achievement of symmetric results with appropriate mechanics. Though diagnosis of certain craniofacial structural variations in transverse dimension is quite simple, some underlying asymmetries may be masked by dental compensations. These undiagnosed transverse discrepancies usually become apparent as treatment progresses, often leading to increased treatment duration, change in treatment plan or compromised result. The management of transverse discrepancies has been universally recognized as one of the most challenging aspects of orthodontic therapy, and this chapter comprehensively deals with the development, differential diagnosis and treatment of such problems.

DEVELOPMENT OF A TRANSVERSE PROBLEM

Dentofacial asymmetric relationships can result mainly from genetic alterations in the mechanism that is responsible to establish symmetry, and various environmental factors producing differences in right and left halves.[1,2] Some of the most severe facial asymmetries are observed in individuals with craniofacial syndromes. Hemifacial microsomia, clefting syndromes and craniosynostoses are some of the examples characterized by significant facial asymmetries. Some clefts of the lip and/or palate are genetically influenced leading to significant facial abnormality associated with collapse of the maxillary dental arch.[2] In certain situations, although some of the facial imbalance is found primarily in the soft tissue, skeletal contributions can be significant. The glenoid fossa position is determined by the growth of the cranial base, and any variation in this growth leads to asymmetrical positions of the glenoid fossae, producing rotation of the mandible with respect to the maxilla. Under these circumstances, even if the maxilla and the mandible are not asymmetric in form, the resultant occlusion exhibits a Class III relationship on the side of the anteriorly positioned fossa and a Class I relationship on the contralateral side. In the absence of dental compensations, this often produces midline deviations. Even if the glenoid fossae are symmetrically positioned, the maxilla can undergo certain degree of rotational growth change relative to the cranial base with resultant asymmetric occlusal relationship.

In addition to asymmetric mandibular positioning, morphological variations between the right and left sides of the mandible, like differences in the length of the body of the mandible or height of the developing ramus, can lead to asymmetries. Moulding of the parietal and facial bones due to intrauterine pressure during pregnancy and significant pressure in the birth canal during parturition can result in facial asymmetry. These changes are usually considered as transient which undergo rapid restoration of the normal skull relationships within a few weeks to several months.[3]

Trauma and/or infection within the temporomandibular joint can cause ankylosis of the condyle to the temporal bone.[4] The loss of muscle function and tone as a result of damage to a nerve may indirectly lead to asymmetry. Various pathological conditions, not necessarily congenital in nature, cause craniofacial asymmetries. Osteochondroma of the mandibular condyle leads to facial asymmetry, mandibular deviation and open bite on the involved side.[5]

Asymmetries within the maxillary or mandibular arch lead to significant differences in the interarch relationships on the right and left sides. When primary molars are ankylosed, the adjacent teeth continue to erupt as a part of dentoalveolar development and appear to tip over the crown of the ankylosed tooth. This results in a loss of space and asymmetric axial inclinations of the adjacent teeth and subsequent asymmetric molar occlusion. Since the leeway space is larger in the mandibular arch than in the maxillary arch, a combination of permanent molar drift into the leeway space and differential growth of the mandible relative to the maxilla allows spontaneous correction of the end-to-end relationship into a normal molar relationship. Any unilateral partial loss of the leeway space results in an asymmetric molar relationship. Such molar occlusion is often encountered in patients with arch length loss as a result of interproximal caries or premature loss of a primary or permanent tooth.

Congenitally missing teeth, supernumerary teeth or ectopic eruptions are common causes for developing occlusal asymmetries. Asymmetries in archform, which can also be characterized by midline discrepancies, are often produced by habits. Transverse discrepancies are also caused by functional mandibular shifts due to centric prematurities leading to a lateral mandibular displacement in habitual occlusion. Temporomandibular joint disorders, like articular disc dislocation or fossae changes, are often associated with asymmetries involving off-centred midline.

DIAGNOSIS OF TRANSVERSE PROBLEMS

Contemporary orthodontic diagnostic process must involve an assessment of problems in the transverse dimension. Minor asymmetries that are often neglected, or underlying asymmetries that are masked by dental compensations, if undiagnosed at the beginning of treatment, usually become apparent as treatment progresses, especially during the finishing stage. This prolongs the treatment duration, causes certain alterations or changes in treatment direction, or it will ultimately leave the patient with a compromised result. To avoid this untoward situation, every clinician should make a conscious effort to assess dentofacial abnormalities in the transverse plane.

Types of transverse discrepancies

Facial asymmetries or transverse discrepancies can be broadly grouped into following categories:

1. Dental asymmetries in one or both arches
2. Skeletal asymmetries involving maxilla and/or mandible
3. Functional mandibular shifts causing asymmetric maxillomandibular relationships
4. Muscular asymmetries

Dental asymmetries

Transverse discrepancies that are dental in nature are mainly caused by local factors, like premature loss of deciduous teeth, congenitally missing single tooth or group of teeth and certain habits, e.g. thumb sucking or tongue thrusting. These dental asymmetries essentially involve midline deviations, asymmetric posterior tooth positions, asymmetric archforms and diverging occlusal planes.

Midline deviations

Quite often, most individuals presenting for orthodontic treatment do not exhibit coincident maxillary and/or mandibular dental midlines with each other or with the facial midline. This may be because of displacement or distortion of the maxillary or mandibular dental arches, tooth rotations, tooth size discrepancies, asymmetric crowding or spacing, etc.[6,7] Midline deviations certainly warrant special consideration in the orthodontic diagnosis and treatment planning. However, aesthetic acceptability of dental midline discrepancies depends on individual factors, including the transverse discrepancies associated with other facial midline structures. It has been found that overjet and dental crowding or spacing were considered to be more significant factors than midline deviations in determining self-satisfaction with dental appearance.[8] In contrast, another study found that symmetry was one of the most important factors in defining an attractive smile.[9] Generally, a dental midline deviation of 2 mm or more is considered to be easily detectable by most individuals, and therefore, warrants its consideration in treatment planning process. Individuals with midline discrepancies present with a variety of clinical situations where maxillary midline is coincident with facial midline and the mandibular dental midline is shifted either to the left or right side; mandibular midline is normally positioned, but the maxillary midline is deviated to the left or right side or it could be the combination of both (Fig. 6.1).

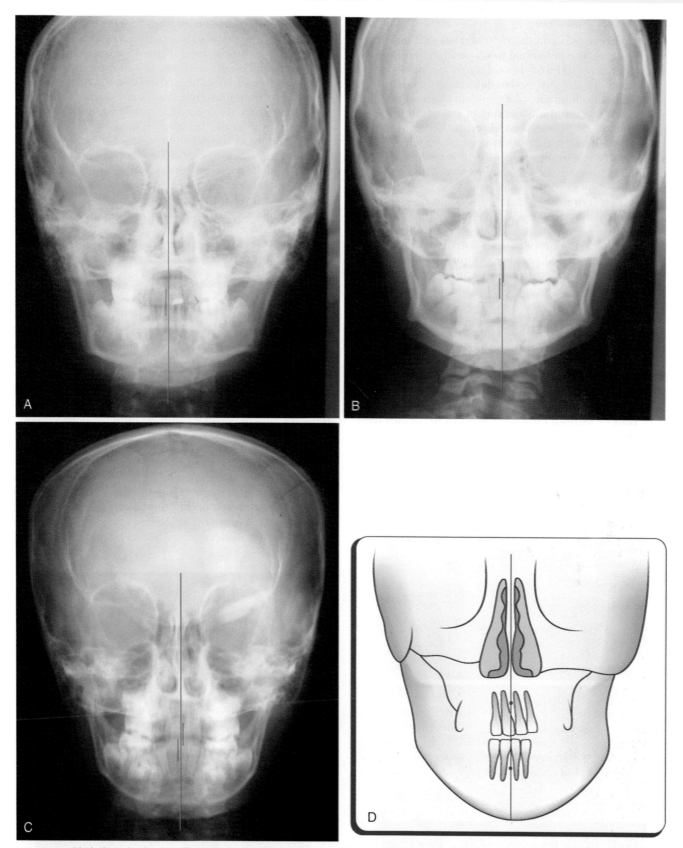

Figure 6.1 Variations in the maxillary and mandibular dental midlines. **(A)** Maxillary and mandibular dental midlines are coincident but are deviated to the right side when related to the mid-sagittal reference plane. **(B)** Maxillary dental midline is coincident with the mid-sagittal plane while the mandibular dental midline is shifted to the right side. **(C)** Maxillary dental midline deviated to the left and the mandibular to the right side of the mid-sagittal plane. **(D)** Maxillary dental midline deviated to the left without apical base discrepancy.

Posterior tooth position

The buccal occlusion on the right and left sides should be evaluated, and the individual tooth positions with respect to their mesiodistal and buccolingual inclinations and rotation be properly assessed to determine their contribution to the development of a problem. Although abnormal mesiodistal axial inclinations of the posterior teeth are sagittal discrepancies, but when assessed with respect to the opposite side, they result in an asymmetric buccal occlusion. In individuals with normal growth, the maxillary molars have a distal axial inclination. With continued favourable growth of the facial complex, the molar will erupt with a more mesial axial inclination.[10] Abnormalities in buccolingual axial inclinations of the posterior teeth may be present in individuals with or without posterior crossbite. Their proper assessment helps the clinician to differentiate dental problems from the skeletal ones. Rotations of the posterior teeth form an important part of transverse dental problems. Mesial migration with forward tipping of the permanent molar is usually accompanied by rotation (mesial-in) of the tooth, leading to a significant space loss in the posterior dental arch. This results in Class II molar relationship on the affected side.

Archform distortions

Abnormal positions of the posterior teeth, either in the buccal or the lingual side, symmetrically or asymmetrically, with or without crossbite, result in deviations from normal configuration of the archform (Fig. 6.2). These distorted archforms are either because of displacement

of a single or group of teeth or because of an underlying skeletal discrepancy, and it is critical to establish differential diagnosis. Since skeletal discrepancies contributing to such problems is common, it is important to understand the role of buccolingual axial inclination compensations in the dental arch that occur naturally to mask the discrepancy. It should be recognized that natural compensation in the form of changes in the buccolingual axial inclinations of the teeth, influencing the arch width, minimizes the magnitude of a problem and makes it to appear less severe clinically. It has been observed that some malocclusions involving transverse component, presenting with a centric relation–centric occlusion discrepancy, are symmetric in centric relation and asymmetric in centric occlusion.[11] Therefore, an assessment of occlusion in centric relation and centric occlusion is the key to differentially diagnose these conditions.

Occlusal plane considerations

Occlusal plane is the line along which the teeth function and is considered to be an important reference plane to achieve functional balance. Occlusal plane, when viewed from the frontal aspect, is an expression of vertical position of teeth on right and left sides of dental arch. Therefore, when vertical relationship of teeth along this plane on one side of the arch is assessed with respect to the other, it forms an integral part of transverse assessment to determine the cant of occlusal plane. As most malocclusions are often the result of a dysplasia in the vertical dimension, every clinician should make an effort to better evaluate function as relates to vertical growth. Occlusal plane changes in transverse dimension are true reflection of relative vertical heights of the segments of teeth on the left and right sides, as a result of differential vertical dentoalveolar growth, vertical eruption of teeth on one side of the arch or underlying skeletal discrepancy (Fig. 6.3). Canted

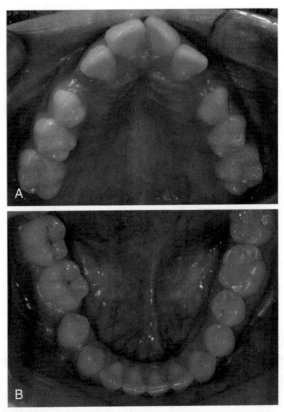

Figure 6.2 Archform distortions. **(A)** Maxillary skeletal constriction and V-shaped archform. **(B)** Asymmetric mandibular archform due to mesiolingual drifting of the mandibular right buccal segment.

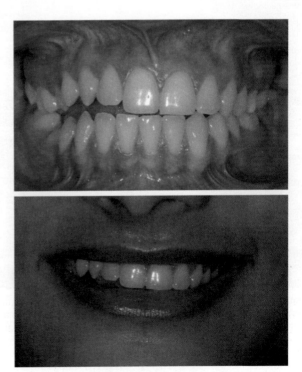

Figure 6.3 Canted maxillary anterior occlusal plane.

occlusal plane may involve both upper and lower arches; however, in majority of the patients, the problem is limited to either the upper or lower arch or isolated to anterior or posterior segment.

Skeletal transverse discrepancies

Transverse skeletal discrepancies may involve either the maxilla or the mandible or a combination of both. The maxillary problems in a transverse dimension usually result from a symmetric or an asymmetric constriction of the basal arch, with or without posterior crossbite depending upon the severity of the condition. The maxilla can undergo some rotational changes relative to the cranial base producing an asymmetric occlusal relationship (Fig. 6.4A).

Most people have some facial asymmetry, and asymmetric development of the jaws, though rare, does produce transverse problems. Severe skeletal problems in a transverse dimension are often produced by some congenital anomalies, like facial clefts, and trauma or infection. Patients with cleft lip and palate pose a unique problem, requiring extensive and prolonged orthodontic care. Individuals with a lateral cleft typically exhibit lingually collapsed maxillary posterior segments and labially displaced premaxillary segment, leading to extreme distortion of the maxilla. The surgical repair of the lip and palate carried out an early stage for aesthetic and functional reasons often results into some degree of lateral constriction of the palate and constriction across anterior segment of the maxillary arch in the early and late mixed dentition.

Transverse mandibular problems result from both asymmetric positioning and asymmetric morphology of the mandible (Fig. 6.4B and C). An abnormal growth of the cranial base may lead to asymmetries in the positions of the glenoid fossae and subsequent rotation of the mandible relative to the maxilla. Mandibular asymmetries significantly contribute to the facial asymmetries, and it is important for the clinician to identify whether a resultant problem is due to a congenital anomaly or a trauma.

There is an absence of tissue in the mandibular condylar region in patients with a congenital anomaly of hemifacial microsomia with a diminished growth on the affected side leading to asymmetry. An injury to the mandibular condyle often produces scarring and fibrosis of the affected area, leading to an apparently similar situation of slower growth and resultant asymmetry. Hemifacial microsomia is characterized by the absence of growth potential due to a lack of tissue; while in a post-traumatic situation, the fibrotic tissue causes restriction of condylar movement and subsequent interference with normal expression of growth, but there is potential for normal growth. In addition to deficient condylar growth, mandibulofacial asymmetries can also be caused by excessive growth of the mandibular condyle on one side. Unilateral overgrowth of the mandibular condyle may be expressed as an enlargement of the whole half of the mandible, with associated prognathism. The gonial and ramal overgrowth hypertrophy may manifest itself as a more localized enlargement of the mandible.

Certain infections and inflammations, especially the ones that originate from middle ear, often leading to ankylosis of the temporomandibular joint, were earlier regarded as important factors contributing to the development of mandibulofacial transverse problems. However, such incidences have significantly reduced owing to advances in diagnostic and therapeutic medicine.

Considerable changes in mandibular function and structure as a result of destruction of the surfaces of the temporomandibular joint and the disc are commonly observed in children suffering from rheumatoid arthritis.

Muscular asymmetries

Any deviation from normal muscle function plays an important role in the development of skeletal and dental transverse discrepancies.[12] Muscular asymmetry, as commonly observed in hemifacial atrophy or cerebral palsy, is one of the factors responsible for facial disproportions and midline discrepancies.[13] Sometime facial transverse

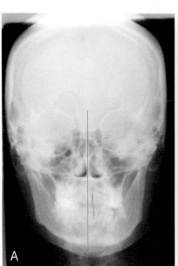
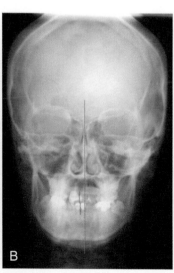
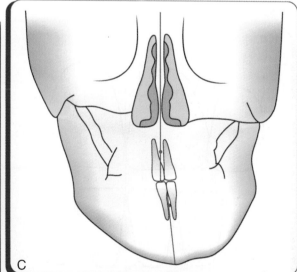

Figure 6.4 Transverse skeletal problems. **(A)** Maxillary and mandibular asymmetry exhibiting symphysis deviation to the left and canted occlusal plane. **(B)** Mandibular asymmetry without occlusal plane distortion. **(C)** Dental midlines coincident. Apical base discrepancy is masked by compensatory tipping of the maxillary and mandibular incisors.

problems are confined mainly to the soft tissues due to disproportionate muscle size as seen in masseter muscle hypertrophy.[14]

Functional transverse problems

Functional transverse discrepancies are often caused by deflections of the mandible due to occlusal interferences.[7,12] During mandibular closure, the abnormal initial tooth contact in centric relation results in subsequent mandibular displacement laterally or anteroposteriorly, leading to asymmetric maxillomandibular relationship (Fig. 6.5). The functional mandibular deviations are caused by a malposed tooth or by a symmetric or an asymmetric constricted maxillary arch.

Sometimes temporomandibular joint disorders, especially an anterior disc displacement without reduction, may lead to midline discrepancy during opening as the displaced disc interferes with the normal forward mandibular translation as on the unaffected side.

Assessment of transverse problems

The diagnosis of transverse discrepancies should be accomplished by a thorough clinical examination and an analysis of various diagnostic records to determine the extent of involvement of dental, skeletal, soft tissue and functional components. The goal of these diagnostic procedures is to identify the causative factor and determine the location and extent of the transverse problem. The differential diagnosis of transverse discrepancies is critical to formulate proper treatment plan.

Clinical examination

One of the challenges in treatment planning and treatment of transverse problems is the proper alignment of maxillary and mandibular dental midlines. Not only should they be coincident with each other, but they must also exhibit a definite relationship with the face. The clinical examination is of vital importance as it enables the clinician to carry out dynamic assessment of these discrepancies. To establish differential diagnosis of midline discrepancies, the dental midlines should be evaluated in different mandibular positions: mouth open; in centric relation; at initial teeth contact and in centric occlusion. Functional transverse problems due to occlusal interferences lead to a mandibular functional shift following initial tooth contact. These functional mandibular shifts may accentuate or mask the midline discrepancy depending upon the direction of shift—in the same or opposite direction of the dental or skeletal discrepancy. Maxillary and mandibular dental arches should be thoroughly examined for arch symmetry and their coordination and for a more localized factor, like malposed or displaced tooth. Clinical assessment of the patient must involve the examination of temporomandibular joint and associated musculature since certain temporomandibular joint disorders causing interferences in normal mandibular translation result in mandibular deviations.

The facial midline is an important component of facial aesthetics, and its proper clinical evaluation must become an integral part of the clinical examination. A common procedure adopted by most clinicians to evaluate the facial midline is to use a dental instrument handle/shaft or a piece of dental floss to connect soft tissue points at nasion, subnasale and pogonion. The author does not consider this approach reliable, since it is difficult to accurately identify these points; and in the presence of mandibular asymmetry, these points would not correspond. For this reason, the philtrum is considered to be a reliable midline structure, and in most instances, can be used as the basis for midline assessment.[15] Another approach is to observe the distance between the canine or first premolar and the corner of the mouth.[12] In the presence of midline deviation, the patient will notice unequal amount of tooth exposure on the right and left side. In clinical examination, the clinician must record the extent to which the maxillary midline is deviated from the facial soft tissue midline, since the orthodontic treatment goal is to position the two midlines

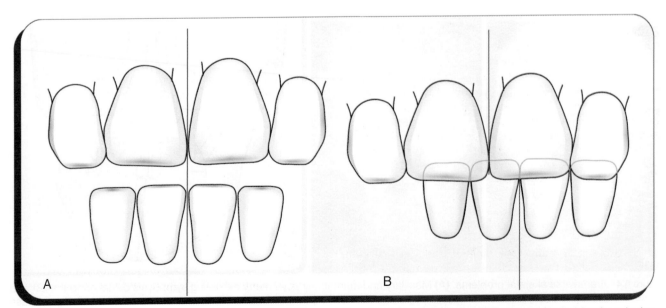

Figure 6.5   Mandibular functional shift. **(A)** Transverse incisor relationship at rest. **(B)** Incisor relationship in habitual occlusion.

and the mandibular midline so they are aligned with each other.

Radiographic examination

While clinical examination is an important step in diagnostic procedures for the orthodontist to assess dynamic relationships of orofacial complex, certain radiographic projections provide valuable information to differentiate between various types of transverse discrepancies. A number of radiographic projections are available for accurate identification of the location and aetiopathology of transverse problems.

The lateral cephalometric radiograph provides little useful information on transverse discrepancies; however, it is a valuable diagnostic tool to locate and quantify associated vertical and sagittal problems in the craniofacial complex. To certain extent, this view enables the clinician to assess ramal height, gonial angle and mandibular length, but due to the inherent characteristics of this projection, like superimposition of the right and left structures and variations in their magnifications as a result of their different distances from the film and X-ray source; its interpretation in diagnosing transverse problems is of limited value.

The panoramic radiograph is a useful view for an overall examination of the dental and bony structures of the maxilla and the mandible. Certain conditions, like missing or supernumerary teeth, impacted teeth, the presence of gross pathology, etc., can be assessed. It also provides valuable information on comparison of some structures, such as mandibular ramus, condyles and configuration of inferior border of the mandible on both sides.

Posteroanterior cephalogram

For cephalometric assessment of orthodontic problems, the routinely prescribed radiograph is the lateral cephalogram. Only when a transverse problem or an asymmetry of face is detected, then the clinician asks for a frontal radiograph. It is a valuable tool in the assessment of the right and left structures of the dentofacial complex. Since these structures are located at relatively equal distances from the film and X-ray source, the unequal enlargement by the diverging rays and the distortion as in lateral cephalogram are significantly reduced. This promotes proper registration and evaluation of the facial and dental midlines and an accurate comparison between the sides to determine the extent of the asymmetry present. The use of posteroanterior cephalogram is fraught with inherent problems: difficulty in reproducing head posture; difficulty in identifying landmarks because of superimposed structures or poor radiographic technique; and concern about exposure to radiation.[16]

Despite these disadvantages, numerous frontal cephalometric analyses have been used for several decades for surgical application as well as orthodontic use. Figure 6.6A illustrates the commonly used frontal cephalometric points. In orthodontic usage, frontal cephalometric assessment serves two primary purposes:

1. To determine transverse skeletal and dentoalveolar dimension and assess skeletal and dental inter-arch relation and quantify the discrepancy, if any.
2. To detect, localize and quantify any skeletal or dentoalveolar asymmetry and midline shifts.

The selection of a reliable vertical reference line is pivotal in carrying out frontal cephalometric assessment. Grummons and Van De Coppello suggested a mid-sagittal reference plane running vertically from crista galli through anterior nasal spine to the chin area. This plane will typically be nearly perpendicular to the Z plane (the plane connecting the medial aspects of the zygomaticofrontal suture).[16]

1. If the location of crista galli is in question, an alternative method of constructing the mid-sagittal reference plane is to draw a line from the midpoint of the Z plane through ANS.[16]
2. If there is upper facial asymmetry, the mid-sagittal reference plane can be drawn as a line from the midpoint of the Z plane through the midpoint of an Fr-Fr line[16] (Fr—foramen rotundum on either sides).

Ricketts suggested a mid-sagittal reference plane through the top of the nasal septum or crista galli, perpendicular to the line through the centres of the zygomatic arches.[17]

The following data should be obtained when performing frontal cephalometric assessment (Fig. 6.6B and Table 6.1):

1. The effective nasal cavity width is measured as it is important to determine the normalcy of respiration in orthodontic patients. The fact that the growth of the nasal capsule influences the mid-facial development and that it can be affected by timely introduction of orthopaedic treatment makes this a very vital data to be obtained.
2. The maxillary width is evaluated relative to the mandible. The *frontal facial lines*, constructed from the inside margins of the zygomaticofrontal sutures to the antegonial (Ag) points, on either sides are related to the point jugale (*J* point—defined as the crossing of the outline of the tuberosity with that of the jugal process) to assess maxillomandibular transverse skeletal relation.
3. The basal mandibular width is best indicated by the width of the mandible at the antegonial notch.
4. The arch width at the level of the first permanent molar is assessed by measuring the distance between the buccal surfaces of the lower first permanent molars on either side.
5. The distance between the tips of the lower cuspids indicates the intercanine arch width. The cuspids change relationships during the process of eruption and hence require the appraisal of age effects.
6. The harmony between the lower dental arch width and the skeletal (basal bone) arch width should be assessed. This is done by relating the buccal surface of the lower molar to the 'Fronto Denture Plane' (J-Ag).
7. Width differences between upper and lower molars are useful in identifying actual and potential crossbites as well as asymmetries. The measurement is made at the most prominent buccal contour of each tooth as seen in the P-A view, and recorded as the buccal overjet of right and left upper molars.

To detect and assess asymmetries, the following evaluations can be done (Fig. 6.6C and Table 6.2).

1. Four horizontal planes are drawn to show the degree of parallelism and symmetry of the facial structures:
   a. Plane connecting the medial aspects of the zygomaticofrontal sutures (Z point) on either sides (Z plane)

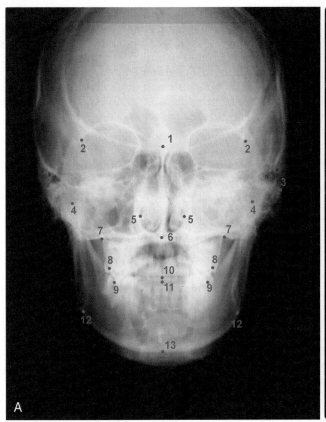

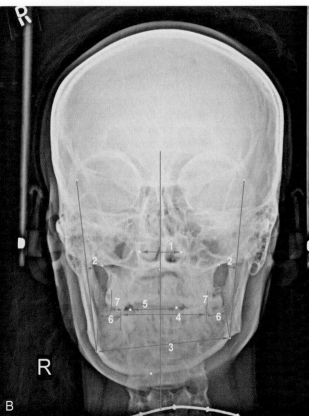

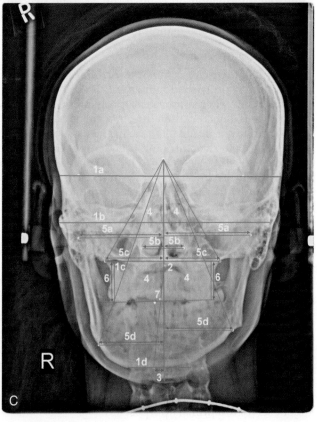

Figure 6.6   (A) Frontal cephalometric points. 1, Crista galli (Cg). 2, Point at the medial margin of the zygomaticofrontal suture (left and right) (Z points). 3, Point at the most lateral border of the centre of the zygomatic arch (left and right) (ZA points). 4, Most superior point on condylar hand (left and right)—condylion (Cd). 5, Most lateral aspect of the piriform aperture (left and right) (NC). 6, Anterior nasal spine (ANS). 7, The intersection of the lateral contour of the maxillary alveolar process and the lower contour of the maxillo-zygomatic (jugal) process of the maxilla (left and right)—point Jugale (J points). 8, The most prominent lateral point on the buccal surface of the first permanent maxillary molar (left and right) (A6). 9, The most prominent lateral point on the buccal surface of the first permanent mandibular molar (left and right) (B6). 10, The midpoint between the mandibular central incisors at the level of the incisal edges—incision inferior frontale (iif). 11, The midpoint between the maxillary central incisors at the level of the incisor edges—incision superior frontale (isf). 12, The highest point in the antegonial notch (left and right)—antegonion (Ag). 13, Menton (Me). **(B)** Frontal cephalometric assessment. 1, Nasal cavity width—distance between NC points. 2, Maxillary relation (maxillary concavity)—distance from J point to frontal facial plane (Z-Ag) on either sides. 3, Mandibular width—distance between Ag points. 4, Intermolar width—distance between buccal surfaces of mandibular first molars. 5, Intercuspid width—distance between incisal cusp tips of mandibular canines. 6, Lower molar to frontodenture plane (B6 to J-Ag) on either sides. 7, Buccal surface of upper molar to lower molar. **(C)** Assessment of asymmetry. 1, Four horizontal planes—a, connecting medial aspects of the zygomaticofrontal sutures (Z-Z); b, connecting the centres of the zygomatic arches (ZA-ZA); c, connecting the medial aspects of the jugal processes (J-J); d, plane parallel to Z plane at menton. 2, Distance from ANS to mid-sagittal plane. 3, Distance from Pog to mid-sagittal plane. 4, Two pairs of triangles, each pair bisected by mid-sagittal plane—one pair from Cg to J to MSR on either sides, one pair from Cg to Ag to MSR on either sides. 5, Linear distances to the mid-sagittal plane from bilateral points—a, condylion; b, nasal cavity; c, J point; d, antegonion. 6, Distance from the buccal cusps of the upper first molars (on the occlusal plane) along the J perpendiculars. 7, Distance between incision inferior frontale and ANS-Me plane and distance between incision superior frontale and ANS-Me plane.

Table 6.1   Frontal cephalometric assessment

No.	Parameter	Description	Value	Age appraisal
1.	Effective nasal cavity width	Linear distance from NC to NC	24.5 ± 2 mm (at 8 years of age)	Increases 0.5 mm each year; 22 mm at age 3; 29.5 mm at age 18
2.	Maxillomandibular transverse relation	Perpendicular distance from J point to Z-Ag plane	10 ± 1.5 mm (on either sides)	None
3.	Effective mandibular width	Linear distance from Ag to Ag	68.25 ± 3 mm (at 3 years of age)	Increases 1.25 mm each year; 75 mm at age 8; 88.5 mm at age 18
4.	Arch width at first permanent molar	Linear distance between buccal surfaces of first molars	56 ± 2 mm	May narrow slightly with mesial drift but essentially no change
5.	Arch width at lower cuspids	Linear distance between lower canines incisal tips	Age 3 = 25 mm; age 8 = 22.5 ± 2 mm; age 13 = 26 ± 1.5 mm	Crowns converge, then diverge in eruption
6.	Harmony of arch width with jaws	Perpendicular distance from buccal surface of lower molar to J-Ag plane	6 ± 2 mm (at 8 years of age)	Increases by 0.8 mm each year; age 6 = approximately 5 mm, age 13 = 10 mm and age 18 = 14.2 mm
7.	Indicator for molar crossbite	Buccal surface of upper molar to lower molar	Upper more buccal by 1 ± 1 mm	None

Table 6.2   Assessment of asymmetry

No.	Parameter	Description	Value
1.	a. Z plane; b. ZA-ZA plane; c. J point–J point; d. plane at Me parallel to Z plane	Four horizontal planes to assess the degree of parallelism and symmetry of the facial structures	
2.	Maxillary skeletal symmetry	ANS to MSR	0 mm
3.	Mandibular skeletal symmetry	Pog to MSR	0 mm
4.	Cg-J-MSR (perpendicular to MSR through J on either side); Cg-Ag-MSR (perpendicular to MSR through Ag on either side)	This produces two pairs of triangles, each pair bisected by mid-sagittal reference plane	If perfect symmetry is present, the four triangles become two, J-Cg-J and Ag-Cg-Ag.
5.	a. Co to MSR; b. NC to MSR; c. J point to MSR; d. Ag to MSR	Linear distances measured on either sides	Linear distances should be equal on either sides in case of perfect symmetry.
6.	Cant of functional posterior occlusal plane	Distances are measured from the buccal cusps of the upper first molars (on the occlusal plane) along the J perpendiculars on either sides	Either sides should be equal, if there is no cant of occlusal plane
7.	isf to A-Pog; iif to A-Pog	The midline drifts of the upper and lower incisors	0 ± 1 mm; 0 ± 1 mm

b. Plane connecting the centres of the zygomatic arches

c. Plane connecting the medial aspects of the jugal processes at their intersection with the outline of the maxillary tuberosities (J point)

d. Plane drawn at the menton parallel to the Z plane.

2. By relating the ANS to the mid-sagittal plane, maxillary skeletal symmetry is assessed.

3. By relating pogonion point to the mid-sagittal plane, mandibular skeletal symmetry is assessed.

4. Perpendiculars are drawn to the mid-sagittal plane from J point and Ag point and connecting lines from crista galli to J and Ag. This produces two pairs of triangles, each pair bisected by mid-sagittal reference plane. If perfect symmetry is present, the four triangles become two, J-Cg-J and Ag-Cg-Ag. This is a quick and easy method to assess symmetries in both jaws.

5. To quantify asymmetries of facial structures, linear measurements are made to the mid-sagittal reference line. Also the amount of vertical offset on the mid-sagittal

reference line indicates the degree of asymmetry in the vertical plane. The points evaluated are condylion (Co), lateral piriform aperture (NC), J and antegonial notch (Ag).

6. To assess cant of the functional posterior occlusal plane, a 0.014″ wire is placed across the mesio-occlusal areas of the maxillary first molars. Distances are measured from the buccal cusps of the upper first molars (on the occlusal plane) along the J perpendiculars. The Ag plane, MSR and the ANS–Me plane are also drawn to depict the dental compensations for any skeletal asymmetries in the horizontal or vertical planes (maxillomandibular imbalance).

7. The midline drifts of the upper and lower incisors should also be assessed (relative to the A-Pog line). Ideally, they should be coincident with the mid-sagittal plane.

TRANSVERSE DISCREPANCIES: THEIR RELATIONSHIP WITH SAGITTAL AND VERTICAL DIMENSIONS

It should be recognized that there is an inter-relationship among the sagittal, vertical and transverse dimensions; and quite often, discrepancies in one plane affect the other. When an individual presents with abnormalities in all three planes, the correction of sagittal discrepancy is generally considered to be a common goal for both the patient and the clinician. However, a successful treatment outcome is also dependant on an accurate diagnosis and clinical management of the vertical and transverse discrepancies. Any treatment-induced change in the patient's increased or decreased anterior vertical dimension influences the intermaxillary relationship in the sagittal dimension. Similarly, an alteration in the patient's sagittal jaw relationship also impacts the dental and skeletal relationships in the transverse dimension. In a patient with sagittal discrepancy having Class II molar relationship and an increased overjet, an advancement of the mandible into a Class I molar relationship to eliminate the overjet may result into a posterior crossbite. In a patient with constricted maxillary arch resulting in a unilateral or bilateral posterior crossbite, forward posturing of the mandible will make it more pronounced clinically. Conversely, the sagittal maxillary discrepancy expressed clinically as a Class III malocclusion in a growing patient usually benefits from growth modification therapy by maxillary protraction and also improves the associated transverse discrepancy as the wider part of the maxilla articulates with the narrower part of the mandible. Therefore, in case of a skeletal Class II or Class III malocclusion in which treatment is primarily focused at resolution of the sagittal discrepancy alone may either improve or exaggerate the associated transverse problem. Similarly, orthodontic intervention mainly targeted at correcting the vertical dimension alone in skeletal Class II or Class III malocclusion may either improve or aggravate the associated transverse discrepancy due to sagittal mandibular repositioning. Therefore, it is not only important to identify various components contributing to the development of a malocclusion, but also to understand the interaction of the transverse, vertical and sagittal dimensions that plays an important role in orthodontic diagnosis and treatment planning.

TREATMENT PLANNING CONSIDERATIONS

The treatment of transverse discrepancies in orthodontics is generally considered to be a challenging task for the clinician. Depending upon the nature of the problem, whether dental or skeletal in origin, and its severity; several treatment options are available to resolve the problem. In addition to the findings derived from the clinical examination including functional assessment, a detailed study of the various diagnostic records is necessary to determine the aetiology, location and the magnitude of a transverse problem. This is essential to formulate the proper treatment plan. For the effective and efficient resolution of these abnormalities, they must be differentially diagnosed to determine their nature—dental, skeletal, muscular or functional and severity. It is essential to compare the extent of transverse discrepancies between centric relation and centric occlusion.

- Age of the patient plays an important role in treatment planning process, as early resolution of dental or functional asymmetries prevents subsequent development of skeletal problems. It also dictates the type of treatment modality to be used, whether orthopaedic, orthodontic, a combination of both or surgical intervention.

- Dental asymmetries due to congenital absence of teeth, usually the lateral incisor or second bicuspid, are treated orthodontically. The treatment mechanics usually involve differential molar distalization, asymmetric extractions and use of elastics in various configurations, like Class II on one side and Class III on the other with or without anterior oblique elastics. Abnormalities in the transverse dimension caused by disproportionate crown widths are corrected by a combination of asymmetric treatment mechanics and prosthodontic restorations or composite buildups to restore normal proportions.

- An individual with a midline deviation between the maxillary and mandibular arches without apical base discrepancy requires simple mechanics to tip teeth in a predetermined direction. However, the presence of a true apical base discrepancy requires translatory mechanics to correct the midlines, which is more difficult having limitation to the amount of mesiodistal tooth movement.[18] The clinician must properly assess the mesiodistal and buccolingual axial inclinations of the posterior teeth for a gross differentiation of dental from skeletal problems. Consideration of mesiodistal or buccolingual tipping as a part of dental problem is not always true since migration of a tooth may occur in the early stages of its eruption, leading to mild or no tipping. During different treatment planning processes, the clinician should determine whether compensatory axial inclinations as a result of underlying skeletal discrepancy should be maintained or corrected.

- The posteroanterior radiographic projection is a valuable tool in quantitatively and qualitatively evaluating the extent of the skeletal asymmetry present. The existing skeletal problem should be further assessed to determine the nature and its severity that guides the clinician to select an effective treatment modality. In growing patients with transverse skeletal problems, orthopaedic appliances are used either to improve or correct the problem, followed by fixed appliance therapy to fine-tune the dentition. However, severe skeletal problems require a complex treatment approach involving surgical repositioning of the maxilla or mandible or both and orthodontic treatment. If for some reason, the surgical treatment is turned down by the patient and orthodontics is the only treatment option available to address the skeletal problem, certain associated compromises must be explained to the patient before treatment is initiated. The primary goal of presurgical orthodontics should be to eliminate the dental compensations for the skeletal problems in all three planes of space. Transverse deformities that are confined to the soft tissues can be treated by augmentation or reduction surgery. These surgical procedures include the use of bone grafts and implants in the desired areas of the face that require recontouring.[19]

- There are various treatment options to address transverse discrepancies due to functional mandibular shifts. Mild deviations can be corrected with minor occlusal adjustments, while more severe problems require orthodontic treatment. Certain functional transverse problems may be the result of underlying skeletal asymmetry and can be managed by rapid maxillary expansion, orthognathic surgery and orthodontic treatment.

TREATMENT OF TRANSVERSE DISCREPANCIES

Once the diagnosis of transverse discrepancies is established, specific goals of treatment are defined and a final treatment plan is formulated. Patients with transverse problems may present with some of the most biomechanically challenging situations to the clinician. Depending upon its severity and whether the abnormality in transverse dimension is primarily dental or skeletal in nature, a number of treatment options are available to address the problem; these may be broadly divided into four major treatment methods: an early resolution of transverse discrepancies involving the elimination of mandibular functional shifts, and orthopaedic approach to correct the developing skeletal imbalance; orthodontic treatment mechanics to address problems that are dental in nature; a combination of orthodontic and surgical treatment for severe skeletal discrepancies; and orthodontic camouflage in case of mild skeletal involvement.

Early resolution of transverse problems

The selection of appropriate treatment strategy for early resolution of transverse problems is based upon the findings of the evaluation of path of mandibular closure from postural rest to habitual occlusion in the transverse plane. Individuals with transverse problems, expressed clinically as posterior crossbites resulting from a narrow upper jaw, are relatively common in the primary dentition (Figs 6.7 and 6.8). The local environmental factors, like sucking habits, generally, tend to produce some constriction of the upper arch, especially in the primary canine region. This results in the development of occlusal interferences, which may then lead to a functional shift of the mandible. Observing the behaviour of the mandibular midline during the mandibular closure from rest position to habitual occlusion is important to establish the differential diagnosis of transverse problems. Patients with coincident maxillary and mandibular midlines in postural rest position of the mandible and mandibular midline shift in the occlusal position indicate the presence of functional transverse discrepancy. A unilateral posterior crossbite almost always results from a functional mandibular shift and rarely from a true skeletal or dental asymmetry.

Transverse discrepancies associated with a mandibular shift should be treated as soon as they are diagnosed (Figs 6.7–6.11). They are considered to be among the few conditions requiring immediate intervention. If untreated, they can produce asymmetric jaw growth and dental compensations leading to a skeletal discrepancy at a later stage. Various treatment modalities to address functional transverse discrepancies as a result of mandibular shifts at an early age include occlusal equilibration to eliminate prematurities during mandibular excursion; expansion of a constricted maxillary arch, particularly in

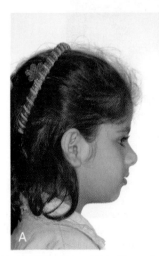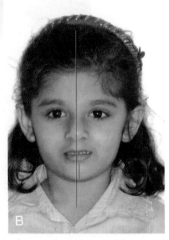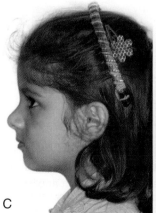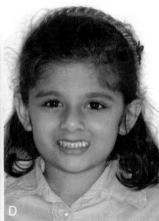

Figure 6.7 Case YM. **(A and C)** Extraoral photographs of a 4-year-old patient showing straight profile. **(B)** Significant facial asymmetry due to deviated chin to the left side. **(D)** Smile exhibiting coincident maxillary dental midline with the facial midline while the mandibular midline is shifted to the left side.

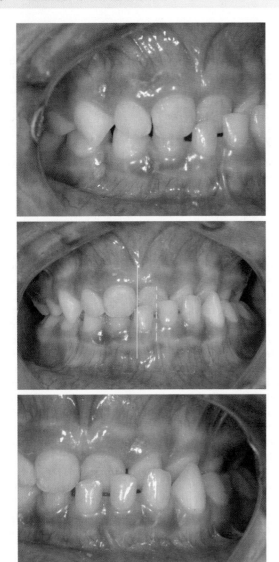

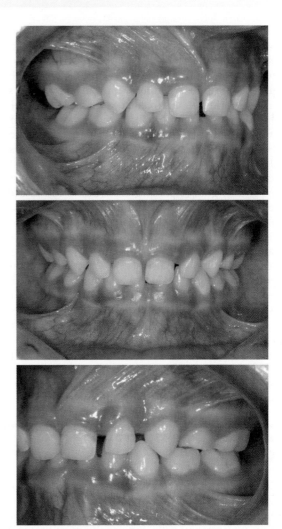

Figure 6.10 Case YM. Post-treatment intraoral photographs showing substantial improvement in midline discrepancy and correction of anterolateral crossbite as a result of mandibular repositioning.

Figure 6.8 Case YM. Pretreatment intraoral photographs demonstrate significant midline discrepancy and lingual cross-bite of the entire left half of the maxillary arch. Constriction of the maxillary arch and occlusal interferences in the canine region resulted in an anterolateral functional shift of the mandible.

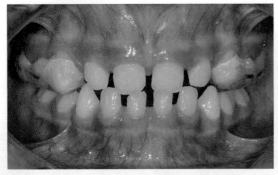

Figure 6.9 Case YM. Bonded maxillary expansion appliance to resolve maxillomandibular arch width discrepancy and to eliminate occlusal interferences.

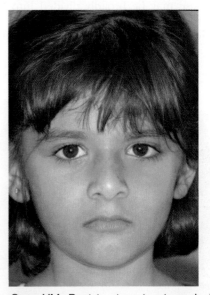

Figure 6.11 Case YM. Post-treatment extraoral photograph showing the chin aligned with the facial midline.

the primary canine region and repositioning of individual teeth to address intra-arch transverse problems.

If a child exhibits normal intermolar width, minor occlusal adjustments to eliminate deflective contacts may be the only treatment procedure required. A bilateral maxillary constriction of a lesser magnitude produces dental interferences, forcing the mandible to acquire a new position for maximum intercuspation. Usually, a maxillary constriction of a greater degree does not lead to a mandibular shift as it allows the maxillary arch to occlude inside the mandibular arch. Both of these clinical situations, once diagnosed, should be resolved in the primary dentition. This correction is considered to be stable and does influence the position of the bicuspids.[20,21] If the permanent first molars are expected to erupt within 6 months, the treatment is delayed till their eruption to facilitate their correction. There are several appliances available for correction of maxillary dental constriction. Both the W-arch and the quad-helix appliances require little patient cooperation and are reliable and easy to use.

Therefore, the goal of a posterior unilateral crossbite correction in the primary dentition is to allow the permanent successors to erupt into a normal occlusal relationship along with the elimination of a mandibular functional shift. It is suggested that delaying the interceptive treatment till the eruption of permanent successors will establish the permanent dentition in a deflected occlusal plane. In the mixed dentition stage, the transverse discrepancies are generally identified as skeletal or dental in nature and of different magnitude. A common problem observed in the transverse dimension is either unilateral or bilateral posterior crossbite due to skeletal maxillary constriction. This may result from maxillary constriction or mandibular expansion, involving single or a group of teeth. Therefore, the clinician should make sure that a systematic diagnostic approach has identified the skeletal and dental components contributing to development of the problem.

Mandibular deviation

If the maxillary arch is relatively narrow or the mandibular arch is wider, it is likely that a child may shift the jaw laterally upon closure to get maximal occlusal interdigitation, producing an apparent unilateral crossbite. If this mandibular shift is not corrected in the primary dentition, those factors that modify and redirect normal growth may cause the mandible to grow asymmetrically. The resultant new occlusion is a consequence of the ac-

quired mandibular skeletal asymmetry and associated dental compensations. Quite often, the mandibular shift may occur in anterolateral position, producing both anterior and unilateral posterior crossbites. Delaying the treatment for all the permanent teeth to erupt before correcting the crossbite and the functional shift makes the condition more severe due to continued unfavourable mandibular growth. Such clinical situations should be diagnosed and treated early with orthopaedic treatment to avoid creating severe skeletal discrepancies.

The management of a patient with mandibular prognathism and deviation in a mixed dentition stage is illustrated in Figures 6.12–6.17.

Patient's dentofacial features were characterized by concave profile due to mandibular prognathism, facial asymmetry due to mandibular deviation, unilateral posterior crossbite and mandibular midline shift (Figs 6.12 and 6.13). Early orthopaedic correction was planned with the U bow activator of Karwetzky to resolve both transverse and sagittal discrepancies and establish favourable environment to promote normal future growth.

The Karwetzky appliance consists of maxillary and mandibular active plates that are joined together by a U bow in the region of the first permanent molars[22] (Fig. 6.14). These plates are extended to cover lingual and occlusal aspects of all teeth and lingual soft tissues—gingival and alveolar mucosa. The appliance is usually made using interocclusal space or clearance as the height of the construction bite; and anteroposteriorly, the most posterior positioning of the mandible in postural rest.

During the construction of the appliance, care should be taken to make sure that the occlusal aspects of maxillary and mandibular plates are flat, well polished and are in contact with each other evenly. These two components are then joined together with the U bow made from 1.1 mm hard round stainless steel wire, having one longer and one shorter leg in the region of the first permanent molars.

The shorter leg of the U bow is incorporated in the upper appliance, while the longer leg is attached to the lower plate. Various types of Karwetzky appliance are created, each for a different treatment purpose depending on the placement of the end of the U bows.

Type I appliance is used for the treatment of Class II division 1 and division 2 malocclusions, incorporating posteriorly placed longer legs of the U bow. By constricting the U bow, the mandible is guided anteroposteriorly in a forward position.

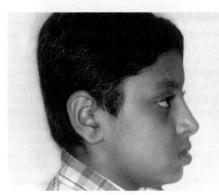
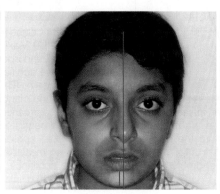
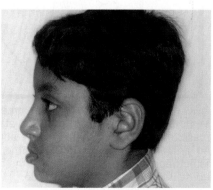

Figure 6.12   Case RS. Facial photographs of an 11-year-old male patient exhibiting concave profile, protruded lower lip, prominent chin and facial asymmetry (chin deviated to the right).

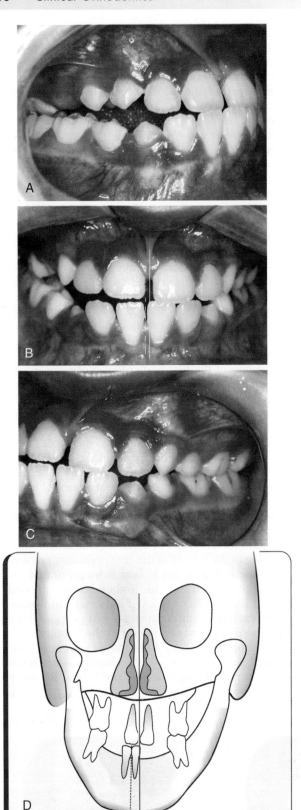

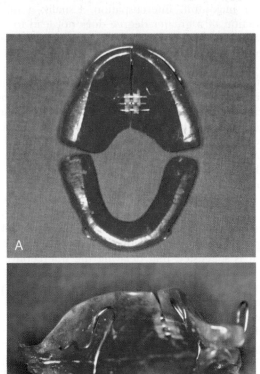

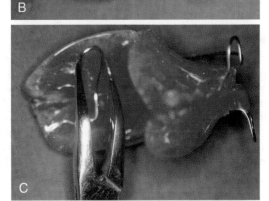

Type II appliance is indicated for the treatment of Class III malocclusion, in which longer legs of the U bow are positioned anteriorly. As the U bows are constricted, the lower half of the appliance gets displaced posteriorly, exerting a retrusive force on the mandible.

In individuals with transverse discrepancy, characterized by mandibular deviation to one side, type III appliance is

Figure 6.14 Case RS. Karwetzky appliance and its clinical management. **(A)** Maxillary and mandibular plates—midline expansion screw incorporated in the maxillary component and both plates have acrylic extensions on the occlusal and incisal surfaces of teeth. **(B)** The lingual view of the appliance showing maxillary and mandibular components held together by a U bow in the first permanent molar region. The stage 1 treatment with this appliance consisted of correction of transverse discrepancy by creating an appliance with a U bow configuration, having its longer leg mesially on the left side and distally on the right side. **(C)** The appliance activation is done by constricting the U bow that tends to displace the mandible to the left.

Figure 6.13 Case RS. **(A–C)** Pretreatment intraoral photographs showing late mixed dentition stage, right posterior crossbite, mandibular dental midline shift to the right side and anterior crossbite. **(D)** Pretreatment frontal cephalometric tracing showing deviation of the mandibular skeletal and dental midlines to the right side.

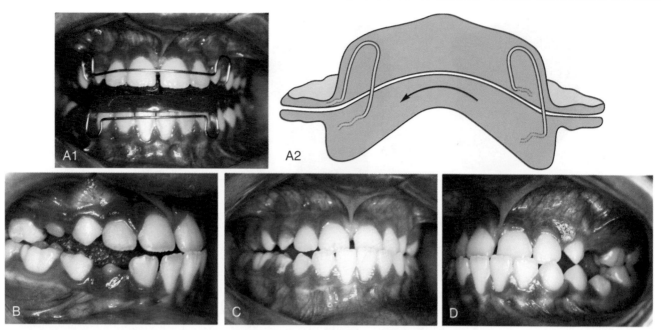

Figure 6.15   Case RS. The stage 1 treatment to resolve transverse discrepancy. **(A1)** Photograph showing the use of the appliance at the beginning and end of stage 1 treatment. **(A2)** Mechanism of action of the appliance. **(B–D)** The correction of maxillomandibular transverse discrepancy. Note the presence of sagittal discrepancy which was not attempted during this stage.

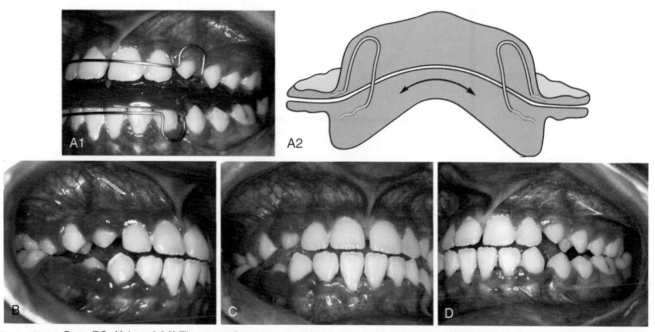

Figure 6.16   Case RS. **(A1 and A2)** The stage 2 treatment with this appliance was aimed at the correction of sagittal discrepancy by changing the U bow configuration that facilitates gradual retrusion of the mandible. **(B–D)** Photographs showing the sagittal correction.

used to influence the mandibular position in a transverse than a sagittal plane. This appliance typically incorporates the longer leg of the U bow attached to the lower plate anteriorly on one side and posteriorly on the other side. Constricting the bow will tend to displace the mandible away from the side where the longer leg of the bow is positioned posteriorly, thereby promoting transverse mandibular position correction (Fig. 6.15A2). Appliance activations are done by constricting U bows with flat-nosed, grooved pliers. In a situation where patient has

both transverse and sagittal discrepancies due to mandibular deviation and prognathism, the transverse discrepancy is addressed first by type III appliance, and the sagittal correction is achieved by converting the same appliance into a type II appliance by changing the U bow position to facilitate retrusive effect on the mandible. It is important to keep the appliance as simple as possible and resist the temptation to accomplish too many things at the same time. The author feels that this appliance is very versatile having many inherent advantages. The mobility of the

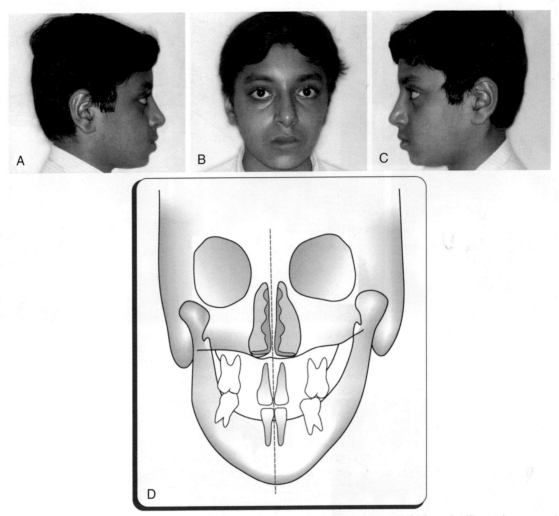

Figure 6.17 Case RS. **(A–C)** Post-treatment (orthopaedic) extraoral photographs exhibiting significant improvement in the facial profile and symmetry. **(D)** Post-treatment frontal cephalometric tracing exhibiting symmetric configuration of dental and skeletal components.

upper and lower parts allows various mandibular movements, facilitates the gradual and sequential mandibular positioning, exerts delicate forces optimal to reinforce functional stimuli and exerts a delicate influence on the dentition and temporomandibular joints.

Maxillary constriction

Maxillary skeletal deficiency in the transverse plane of space is characterized by narrow width of the palatal vault and often accompanies excessive vertical growth. The correction of this problem in preadolescent patients can be accomplished by opening the mid-palatal suture, thereby increasing the transverse dimension of the maxilla, and widening the roof of the mouth and the floor of the nose. It should be recognized that the mid-palatal suture is an important growth site contributing to the normal width of the maxilla, which is active until the late teens. With increasing age, the two halves of the maxilla get tightly interdigitated at this suture, eventually making it difficult to open. The author has been able to obtain significant increments in transverse dimension of the maxilla by mid-palatal suture opening up to the age of 16 to 17 years.

In patients with constricted maxilla, normal transverse dimension of the maxilla is best achieved by orthopaedic

expansion that involves the use of a heavy force applied across the mid-palatal suture to move both halves away from each other. This may be accomplished with hyrax-type expansion screw (Fig. 6.18), by turning it twice a day, producing 0.5 mm of opening per day and delivering a force of 5 to 7 pounds, with an active treatment period of 2–3 weeks.[23] As many maxillary teeth as possible should be ideally included in the anchorage unit. The concept of rapid maxillary expansion is based upon the fact that the forces are applied to the anchorage teeth at a rate and magnitude beyond their capacity to respond. With this rate of movement, as the suture is separated faster than the bone can be deposited, the space established at the mid-palatal suture is filled initially by tissue fluids and haemorrhage. The movement of right and left halves of the maxilla away from each other becomes clinically evident by the appearance of a large diastema between the central incisors. Typically, the suture opens more anteriorly than posteriorly, probably due to the buttressing effect of the other maxillary sutures in the posterior region (Fig. 6.18C). After the desired amount of expansion—in most instances, it is over expanded until the palatal cusps of maxillary posterior teeth come in contact with the lingual inclines of the buccal cusps of the mandibular

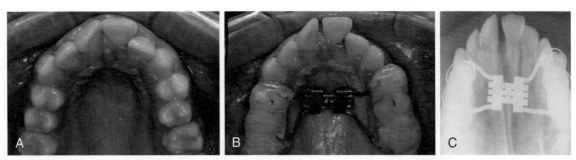

Figure 6.18 **(A)** Transverse maxillary skeletal discrepancy. **(B)** Bonded rapid palatal expansion appliance for orthopaedic expansion. The mid-palatal suture opening becomes clinically evident by the appearance of a median diastema. **(C)** The occlusal radiograph shows fan-shaped (more anterior than posterior) opening of the mid-palatal suture.

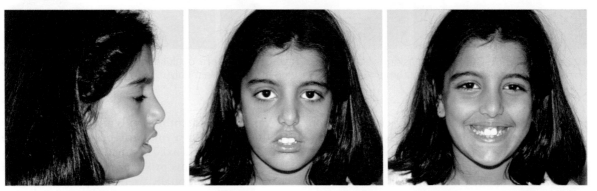

Figure 6.19 Case SW. Pretreatment facial photographs of a 10-year-old female patient showing mild facial convexity and incompetent lips, and the smile displaying dental midline discrepancy, constricted maxillary arch and excessive gingival show.

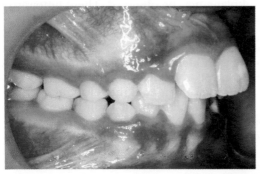

Figure 6.20 Case SW. Pretreatment intraoral photograph exhibiting mixed dentition stage, constricted maxillary arch and upper and lower arch crowding.

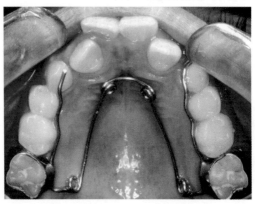

Figure 6.21 Case SW. Optimal maxillary arch expansion achieved with the quad-helix appliance.

posterior teeth—the same appliance can be used as a retainer for a period of 3–4 months. This allows the new bone to be filled in the space at the suture. During this period, every clinician should be aware of another aspect of orthopaedic expansion that orthodontic tooth movement often continues until bone stability is achieved. As the teeth are held with a rigid retainer, the two halves of the maxilla tend to move back towards each other while dental expansion is maintained. The addition of palatal flanges of acrylic to the appliance may reinforce the anchorage to help maintain the skeletal expansion effect.[24] In most instances, therefore, the net treatment effect is a combination of both skeletal and dental expansions.

Slow maxillary expansion can be accomplished by applying a force across the mid-palatal suture more slowly,

in the range of 2 to 4 pounds, depending on the age of the patient[25] (Figs 6.19–6.22). This treatment approach opens the suture at a slower rate that is closer to the speed of bone formation, resulting in almost the same net result with less trauma to the teeth and bone. Certain lingual arch appliances, like W-arch and quad-helix appliance, which deliver approximately 2 pounds of force, have been demonstrated to open the mid-palatal suture in very young patients.[26]

It is apparent that more dental change takes place during the phase of active treatment with expansion lingual arches, while rapid maxillary expansion produces more skeletal effects during the active stage. However, the overall treatment result of rapid versus slow maxillary expansion appears to be similar with slower expansion producing a

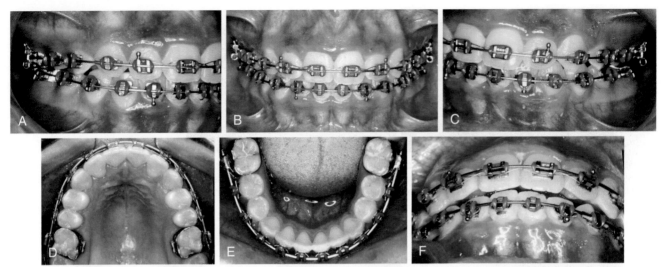

Figure 6.22   Case SW. **(A–C)** Post-expansion fixed appliance therapy to achieve occlusal goals. **(D–F)** Well-coordinated and compatible maxillary and mandibular archforms during the finishing stage of treatment.

more physiologic response. This draws clinician's attention to the fact that individuals with skeletal maxillary constriction associated with some degree of dental constriction, and obviously no pre-existing dental expansion, are the best candidates for these treatment modalities.

Orthodontic correction of dental transverse discrepancies

The treatment planning and design of mechanics for a patient with transverse discrepancies requires the differentiation between dental and skeletal problems. Various types of dental transverse problems are encountered in orthodontic practice, and their correction requires special attention. These include midline deviation with normal left and right buccal occlusion, asymmetric right and left buccal occlusion with or without midline deviation, posterior crossbite, asymmetric archforms, canted occlusal plane, etc.

Transverse problems involving asymmetric buccal occlusion

Asymmetric left and right buccal occlusion can be due to differences in molar relationship between left and right sides in all three planes of space—sagittal, transverse and vertical. Differences in molar relationship in sagittal plane, for example, Class I on one side and Class II on the other, may be associated with normal or abnormal axial inclinations of molars. Depending on the severity of a problem, these clinical situations require asymmetric treatment mechanics with or without extractions. Both non-extraction and extraction treatment approaches essentially involve differential space gaining mechanics, differential anchorage and asymmetric space consolidation mechanics. Since the management of such problems with asymmetric mechanics without producing adverse reciprocal tooth movements is a difficult and challenging task for the clinician, the author feels that the key to manage these problems is to resolve them during early stages of treatment, which allows the clinician to use symmetric mechanics during the remainder of treatment. When non-extraction treatment approach is desired, maintenance and use of leeway space and mechanics to derotate, upright and distalize the molar are helpful in re-establishing arch symmetry.

Various treatment methods are available to the orthodontist to correct asymmetric buccal occlusion resulting from an abnormal axial inclination of the molar unilaterally. To address this problem, unilateral Class II elastics have been traditionally used in association with a continuous archwire; however, this approach may cause undesirable tooth movements. Due to vertical component of the Class II elastic force, extrusion of the mandibular molars and significant canting of the maxillary anterior occlusal plane may be observed. These untoward effects essentially depend on the magnitude of force, point of force application and the duration of elastic wear. If the use of unilateral Class II elastics is the method of choice to resolve a problem, the associated unfavourable effects may be controlled by reducing the magnitude of elastic force, duration of wear and the selection of appropriate point of force application that will generate more of a sagittal and less of a vertical force vector.

Unilateral tip-back bends incorporated in the archwire have been advocated for the correction of axial inclination of molars. However, it should be noted that although a unilateral tip-back moment at the molar on the side of the tip-back bend uprights the mesially inclined molar, it also produces a unilateral intrusive force on the anterior segment of the arch, resulting in a cant of the anterior occlusal plane. This can be prevented by using a lingual or palatal arch made from 0.032″ TMA or 0.032 × 0.032″ TMA wire, which is activated to deliver a tip-forward moment on the Class I side and a tip-back moment on the Class II side, which can be easily countered by using a rigid continuous archwire in the remaining teeth.[27,28]

Asymmetric posterior occlusion caused by bodily displacement of the molars without abnormal axial inclinations or mesial drifting of molars with associated tipping that is of greater magnitude (greater than 2.0 mm) can be best managed by unilateral molar distalization. Bilateral Class II molar relationship of unequal magnitude resulting in an asymmetric buccal occlusion can be corrected by differential maxillary molar distalization to gain optimal space on both sides to create symmetric posterior occlusion and to correct associated midline deviation (Figs 6.23–6.28).

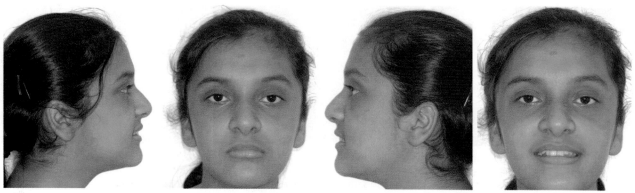

Figure 6.23 Case PM. A 15-year-old female patient exhibiting incompetent lips and no significant facial disproportions.

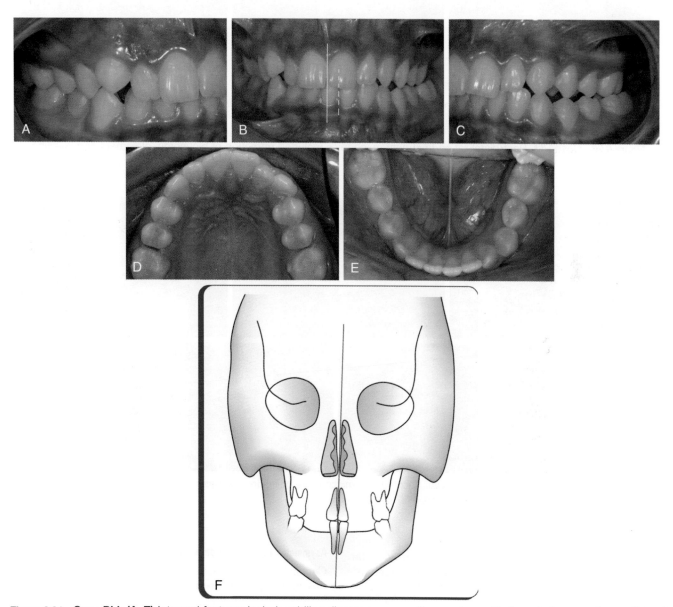

Figure 6.24 Case PM. **(A–E)** Intraoral features include midline discrepancy, maxillary and mandibular anterior crowding, unilateral posterior crossbite and Class II molars on the left side and well-developed upper and lower arches. **(F)** Pretreatment frontal cephalometric tracing showing dental midline discrepancy.

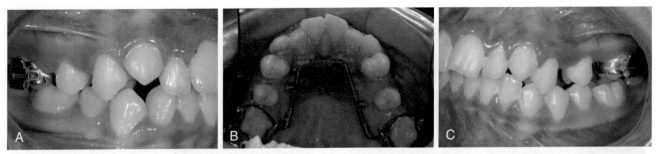

Figure 6.25 Case PM. Treatment plan included maxillary molar distalization mechanics for differential space gain to resolve anterior crowding and midline discrepancy. **(A–C)** Maxillary molars are distalized in super Class I relationship. Note the distal and buccal force direction on the left side to simultaneously distalize and to correct the molar crossbite.

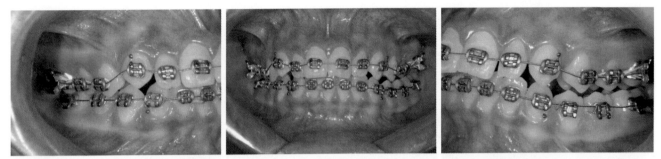

Figure 6.26 Case PM. Post-distalization treatment mechanics included retraction of bicuspids, alignment and levelling.

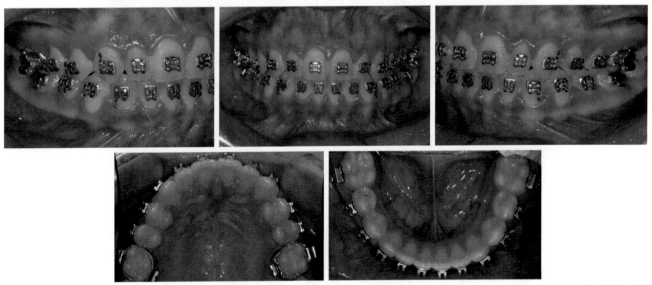

Figure 6.27 Case PM. Predebonding clinical evaluation. Dental midlines are coincident, molars and canines are in Class I relationship, proper torque, tip overbite and overjet relationship.

It is certainly true that individuals with dentoalveolar asymmetries can present some of the most biomechanically challenging situations to the clinician. It is crucial to determine whether it is a buccal segment asymmetry or an uneven crowding in the arches, which is primarily responsible for a midline deviation. One of the treatment modalities for manageing such problems with crowding is to extract a combination of teeth that will simplify intra-arch and inter-arch mechanics (Figs 6.29–6.34).

Asymmetric buccal occlusion without midline deviation

Certain local factors, like premature loss of the deciduous molar, palatal displacement of second premolars or ectopic eruption of teeth, often produce asymmetric posterior occlusion. This clinical situation is not always associated with midline deviation. The mesiopalatal rotation of the permanent molar usually accompanies its mesial migration with anterior tipping, resulting in a space loss in the posterior segment of the dental arch.

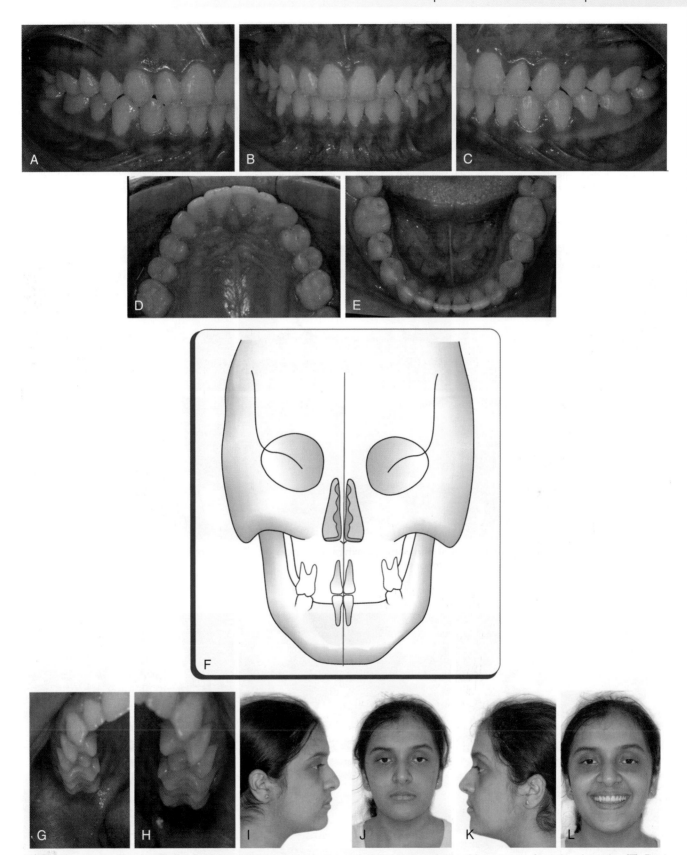

Figure 6.28 Case PM. **(A–E)** Post-treatment intraoral photographs demonstrating achievement of occlusal goals. **(F)** Post-treatment frontal cephalometric tracing showing dental symmetry. **(G and H)** Maxillary arch posterior segmental views showing optimal buccal root torque and its effect on the vertical position of buccal and palatal cusps. **(I–L)** Post-treatment facial views exhibiting normal facial proportions and pleasing smile.

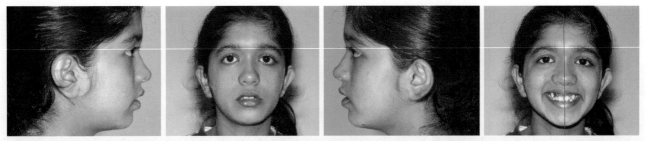

Figure 6.29 Case FM. Extraoral features of a 16-year-old female patient showing normal facial profile and proportions. Pretreatment smile displays maxillomandibular dental midline discrepancy, asymmetric vertical positioning of canines and mild cant of upper anterior occlusal plane with incisal edges of the right central and lateral incisors more incisally positioned than the left side.

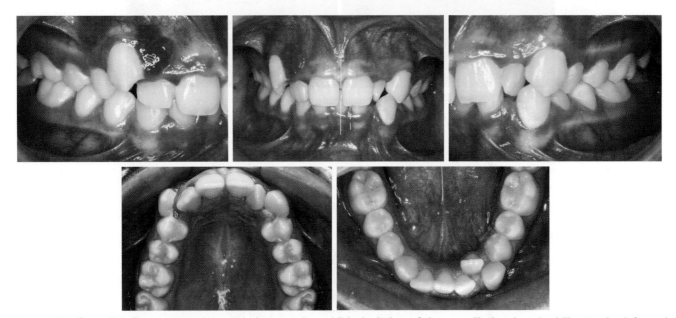

Figure 6.30 Case FM. Pretreatment intraoral photographs exhibit deviation of the mandibular dental midline to the left, and crowding of the maxillary and mandibular anterior teeth.

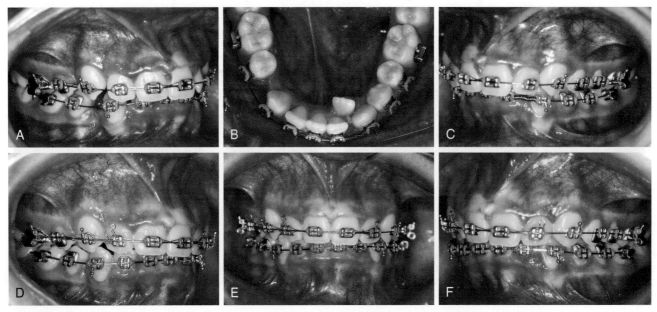

Figure 6.31 Case FM. Treatment plan involved the extraction of first bicuspids unilaterally (right side), despite the heavy crowding on the left side, to resolve midline discrepancy and crowding. **(A–F)** Asymmetric orthodontic treatment mechanics.

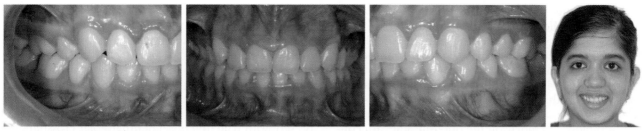

Figure 6.32 Case FM. Post-treatment intraoral photographs demonstrate proper alignment of maxillary and mandibular dental midlines, symmetric vertical positioning of maxillary canines and symmetric posterior occlusion. However, the smile exhibits excessive gingival display.

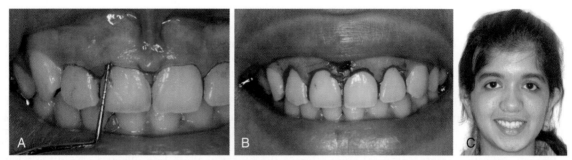

Figure 6.33 Case FM. **(A and B)** To reduce gingival display upon smile and to establish normal gingival architecture, gingivoplasty was performed in the maxillary anterior segment. **(C)** Post-gingivoplasty, smile displays optimal amount of dental and gingival components.

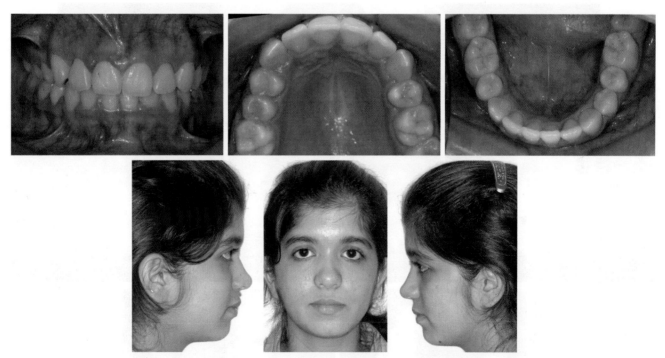

Figure 6.34 Case FM. Post-treatment intraoral and extraoral photographs.

A mild anterior tipping associated with a mesiopalatal rotation of the maxillary permanent first molar, and distal tipping of the first bicuspid, following a palatal displacement of the second bicuspid can be effectively managed by the reciprocal forces generated from the open coil spring. This also facilitates derotation of the first molar since the force is applied away from the centre of resistance of a tooth in a transverse plane. However, it is emphasized that this approach is limited to mild discrepancies, and the key is to use ultra-light forces to prevent undesirable tooth movements. If it is desired to limit the anterior movement of the first bicuspid, it can be best achieved by the use of a Nance palatal button to reinforce the anchorage. A mesial-in rotation of the maxillary first molar, of a greater magnitude, should be effectively corrected by a transpalatal arch. A transpalatal arch is made from 0.032″ TMA or 0.030″ stainless steel wire, and placed with the unilateral first-order activation. Undesirable tooth movements associated with this mechanics, like mesial tipping of the rotated molar and distal tipping of the molar on the opposite side, are controlled by including a large number of teeth in the anchorage unit, which receive a rigid segment of wire (0.017″ × 0.025″ stainless steel) from the premolar on the affected side extending to the molar on the opposite side of the dental arch.

Posterior crossbites

Dentoalveolar crossbites are caused by the displacement of a tooth or group of teeth within the dental arches or by a constriction of the arch. True unilateral posterior crossbites result from an intra-arch asymmetry; however, in most instances, these conditions are usually found, on closer examination, to be caused by a bilateral constriction of the maxillary arch and subsequent shift of the mandible to one side upon closure in habitual occlusion. Before designing definitive treatment mechanics, the clinician is required to make the appropriate distinctions between these two versions and determine the severity of the problem. More severe constriction may result in a bilateral crossbite without mandibular shift.

Various treatment modalities that are available to address these problems include heavy labial expansion arch made from 0.032″ stainless steel wire inserted in the headgear tubes, along with the main archwire in the brackets; expansion lingual arch, cross elastics and split plate–type removable appliance. Some individuals do present with true unilateral dentoalveolar crossbites that are diagnosed by making sure that unilateral crossbite exists both in centric relation and in maximum intercuspation without a mandibular shift. The best approach to deal with this situation is to move teeth in the constricted segment of the arch, involve maximum number of remaining teeth in the anchorage unit and modify the appliance accordingly.

For some reason, if the patient requires bite plate to be used along with the fixed appliance, a jackscrew may be incorporated in the appliance at the desired location to generate optimal force to move affected teeth buccally (Figs 6.35–6.40). This appliance also helps in relieving the posterior occlusion, thereby eliminating the interferences in the buccal movement of teeth. The removable appliance expands the arch almost entirely by tipping the posterior teeth buccally and causing overhanging of palatal cusps. Therefore, it is critical to establish proper buccal root torque during the finishing stage of fixed

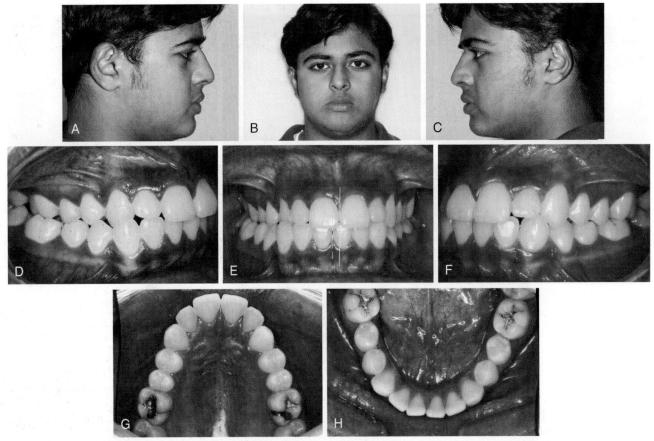

Figure 6.35 Case CK. **(A–C)** A 17-year-old male patient exhibiting normal facial proportions. **(D–F)** Pretreatment intraoral features include dental midline discrepancy (mandibular midline shifted to the right), unilateral posterior crossbite on the right side, Class I molar relationship on the right side and super Class I on the left. **(G and H)** The mandibular archform is normal; however, the maxillary archform is relatively narrow.

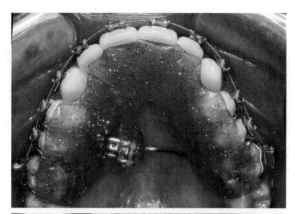

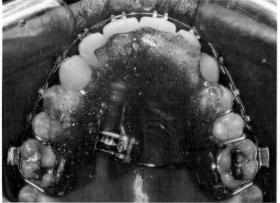

Figure 6.36 Case CK. Non-extraction treatment was planned to correct transverse discrepancies and achieve maximum intercuspation at the conclusion of treatment. Posterior biteplate with expansion screw was used by the patient to relieve the posterior occlusion and eliminate interference in the buccolingual tooth movement.

appliance therapy that will ultimately promote the maximum intercuspation and will also eliminate occlusal interferences.

Both the W-arch and the quad-helix appliance are effective, reliable and easy to use. However, the author prefers quad-helix since the extra wire incorporated in this appliance in the form of anterior and posterior helices gives it greater range of action than the W-arch. It is constructed from 0.038″ stainless steel wire and activated by widening it by 3–5 mm to produce optimal forces. Some of the salient features for effective and efficient management of bilateral dentoalveolar crossbites with the quad-helix appliance include proper appliance construction, precision in appliance activation, attention to soft tissue irritation, mild overcorrection and approximately 3 months of retention with the same appliance.

Transverse occlusal plane considerations

The goal of orthodontic treatment is to have the occlusal plane, as evaluated from the frontal view, parallel to certain facial structures and parameters, like interpupillary line. Any deviation from this relationship results in a canted anterior occlusal plane that significantly impairs the dentofacial aesthetics.

Establishing differential diagnosis of this problem is an important step before the final treatment strategy is formulated. Both maxillary and mandibular dental arches are carefully examined to find out whether the problem is limited to upper, lower or both arches, and whether it is present in the anterior or posterior segment. If both the maxillary and mandibular arches exhibit equally diverging occlusal planes in transverse direction, the use of vertical interarch elastics to extrude the abnormally positioned teeth will help in establishing the normal

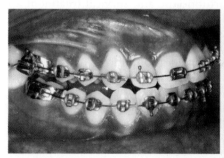
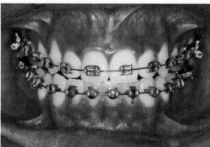
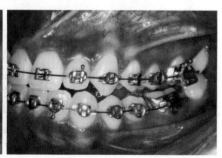

Figure 6.37 Case CK. The biteplate was discontinued after 4 months of its use. At this stage, the posterior occlusion on both the sides demonstrates an open bite that needs to be carefully settled.

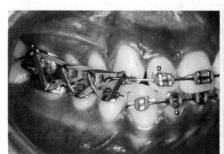
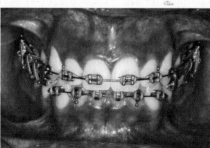
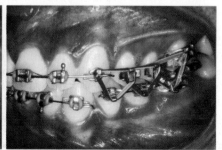

Figure 6.38 Case CK. During the finishing stage, the mandibular archwire was cut distal to cuspids on both sides and vertical elastics were employed to reduce the open bite. Later, the maxillary archwire was cut distal to the canines bilaterally and the posterior segments of the archwire were removed. Posterior vertical settling elastics were used to achieve maximum intercuspation.

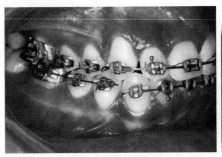
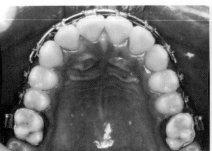
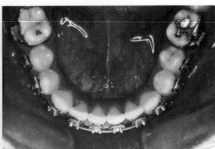

Figure 6.39 Case CK. Prebonding evaluation shows normal posterior occlusion, good intercuspation and well-coordinated and compatible maxillary and mandibular archforms.

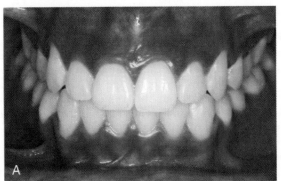

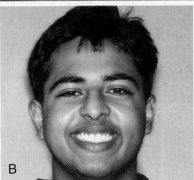

Figure 6.40 Case CK. **(A)** Post-treatment intraoral frontal view exhibits well-aligned maxillary and mandibular dental midlines and normal occlusion. **(B)** Post-treatment pleasing smile.

Skeletal transverse problems in adults

For some individuals whose transverse skeletal problems, for some reason, were not attended at an early stage of their development; or whose transverse discrepancies are so severe that neither orthopaedic correction nor camouflage offers a solution, combined orthodontic and surgical correction is the only treatment approach. Optimal correction of these problems requires a team approach and skills of the orthodontist and maxillofacial surgeons from the treatment planning process through the completion of treatment and post-treatment follow-ups.

As compared to the maxilla, the mandible provides maximum soft tissue support and plays a larger role in the development of dentofacial asymmetries.[30] In majority of cases, maxillary asymmetry is secondary to asymmetric mandibular growth, with the maxillary dental midline and the cant of the frontal occlusal plane being the parameters to measure.

An integrated orthodontic and surgical treatment approach for the correction of transverse skeletal problems essentially consists of presurgical orthodontics, surgery and postsurgical orthodontics; and neither the presurgical nor the postsurgical orthodontic treatment differs significantly from the same in other types of problems. The presurgical orthodontic treatment mechanics consisting mainly of alignment, levelling, space closure, arch width compatibility and torque control must be accomplished based upon surgical goals. One of the goals of presurgical orthodontics is to eliminate existing dental compensations for the skeletal deformity. In the transverse maxillomandibular asymmetric relationship associated with mandibular deviation, it is common to observe the maxillary dental midline shift to the deviated side of the chin and the mandibular dental midline shift to the opposite side, making the intraoral clinical condition to appear less severe.

Changes in the transverse dimension of the maxilla, either maxillary constriction or expansion, can be accomplished surgically in the course of Le Fort I downfracture surgery with relative ease and stability. Another approach to deal with skeletal maxillary constriction in adults is surgically assisted rapid palatal expansion. This procedure involves the use of bone cuts to reduce the resistance of the mid-palatal and lateral maxillary sutures without totally freeing the maxillary segments. The range of expansion or constriction, surgically, is limited

occlusal plane. However, if a canted maxillary anterior occlusal plane is due to extrusion of a group of teeth, it should be corrected with intrusion mechanics. If only one side of the anterior segment required extrusion as a part of levelling of the occlusal plane, the cantilever arch, made from 0.17″ × 0.025″ TMA, is inserted into the auxiliary tube on the first molar and tied to the anterior teeth requiring extrusion.[29] A force of approximately 30 g is considered to be optimal. Canted maxillary anterior occlusal plane due to extrusion of teeth and deep overbite can be corrected by the intrusion arch made from 0.017″ × 0.025″ TMA wire, which is tied to the segmental arch in the region of the extruded teeth.[29] A force of approximately 60 g for four maxillary incisors and approximately 50 g or less for four mandibular incisors is optimal for intrusion.

because of the temporomandibular joint articulation and problems with soft tissue management. An important decision the clinician has to make is the extent to which surgical procedure is used to correct the underlying skeletal deformity. If the mandibular asymmetry is due to unequal ramus heights, the goal of surgical procedure is to establish equal ramus lengths that are a main cause of the deformity. It has been universally acknowledged that individuals are much more concerned about the position of the chin than the mandibular angle. Based on this, an alternative approach to deal with this clinical situation is to leave unequal ramus heights untreated, and just correct a deviated chin position by inferior border osteotomy.

Individuals with skeletal Class III due to mandibular prognathism, associated with deviated chin, can be managed by differential manipulation of bony parts with bilateral sagittal split osteotomy (Figs 6.41–6.45). Since the introduction of this surgical technique by Obwegeser in 1960s, it has undergone several modifications with

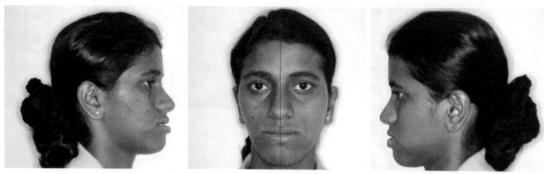

Figure 6.41 Case HC. A 19-year-old female patient with concave profile, prominent chin, mild deviation of the chin to the left and increased lower anterior face height.

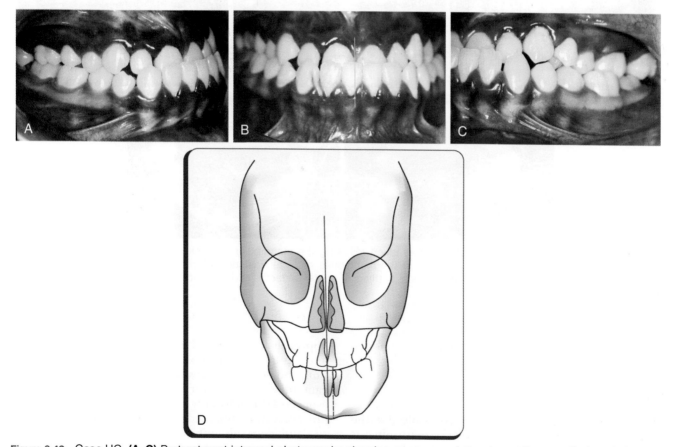

Figure 6.42 Case HC. **(A–C)** Pretreatment intraoral photographs showing reverse overjet and overbite, mandibular midline shift to the left, asymmetric posterior occlusion—Class III molar relationship on the right side is more severe than on the left—and bilateral posterior crossbite. **(D)** Pretreatment frontal cephalometric tracing showing mandibular skeletal asymmetry. This is an example of a patient demonstrating problems in all three planes of space—sagittal, vertical and transverse dimension.

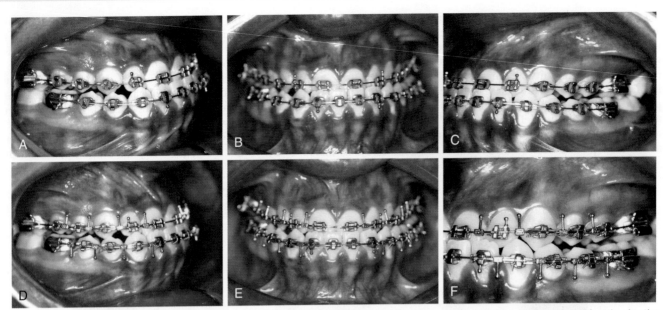

Figure 6.43 Case HC. It was decided to correct the skeletal problem in this adult patient by a combination of orthodontics and surgery. **(A–F)** Presurgical orthodontic procedures to eliminate dental compensations.

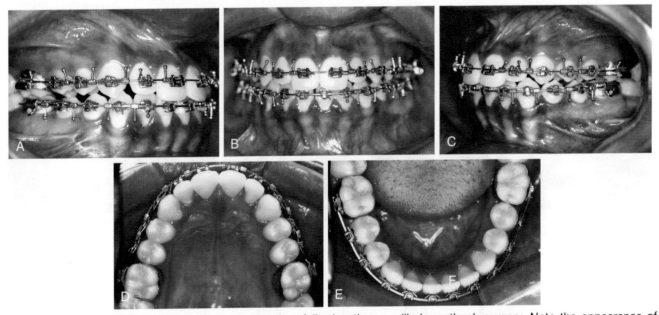

Figure 6.44 Case HC. **(A–E)** These pictures were taken following the mandibular setback surgery. Note the appearance of bilateral posterior open bite and overcorrection of the mandibular midline. Postsurgical orthodontic procedures were aimed at fine-tuning the occlusion, especially the vertical settling of posterior teeth, midline discrepancy correction and achieving normal overjet and overbite.

newer methods of reduction, stabilization and fixation of the bony segments.

Camouflage

The goal of treatment planning process involved in the management of patients with dentofacial deformities is to develop a plan that will maximize benefit to the patient. As a treatment possibility for transverse discrepancy, the clinician has to consider two important aspects of treatment—one is the comprehensive treatment

approach that is aimed at establishing normal skeletal and dental relationships for optimum aesthetics, function and long-term aesthetics; other approach is the camouflage that is directed to correct the most obvious aspects of the deformity as perceived by the society without correcting the underlying problem. The goal of camouflage treatment may emphasize the appearance rather than function and dental occlusion. For some reason, if growth modification is not possible and surgery is not considered by the patient, orthodontic and/or surgical camouflage may be considered to achieve

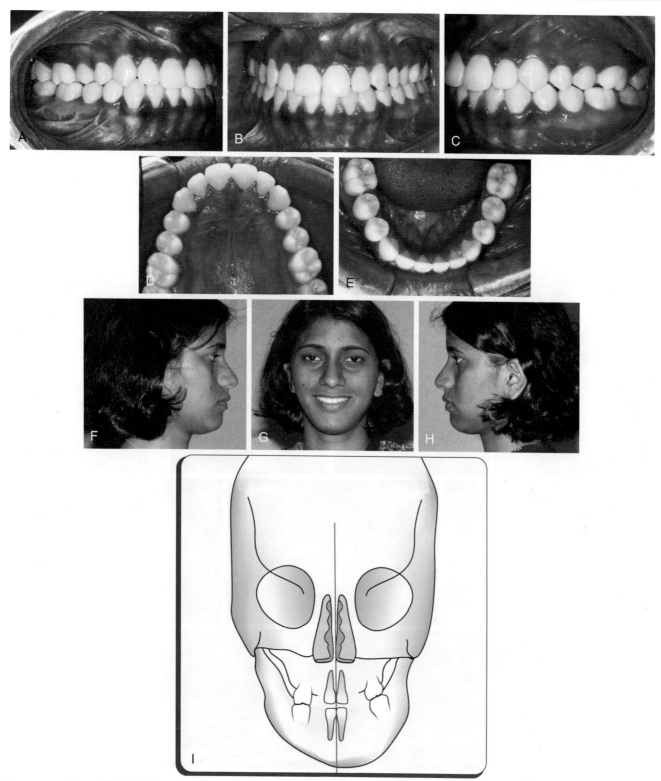

Figure 6.45 Case HC. **(A–E)** Post-treatment intraoral photographs showing normal occlusal relationship and good archforms. **(F–H)** Post-treatment facial photographs exhibit normal sagittal, vertical and transverse facial proportions. **(I)** Post-treatment frontal cephalometric tracing demonstrating dental and skeletal symmetry.

reasonable facial aesthetics (Figs 6.46–6.48). One of the important aspects of this approach is the necessity to predict the treatment outcome and whether it would be satisfactory. Surgical camouflage has been viewed as having similar goals as orthodontic camouflage to achieve reasonable aesthetics without eliminating the underlying skeletal problem. Patients with facial asymmetry exhibit considerable amount of dental compensation, to bring the dental midlines closer together than the skeletal midlines. In most instances, the deformity lies in the mandible, making the chin to deviate on the right or left side, and is often associated with the nose deviating in the same direction. Since the transverse position of the maxillary teeth is obvious, and

therefore, aesthetically important, the emphasis of camouflage treatment must be on correcting the maxillary dental midline. The correction of skeletal midlines is possible only with jaw surgery, and the mandibular midline, in contrast, is seen only on close observation. Surgical camouflage procedures, like genioplasty to reposition the chin laterally and rhinoplasty to correct nasal deviation, are performed to conceal the underlying jaw deformity. As these procedures involve minimal surgery, when compared with bilateral mandibular ramus osteotomy or a Le Fort I osteotomy, they are considered a part of surgical camouflage. The key to this treatment modality is the clinician's judgment as to whether the best treatment plan is to correct the underlying deformity or just conceal it.

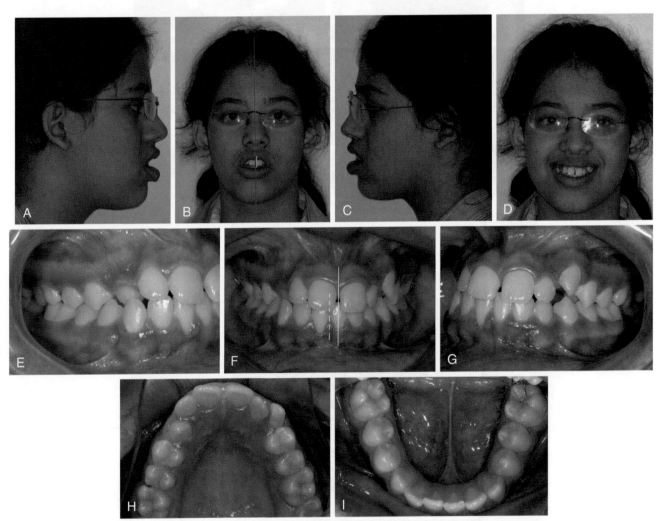

Figure 6.46 Case MR. **(A–D)** Pretreatment extraoral photographs demonstrating incompetent lips, significant increase in lower anterior facial height and deviation of the chin to the right side. **(E–I)** Pretreatment intraoral photographs exhibit mandibular dental midline shift to the right side, maxillary right canine in crossbite, maxillary left canine high labially placed and mild crowding of the upper and lower anterior teeth.

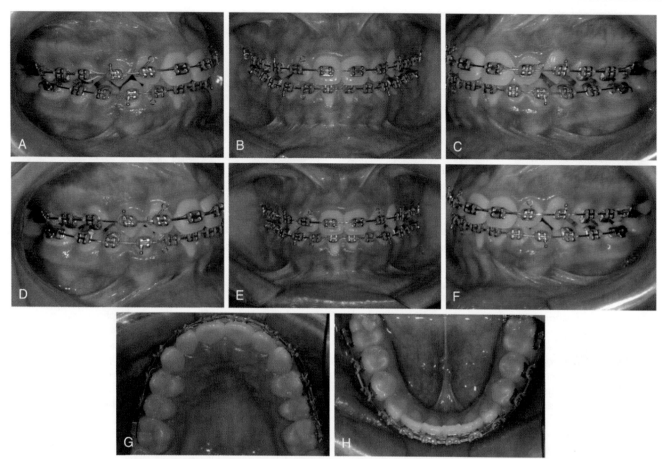

Figure 6.47 Case MR. As the patient was not keen to undergo any surgical procedure to resolve the underlying skeletal discrepancy, orthodontic camouflage was considered to be the final treatment plan. The treatment goals were to align maxillary dental midline with the facial midline, correct canine crossbite, align teeth and position the mandibular dental midline as close to the facial midline as possible. **(A–C)** Transitional orthodontic treatment. **(D–H)** Finishing stage.

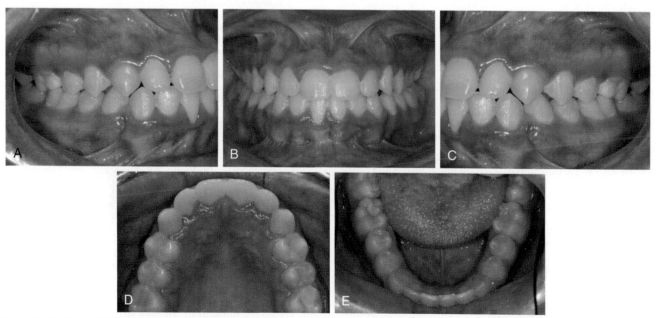

Figure 6.48 Case MR. **(A–E)** Post-treatment intraoral photographs showing considerable improvement in the occlusal relationships of teeth and well-coordinated maxillary and mandibular archforms.

Continued

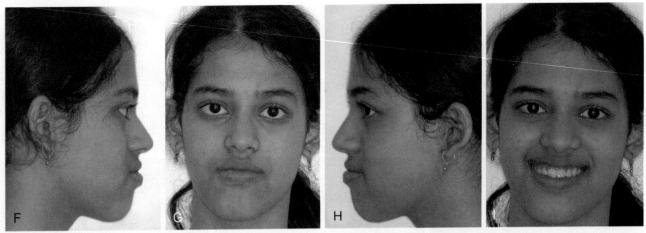

Figure 6.48, cont'd   (F–I) Post-treatment facial photographs showing significant improvement in facial aesthetics.

CONCLUSION

Transverse discrepancies warrant special consideration in the orthodontic diagnosis and treatment planning. Patients with these problems pose special diagnostic and biomechanical challenges to the clinician. Determination of the underlying cause of the asymmetric or symmetric transverse problem must be an important ingredient in the process of formulation of an appropriate treatment plan. Depending upon the structures involved, these problems may be primarily dental, skeletal or functional in origin or may even have a combination of these factors present. It is equally important to determine the relationship of the transverse discrepancy with the sagittal and vertical problems, which often have a significant impact on designing a treatment strategy. Various treatment options that are available to address broad spectrum of transverse discrepancies include early elimination of deflective contacts causing mandibular shift in functional problems, orthopaedic correction of skeletal discrepancies, extraction or non-extraction treatment modalities to resolve dental problems, orthosurgical approach for the correction of severe skeletal problems in adults and orthodontic and/or surgical camouflage. The appliance design must be based on sound biomechanical principles, and it should utilize the appropriate force system to address the transverse discrepancy while simultaneously preventing undesirable tooth movements.

REFERENCES

1. Lundstrom A. Some asymmetries of the dental arches, jaws and skull, and their etiological significance. Am J Orthod 1961; 47:81–106.
2. Vagervik K. Orthodontic management of unilateral cleft lip and palate. Cleft Palate J 1981; 18:256–269.
3. Boder E. A common form of facial asymmetry in the newborn infant: its etiology and orthodontic significance. Am J Orthod 1953; 39:895–910.
4. Erickson GE, Waite DE. Mandibular asymmetry. J Am Dent Assoc 1974; 89:1369–1373.
5. Keen RR, Callahan GR. Osteochondroma of the mandibular condyle: report of case. J Oral Surg 1977; 35:140.
6. Nanda R, Margolis MJ. Treatment strategies for midline discrepancies. Semin Orthod 1996; 2:84–89.
7. Lewis PD. The deviated midline. Am J Orthod 1976; 70:601–616.
8. Graber LW, Lucker GW. Dental esthetic self-evaluation and satisfaction. Am J Orthod 1980; 77:163–173.
9. Hulsey CM. An esthetic evaluation of lip-teeth relationships present in the smile. Am J Orthod 1970; 57:132–144.
10. Burstone CJ. Distinguishing developing malocclusion from normal occlusion. Dent Clin North Am 1964; July: 479–491.
11. Faber RD. The differential diagnosis and treatment of crossbites. Dent Clin North Am 1981; 25:53–68.
12. Persson M. Mandibular asymmetry of hereditary origin. Am J Orthod 1973; 63:1–11.
13. Bart RS, Kopf AW. Tumor Conference #20: hemifacial atrophy. J Dermatol Surg Oncol 1978; 4(12):908–909.
14. Eubanks RJ. Surgical correction of masseter muscle hypertrophy associated with unilateral prognathism: report of case. J Oral Surg 1957; 15:66.
15. Arnett WG, Bergman RT. Facial keys to orthodontic diagnosis and treatment planning – part II. Am J Othod Dentofac Orthop 1990. 103:395–411.
16. Grummons DC, Kappeyne Van De Coppello MA. A frontal asymmetry analysis. JCO 1987; 21(7):448–465.
17. Ricketts RM. Perspectives in the clinical application of cephalometrics. Angle Orthod 1981; 51(2):115–150.
18. Burstone CJ. Diagnosis and treatment planning of patients with asymmetries. Semin Orthod 1998; 4:153–164.
19. Gorney M, Harries T. The preoperative and postoperative consideration of natural facial asymmetry. Plast Recontsr Surg 1974; 54:187.
20. Schroder I, Schroder U. Early treatment of unilateral posterior skeletal crossbite in the primary dentition. J Dent Res 1981; 60:516.
21. Kutin G, Hawes R. Posterior cross-bites in the deciduous and mixed dentitions. Am J Othod 1969; 56:491–504.
22. Graber TM, Neumann B. The activator: use and modifications. In: Graber TM, Neumann B, eds. Removable orthodontic appliances. 2nd edn. Philadelphia: W.B. Saunders; 1984. 198–243.
23. Proffit WR, Fields HW. Treatment of skeletal problems in preadolescent children. In: Proffit WR, Fields HW, eds. Contemporary orthodontics. St Louis: C.V. Mosby; 1986. 354–398.
24. Haas AJ. The treatment of maxillary deficiency by opening the midpalatal suture. Angle Orthod 1965; 35:200–217.
25. Hicks EP. Slow maxillary expansion: a clinical study of the skeletal versus dental response to low-magnitude force. Am J Orthod 1978; 73:121–141.
26. Bell R, Lecompte E. The effects of maxillary expansion using a quad helix appliance during the deciduous and mixed dentitions. Am J Orthod 1981; 79:152–161.
27. Burstone CJ. Precision lingual arches, active applications. J Clin Orthod 1989; 22:101–109.
28. Romeo DA, Burstone CJ. Tip back mechanics. Am J Orthod 1977; 72:414–421.
29. van Steenbergen E, Nanda R. Biomechanics of Orthodontic correction of dental asymmetries. Am J Orthod Dentofac Orthop 1995; 107:618–624.
30. Legan Harry L. Surgical correction of patients with asymmetries. Semin Orthod 1998; 4:189–198.

Surgical Orthodontics

7

NR Krishnaswamy and Prasanna K Shivapuja

People today usually recognize irregular teeth or obvious jaw deformities and seek treatment from an orthodontist, who can improve teeth alignment, function and facial aesthetics. More severe deformities that cannot be addressed with orthodontics alone will require a combination of surgical and orthodontic corrections and are called dentofacial deformities. These deformities can affect facial aesthetics and function in several ways and would require combined orthodontic and orthognathic surgical treatment.

Several factors presenting either collectively or individually may indicate the need for combined orthodontic and surgical treatment. They include impaired mastication, temporomandibular pain and dysfunction, oral respiration due to lack of lip competency, impaired speech and susceptibility to caries and periodontal disease. Although the functional impediment is important, the most common reason for patients seeking surgical correction and the most important indication of the need for orthognathic surgery are usually the psychosocial effects resulting from the unaesthetic appearance from the dentofacial deformity.

Because of rapid advances in both orthodontics and maxillofacial surgery, it is now possible to treat patients with dentofacial deformities to produce outstanding results that are aesthetically and functionally efficient. This, with the advent of modern computing skills and with the availability of more reliable video and computer imaging softwares, makes it not only possible for the surgeon and the orthodontist to interact better but also facilitates the patient to perceive the outcome of the treatment procedure, making the patient a partner in the treatment planning processes.

Ackerman and Proffit[1] have further recommended that the clinician might ignore the limitations of the soft tissue in guiding the treatment planning processes.

These constraints include the pressure exerted on the teeth by the surrounding soft tissue envelope and the tongue, the temporomandibular joint including the muscles that play a major role in function and the periodontal apparatus. Superimposed on all these is the dynamic soft tissue integrity of the entire face.[1]

There are only three alternatives for treating patients with severe skeletal or dentofacial deformity.[2]

1. *Growth modification in a growing child:* Although recent outcome studies[3] of growth modification using orthopaedic forces and functional appliances are skeptical about the quantum of additional growth that can be obtained by using this approach, it is still a popular choice because the direction and expression of growth can be reasonably modified (Fig. 7.1).
2. *Orthodontic camouflage:* In non-growing individuals, where the skeletal dysplasia is not very severe, the axial inclination of the teeth can be modified to mask the severity of the underlying malocclusion (Fig. 7.2).
3. *Orthognathic surgery:* Once growth is complete, orthognathic surgery in conjugation with orthodontics becomes the only option to correct the severe jaw discrepancy (Fig. 7.3). It is indicated in those patients who have

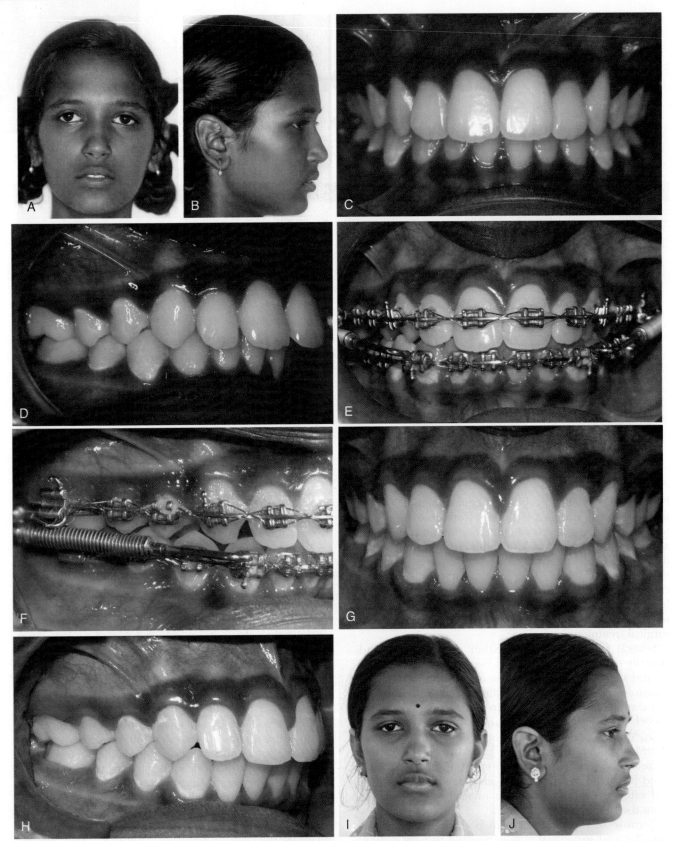

Figure 7.1 Case VP. Growth modifications in a growing child with a retrusive mandible. (**A** and **B**) Pretreatment facial photographs. (**C** and **D**) Pretreatment intraoral photographs. (**E** and **F**) Fixed functional device to modify mandibular growth. (**G** and **H**) Post-treatment intraoral photographs. (**I** and **J**) Post-treatment facial photographs.

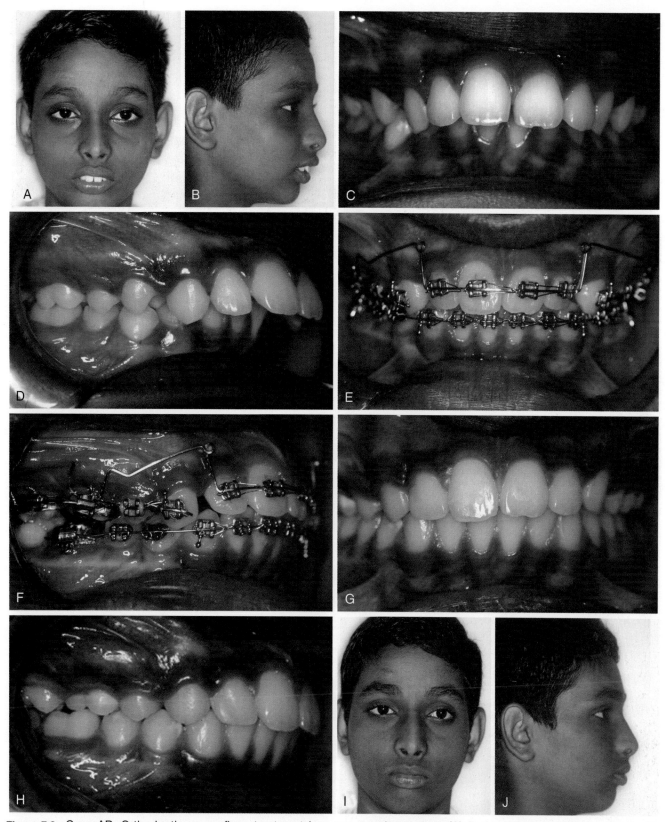

Figure 7.2 Case AR. Orthodontic camouflage treatment in a non-growing patient. **(A)** Pretreatment frontal view. **(B)** Profile view. **(C and D)** Occlusion. **(E and F)** The dentition was compensated to camouflage the skeletal malocclusion. **(G and H)** Post-treatment occlusion reveals good reduction in overjet with molars in Angle Class II and canines in Class I relationship. **(I and J)** Post-treatment facial view revealing good soft tissue balance despite a convex profile.

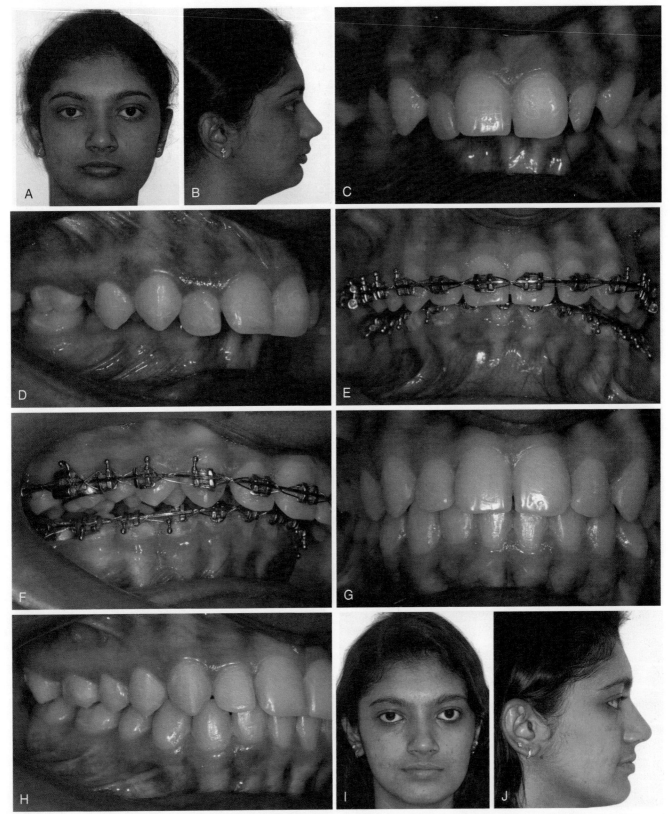

Figure 7.3 Case EN (21 years 4 months). (**A** and **B**) Facial view prior to treatment showing short vertical facial height and anteroposterior deficiency of the mandible. (**C** and **D**) Pretreatment occlusion revealing 100% deep overbite and increased overjet. (**E** and **F**) Presurgical orthodontic preparation to decompensate the dentition. (**G** and **H**) Occlusion at the completion of treatment. (**I** and **J**) Facial view at the completion of mandibular advancement surgery; note the increase in facial height, reduction in facial convexity and improvement in soft tissue balance.

completed growth phase, in whom growth modification becomes unviable or in those patients with severe skeletal discrepancy wherein orthodontic camouflage will not mask the severity of the skeletal disproportion.

While the choice between growth modification and orthognathic surgery depends upon the growth status of the individual, the choice between camouflage and combined orthodontics and orthognathic surgery depends not only on the severity of the jaw discrepancy but also on other aesthetic parameters. Ackerman and Proffit[4] have enumerated some common denominators of relative dentofacial attractiveness or unattractiveness, which can be used as a guideline to decide between surgery and camouflage. These parameters include the following:

1. It is permissible to procline the upper and lower incisors in patients who have a large nose or a large chin, provided the labiomental fold does not become excessive.
2. Moderate mandibular deficiency is well accepted by the lay public, and the mandibular deficiency can be camouflaged by orthodontic treatment, thereby avoiding mandibular advancement.
3. The prominence of the upper lip is influenced by the position of the upper incisors. Retracting of maxillary incisors reduces the prominence of the upper lip, and an important guideline for orthodontist is that the maxillary incisors should not be retracted to a point that the inclination of the upper lip to true vertical line (TVL) becomes negative. Hence, in patients who already have a retrusive upper lip, it is better to procline the incisors, even if it involves orthognathic surgery to correct the malocclusion.
4. Displaying moderate amount of gingiva adds to the attractiveness of the smile. Orthodontic camouflage should not be undertaken, if the quantum of incisor retraction will lead to excessive gingival display. Orthognathic surgery would be a better option in patients with vertical maxillary excess.
5. Patients who have lower lip trap, resulting in a curled or everted lower lip, can often be treated with orthodontics alone by retracting the upper incisors.
6. A concave profile with thinning of upper lip and lack of vermilion show is an unaesthetic trait and can be corrected by proclining the upper incisors, as proclination of upper incisors will lead to creating fuller lips that is perceived to be more attractive.
7. While moderate midface deficiency can be camouflaged with orthodontics, severe midface deficiency or severe mandibular prognathism creates unattractive lip position and affects throat form. These conditions are best addressed by surgery and orthodontics.
8. Bidental proclination is an unaesthetic trait resulting in excessive lip protrusion; extraction of premolar and orthodontic retraction of incisors will often result in dramatic reduction of lip protrusion.

In general, patients in whom growth is completed, with a reverse overjet of greater than 3 mm, or Class II patients with an overjet of greater than 10 mm, a mandibular body length of less than 70 mm or a facial height of greater than 125 mm can be treated only by orthognathic surgery.

DIAGNOSIS AND TREATMENT PLANNING

Orthognathic surgery is the art and science of diagnosis, treatment planning and execution of treatment by combining orthodontics and oral and maxillofacial surgery to correct skeletal, dental and soft tissue deformities of the jaws and associated structures. Problem-oriented diagnosis and treatment planning approach is a well-established approach in orthodontics and maxillofacial surgery and can be used in patients who are candidates for orthognathic surgery. The method involves collecting adequate information about the patient and distilling from it. The information can then be used to generate a problem list and outline the treatment strategy. The sequence of database collection and treatment planning is outlined in Flowchart 7.1.

Patient's chief concern

A patient's ultimate satisfaction with treatment outcome depends on attention to the patient's chief concern. Understanding the patient's concern, motivations and expectations will help define treatment parameters. It will also help in identifying patients with unrealistic expectations. It is important that patients thoroughly understand all treatment options, expected outcomes and potential risks and complications. Situations in which a patient is uninformed or has unrealistic expectations often result in dissatisfaction.

General patient evaluation

Orthognathic surgery is usually performed on healthy patients. This does not, however, diminish the importance of presurgical evaluation, including medical and dental histories, physical examination and appropriate investigations. Patient examination should rule out or identify patients with airway problems, autoimmune diseases, bleeding disorders or other pathological conditions that may complicate the surgery.

Psychological evaluation

A major reason that patients seek treatment for dentofacial problems is to overcome social handicaps resulting from an abnormal facial appearance. Most often, the motive for patients seeking treatment is due to their feeling of inadequacy and discontent that their facial appearance creates for them.

It is well recognized that physical attractiveness is associated with socially desirable characteristics. In general symmetric faces, straight profile and facial proportions that are close to the population average are considered to be attractive. Women are judged less attractive, if their faces are skeletal Class III, and men are judged more negative, if their faces are skeletal Class II. An individual's response to facial appearance depends on a complex interplay of behaviours, attitudes and beliefs. Because of these strong psychosocial issues, it is imperative that the clinician makes an attempt to

Planning for Orthognathic Surgery

```
                    ┌─────────────────────────┐
                    │  Patient's Chief Concern │
                    └─────────────────────────┘
                                 │
  ┌──────────────────┐          ▼                      ┌──────────────┐
  │ General Patient  │◄─────────────────────────┬─────►│   Frontal    │
  │   Evaluation     │     ┌──────────────┐      │      └──────────────┘
  └──────────────────┘     │    Facial    │──────┤      ┌──────────────┐
           │               │ Examination  │      └─────►│   Profile    │
           ▼               └──────────────┘             └──────────────┘
  ┌──────────────────┐            │
  │   Medical and    │            ▼                      ┌──────────────┐
  │ Dental History   │     ┌──────────────┐      ┌──────►│   Maxillary  │
  └──────────────────┘     │   Intraoral  │──────┤       └──────────────┘
                           │ Examination  │      ├──────►│  Mandibular  │
                           └──────────────┘      │       └──────────────┘
                                  │              └──────►│   Interarch  │
                                  ▼                      └──────────────┘
                           ┌──────────────┐
                           │  Functional  │
                           │ Examination  │
                           └──────────────┘
                                  │
                                  ▼
                        ┌──────────────────┐
                        │  Gnathological   │
                        │   Examination    │
                        └──────────────────┘
```

Flowchart 7.1 Sequence of database collection and planning treatment.

evaluate the psychology of the patient during the initial examination.

Facial evaluation

The clinical assessment of the face is probably the most valuable of all diagnostic procedures.[5] Primary emphasis should be placed on frontal aesthetics, since this is how people see themselves. Balance and proportions between the various facial structures in the individual are more important than numeric values. The patient should be examined in natural head posture,[6] with the teeth in centric occlusion and lips relaxed (Fig. 7.4).

Frontal analysis

From the frontal view, it is particularly important to assess facial form, transverse dimensions, facial symmetry and the vertical relationship in the upper, middle and lower thirds of the face and the lips. Normative values for selected facial dimensions are provided in Table 7.1.

Facial form

The relationship between the facial width and the facial height has a strong influence on facial harmony. The height to width proportion is 1.31 for females

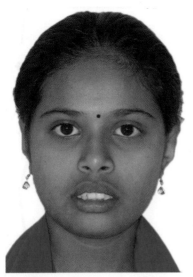

Figure 7.4 Frontal facial evaluation should be done with the patient adopting a natural head posture, with the teeth in centric occlusion and the lips in relaxed posture.

Table 7.1   Normal values for selected facial dimensions

Parameters	Male	Female
Zygomatic width (zy–zy; mm)	137 (4.3)	130 (5.3)
Gonial width (go–go)	97 (5.8)	91 (5.9)
Intercanthal distance	33 (2.7)	32 (2.4)
Pupil–midfacial distance	33 (2.0)	32 (1.8)
Nasal base width	35 (2.6)	31 (1.9)
Mouth width	53 (3.3)	50 (3.2)
Face height (N–gn)	121 (6.8)	112 (5.2)
Lower face height (subnasal–gn)	72 (6.0)	66 (4.5)
Upper lip vermilion	8.9 (1.5)	8.4 (1.3)
Lower lip vermilion	10.4 (1.9)	9.7 (1.6)
Nasolabial angle (degrees)	99 (8.0)	99 (8.7)
Nasofrontal angle (degrees)	131 (8.1)	134 (1.8)

N – nasion; gn – gnathion.

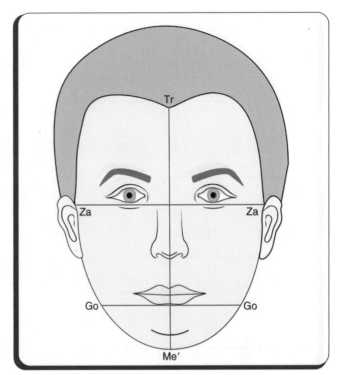

Figure 7.5 Facial form. The facial height (trichion to soft tissue menton and bizygomatic width [Za–Za]) should be 1.3:1 in females and 1.35:1 in males. Bigonial width (Go–Go) should be approximately 30% less than the bizygomatic width.

lines at the hairline, glabella, nasal base and the menton (Fig. 7.6). Orthognathic surgery does not alter the upper one-third, but the structures in the middle and lower thirds influence the facial aesthetics and are affected by surgery.

2. *Middle third:* The nose and the centre of the lips should fall along a TVL that coincides with the chin in the lower third of the face. Generally, no sclera is seen above or below the iris. However, patients with midface deficiency tend to show sclera below the iris. Sequential evaluation of the cheekbones, paranasal areas and alar eminences should be performed and correlated to the upper lip. The cheek bone–nasal base–lip contour is a convenient contour line to evaluate the harmony of the structures of the midface (zygoma, maxilla and nasal base) with the paranasal area and the upper lip (Fig. 7.7). This line starts just anterior to the ear, extends forward through the cheek bone and then runs anteroinferiorly over the maxilla adjacent to the alar base of the nose, ending lateral to the commissure of the mouth. The line should form a smooth, continuing curve (Fig. 7.8). An interruption of the curve may be an indication of an apparent skeletal deformity. Interruption of the line in the maxillary area denotes a maxillary anteroposterior deficiency, while an interruption in the lower portion of the curve usually occurs in patients with mandibular excess.

Lower third of the face

The middle third to lower third vertical height of the face should have a 5:6 ratio. The upper lip length should make up one-third of the lower third facial height.

and 1.351 for males. The bigonial width should be approximately 30% less than the bizygomatic dimension (Fig. 7.5).

Short square facial types are often associated with a Class II deep bite malocclusion, vertical maxillary deficiency, masseteric hyperplasia and macrogenia, while long narrow facial types are often associated with vertical maxillary excess, narrow nose, mandibular anteroposterior deficiency, microgenia and anterior open bite malocclusion.

Vertical dimension

1. *Facial thirds:* The ideal face in both males and females is divided vertically into equal thirds by horizontal

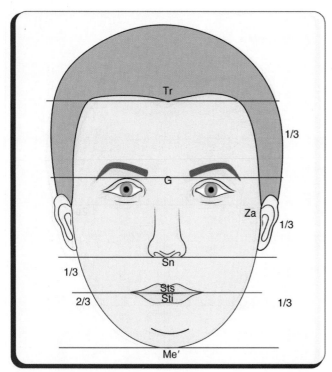

Figure 7.6 Facial third. The distance from trichion (Tr) to glabella (G), G to subnasale (Sn) and Sn to soft tissue menton (Me') should be even. The lower third can be divided into upper one-third, from Sn to stomion superioris (Sts), and lower two-thirds, from stomion inferioris (Sti) to Me'.

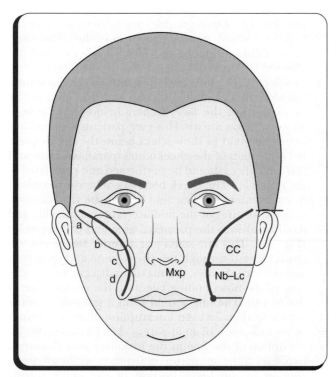

Figure 7.7 Cheek bone–nasal base–lip contour. Cheek bone area can be further divided into three parts: (a) Zygomatic area, (b) Middle area and (c) Subpapillary area. Mxp—the maxillary point is the most medial point in the curvature. The nasal base–upper lip contour (Nb–Lc) extends from Mxp. The line should curve gently without interruption, ending lateral to the contour of the mouth.

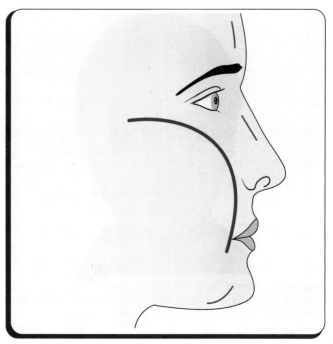

Figure 7.8 The line should form a smooth continuing curve; it starts anterior to the ear and ends lateral to the commissure of the mouth.

Normal upper lip length is 20 ± 2 mm for females and 22 ± 2 mm for males when measured from subnasale to upper lip inferior. Lower lip length is 40 ± 2 mm for females and 44 ± 2 mm for males when measured from lower lip superior to soft tissue menton.

In the middle third, philtrum height is important, especially in its relationship with the upper incisor and the commissure of the mouth. Commissure height normally is not more than 2–3 mm greater than the philtrum height in adults, but in adolescents, the philtrum height may be several millimetres shorter.

Tooth-to-lip relationship

As a general guideline in adolescents, the entire clinical crown of the upper incisor and some gingiva should be visible on smile, while at rest 3–4 mm of maxillary incisor should be displayed[7] (Fig. 7.9). Excessive tooth display may be a result of both hard and soft tissue factors and could be due to: (a) short philtrum height, (b) vertical maxillary excesses, (c) excessive crown height and (d) lingually tipped maxillary incisors. While inadequate incisor display is caused due to: (a) excessive philtrum height, (b) vertical maxillary deficiency, (c) inadequate crown height and (d) flared maxillary incisors.

The incisor display must be correlated with the age of the patient. Due to the difference in the underlying skeletal growth, the lip separation and consequently the quantum of incisor display at rest and smile tends to change with age.

It is normal for children to exhibit lip separation at rest since the soft tissue growth is incomplete. Lips grow earlier in girls than in boys with a cephalocaudal gradient growth in the soft tissue as in the skeleton.

According to Nanda,[8] during childhood and adolescence, the soft tissues of the lower face grow more and

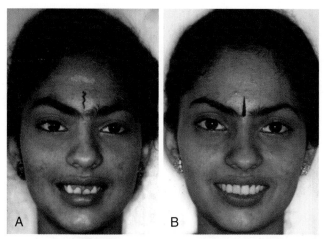

Figure 7.9 Case RA. Optimal tooth to lip relationship **(A)** Excessive incisal and gingival display at rest. **(B)** Posttreatment photograph revealing optimal tooth and lip relationship.

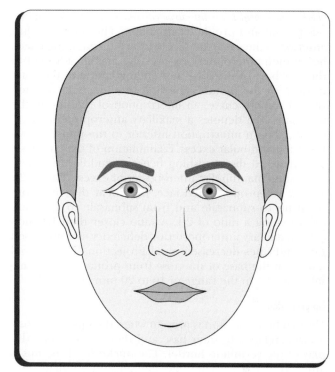

Figure 7.10 Rule of fifth. The transverse relationship of the face is best described by the rule of fifth. The rule emphasizes the total dentofacial area and is based on proportional relationship and not on absolute values.

for a longer time than those of the upper face. Most of the vertical growth of the upper lip is achieved in females by the age of 14 years, whereas the lower lip continues to grow vertically till the age of 16 years. In males, growth of both the upper and the lower lips continues into late teens with more growth of the lower lip.

Transverse dimension

The transverse relationship of the face is best described by the 'rule of fifths'. The face is divided sagittally into five symmetric and equal parts; from helix to helix of the outer ears, each approximating the width of the eye. The outer fifth is measured from the centre helix of the ears to the outer canthus of the eyes. The medial two-fifths of the face are measured from the outer to the inner canthus of the eyes.

The outer border should coincide with the gonial angle of the mandible. Within the medial fifths, it should be noted that the width of the mouth should approximate the distance between the inner margins of the irides of the eyes (Fig. 7.10).

The middle fifth is delineated by the inner canthus of the eyes. The ala of the nose should coincide with these lines. For patients in whom maxillary advancement and superior repositioning are considered and the ala falls outside of the lines, control of alar width is indicated.

Profile analysis

It is helpful to focus on the middle and lower thirds of the face alone in profile since orthognathic surgery does not influence the upper third of the face. A systematic examination of the lower third of the face includes evaluation of the following.

Nose and paranasal areas

The nose is the dominant structure in the profile, and its size and projection must be considered in the context of lip and chin projection[9] (Fig. 7.11). The dorsum is normal, convex or concave. The projection of the nasal bridge should be anterior to the globus (5–8 mm). The nasal tip must be slightly triangular with a distinct break

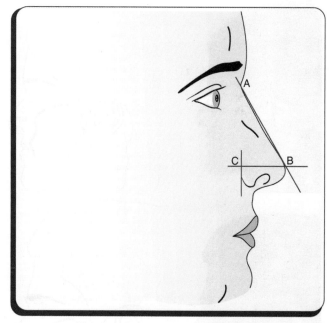

Figure 7.11 The nasal tip projection. If BC is greater than 55–60% of AB, the the nasal tip is considered disproportionate (method of Goode).

in contour between the supratip and the infratip and the columella.

It is important to note the prominence of the paranasal area of the maxilla. The cheeks should exhibit a general convexity from cheek bone apex to the commissure of the mouth. This line of convexity, referred to as *cheek bone–nasal bone–lip curve contour* requires simultaneous frontal and profile examination. The line starts just anterior to the ear, extending forward through the cheek bone, then anteroinferiorly over the maxilla adjacent to the alar base of the nose and ending lateral to the commissure of the mouth. The line should be an uninterrupted smooth curve; an interruption of the line in the maxillary area denotes a maxillary anteroposterior deficiency, and an interruption inferior to the upper lip denotes a mandibular excess. Examination of the paranasal area helps in distinguishing between middle third deficiency and mandibular anteroposterior excess (Fig. 7.12).

In a well-proportioned face, the linear distance from nasal tip to subnasale and from subnasale to alar base must exhibit a ratio of 2:1. A ratio closer than 1:1 indicates maxillary anteroposterior deficiency. An increased ratio indicates decreased nasal projection. The normal length of the base of the nose from pronasale to subnasale must be in the range of 16 to 20 mm (Fig. 7.13).

Lip projection

Normal lip projection is present when the lips are slightly everted relative to their base and there is adequate display of the vermilion border. The thickness of the lips is affected by the patient's age, gender and ethnicity. Further, the hard tissue support of the lips is a recognized determinant of lip position; the current standard is that,

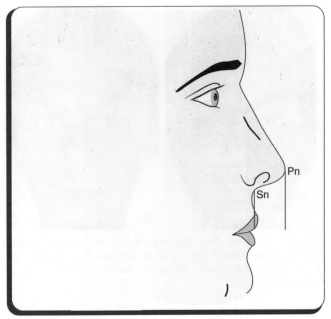

Figure 7.13 Nasal projection. The projection of the nose is measured horizontally from pronasale to subnasale. The normal value is 16–20 mm.

dental protrusion is not excessive unless the lips are both everted and separated at rest.

The anteroposterior lip position may be assessed with the help of a line from subnasale to pogonion, which is referred to as the *lower facial plane*. The lower facial plane is an important guide in assessing the lip position and planning the orthodontic and surgical positioning of the incisors, as well as the surgical positioning of the chin. The upper lip should be 3 ± 1 mm ahead of this plane, and the lower lip should be 2 ± 1 mm ahead of this plane. This assessment is also influenced by the anteroposterior position of the chin and the soft tissue thickness of the lips (Fig. 7.14).

Labiomental fold

The lower lip–chin contour should have a gentle 'S' curve, with a lower lip–chin angle of at least 130° (Fig. 7.15). In Class II cases with mandibular deficiency, the angle is acute because of impingement of the maxillary incisors on the lower lip or macrogenia. The angle is flattened in individuals with microgenia or lower lip tension caused by Class III malocclusion. The assessment of the labiomental fold is very crucial in deciding on genioplasty.

Nasolabial angle

The nasolabial angle, measured between the inclination of the columella and the upper lip, should be in the range of 85°–105° (Fig. 7.16). Larger nasolabial angles in females and smaller nasolabial angles in males are considered to be aesthetically pleasing. In patients with Class III relationship, the angle is acute and tends to be obtuse in patients with Class II sagittal relationship. Retraction of upper incisors should be avoided in individuals with large nasolabial angle and surgical repositioning of the maxilla also affects the nasolabial angle. In general, the maxilla should never be moved posteriorly, especially in combination with superior repositioning. This surgical movement will result in loss of lip support, increase in nasolabial angle, increase in nasal projection and flaring of the nasal base.

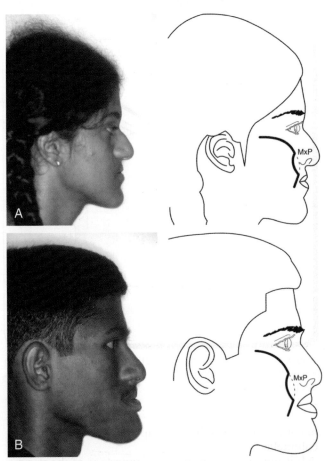

Figure 7.12 Cheek bone–nasal bone–lip curve contour. The line should be an uninterrupted smooth curve. **(A)** Interruption of the line in the maxillary area denotes maxillary anteroposterior deficiency. **(B)** Interruption inferior to the upper lip denotes mandibular excess.

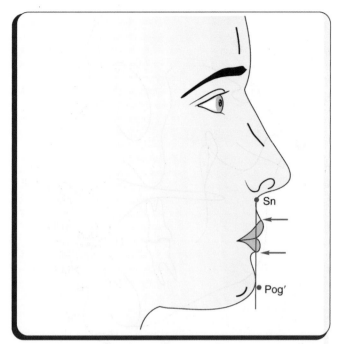

Figure 7.14 Lip projection. The position of the lip is assessed from drawing a line, from Sn to Pog'; ideally, the upper lip must be 3 ± 1 mm ahead of the line and the lower lip must be 2 ± 1 mm ahead of this line.

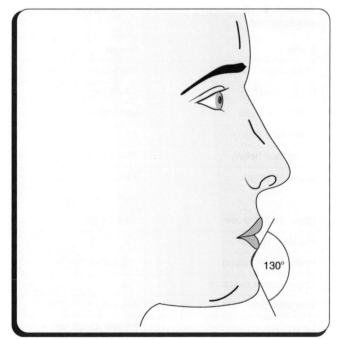

Figure 7.15 Labiomental fold. The labiomental fold depicts the relationship between the lower lip and the chin and should be at least 130°.

Chin projection

Chin projection is determined by the combination of bony chin and the amount of soft tissue covering it. The chin should be assessed in all three dimensions. The width of the chin should be assessed in relation to the overall facial shape. The labiomental fold, chin shape, relation to the dental midline, symmetry and cant of the lower border should be considered.

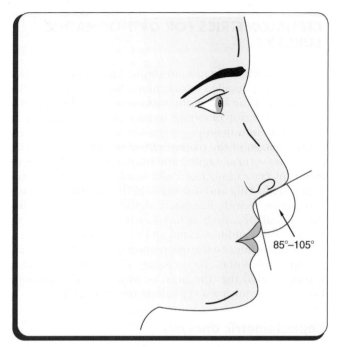

Figure 7.16 Nasolabial angle. The nasolabial angle measures between the columella and the upper lip. It should be in the range of 85°–105°.

Chin–throat angle

The angle between the lower lip, chin and the deepest point along the chin–neck contour should be approximately 90°. The angle tends to become obtuse with advancing age and can be unaesthetic. Deficient chin, retropositioned mandible, lower lip procumbency and excessive fat in the submental area are all factors that make the angle obtuse, resulting in an unaesthetic appearance (Fig. 7.17).

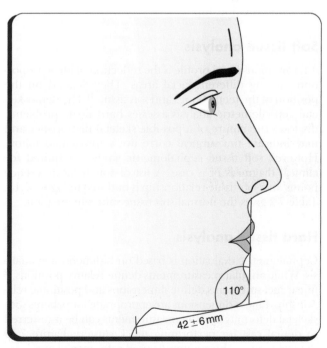

Figure 7.17 Chin–throat angle. The angle between the lower lip, chin and the deepest point in the chin–neck contour should be between 90° and 110°.

CEPHALOMETRICS FOR ORTHOGNATHIC SURGERY

Cephalometric evaluation in surgical patients is essential for obtaining detailed information about the spatial relationship and the size of the various parts of the dentofacial complex, for planning treatment and for assessing the treatment outcome.

Orientation of the patient's head on three converging planes, viz vertical, sagittal and transverse, is important to avoid any errors associated with head rotation, which will result in blurring and distortion of the craniofacial structures. Patients with dentofacial deformity may have structural imbalance, such as facial asymmetry, difference in height of the auditory canal and mandibular asymmetry, which will influence the orientation of the patient's head on the cephalostat. To overcome these influences, it is recommended that the head be in a natural head position when acquiring a cephalometric radiograph.[6]

Cephalometric analysis

Cephalometric analysis based on hard tissue structures has been the main stay in diagnosis and planning for orthognathic surgery for several decades. However, it is now well recognized that soft tissue variations can mask or exaggerate the bony relationship, and surgical predictions based on hard tissue cephalometric landmarks are inaccurate in estimating the soft tissue aesthetics outcome.[10] Moreover, it is now well established that the cranial base can have marked inclination, and cephalometric analysis based solely on cranial base inclination will not accurately depict the spatial relationship of the jaw bases.

Modern cephalometric analysis will involve orienting the head as it is in life, viz the natural head position using extracranial landmarks, and employ both hard and soft tissue parameters to ascertain the skeletal, dental and soft tissue relationship.

Soft tissue analysis

A harmonious facial profile is the reflection of ideal proportions among different facial areas. They depend on the position of the teeth, bones and soft tissue.[11] The dentoskeletal cephalometric analysis assesses hard tissue problems, discloses the nature of a possible skeletal discrepancy and may indicate the surgical corrective approach to follow. However, soft tissue cephalometric study is required for clinical diagnosis of a case. A list of soft tissue reference points and soft tissue relationship is outlined in Figure 7.18. Table 7.2 gives the normal soft tissue values in an adult.

Hard tissue analysis

Cephalometric evaluation is based on bidimensional analysis. While angular measurements define relative positions,[12] linear measurements define dimensions and positional relationship. Linear dimensions are appropriate for patients with skeletal deformity and the measurements can be transferred to dental cast for performing mock surgery. Figure 7.19 depicts some of the commonly used reference planes.

Table 7.3 outlines the normal hard tissue values in an adult.

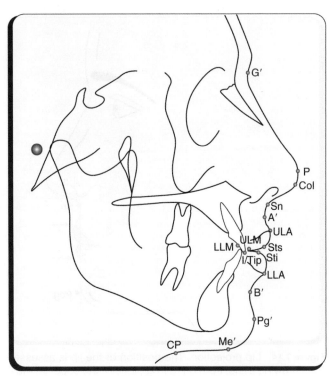

Figure 7.18 Commonly used soft tissue reference points.

Table 7.2   Normative values for soft tissue assessment

Traits	Norms
Facial angle	165°–173°
Nasal projection	13–18 mm
Nasolabial angle	94°–110°
Lower face (%)	53–56%
Lower face height	57–74 mm
Upper lip length	Female 18–22 mm
	Male 22–25 mm
Upper lip thickness	10–14 mm
Maxillary sulcus	127°–147°
Upper lip protrusion	3 ± 1 mm
Upper incisor exposure	1–5 mm
Interlabial gap	1–5 mm
Lower lip–chin length	Female 43–50 mm
	Male 45–54 mm
Lower lip thickness	11–55 mm
Mandibular sulcus	110°–134°
Lower lip protrusion	2 ± 1 mm
B'–SnPg' line	4 ± 1 mm
Lower face–throat angle	96°–110°
Throat length	51–63 mm

B' – soft tissue Point B; SnPg' – subnasale to soft tissue pogonion.

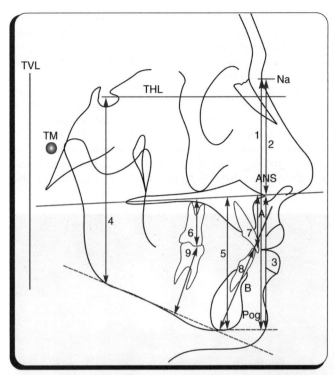

Figure 7.19 Commonly used hard tissue reference planes.

Table 7.3   Hard tissue relationship

Parameters	Male	Female
Maxillary length (TM–ANS)	114 (14)	105 (3)
Mandibular length (TM–Pg)	127 (5)	119 (4)
Total face height (Na–Me)	137 (8)	123 (5)
Upper face height (Na–ANS)	60 (4)	55 (2)
Lower face height (ANS–Me)	80 (6)	69 (5)
Ethmoid point–PNS	55 (4)	50 (3)
Sella–PNS	56 (4)	51 (3)
Posterior face height (S–go)	88 (6)	79 (4)
Palatal plane–menton	76 (6)	67 (4)
Palatal plane–upper molar	28 (3)	25 (2)
Palatal plane–upper incisor	33 (3)	30 (3)
PNS–ANS	62 (4)	57 (4)
Mandibular plane–lower incisor	49 (3)	42 (3)
Mandibular plane–lower molar	38 (3)	33 (3)
PTM vertical	18	18

TM – temporomandibular point; ANS – anterior nasal spine; Pg – pogonion; Na –nasion; Me – menton; PNS – posterior nasal spine; S – sella; go – gonion; PTM – pterygomaxillary vertical.

Soft tissue profile alterations

In orthognathic surgery, dentoskeletal positional alterations induced by osteotomies do not always correlate dimensionally with soft tissues.[13] Therefore, it is necessary to weigh the proportional relationship between the modifications of hard tissue changes and the soft tissue-related responses. Accurately predicting the soft tissue response to hard tissue movement is impossible because individual's response to identical procedures vary, particularly with reference to the lips. However, some common soft tissue reactions to surgical procedures are outlined in Table 7.4.

Table 7.4   Soft tissue reaction to various surgical procedures

Procedures	Effects
Maxillary advancement	Widens nasal base
	Highlights paranasal areas
	Reduces nasal prominence
	Raises tip of the nose
	Highlights upper lip
	Shades the chin
Maxillary setback	Retracts paranasal areas
	Increases upper lip length
	Decreases interlabial gap
	Lowers tip of the nose
	Highlights chin
Maxillary impaction	Widens nasal base
	Highlights paranasal areas
	Raises tip of the nose
	Reduces upper teeth show
	Shortens lip and causes vertical reduction of the lower third
	Increases chin prominence
Down graft	Lowers tip of the nose, columella and alar bases
	Lengthens upper lip
	Retracts upper lip and paranasal areas
	Increases nasolabial angle
Mandibular advancement	Increases height of the lower third
	Increases chin projection
	Reduces lower lip eversion
	Increases lower lip protrusion
	Decreases mentocervical angle
	Increases mentocervical sharpness
Mandibular setback	Increases lower lip show
	Reduces height of the lower third
	Reduces chin prominence
	Reduces lower lip eversion
	Reduces lower lip protrusion
	Highlights paranasal areas

Dental cast

Dental cast is a permanent record of the patient's condition before treatment and is the essential component of the diagnostic records. The study cast can be used to view the dental relationship, the shape of the teeth and arches and for performing arch length and tooth-size discrepancy analyses.

For patients who are candidates for orthognathic surgery, the dental casts are essential for trial treatment wherein the movement of the teeth and jaws can be simulated (mock surgery). Mounting of dental casts on an anatomical articulator is particularly useful in patients who have a discrepancy between centric relation and maximal intercuspal position. In these patients, mounted models help in identifying the occlusal prematurity that contributes to a functional shift (Fig. 7.20).

Mounting of models is essential in patients who have temporomandibular joint problems. In these patients, a muscle deprogramming splint must be employed to eliminate muscle spasm and allow the condyle to seat in the fossa. Articulator mounting of models is essential in patients in whom the vertical position of the maxilla will be altered. In these patients, the auto-rotation of the

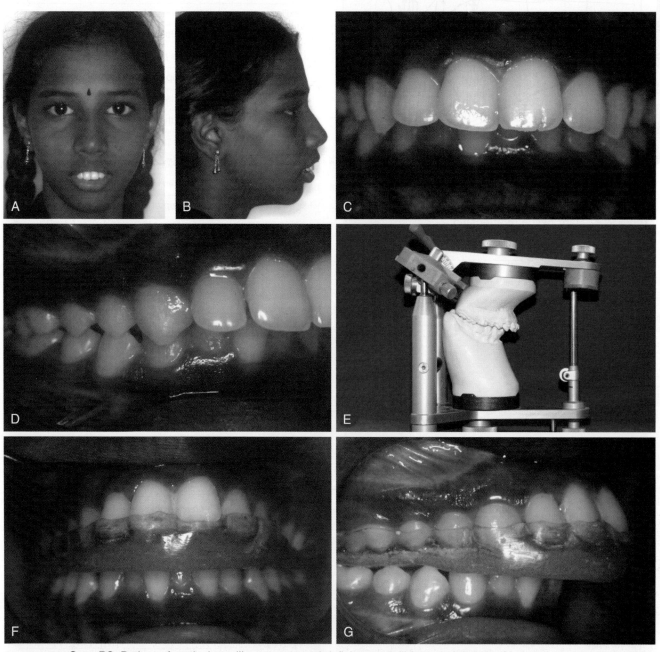

Figure 7.20   Case RS. Patient of vertical maxillary excess and deficient mandible and chin, with Class II dentoalveolar relationship and temporomandibular disorder, treated with deprogramming splint, orthodontics and orthognathic surgery. (**A** and **B**) Pretreatment facial photograph; note increased incisor exposure at rest, increase in lower facial height, convex profile, retrusive mandible and chin. (**C** and **D**) Intraoral photograph; note increased overjet, deep overbite, Class II molar and canine relationship. (**E**) Semi-adjustable articulator for assessing maxillomandibular relationship. (**F** and **G**) Deprogramming splint to eliminate muscle spasm and allow the condyle to seat in the fossa.

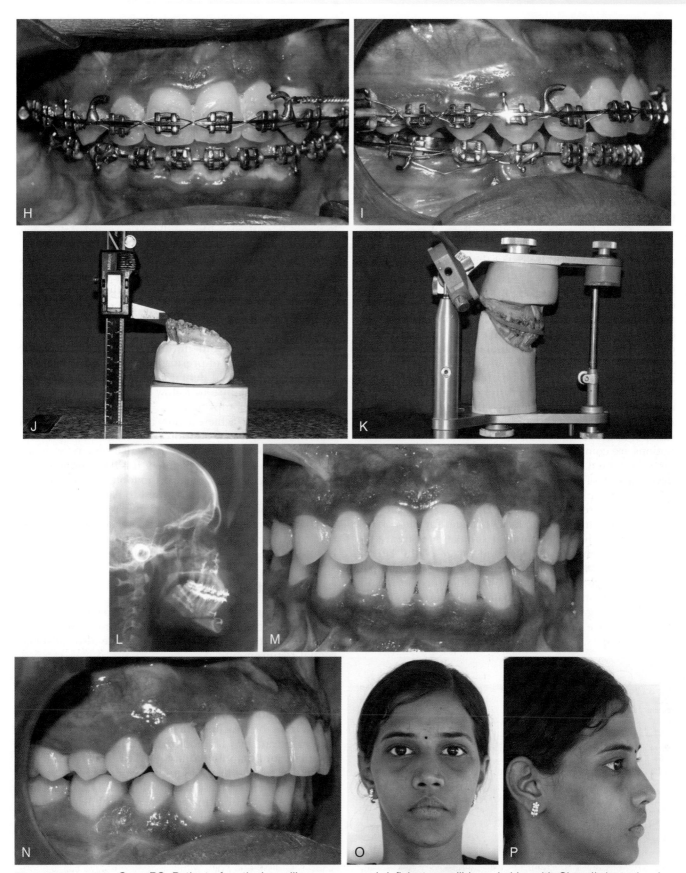

Figure 7.20, cont'd   Case RS. Patient of vertical maxillary excess and deficient mandible and chin, with Class II dentoalveolar relationship and temporomandibular disorder, treated with deprogramming splint, orthodontics and orthognathic surgery. (**H** and **I**) Presurgical decompensation. (**J**) Ericson model platform for mock surgery. (**K**) Surgical splint constructed on a semi-adjustable articulator. (**L**) Cephalometric depicting maxillary impaction, mandibular advancement and augmentation genioplasty. (**M** and **N**) Post-treatment occlusion. (**O** and **P**) Post-treatment extraoral photographs.

mandible that follows maxillary vertical repositioning cannot be assessed by hand-held models.

Whenever articulator mounting is decided, it must be performed after obtaining a facebow transfer and occlusal bite, which are essential to mount the model on a semi-adjustable articulator.

Prediction for treatment planning

For individuals who are candidates for orthognathic surgery, the outcome of various surgical procedures can be predicted prior to initiating treatment.[14] Conventionally, cephalometric tracings and dental casts were employed to simulate the effects of orthodontic and surgical treatments. Cephalometric prediction allows direct evaluation of both dental and skeletal movements whereas cast prediction shows in more detail the dental relationship that indirectly reflects the underlying skeletal changes. Manual cephalometric prediction, using the tracing overlay approach is a time tested method of predicting the outcome. The limitation of this approach is that it does not incorporate the patient's facial structures, and consequently, the patient cannot be involved in the decision making process. With the advent of computer imaging, the patient's image can be predicted.

David Sarver,[15] popularized the computer-assisted cut and paste movements to describe the anticipated profile resulting from the dental and osseous movements. Surgical options are simulated on the screen and the treatment options are compared and the hard copies of several options presented serve as a visual aid in discussion. As a development of the true imaging software programme, effort was made to quantify the movements produced on a computer screen to allow the planes to correlate the required movement to the facial changes for the correction of malocclusion. Treatment simulation software allows the blending of the digitized image of the lateral cephalometric tracing with the photo image of the patient. Currently, several computerized procedures and software are commercially available, which are reasonably accurate, saving valuable operator time by greater speed, multiple choice of analysis, rapid superimposition of serial radiographs, storage and retrieval of multiple records

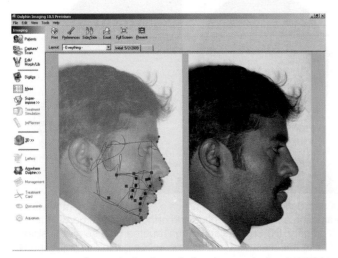

Figure 7.21 Computerized prediction for surgical outcome.

and generate life-like representation of the final outcome (Fig. 7.21).

ORTHODONTIC PREPARATION

Patients with dentofacial deformity have dentoalveolar compensation to mask the skeletal imbalance, and this is nature's accommodation to facilitate function. In Class II skeletal deformity, the nature of the dentoalveolar compensation is characterized by retrusive maxillary and protrusive mandibular incisors; and in Class III skeletal deformity, the compensation is characterized by proclined maxillary incisors and retroclined mandibular incisors. In patients with maxillary transverse deficiency, the maxillary posteriors are buccally inclined and the mandibular posteriors may be lingually inclined. Patients who are candidates for combined orthodontic and surgical correction must at first have this dentoalveolar compensation eliminated to facilitate the surgeon to optimally align the jaw bones. The preoperative positioning of teeth dictates the nature and the extent of the surgical procedure and influences the final aesthetic results. Poor or lack of presurgical orthodontic preparation with any residual dental compensation for skeletal discrepancy or failure to follow the treatment plan will lead to surgical compromise.

In an attempt to achieve a more acceptable and functional aesthetic result, it may also force the surgeons to perform adjunctive procedures, such as segmental surgery or genioplasty that was not initially planned. It is thus important for the surgeons to understand the orthodontic decision making processes as it is for the orthodontist to have a good understanding of the presurgical orthodontic requirements. The orthodontic treatment objectives, extraction patterns and mechanics used in surgical orthodontic cases differ or may be in opposite to those used in nonsurgical cases.

Presurgical orthodontics

The goal of presurgical orthodontics is to decompensate for dentoalveolar compensation and to position the teeth upright over the basal bone, while also satisfying spatial requirements.

Horizontal plane

In patients with Class II deformity, the objective of presurgical orthodontics is to procline the maxillary incisors and retract the proclined mandibular incisors. The decision to extract may be modified by different goals in the maxillary and mandibular arches. This may result in extraction of second bicuspid in the upper arch to alleviate crowding and first bicuspid in the lower arch to align and retract lower incisors to facilitate mandibular advancement. These extraction choices are opposite to those performed in conventional orthodontic compensation for Class II discrepancy where the upper first and lower second bicuspids are preferred (Fig. 7.22).

The reverse would be true for skeletal Class III discrepancy where lower second and upper first, or at times, only upper first premolars would be extracted to create sufficient negative overjet to facilitate maxillary advancement and mandibular setback or both (Fig. 7.23).

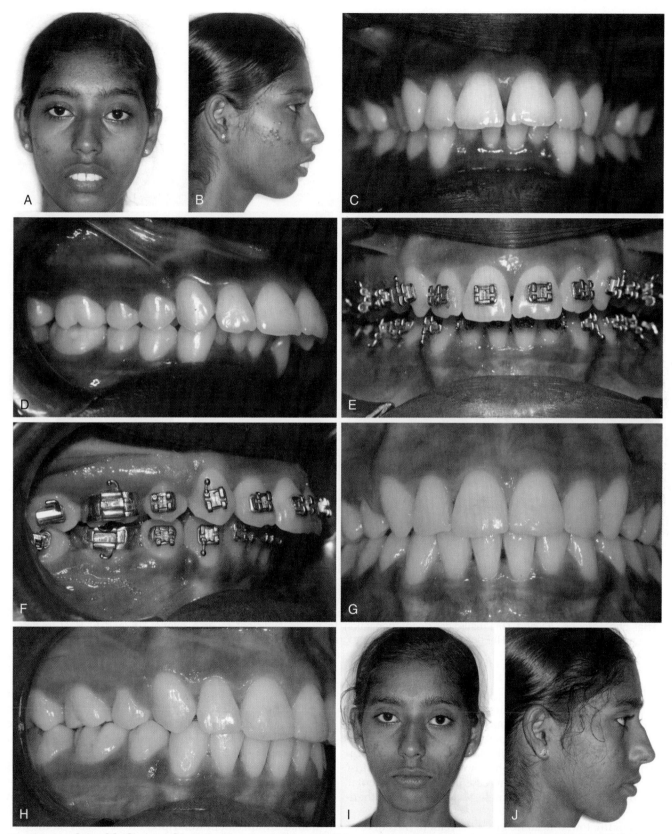

Figure 7.22 Case SS. Skeletal Class II with retrognathic mandible, treated with mandibular advancement. (**A** and **B**) Pretreatment facial photographs. (**C** and **D**) Intraoral photographs. (**E** and **F**) Presurgical decompensation to upright the lower incisors and increase the overjet. (**G** and **H**) Postsurgical intraoral photographs. (**I** and **J**) Postsurgical facial photographs after mandibular advancement.

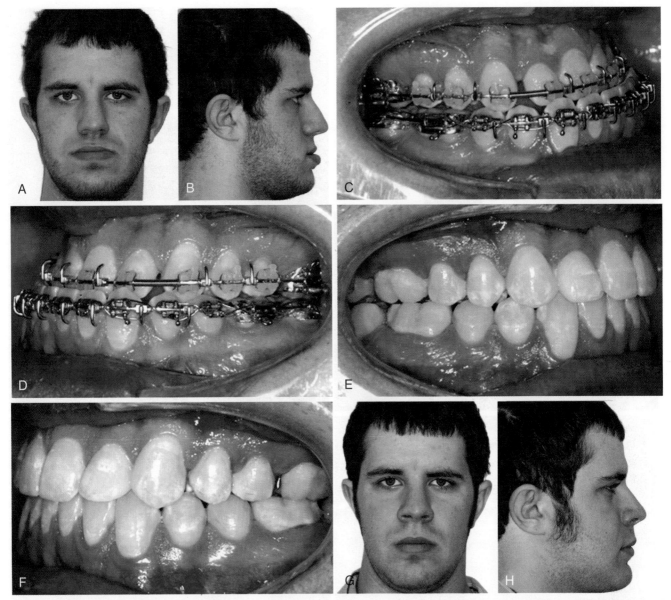

Figure 7.23 Case DY. Skeletal Class III with retrusive maxilla, treated with maxillary advancement. (**A** and **B**) Pretreatment facial photographs. (**C** and **D**) Presurgical decompensation to create sufficient reverse overjet. (**E** and **F**) Post-treatment intraoral photographs. (**G** and **H**) Post-treatment facial photographs.

Vertical plane

A dental compensation in the vertical dimension affects both maxillary and mandibular incisors; patients with skeletal anterior open bite pattern have excessive eruption of maxillary and mandibular incisors, which compensate for the increase in the lower facial height. Most often, this may result in an increase in the upper alveolar height leading to a gummy smile, which may be aesthetically objectionable.

When the lower facial height is decreased, the curve of Spee is excessive in the lower anterior with both infraocclusion of the posteriors and supraeruption of the anteriors. The presurgical preparation to decompensate the dentition in the vertical plane depends upon the anterior facial height.

In patients with skeletal open bite, which would require segmental osteotomy in the maxilla, presurgical

orthodontic preparation should maintain two different occlusal planes; the anterior segment from canine to canine and the posterior segment distal to the canine should be levelled independently by using a segmental archwire (Fig. 7.24).

When the lower facial height is reduced as in patients with skeletal Class II with deep overbite, the dental arches are not levelled presurgically. The purpose is to maintain the curve of Spee before surgery, so that the surgical mandibular advancement will tripod the occlusion on the incisors and molars. This will result in an increase in the lower anterior facial height by the virtue of the mandibular incisor teeth being in an edge-to-edge incisor relationship. The arch can then be levelled postsurgically, primarily by extruding the buccal segments with intermaxillary elastics in order to level the curve of Spee, while maintaining the lower facial height (Fig. 7.25).

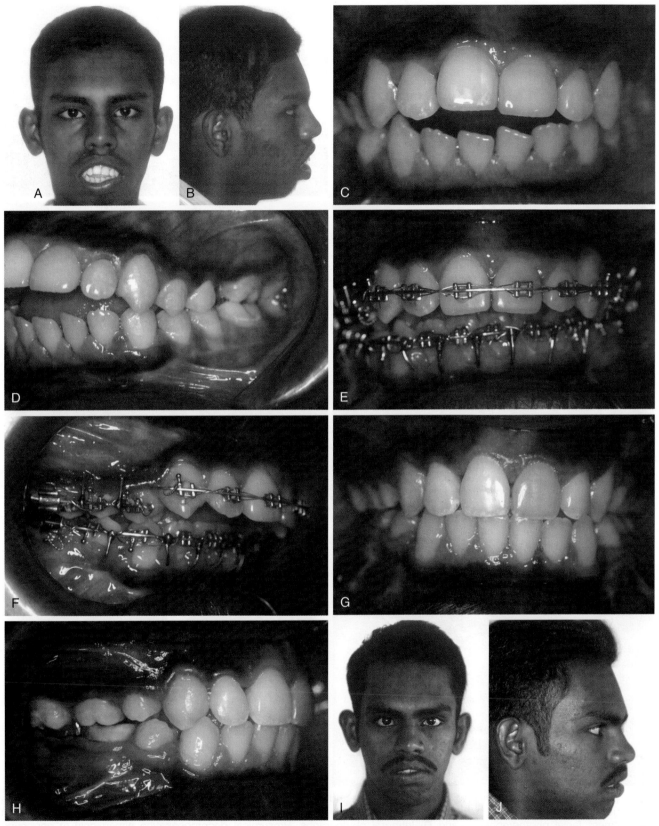

Figure 7.24 Case IA with skeletal open bite. (**A** and **B**) Pretreatment facial photographs. (**C** and **D**) Intraoral photographs. (**E** and **F**) Presurgical decompensation; note the segmental mechanics for maintaining two independent occlusal planes in the upper arch. (**G** and **H**) Post-treatment intraoral photographs following two-piece maxillary osteotomy. (**I** and **J**) Post-treatment facial photographs.

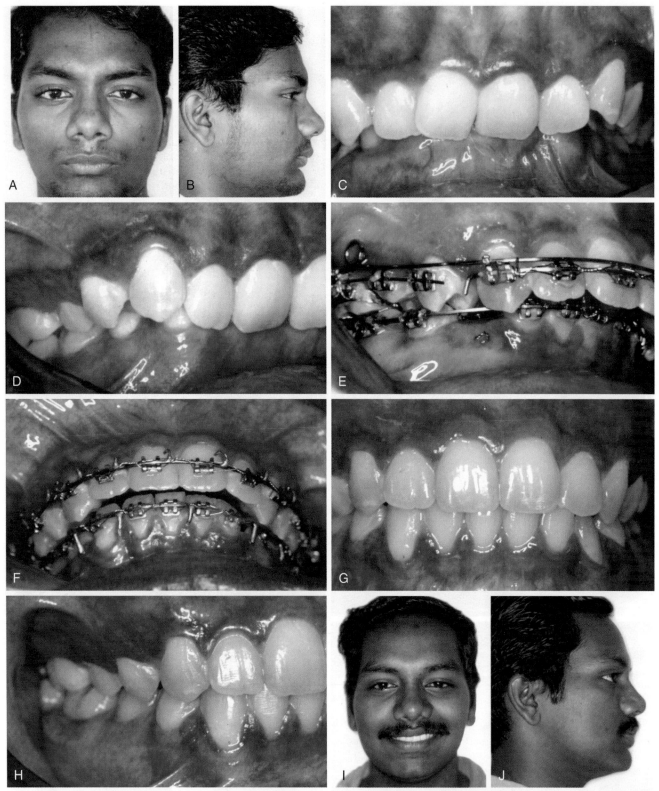

Figure 7.25 Case MD with decreased lower facial height and skeletal deep bite. Intraoral Class II Div 2 malocclusion with retroclined incisors treated with mandibular advancement to reduce facial convexity and increase facial height. (**A** and **B**) Pretreatment facial photographs. (**C** and **D**) Intraoral photographs. Presurgical decompensation aimed only at correcting the axial inclination of the incisors. (**E** and **F**) Levelling of curve of Spee is best achieved following surgery. (**G** and **H**) Post-treatment intraoral photographs. (**I** and **J**) Post-treatment facial photographs.

Transverse considerations

In skeletal Class II malocclusion, the maxillary arch is constricted; while in Class III malocclusion, the mandibular arch is tapered. The archforms are corrected presurgically, and then the arches are coordinated with full-size rectangular archwires during presurgical orthodontics.

In skeletal Class III patients with transverse maxillary deficiency, either a surgically assisted RPE or a multiple piece Le Fort I osteotomy can be performed. These two surgical procedures do not require presurgical arch coordination that is best accomplished during postsurgical orthodontics.

ORTHODONTICS FOR SURGICAL PATIENTS

Presurgical orthodontics

1. Aligning and levelling by extrusion
2. Archform coordination
3. Opening space to facilitate osteotomy cuts

Postsurgical orthodontics

1. Levelling by extrusion
2. Root paralleling
3. Finishing and detailing

SURGICAL PROCEDURES

Surgical treatment for dentofacial deformity consists of both orthognathic procedures to correct jaw relationship and adjunctive procedures to correct hard and soft tissue contours. The choice of surgical procedure is dictated by the aesthetic goals that are determined by the patient's main concern.

Surgical treatment for skeletal Class II malocclusion

Most Class II skeletal malocclusions are corrected by altering the position of the mandible and chin unlike in the past, where excess overjet was addressed by performing a maxillary anterior osteotomy by setting the premaxilla back following premolar extraction. In view of the better understanding of the soft tissue maturity following ageing and the soft tissue response following maxillary repositioning, surgery to set the premaxilla is now avoided. This procedure has the potential to flatten the middle third of the face and reduce the prominence of the lip, thereby accelerating the effect of ageing process.

The mandible can be predictably brought forward to reduce the facial convexity. The surgical technique of choice is the bilateral sagittal split ramus osteotomy wherein the distal (tooth bearing) segment of the mandible is brought forward to obtain maximal intercuspation with the maxillary dentition. The position of the maxillary and mandibular incisors controls the amount the mandible can be advanced, as well as the facial aesthetics after surgery.

In some patients, the chin may appear deficient after advancement of the mandible and an advancement genioplasty may be indicated to improve the final aesthetics.

Surgery for Class III skeletal dysplasia

Till the early 1980s, most Class III skeletal pattern was thought to be due to excessive anteroposterior growth of the mandible and most were corrected by mandibular setback procedures. It was later recognized that a majority of Class III patients have a significant anteroposterior deficiency of the maxilla.

Therefore, the clinician must determine whether one jaw is primarily at fault or a combination of maxillary deficiency and mandibular excess is causing the malocclusion.

In patients with isolated mandibular excess, bilateral sagittal split osteotomy and mandibular setback is the procedure of choice, although a transoral vertical ramus osteotomy may be indicated in cases requiring larger setbacks. On rare occasions, procedures, such as body osteotomies or segmental subapical osteotomies, are indicated. A genioplasty may at times be necessary for aesthetic positioning of the chin.

The treatment of maxillary anteroposterior deficiency is accomplished by advancing the maxilla by means of Le Fort I osteotomy. This versatile procedure enables the surgeon to correct the discrepancies in the vertical, transverse and occlusal planes.

Most cases of maxillary anteroposterior deficiency also exhibit a transverse deficiency and the decision has to be made whether a surgically assisted rapid palatal expansion or multiple piece Le Fort I osteotomy is to be employed for correcting the transverse deficiency.

Surgery for vertical problems

Maxillary vertical deficiency

Maxillary anteroposterior deficiency is often associated with maxillary vertical deficiency. It is common in patients with cleft lip and palate because overclosure of the mandible makes patients with maxillary vertical deficiency appear clinically similar to those with mandibular anteroposterior excess. The clinician must determine whether it is an anteroposterior or a vertical problem. In patients with maxillary vertical deficiency, the maxilla can be repositioned inferiorly by a Le Fort I down grafting procedure. This is one of the least stable of all surgical procedures and rigid fixation must be employed to improve the stability.

Maxillary vertical excess

There is no alternative to surgery for adult patients with vertical maxillary excess. The orthodontic preparation and surgical execution must be very accurate. To correct the vertical excess, the maxilla must be superiorly repositioned with a Le Fort I osteotomy. The position of the mandible will be altered following maxillary impaction. If the overjet continues to be in excess after maxillary impaction, a sagittal split osteotomy of the mandible must be performed to reduce the facial convexity. If the overjet is optimal and the facial height continues to be disproportionate or if there is persistent facial convexity, then a vertical genioplasty to reduce the vertical height of the chin or an augmentation genioplasty to improve the facial profile must be contemplated.

Postsurgical orthodontics

Postsurgical orthodontics can begin 6–8 weeks after surgery or when the surgeon thinks the healing has reached the point of satisfactory clinical stability. The first step in postsurgical orthodontics is the removal of the splint and the stabilization of the archwires, which is followed by the repairing of the appliance that usually gets damaged during surgery; following repair of the appliance, light archwire and elastics are employed to settle the occlusion.

The elastics, in addition to promoting the settling of occlusion, override the patients proprioceptive drive towards positioning the mandible in maximum intercuspation; this will help the patients in maintaining proper centric relation and occlusion. The vector of elastics depends on the type of surgery. It is customary to run elastics in Class II vector in patients who have had mandibular advancements and in Class III vector in patients who have had maxillary advancement or mandibular setback or both. Care must be taken to avoid tooth movement that may promote relapse tendency of the surgical correction, like aligning a second molar in a patient who has had a surgery to correct a skeletal open bite.

Special consideration must be given for patients who have had transverse correction, since there is a very strong relapse tendency for patients who have had transverse expansion of the maxilla, a rigid overlay archwire (36 mil or heavier) should be maintained at least for 6 months. Generally, postsurgical orthodontics should not be performed for more than 3–4 months and an optimum occlusion must be achieved within this period. Debonding the appliance and inserting the retainers should follow the same principles as in conventional orthodontics.

Stability following orthognathic surgery

Current data make it clear that, although modern orthognathic surgery can move the jaws and dentoalveolar segments, within limits, in any desired direction, there are major differences in stability and predictability. Tanya Bailey[16] introduced the concept of hierarchy of stability and grouped procedures into four major categories.

Superior repositioning of the maxilla is the most stable orthognathic procedure, closely followed by mandibular advancement in patients with short or normal face height and less than 10 mm advancement.

Both these procedures can be highly stable and exhibit a more than 90% chance of less than 2 mm change at landmarks and almost no chance of more than 4 mm change during the first postsurgical year. Surgical repositioning of the chin via lower border osteotomy, the most prevalent adjunctive procedure, also is highly stable and predictable.

Advancement of the maxilla falls into the second category and can be described as stable. With forward movement of moderate distances (<8 mm), there is an 80% chance of less than 2 mm change, a 20% chance of 2–4 mm relapse and almost no chance of more than 4 mm change.

Downward movement of the maxilla is in the problematic category; if the maxilla is moved both forward and down, the vertical component is likely to relapse, although the horizontal component has a good chance of being retained. Correcting maxillary asymmetry usually involves moving one side up to correct a canted occlusal plane and usually is done in conjunction with mandibular surgery. The maxillary component of asymmetry surgery also can be judged to be stable by the same criteria.

CONCLUSION

Orthognathic surgery is indicated for those patients seeking changes in aesthetics and function of a magnitude that is not possible with orthodontics alone. Careful planning and good communication between the orthodontist, surgeon and the patient is essential to avoid any complications.

Current technology allows the clinician to simulate treatment and plan for optimum aesthetics and function. However, despite all this, complications could occur and the clinician should be knowledgeable enough to recognize and respond effectively.

REFERENCES

1. Ackerman JL, Proffit WR. Soft tissue limitations in orthodontics. Angle Orthod 1997; 67:327–336.
2. Proffit WR. Contemporary orthodontics. 4th edn. St.Louis, Mosby.
3. Tulloch C, Profit WR. Outcomes in a 2-phase randomized clinical trial of early treatment. Am J Ortho 2004; 125:657–667
4. Ackerman JL. Orthodontics: art, science or trans-science? Angle Orthod 1974; 44:243–250.
5. Arnett GW, Bergman RT. Facial keys to orthodontic diagnosis and treatment planning. Part I. Am J Orthod Dentofacial Orthop 1993; 103:299–312.
6. Moorrees CF, Kean MR. Natural head position: a basic consideration of the interpretation of cephalometric radiographs. Am J Phys Anthropol 1958; 16:213–234.
7. Zachrisson BU. Esthetic factors involved in anterior tooth display and the smile: vertical dimension. J Clin Orthod 1998; 32:432–445.
8. Nanda RS, Kapila S, Hanspeter Meng, et al. Growth changes of the soft tissue profile. Angle Orthod 1990; 60:177–190.
9. Powell N, Humpherys B. Proportions of the aesthetic face. New York: Thieme-Stratton; 1984.
10. Arnett GW, Bergman RT. Facial keys to orthodontic diagnosis and treatment planning. Part I. Am J Orthod Dentofacial Orthop 1993; 103:395–411.
11. Holdaway RA. A soft tissue cephalometric analysis and its use in orthodontic treatment planning. Part I. Am J Orthod Dentofacial Orthop 1983; 84:1–28.
12. Burstone CJ, James RB, Legan H, et al. Cephalometrics for orthognathic surgery. J Oral Surg 1978; 36:269–277.
13. Bennet MA, Wolford LM. Maxillary surgery technical considerations. In: Bell W, Proffit W, White R, eds. Surgical correction of dentofacial deformities, vol. 3. Philadelphia: WB Saunders Company; 1985. 45–52.
14. Hill SC. Prediction tracing. In: Bell WH, Proffit WR, White RP, eds. Surgical correction of deformities, vol. 3. Philadelphia: WB Saunders Company; 1985. 210–217.
15. Sarver DM. Esthetic orthodontics and orthognathic surgery. St Louis: Mosby; 1998.
16. Bailey LJ. Stability and predictability of orthognathic surgery. Am J Orthod Dentofacial Orthop 2004; 126:273–277.

Role of Skeletal Anchorage in Modern Orthodontics

8

Sung-Hoon Lim and Ki Beom Kim

Skeletal anchorage is frequently used in the orthodontic treatments to reinforce anchorage during closure of extraction space or to generate various orthodontic force systems. By the use of skeletal anchorage, many tooth movements that were previously thought almost impossible became more feasible. Also, unwanted tooth movement can be minimized by using skeletal anchorage. Although skeletal anchorage gives freedom in the design of force system and overcomes patient compliance issues, this does not expand the anatomic limit of tooth movement. Skeletal anchorage should be planned based on the careful evaluation of the required force systems and anatomic limits. In this chapter, various types of skeletal anchorage were explained with an emphasis on the palatal mini-implant system.

VARIOUS SKELETAL ANCHORAGE USED IN MODERN ORTHODONTICS

Orthodontic mini-implant

Orthodontic mini-implants and bone plates are the most popular types of skeletal anchorage. Skeletal anchorage is most frequently used as anchorage reinforcement during space closure in premolar extraction cases. For this purpose, mini-implants are more frequently used than bone plates because the surgical procedure does not include flap elevation and the patient's discomfort is less. Mini-implants for anchorage reinforcement are commonly placed at the buccal interdental alveolar bone between second premolar and first molar or between first and second molars (Fig. 8.1). Mini-implants placed at the interdental alveolar bone can also be used for 1–2 mm distalization of molars[1, 2] and intrusion of molars. The success rates of mini-implants placed at buccal interdental alveolar bone were reported to be around 90%,[3–5] and can bear a tipping moment less than 900 cN.mm.[6, 7] The width of interdental alveolar bone available for mini-implants placement varies widely among individuals. Therefore, placing mini-implant in the buccal interdental alveolar bone can be difficult in patients whose interdental alveolar bone is too narrow to accommodate a mini-implant. Furthermore, mesial or distal movement of teeth adjacent to mini-implants should not be attempted in these patients, because root contact with a mini-implant can cause severe root resorption.[8] Possibility of root contact during mini-implant placement was reported as 13.5% in an experienced clinician group, and 21.3% in a novice group in a study using a typodont excercise.[9] Also, 20% of the mini-implants placed in the buccal interdental alveolar bone showed root contact in a study using CBCT images taken after placement of the mini-implant.[10] Jung et al[4] reported successful mini-implants were placed 0.49 mm away from roots, whereas the failed mini-implants were

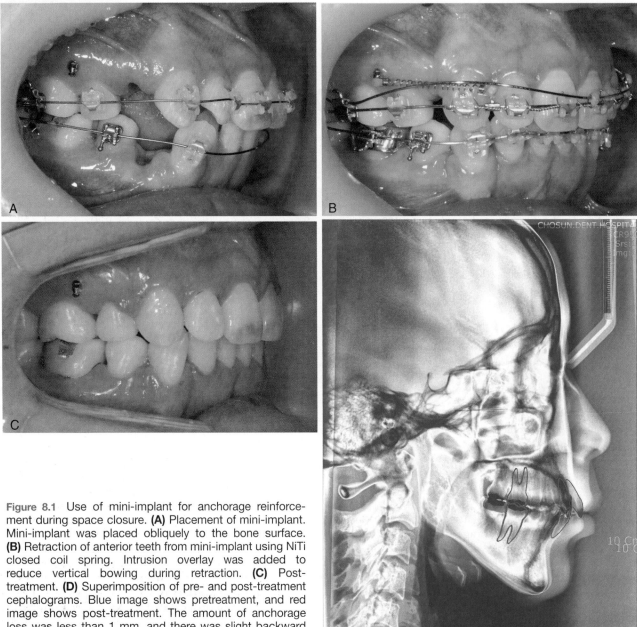

Figure 8.1 Use of mini-implant for anchorage reinforcement during space closure. **(A)** Placement of mini-implant. Mini-implant was placed obliquely to the bone surface. **(B)** Retraction of anterior teeth from mini-implant using NiTi closed coil spring. Intrusion overlay was added to reduce vertical bowing during retraction. **(C)** Post-treatment. **(D)** Superimposition of pre- and post-treatment cephalograms. Blue image shows pretreatment, and red image shows post-treatment. The amount of anchorage loss was less than 1 mm, and there was slight backward rotation of mandible.

only 0.11 mm away from roots. They suggested that root contact is more important than the placement angle or cortical bone thickness.[4] In patients showing very thick buccal alveolar bone, mini-implants can be placed almost vertical to the occlusal plane to avoid root contact. But this condition is not frequently encountered.

Bone plate

Another skeletal anchorage system is bone plate, such as the skeletal anchorage introduced by Umemori et al.[11] Bone plate can be placed in the zygomatic buttress area or mandibular body (Fig. 8.2). The mucosal penetration part of bone plate may cause soft tissue irritation and hyperplasia. To reduce soft tissue irritation, De Clerck et al[12] suggest placing the mucosal penetration part in the attached gingiva and make it a right angle

to the bone surface. Another disadvantages of bone plates are they require incisions during placement and removal.

Palatal implant and plate

Another kind of skeletal anchorage is palatal implants. When implants or mini-implants are placed in the palate, root contact can be avoided and favourable bone support can be achieved without mucosal incision. In 1996, Wehrbein et al[13,14] introduced placement of palatal implants with diameters of 3.3 mm, and lengths of 4 or 6 mm. They connected transpalatal arch to the abutment over the palatal implant to reinforce anchorage during closure of extraction space.[13,14] In a laboratory study,[15] a transpalatal arch made with .032″ × .032″ stainless steel showed 1 mm of deflection when retraction forces of

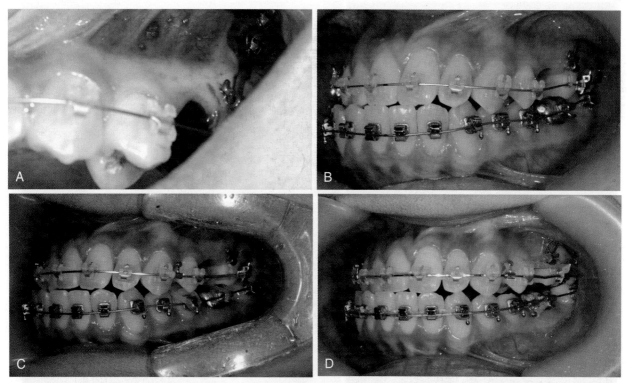

Figure 8.2 Use of mini-plate for intrusion of posterior teeth. **(A)** A mini-plate was placed in the zygomatic buttress area. **(B)** Intrusion of molar was started by applying elastomeric chain. **(C)** Space closure of extraction space using elastomeric chain accompanied with intrusion. **(D)** A cantilever spring was placed at the tube of the mini-plate to intrude the second molar. Posterior open bite was created as a result of intrusion.

200 cN were applied on both sides, indicating there would be 1 mm anchorage loss when this type of indirect anchorage was used. Wehrbein et al[16] reported there was anchorage loss of 0.7 mm on the right side, 1.1 mm on the left side when this type of indirect anchorage was used.

Although Wehrbein et al[13] used implants with a diameter of 3.3 mm, orthodontic mini-implants with a 2 mm diameter can be used similarly (Fig. 8.3). For this purpose,

the transpalatal arch should have a U-shaped loop at the centre to be bonded around the mini-implant head with composite resin. In this application, resin bonding between the mini-implant head and transpalatal arch fails ocasionally and anchorage loss can occur. Although a single palatal mini-implant placed in the mid-palate can be used for maxillary molar distalization by applying elastomeric chain from the mini-implant head to the midpoint of the transpalatal arch attached to first

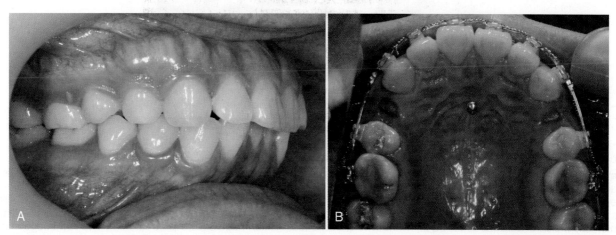

Figure 8.3 Use of single palatal mini-implant as an indirect anchorage for retraction of anterior teeth. **(A)** Pretreatment. **(B)** All first premolars were extracted and a mini-implant was placed in the mid-palate between canine and first premolar.

Continued

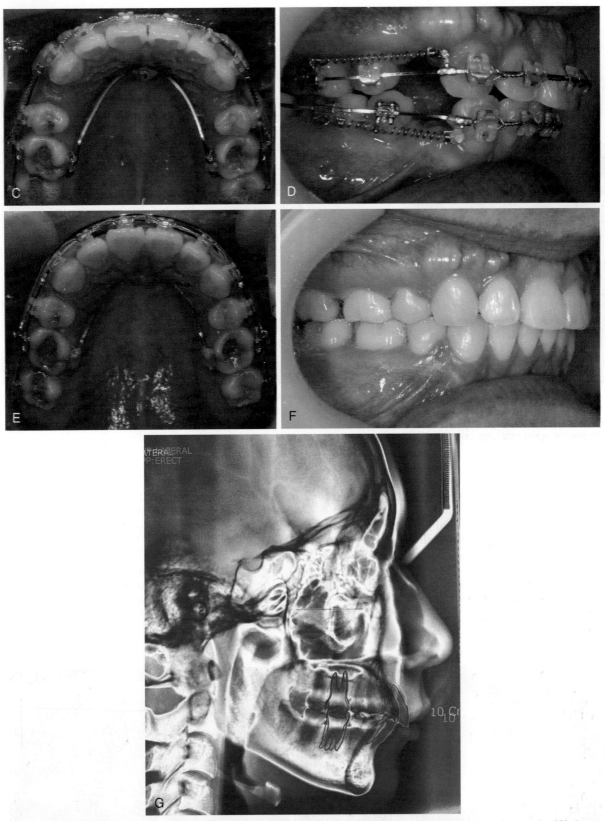

Figure 8.3, cont'd   Use of single palatal mini-implant as an indirect anchorage for retraction of anterior teeth. **(C)** A precision lingual arch with a small U-loop at the midpoint was bonded to the mini-implant head. **(D)** NiTi closed coil spring (100 cN) was applied from a crimpable hook distal to the canine to the first molar. **(E)** An intrusion overlay arch was inserted to the auxiliary tubes of the first molars. **(F)** Post-treatment. **(G)** Superimposition of pre- and post-treatment cephalograms showed that the maxillary incisors were retracted bodily without anchorage loss. Blue image shows pretreatment, and red image shows post-treatment.

molars, this distalization force will cause mesial tipping of maxillary first molars (Fig. 8.4). Therefore, it is desirable to make the distalization force pass through the centre of resistance of the molars to induce translation. To do this, there are two solutions. One solution is to place a mini-implant in the palatal aspect of the alveolar bone at the level of centre of resistance of the molars. Although, the interdental space is wider on the palatal side than the buccal, thick palatal mucosa in this area creates a long distance between cortical bone and the mini-implant head. This induces a larger moment that readily approaches the reported limitation of 900 cN.mm.[6,7] Also, the cortical bone in this area is less dense relative to the mid-palatal suture. As a result, the success rate of mini-implants is less favourable in this region. Another solution is placing bone plates with an extension or lever that can be placed at the level of the centre of resistance of molars. Bone plates can be placed either buccally[12] or palatally.[17]

Chung et al[17] suggested that the bone plate can be placed in the palate without flap elevation when the mucosa is thin. However, Kook et al[18] reported that there was severe soft tissue inflammation and overgrowth around the bone plate that was placed over the mucosa without flap elevation, and suggested modified bone plates with supporting tubes under the bone plate that would prevent it from impinging over the mucosa. To place this modified bone plate, a stent made from the plaster model is required.[18] Although these bone plates can be used to make the orthodontic force pass through the centre of resistance of teeth, bone plates cannot be adjusted according to the actual tooth movement occurred after it has been placed in the bone.

Wilmes and Drescher[19] introduced a palatal mini-implant system where an abutment can be placed over the mini-implant head. Wilems et al[20] also reported that a plate with wires can be placed over the two mini-implant heads and can be fixed by abutment screws. They reported that various tooth movements including molar distalization are possible with this appliance.[19, 20] However, removal and fastening of the abutment for adjustment of the lever can be dangerous to the mini-implant because they both can cause rotation of the mini-implant and induce failure. Therefore, once the abutment is placed, it should not be removed until removal of the mini-implant. Abutments equipped with bracket are available.[19] These abutment brackets can be placed over a single mini-implant, however, the mini-implant cannot resist the moment around its axis.

LIM (lingual irritation-free minimally-invasive) plate system

A skeletal anchorage system that can provide versatile tooth movement and minimize soft tissue irritation was developed by the author (SH Lim) and named as 'LIM (lingual irritation-free minimally-invasive) plate system' (Fig. 8.5). This system is manufactured by Jeil Medical, Seoul, Korea. The plate of LIM plate system is supported

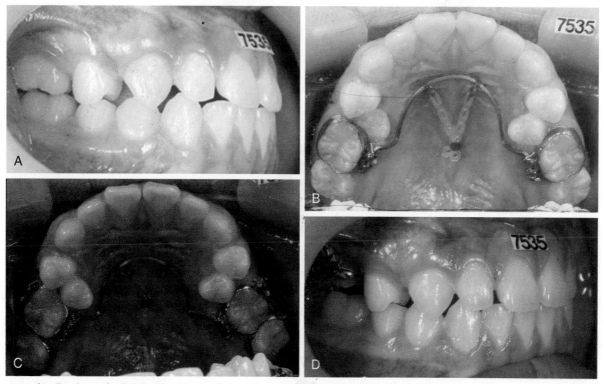

Figure 8.4 Application of distalization force from a mini-implant placed in the mid-palate to the transpalatal arch can cause mesial tipping of molars because the distalization force passes through the apical side of the centre of resistance of first molars resulting in a large moment causing distal movement of the root apex and mesial movement of the crown. **(A)** Pretreatment. **(B)** Placement of palatal mini-implant and elastomeric chains were applied from mini-implant to transpalatal arch. **(C and D)** After six months of distalization, mesial tipping of first molars occurred.

by two mini-implants that have a bolt and nut head structure. The platform of the mini-implant head supports the plate over the mucosa preventing impingement of the mucosa by the plate.

PLACEMENT OF LIM PLATE SYSTEM

Components of LIM plate system

Mini-implants of the LIM plate system have a 2.0 mm diameter and they come in lengths of 6 mm and 8 mm (Fig. 8.5). Nuts have a symmetrical top and bottom structure, therefore, they can be placed in either directions. Nuts and mini-implants are placed using the same driver (Fig. 8.5B). This driver has a pick-up mechanism consisting of balls and elastic rings on its side, which can hold the nut or mini-implant. This driver is sometimes called the 'pick-up driver'. Mini-implants and nuts are made using titanium alloy (ASTM grade V ELI Ti-6Al-4V) to provide good strength and fracture resistance. The screw part of the mini-implant has a self-drilling tip enabling placement of the mini-implant without drilling.

Two types of plates are provided. One is a bracket plate (Fig. 8.6) and the other one is a lever plate (Fig. 8.7). Both plates are fixed by the bolt and nut structures of the mini-implant head. Lever plates are equipped with levers extending bilaterally; bracket plates are equipped with brackets over the plate and do not have levers. The brackets equipped on the bracket plate have a .032" (slot height) × .040" (slot depth) which is similar to the slot size of the precision lingual bracket of Burstone and Manhartsberger.[21] The lever plates cannot be removed for adjustment because there is possibility of rotation of mini-implant during removal or fastening of the nuts. Two lengths of bracket plates are provided. Regular bracket plate can be placed over two mini-implants with centre-to-centre distance of up to 9.4 mm. The lever plate has the same length as the regular bracket plate. Short bracket plates can be placed over two mini-implants with

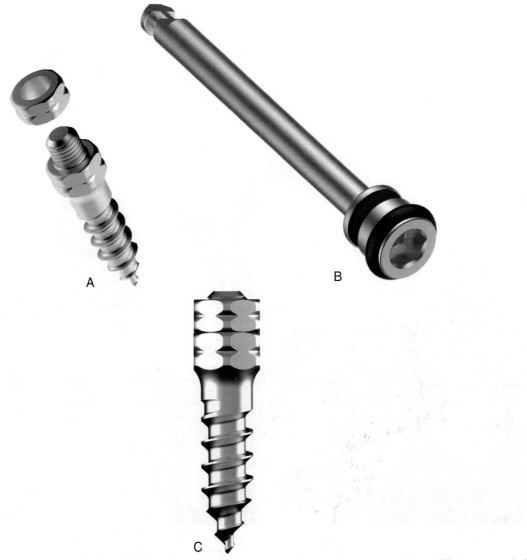

A

B

C

Figure 8.5 Mini-implant and nut used in LIM (Lingual irritation-free minimally-invasive) plate system. **(A)** An expanded view of mini-implant and nut. **(B)** Pickup driver for both the mini-implant and nut of LIM plate system. **(C)** Assembled view of mini-implant and nut.

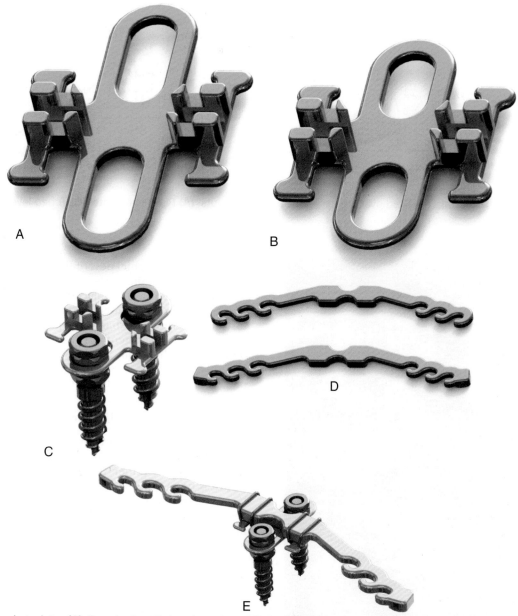

Figure 8.6 Bracket plate. **(A)** Regular length bracket plate. **(B)** Short-length bracket plate. **(C)** Bracket plate was fixed over the mini-implants with nuts. **(D)** Preformed lever (top) and tubed preformed lever with .018" × .025" slot tube at lateral ends (bottom). **(E)** Preformed lever is tied over the bracket plate.

centre-to-centre distance of up to 7.4 mm. All plates and levers are made using commercially made pure titanium.

The bracket on the bracket plate has a slot width of 7.5 mm. To minimize the profile height of the bracket, bracket wings were formed at the same level of the base of the bracket slot. Therefore, the bracket profile is the same as the depth of the bracket slot that is 1.0 mm (.040"). Due to the flat bracket wings, tying each wing separately is more convenient than tying the twin wings with a single ligature wire. Also, serif-like hooks were formed at the end of bracket wings to prevent dislodging of the ligature wires during tying (Fig. 8.6).

When using a bracket plate, a preformed lever covers the entire bracket that can be placed and tied over the bracket plate. Also, a wire lever or spring made with .032" × .032" stainless steel or titanium molybdenum alloy (TMA, Ormco, Glendora, CA) that is used for fabrication of a precision lingual arch[21] can be inserted into the bracket. The lever plate and preformed lever are manufactured from ASTM grade III commercially pure titanium. The bracket plate is manufactured from ASTM grade IV commercially pure titanium for additional strength. The lever plate and preformed lever are also equipped with a .018" × .025" slot tube at the lateral ends.

When mini-implants are placed in the mid-palate, mucosa around the mini-implant frequently grows about 1 mm toward the mini-implant head (Fig. 8.8). Therefore, the plate and the platform of the mini-implant head that supports the plate should be more than 1 mm

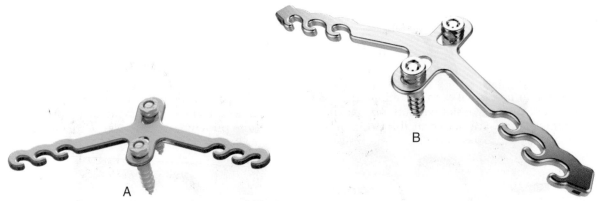

Figure 8.7   Lever plate is fixed over the mini-implant head by nuts. **(A)** Plain lever plate. **(B)** Tubed lever plate.

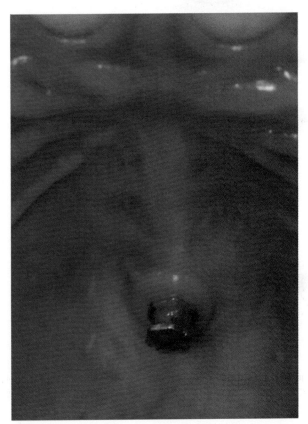

Figure 8.8   Usual thickening of the mucosa after placement of a mini-implant in the palate. Thickening occurs more frequent in younger patients and in patients who have thicker mucosa.

away from the mucosa. The soft tissue thickness at the mid-palate is about 1 mm. The mini-implant of LIM plate system has a 1 mm length of non-threaded transmucosal neck that becomes wider and continued to the hexagonal platform of 1.2 mm. Therefore, if the mini-implant is placed until its threaded part is fully inserted into the bone, there may be 1.2 mm of space between the mucosa and the plate. If the mini-implant is placed obliquely to the bone surface, the space will be slightly more because the threaded length of the mini-implant cannot be fully inserted into the bone. Because the thickness of the plate

is 0.4 mm, and the thickness of the nut is 1.2 mm, the top surface of the nut that is the most superior surface of the LIM plate system will be placed 2.8 mm superior to the mucosa. Most of the patients do not complain of discomfort and there is no change in pronunciation immediately after the placement of LIM plate system. From this observation, the name of LIM (lingual irritation-free minimally-invasive) plate system was coined. It is also named after the name of its inventor (SH Lim).

Placement site of LIM plate system

Two mini-implants are usually placed with one in an anterior position and the other one in a posterior position. If the patient is under the age of 12, the mid-palatal suture is not a good site for placement of mini-implants because the suture would be wide and fibrous. In adolescent patients over the age of 12, the mid-palatal suture may be a good site for placement, but the success rate of mini-implants is lower than in adults. An occlusal view radiograph of the maxilla may be helpful in determining bone density of the mid-palatal suture of adolescent patients. Alternatively, probing of the mid-palatal suture can be used to evaluate bone density. If the mid-palatal suture is wide and fibrous, paramedian area should be selected as a placement site for mini-implants. However, even the paramedian area may have insufficient bone density to support the mini-implant in the patients whose mid-palatal suture is wide and fibrous. In adults, the mid-palatal suture has denser bone than the paramedian area. However, the bone thickness in the mid-palate becomes thinner from an anterior to posterior direction.[22] Therefore, placing mini-implants as anterior as possible is more desirable, especially when the palatal bone is thin. However, the incisive canal in the anterior part of the palate, and which runs in a posterosuperior direction, may limit the possible area for mini-implant placement. Kim and Lim[23] reported that the posterior border of the incisive foramen is located at 6.15 mm posterior to the posterior border of the incisive papilla, and slightly anterior to the plane passing through the lingual cusps of maxillary first premolars and perpendicular to the occlusal plane. This position is the same as 14.8 mm posterior to the interdental gingiva between the central incisors. To avoid involvement of incisive canal during placement of mini-implants, anterior mini-implants should be placed at or posterior to this plane and at least 10 mm posterior to the posterior border of the incisive papilla, or 20 mm posterior to the interdental gingiva between the central incisors. This position is nearly 30 mm posterior to the incisal edge of the central incisors. This position usually takes the position anterior to the distal end of the palatal slope of anterior maxilla. If anterior mini-implants are placed at this position, they should not be placed perpendicular to the mucosa to prevent penetration into the incisive canal.

Kim, Lim, and Gang[22] showed that the lateral cephalogram depicts the palatal bone at 5 mm off-centre from the mid-palatal suture and that the palatal bone thickness at the mid-palatal suture can be estimated from a lateral cephalogram. The mid-palatal bone thickness measured from cone-beam computed tomography was not statistically different from the cephalometric measurements converted to 100% magnification ratio at the premolar region and were only 0.3 mm thicker at mesial surface of first molar and 2.3 mm thicker at distal surface of first molar.[22] These differences in thickness occur due to the rise of the nasal crest.[22]

The best area for mini-implant placement varies according to the thickness of available palatal bone. If palatal bone is thick at first molar area, then placing mini-implants at this region is recommended because two mini-implants can be placed parallel and also perpendicular to the mucosa. When the posterior palatal bone is very thin, more anterior positioning of mini-implants is desirable. To find a mid-palatal position that has thicker bone and distance from the incisive canal, a lateral cephalogram or cone-beam computed tomography can be used to measure the distance from the incisal edge of the central incisor to the ideal mid-palatal position for mini-implant placement. To locate this position in the patient's oral cavity, a ruler or gauge can be used. When the bone thickness posterior to the incisive canal is not sufficient, then two mini-implants can be placed horizontally in the paramedian areas near the canine or first premolar and then a bracket plate can be placed horizontally.

Posterior mini-implants are placed 4.2–7.2 mm posterior to the anterior mini-implant when short-length bracket plates are used. When regular length bracket plates or lever plates are used, posterior-mini-implants are placed 4.2–9.2 mm posterior to the anterior mini-implants. In children or adolescents having fibrous sutures, the paramedian area near the first premolar is recommended for placement of mini-implants.

Placement procedure of LIM plate system

Before mini-implant placement, disinfection and local anaesthesia are required. Infiltration anaesthesia using 0.5–1 cc of lidocaine HCl 2% with 1:100,000 epinephrine is sufficient for anaesthesia. When bicortical anchorage is planned, there may be some pain when the mini-implant is driven into the nasal mucosa. The placement procedures for LIM plate system is explained in Figure 8.9. Pre-drilling is not required. Mini-implants are placed using a motor unit. 50 N.cm of torque with 30 rpm is usually used. Some wireless motor units for orthodontic

mini-implant placement have 30–35 N.cm of maximum torque. This torque level is insufficient to place mini-implants in the mid-palatal suture of adults. In rare cases, a mini-implant may not be fully inserted at 50 N.cm of torque. In this case, the mini-implant should be removed and placed after drilling. Alternatively, mini-implants can be driven manually using the handpiece of an implant motor as a manual wrench while rotating the implant motor to prevent counterclockwise rotation of the driver during manual driving. However, this may cause fracture of the mini-implant tip, if the mini-implant was not inserted deep enough when applying manual driving. Therefore, this can be applied only after almost complete insertion of the mini-implant into the bone.

Anterior mini-implants are usually placed in the mid-palatal area between the lingual cusps of right and left second premolars (Fig. 8.9A). If the anterior mini-implant is placed at the palatal slope of the anterior palate perpendicular to the mucosa and the posterior mini-implant is placed also perpendicular to the mucosa, then these two mini-implants will not be parallel. When the two mini-implants are not parallel, placement of the plate can be difficult. Therefore, two mini-implants should be placed parallel to each other. To do this, the anterior mini-implant should be tipped more anteriorly and not perpendicular to the mucosa of the anterior palate, and should be perpendicular to the posterior palatal surface. Also, the mini-implant heads should be the same height, if possible. Otherwise, bending of the plate will be required to adapt it to the mini-implants. To place mini-implant heads at the same height, the length of mini-implant over the mucosa can be longer in the posterior mini-implant when the anterior mini-implant was placed in the palatal slope of the anterior palate. When two mini-implants are placed in the posterior palate around the first molar, the two mini-implants can be placed parallel and also almost perpendicular to the mucosa.

Two mini-implants of the LIM plate system should be placed with 4.2–7.2 mm (short-length bracket plate) or 4.2–9.2 mm (regular length bracket plate and lever plate) distance between the centres of two mini-implants (Fig. 8.9B). To measure this distance, a periodontal probe is placed behind the implant that was placed first and 5 mm of distance is marked by pressing the explorer or probe against the palatal mucosa (Fig. 8.9B). Because the mini-implant has 2.49–2.73 mm diameter at its hexagonal head, 5 mm distance from the outer surface of the mini-implant will be about 6.3 mm distance between the centres of two mini-implants. During initial insertion of a mini-implant, the implant can slip which can result incorrect distance between the two mini-implants. A 2.1 mm narrowing of the distance and 2.9 mm widening of the distance can be allowed because 4.2–9.2 mm distance can be accepted for the placement of the regular length bracket plate and lever plate. After placement of the mini-implants, the distance between the centre of the bolt structure of the mini-implants is measured. If this distance is within the 4.2–7.2 mm range, then a short bracket plate can be chosen to reduce tongue irritation. When regular length bracket plates or lever plates are chosen, the plates are placed as posterior as possible and the extra area of the plate protruding distally to the mini-implant can be bent down

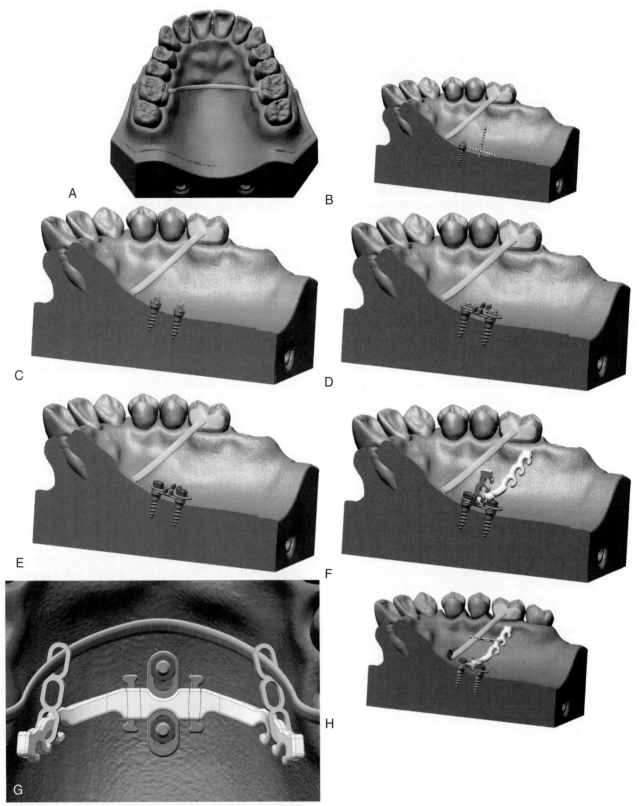

Figure 8.9 Placement procedure of LIM plate system. **(A)** A transpalatal arch is placed. **(B)** Anterior mini-implant is placed at mid-palate between the lingual cusps of the right and left second premolars. Then, mucosal indentation is formed using periodontal probe 5 mm posterior to the distal surface of the anterior mini-implant. **(C)** Posterior mini-implant is placed at the mucosal indentation. **(D)** Bracket plate is placed over the mini-implant head. Bending of the plate is required, if the fit is not good. **(E)** Nuts are fastened over the mini-implant head to fix the mini-plate. **(F)** A preformed lever is placed over the bracket on the bracket plate. **(G)** Tying each wing separately is easier than tying with one ligature wire because wings are flush with the base of the plate. **(H)** Elastomeric chains are connected between the transpalatal arch and the preformed lever.

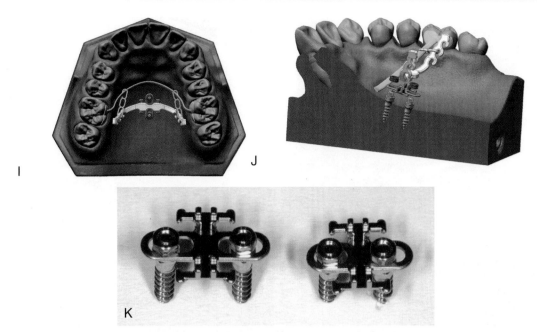

Figure 8.9, cont'd Placement procedure of LIM plate system. **(I)** As molars are distalized, premolars will be distalized by the supracrestal gingival fibres. **(J)** An expanded view of the bracket plate and preformed lever assembly. **(K)** Regular length bracket plate assembly (left) and short-length bracket plate assembly (right).

using a plier or a band pusher to reduce tongue irritation (Fig. 8.10). This procedure also can be performed using a band pusher after placement of nuts to fix the plate.

Bracket plates are more versatile than lever plate. When simple tooth movement is required, lever plates can be used for more convenience. For complex tooth movement, bracket plates are better because the preformed lever or wire lever can be removed to adjust extra-orally, and additional levers or springs can be welded or soldered to the main levers. When titanium molybdenum alloy levers are used, usual electric welding of additional levers or springs provide sufficient bond strength because this alloy has very good weldability.[24] To attach stainless steel wire to the stainless steel lever, soldering or laser welding is required. For intermediate cases, tubed type lever plates can be used, and auxiliary wire levers can be inserted into the tubes at the bilateral end of the lever.

Before placement of the plate, one side margin of an unfolded 2" × 2" gauze is moistened with saline and then the gauze is placed in the palate distal to the posterior mini-implant (Fig. 8.11). This wet gauze acts like a net covering the throat thus preventing the plate from falling into the throat, if the plate is dropped from the plier.

Plates are placed using a utility plier so that two holes are placed over the bolt structures of the mini-implants (Fig. 8.9C). Then, adaptation of the plate over the mini-implant heads is checked. If there is a large gap, the plate should be bent to fit to the mini-implant heads. When the heights of the two mini-implants are not same, a step bend should be bent to accommodate the height differences (Fig. 8.12). When step bending is made near the bracket wing, then placement of preformed wire would be difficult. If a large gap remains, nuts cannot be fastened over the bolt of the mini-implant head (Fig. 8.9D

and E). When there is a small gap, plates can be placed because it can deform and become fitted to the mini-implant head. When placing lever plates, levers should be adjusted to fit closely to the palate. After adjustment of the plate and lever of the lever plate, nut is picked up using the same driver used for mini-implant placement. The nut is fastened with 25 N.cm torque which is sufficient to prevent loosening. 50 N.cm torque can cause rotation of the mini-implant and also the plate, if the opposite mini-implant is not held tightly by the surrounding bone. After placement of the plate, prescription of antibiotics or analgesics is usually not needed. When a preformed lever is used, the lever should be adjusted to fit to the palate using a three-prong plier or other pliers. Although, levers are inserted into the bracket of the bracket plate usually immediately after the placement of plate (Fig. 8.9F and G), impressions can be taken later, if complex wire bending is required. Blocking out the undercuts under the plate using utility wax is required to prevent tearing of the impression material. An analogue for the plate is not required because alginate impressions can capture the slot accurately. Orthodontic forces can be applied immediately after the placement of plate (Fig. 8.9H).

After placement of levers into the bracket of the bracket plate, a ligature tie is preferred to fix the lever. .012" stainless steel ligature wire is preferred. Tying each wing separately is easier than tying two wings by one ligature wire (Fig. 8.6E). When applying heavy forces to the lateral ends of the lever, the lever will be deflected elastically. When distalization forces are applied from the lever to the anteriorly positioned transpalatal arch, the lateral ends of the lever will be deflected mesially and can impinge into the mucosa because the arch becomes narrower anteriorly. These deflections should be considered when adapting the lever to the palate.

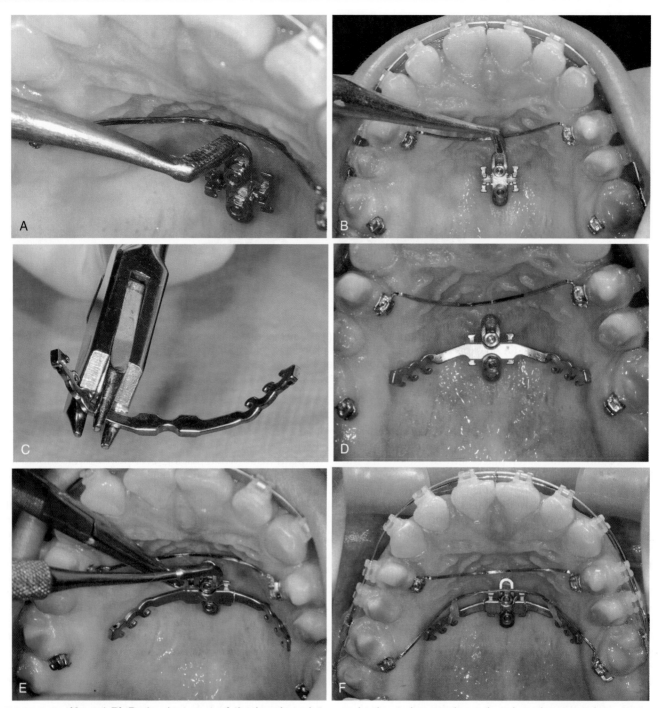

Figure 8.10 **(A** and **B)** Redundant part of the bracket plate can be bent down using a band pusher to reduce tongue irritation. **(C)** Preformed lever is bent according to the palatal curvature using a three-prong plier. **(D)** Preformed lever is placed over the bracket plate. **(E)** Ligature tying of preformed lever. To prevent slippage of ligature wire during tying, a sickle scaler was used. **(F)** After application of an elastomeric chain for distal movement of the maxillary first molars.

Removal of LIM plate system

Removal procedure of LIM plate system does not require anaesthesia. Wireless motor for orthodontic mini-implant placement (Orthonia, Jeil Medical, Seoul, Korea) can be used for removal of the mini-implants. After disinfection and irrigation, nuts should be seated securely into the pick up driver to prevent falling out into the oral cavity. After removal of the nuts, the plate is removed using a utility plier. During removal of nuts and plate, a gauze with margins soaked with saline can be placed posterior to the plate to prevent the nuts or plate from falling into the throat. Mini-implants are

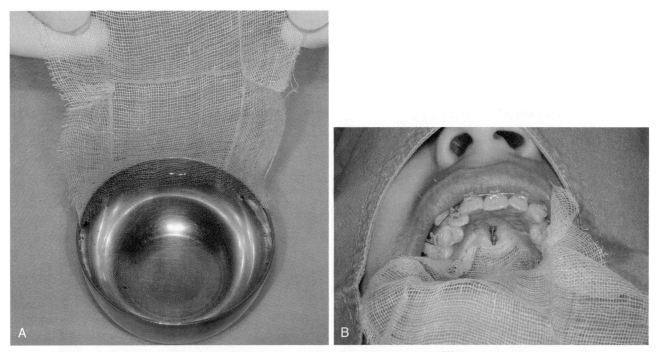

Figure 8.11 **(A)** A 2" × 2" gauze is unfolded and soaked with saline at one margin. **(B)** The soaked margin is attached on the palate posterior to the posterior mini-implant. This gauze drapes down to the tongue and lower lip. If a nut or plate slips from the driver or plier, this gauze mesh prevents the nut or plate from falling into the throat.

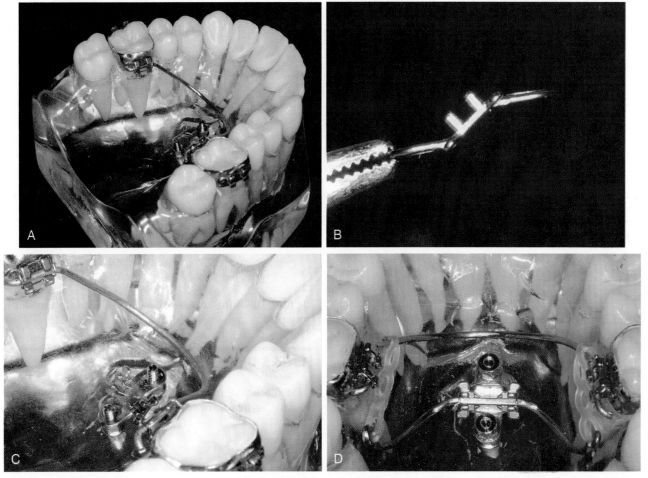

Figure 8.12 Bending of the plate. **(A)** Two mini-implants were placed at different heights. **(B)** Side view of the step bend on the bracket plate. **(C)** Bracket plate with step bend was placed over the mini-implants. **(D)** .032" × .032" precision lingual arch was tied into the bracket. Preformed lever could not be inserted over the bracket due to the interference caused by the bending of the plate.

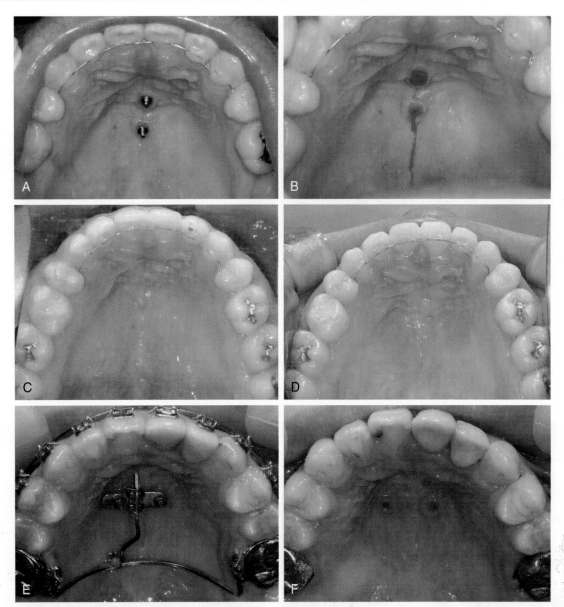

Figure 8.13 Healing of mucosa after removal of mini-implants of LIM plate system. **(A)** Immediately after removal of the bracket plate. 1 mm thickening of the mucosa around the mini-implant is seen. **(B)** Immediately after removal of mini-implants. **(C)** One week after removal of mini-implant. **(D)** Six months after removal of mini-implant. **(E)** Horizontal placement of two mini-implants. **(F)** Immediately after removal of mini-implants.

then removed. A 30 N.cm of torque is sufficient for removal in most cases. Sutures are not required and antibiotics are usually not needed. It is recommended to refrain from hot drinks or food on the day of removal. 1 mm thickening of the mucosa around the mini-implant is usually seen (Fig. 8.13). Due to this mucosal thickening, the plate should be at least 1 mm away from the mucosa. To achieve this, the 1.2 mm height hexagonal head of the mini-implant should not be placed under the mucosa.

CASES USING LIM PLATE SYSTEM

LIM plate system can be used for various purposes. Following figures show clinical cases using LIM plate system.

Molar distalization in non-extraction case (Fig. 8.14)

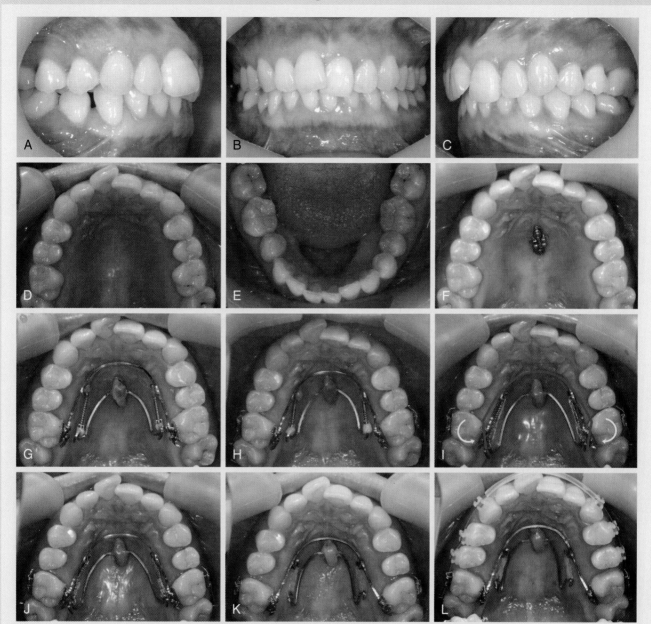

Figure 8.14   Distalization of maxillary molars using LIM plate system. **(A–E)** Pretreatment intraoral photographs of a 30-year-old female whose chief complaint was maxillary incisor crowding. She refused full arch fixed treatment and wanted treatment of the maxillary arch only. Mandibular right second premolar was missing. **(F)** A bracket plate was placed in the mid-sagittal suture. **(G)**, After placement of .032" × .032" stainless steel (SS) wire lever and transpalatal arch, NiTi closed coil springs were inserted between transpalatal arch and wire lever. **(H)** At 3 months of treatment, mesial rotation of maxillary right first molar was observed as a sign for molar distalization. **(I)** At 4 months of treatment, loose contacts between second premolars and first molars were observed. Elastomeric chain was added and **(J)** At 5 months of treatment, spacing between posterior teeth developed. **(K)** At 6 months of treatment, NiTi closed coil springs were replaced with elastomeric chains. **(L)** At 8 months of treatment, brackets were bonded on the maxillary arch except the incisors and a NiTi archwire was inserted.

Continued

Molar distalization in non-extraction case (Fig. 8.14)—cont'd

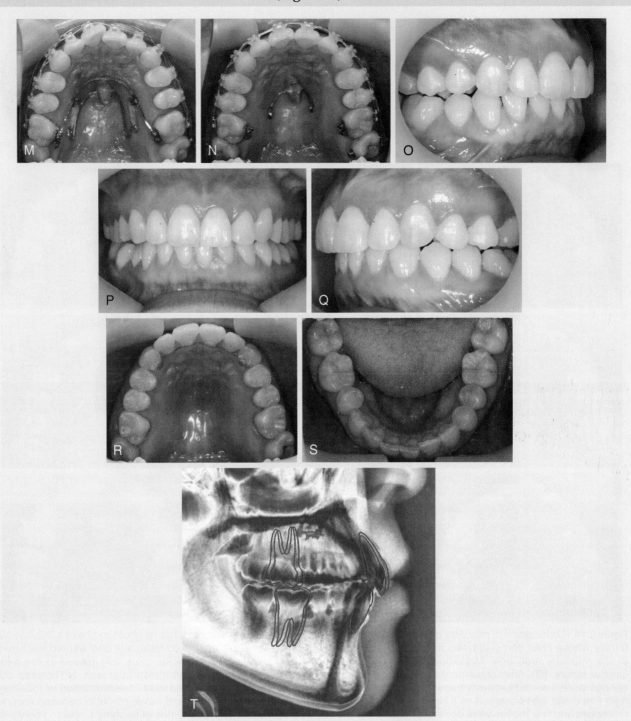

Figure 8.14, cont'd   Distalization of maxillary molars using LIM plate system. **(M)** At 9 months of treatment, brackets were bonded on the incisors and a .016" SS bypass arch and NiTi anterior segment wire were placed. Elastomeric chain was applied to retract canines and premolars. **(N)** At 11 months of treatment, .016" × .022" titanium molybdenum (TMA) finishing archwire was placed. **(O–S)** At 14 months of treatment, debonding and removal of mini-implants were performed. **(T)** Superimposition of pre- (blue) and post-treatment (red) cephalograms. Retraction of maxillary incisors and 2 mm distalization of maxillary molars were shown. Part of molar distalization was lost during closure of space after alignment of maxillary incisors.

Distalization of maxillary molars in extraction case (Fig. 8.15)

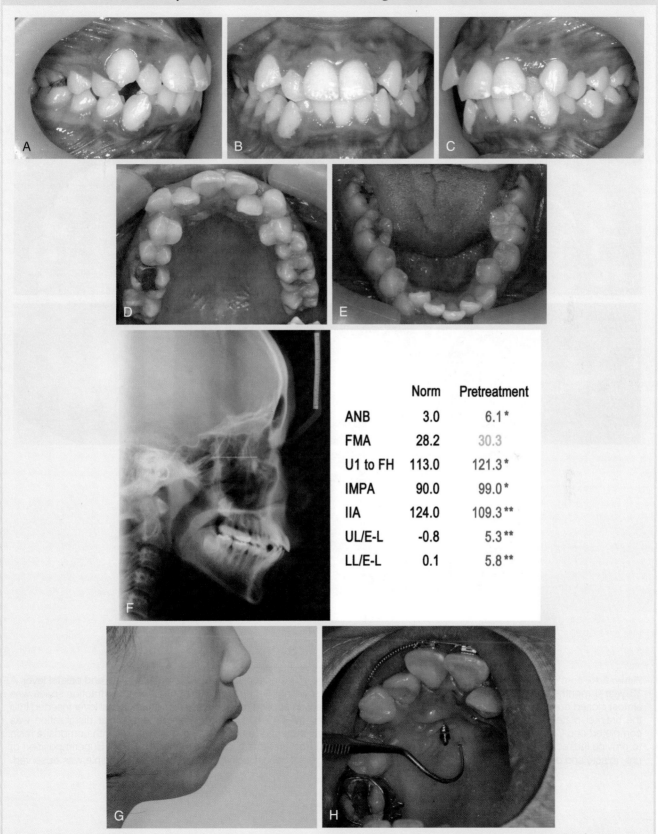

	Norm	Pretreatment
ANB	3.0	6.1*
FMA	28.2	30.3
U1 to FH	113.0	121.3*
IMPA	90.0	99.0*
IIA	124.0	109.3**
UL/E-L	-0.8	5.3**
LL/E-L	0.1	5.8**

Figure 8.15 Distalization of maxillary molars during closure of extraction space using a bracket plate and palatal lever. A 13-year-0-month-old female presented with a chief complaint of crowding. **(A–E)** Pretreatment intraoral photographs. **(F)** Pretreatment cephalogram and cephalometric analysis. **(G)** Pretreatment lateral facial photograph showing hypermentalis activity. **(H)** Two mini-implants were placed in the off-centre area of the mid-palatal suture with 6 mm interval.

Continued

Distalization of maxillary molars in extraction case (Fig. 8.15)—cont'd

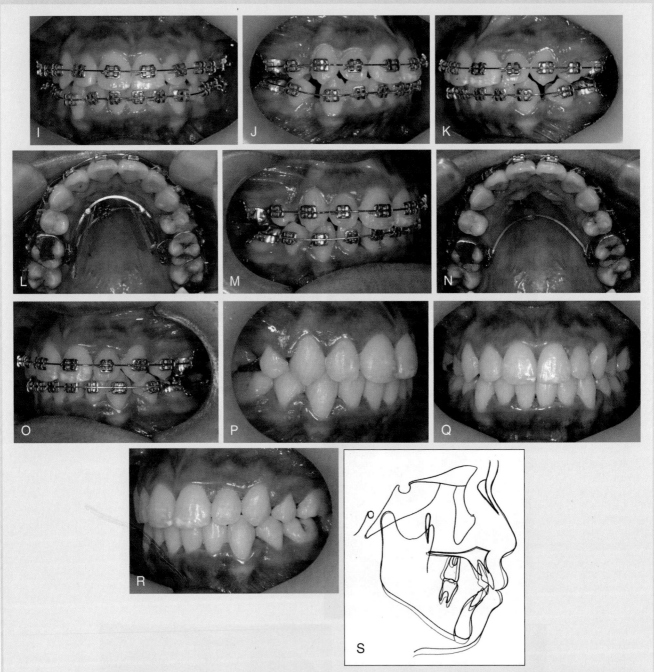

Figure 8.15, cont'd   Distalization of maxillary molars during closure of extraction space using a bracket plate and palatal lever. A 13-year-0-month-old female presented with a chief complaint of crowding. **(I–L)** At 7 months of treatment, extraction space was almost closed during alignment of anterior teeth. Distalization force was applied from the stainless steel palatal lever inserted into the bracket plate to the transpalatal arch attached to first molars. **(M–O)** At 11 months of treatment, molar distalization was completed and Class I molar relationships were achieved. TPA was attached to the posterior mini-implant with composite resin to provide indirect anchorage for retraction of anterior teeth. **(P–R)** Post-treatment intraoral photographs. **(S)** Superimposition of pre- (black) and post-treatment (red) cephalograms registered at cranial base. Backward rotation of the mandible was observed.

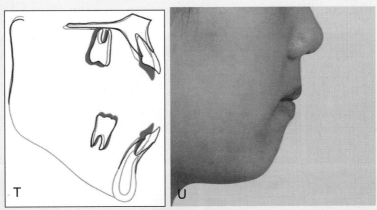

Figure 8.15, cont'd   Distalization of maxillary molars during closure of extraction space using a bracket plate and palatal lever. A 13-year-0-month-old female presented with a chief complaint of crowding. **(T)** Superimposition of pre- (black) and post-treatment (red) cephalograms registered at the mandible. **(U)** Post-treatment lateral facial photograph. Hypermentalis activity was improved, although not completely removed.

Maxillary molar distalization for anteroposterior decompensation (Fig. 8.16)

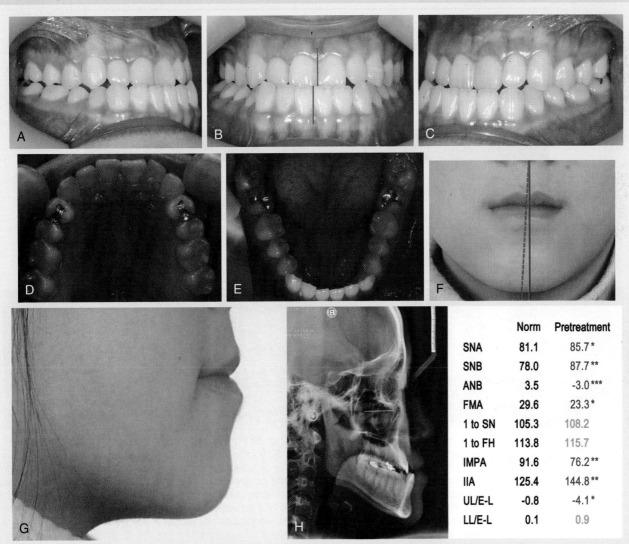

	Norm	Pretreatment
SNA	81.1	85.7 *
SNB	78.0	87.7 **
ANB	3.5	-3.0 ***
FMA	29.6	23.3 *
1 to SN	105.3	108.2
1 to FH	113.8	115.7
IMPA	91.6	76.2 **
IIA	125.4	144.8 **
UL/E-L	-0.8	-4.1 *
LL/E-L	0.1	0.9

Figure 8.16   Distalization of maxillary molars for decompensation of the labioversion of maxillary incisors in a patient needing mandibular setback surgery. A female patient of 18 years 8 months of age presented with a chief complaint of protrusive mandible. **(A–E)** Pretreatment intraoral photographs. **(F and G)** Pretreatment facial photographs. **(H)** Pretreatment cephalogram and cephalometric analysis.

Continued

Maxillary molar distalization for anteroposterior decompensation (Fig. 8.16)—cont'd

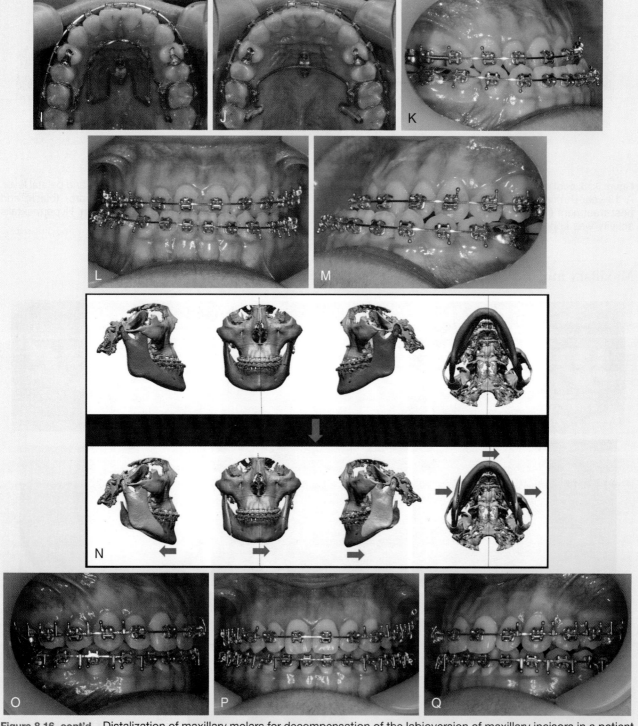

Figure 8.16, cont'd   Distalization of maxillary molars for decompensation of the labioversion of maxillary incisors in a patient needing mandibular setback surgery. A female patient of 18 years 8 months of age presented with a chief complaint of protrusive mandible. **(I),** Bracket plate and wire lever were placed and distalization force was applied from the wire lever to the transpalatal arch using a NiTi closed coil spring. **(J–M)** At 9 months of treatment, presurgical orthodontic treatment was completed. The transpalatal arch made with .032" × .032" titanium- molybdenum wire was used to constrict the maxillary arch for establishment of arch coordination. **(N)** 3D simulation of BSSRO setback surgery. Mandibular setback of 8 mm on the right and 10 mm on the left along with 2 mm shift to the left side were planned. Surgery was performed at 10 months of treatment. **(O–Q)** Intraoral photographs immediately after surgery.

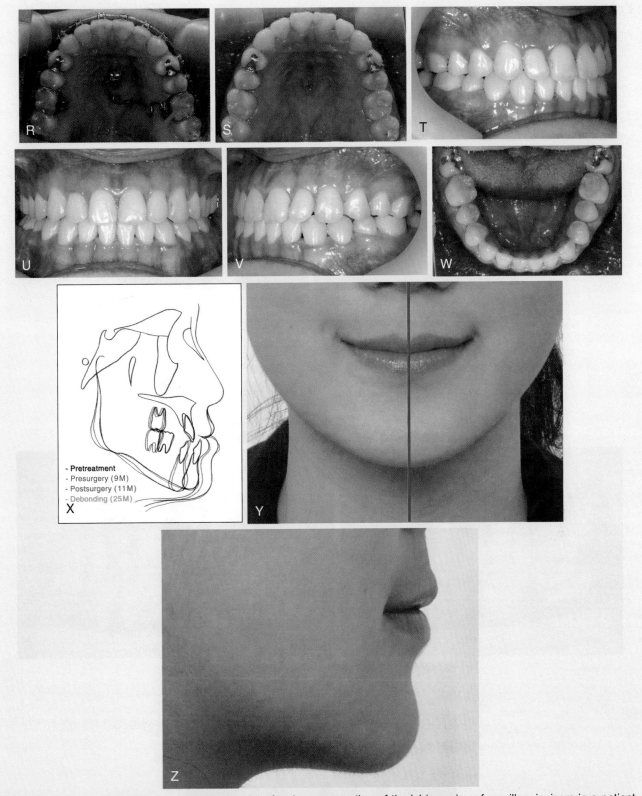

Figure 8.16, cont'd   Distalization of maxillary molars for decompensation of the labioversion of maxillary incisors in a patient needing mandibular setback surgery. A female patient of 18 years 8 months of age presented with a chief complaint of protrusive mandible. **(R)** After surgery, molar distalization resumed on the left side. Lingually directed distalization force was applied to reduce buccal overjet on the left side. **(S–W)** Post-treatment intraoral photographs. **(X)** Superimposition of pre- and post-treatment cephalograms. Maxillary molar distalization and forward rotation of the mandible during postsurgical orthodontic treatment was observed. Despite distalization of molars, linguo-version of maxillary incisors was not satisfactory due to the space gained by distalization was taken up during constriction of maxillary arch. **(Y and Z)** Post-treatment facial photographs.

Protraction of maxillary posterior teeth (Fig. 8.17)

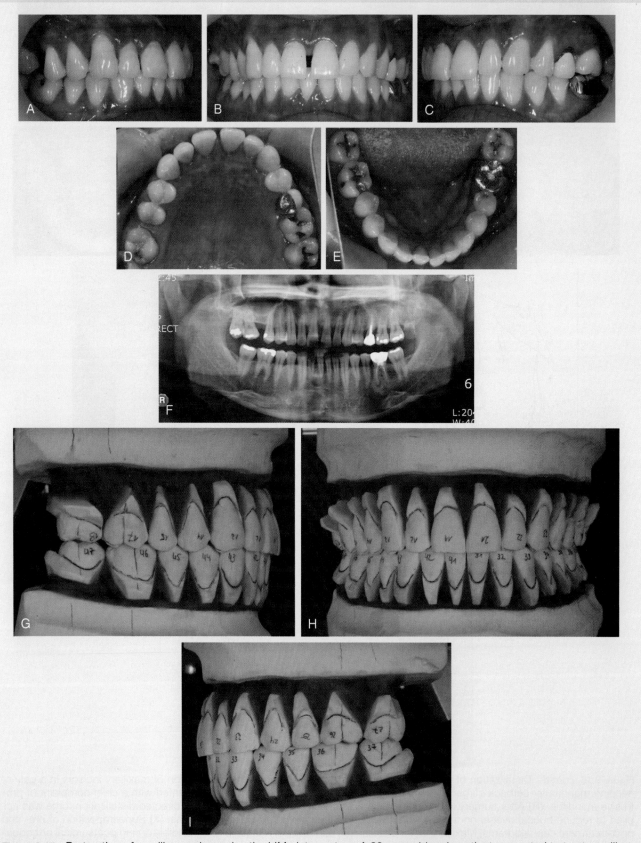

Figure 8.17 Protraction of maxillary molars using the LIM plate system. A 32-year-old male patient presented to treat maxillary diastema that developed after extraction of his maxillary right first molar. **(A–E)** Pretreatment intraoral photographs. **(F)** Pretreatment panoramic radiograph. Mesial tipping of maxillary right second and third molars was observed. Extraction of mandibular right central incisor was planned due to severe mobility. **(G–I)**, Setup models showing occlusion after closure of the diastema and the extraction space of the maxillary right first molar by protraction of the maxillary right second and third molars.

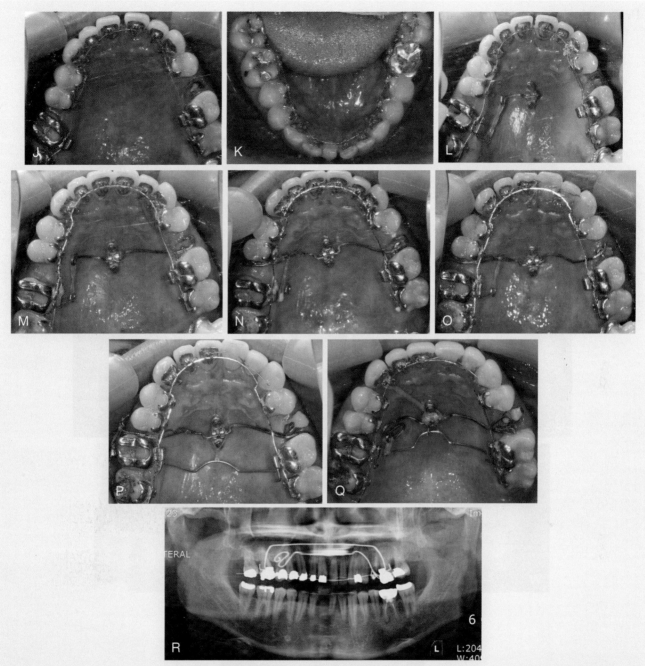

Figure 8.17, cont'd Protraction of maxillary molars using the LIM plate system. A 32-year-old male patient presented to treat maxillary diastema that developed after extraction of his maxillary right first molar. **(J** and **K)**, Customized lingual brackets (Incognito, TOP-Service fürLingualtechnik, Bad Essen, Germany) were bonded. Maxillary left second premolar was fractured and root was left before the start of treatment. Extraction and implant restoration after orthodontic treatment was planned along with forced traction to increase alveolar bone. Mandibular right central incisor was extracted and pontic was placed. **(L)** Bracket plate was placed in the mid-palate. Wire lever was placed on the bracket plate. Another lever was inserted into the lingual sheath of the maxillary second molar. An elastomeric chain was applied between two levers making the protraction force pass at the level of centre of resistance of the tooth. **(M)** Seven months of treatment. Bilateral lever was used to extrude remaining root of the maxillary left second premolar. **(N)** Nine months of treatment. TMA wire segment was welded to the wire lever to extend to the distal surface of the maxillary right second premolar and protraction force was applied to both premolars and molars. **(O)** Eleven months of treatment. Lingual brackets on maxillary left incisors, maxillary left canine, and all mandibular teeth were removed and fixed retainers were bonded due to severe gingival inflammation around the bracket. **(P)** One year and five months of treatment. Transpalatal arch was inserted to correct rotation of maxillary right molars and protraction force was applied at the mid-palate. To prevent protraction of the left first molar, lever contacted maxillary left first molar crown. **(Q)** One year and ten months of treatment. Spring lever was used to protract maxillary right molars. **(R)** Panoramic radiograph at one year and ten months of treatment.

Continued

Protraction of maxillary posterior teeth (Fig. 8.17)—cont'd

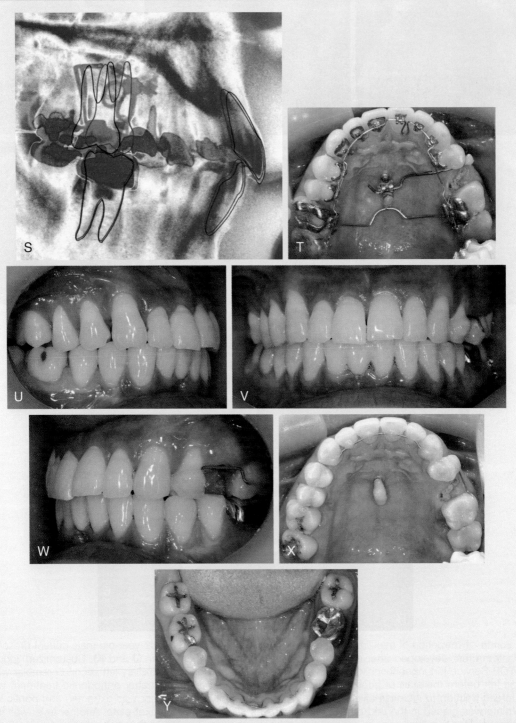

Figure 8.17, cont'd Protraction of maxillary molars using the LIM plate system. A 32-year-old male patient presented to treat maxillary diastema that developed after extraction of his maxillary right first molar. **(S)** Cephalometric superimposition of pretreatment (blue) and at one year and ten months of treatment (red). Maxillary right second molars were drawn and 3 mm protraction of maxillary right molars was observed. **(T)** For final detailing, lingual self-ligating bracket was bonded on maxillary left incisors and canine. Lever was used to protract maxillary left first premolar. **(U–Y)** After two years and four months of treatment, maxillary brackets were debonded. Post-treatment intraoral photographs.

Intrusion of maxillary posterior teeth (Fig. 8.18)

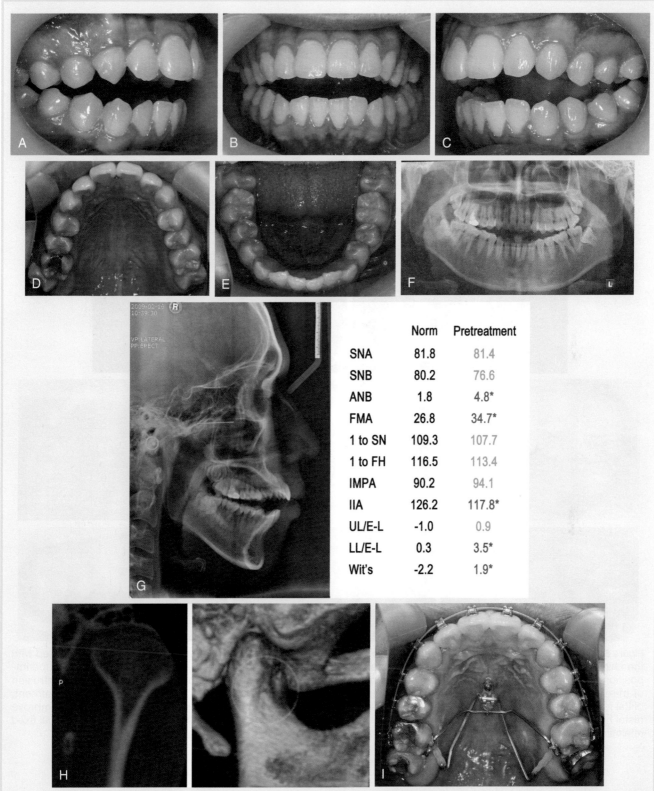

	Norm	Pretreatment
SNA	81.8	81.4
SNB	80.2	76.6
ANB	1.8	4.8*
FMA	26.8	34.7*
1 to SN	109.3	107.7
1 to FH	116.5	113.4
IMPA	90.2	94.1
IIA	126.2	117.8*
UL/E-L	-1.0	0.9
LL/E-L	0.3	3.5*
Wit's	-2.2	1.9*

Figure 8.18 Intrusion and distalization of maxillary molars using LIM plate system. A 20-year-old male presented with the chief complaint of open bite. He had been treated for retrodiscitis and capsulitis of his right TMJ. **(A–E)** Pretreatment intraoral photographs. **(F)** Pretreatment panoramic radiograph. **(G)** Pretreatment cephalometric radiograph and cephalometric analysis. **(H)** There was no progressive bone resorption at the condyle. **(I)** At 8 months of treatment, distally directed intrusive forces were applied to the lingual brackets bonded on the maxillary first molars.

Continued

Intrusion of maxillary posterior teeth (Fig. 8.18)—cont'd

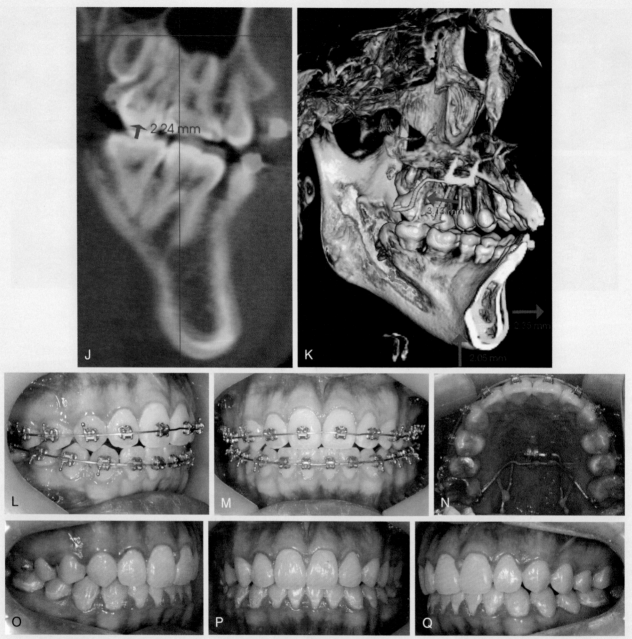

Figure 8.18, cont'd   Intrusion and distalization of maxillary molars using LIM plate system. A 20-year-old male presented with the chief complaint of open bite. He had been treated for retrodiscitis and capsulitis of his right TMJ. **(J and K)** Superimposition of pretreatment (ivory) and 1 year of treatment (blue) cone-beam CT images. 3 mm distalization and 2 mm intrusion of maxillary first molar, and 2 mm superior movement of menton was observed. **(L–N)** At 1 year 6 months of treatment, distal forces passing through the apical side of the centre of resistance of the maxillary first molars were applied to improve distal tipping of the maxillary first molars. **(O–S)** At 2 years 3 months of treatment, debonding was performed and lingual fixed retainers were bonded.

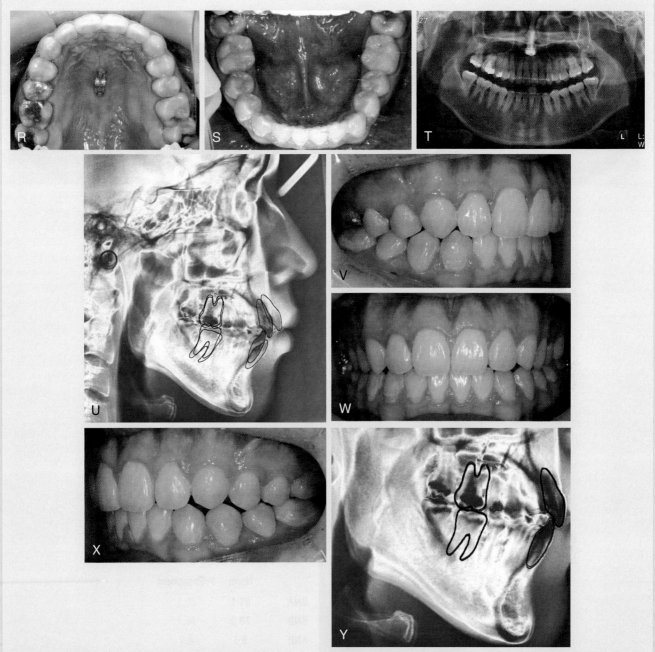

Figure 8.18, cont'd   Intrusion and distalization of maxillary molars using LIM plate system. A 20-year-old male presented with the chief complaint of open bite. He had been treated for retrodiscitis and capsulitis of his right TMJ. **(T)** Post-treatment panoramic radiograph. **(U)** Superimposition of pre- (blue) and post-treatment (red) cephalograms. Forward rotation of the mandible was observed. **(V–X)** 11 months post-treatment. Slight opening of the anterior overbite was observed. **(Y)** Superimposition of post-treatment (blue) and 11 months post-treatment (red) cephalograms showed mild extrusion of the molars and backward rotation of the mandible.

Extrusion of maxillary anterior teeth (Fig. 8.19)

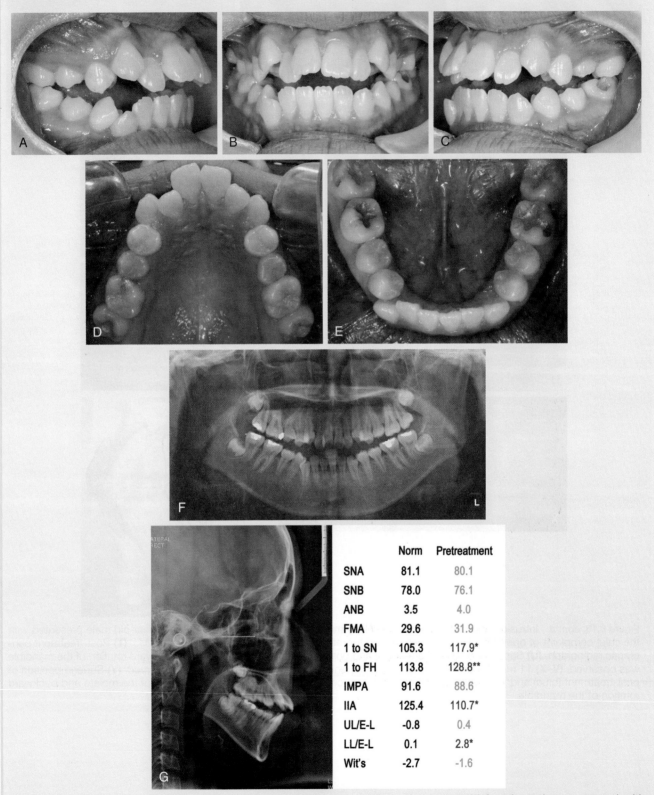

	Norm	Pretreatment
SNA	81.1	80.1
SNB	78.0	76.1
ANB	3.5	4.0
FMA	29.6	31.9
1 to SN	105.3	117.9*
1 to FH	113.8	128.8**
IMPA	91.6	88.6
IIA	125.4	110.7*
UL/E-L	-0.8	0.4
LL/E-L	0.1	2.8*
Wit's	-2.7	-1.6

Figure 8.19 Extrusion of maxillary anterior teeth using LIM plate system. A 14-year-old female patient presented with a chief complaint of crowding and anterior open bite. **(A–E)** Pretreatment intraoral photographs. **(F)** Pretreatment panoramic radiograph. Short roots of maxillary incisors were observed. **(G)** Pretreatment cephalometric radiograph and cephalometric analysis. Extractions of maxillary second premolars and mandibular first premolars were planned.

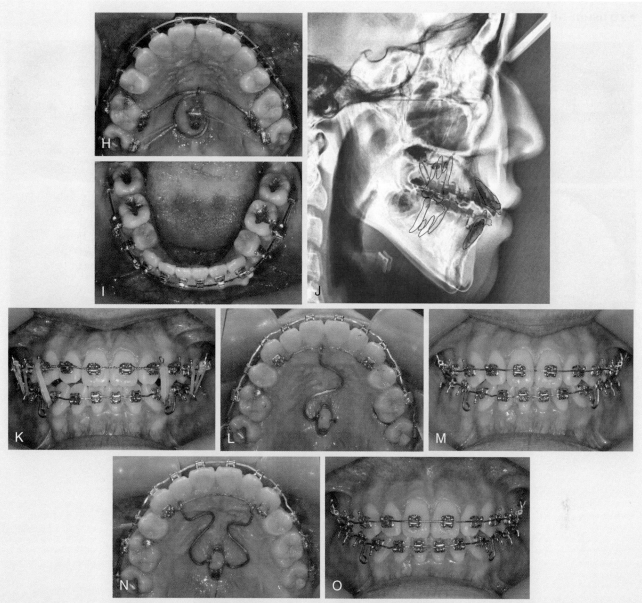

Figure 8.19, cont'd Extrusion of maxillary anterior teeth using LIM plate system. A 14-year-old female patient presented with a chief complaint of crowding and anterior open bite. **(H** and **I)** Intrusion spring was placed over the TPA and elastic thread was used to intrude maxillary second molars. **(J)** Superimposition of pretreatment (blue) and 2 years of treatment (red) cephalograms showed intrusion of the maxillary molars and forward rotation of the mandible. Differential growth of mandible was also seen. **(K)** Although wearing of vertical elastics was instructed, patient's compliance was not sufficient. **(L** and **M)** Wire lever from the bracket plate was hooked to the lingual arch between canines was applied to extrude the maxillary anterior teeth. **(N** and **O),** Wire levers were hooked near the lingual brackets of maxillary canines. Bite was deepened.

Continued

Extrusion of maxillary anterior teeth (Fig. 8.19)—cont'd

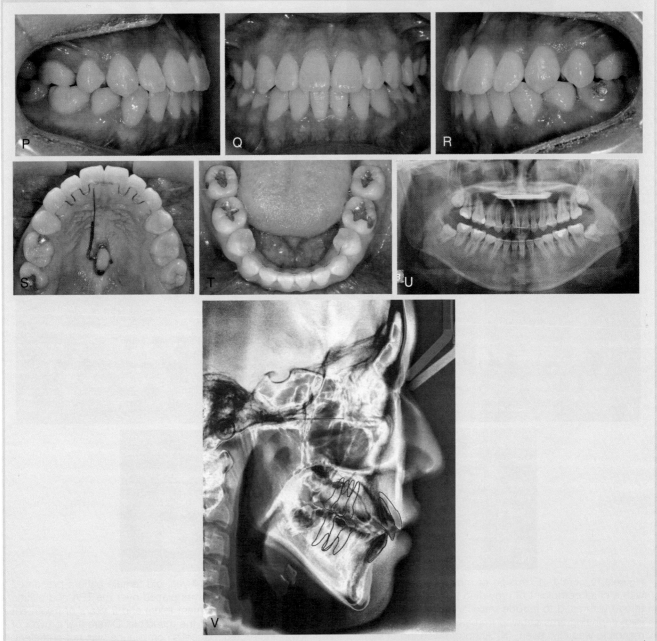

Figure 8.19, cont'd   Extrusion of maxillary anterior teeth using LIM plate system. A 14-year-old female patient presented with a chief complaint of crowding and anterior open bite. **(P–T)** Post-treatment intraoral photographs. Maxillary fixed retainer with interproximal U-loops was made using .016" TMA wire. A wire lever made with TMA was welded to this fixed retainer to prevent relapse of extruded incisors. **(U)** Post-treatment panoramic radiograph. **(V)** Superimposition of pre- (blue) and post-treatment (red) cephalograms. Although FMA was reduced, growth of the mandible masked the effect of forward rotation. Extrusion of maxillary incisors was observed.

Traction of impacted canine (Fig. 8.20)

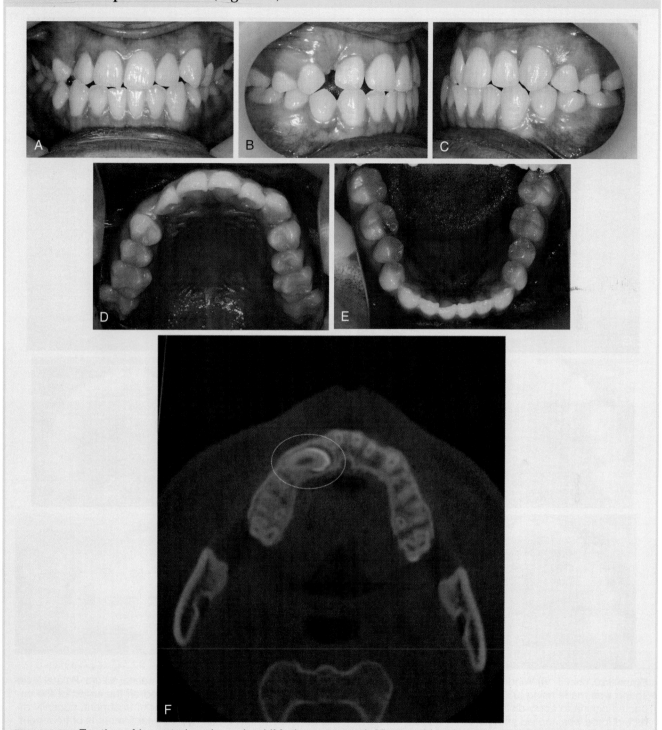

Figure 8.20 Traction of impacted canine using LIM plate system. A 25-year-old male was referred from a local clinic for evaluation and treatment of his impacted maxillary right canine. **(A–E)** Pretreatment intraoral photographs. **(F–H)** Pretreatment CBCT images. Circles indicate impacted maxillary right canine.

Continued

Traction of impacted canine (Fig. 8.20)—cont'd

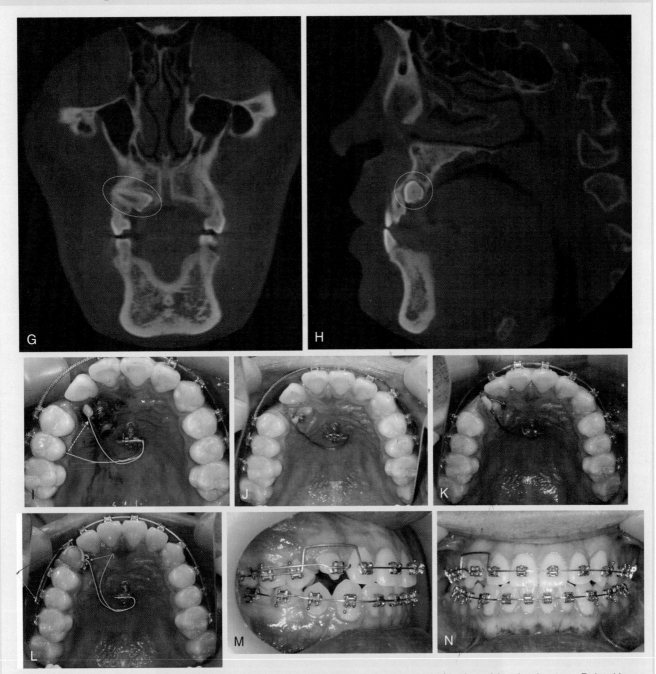

Figure 8.20, cont'd **(I)** Window opening was performed and bracket plate was placed in the mid-palatal suture. Palatal lever spring was made using .032" × .032" titanium molybdenum alloy and tied to the button bonded on the crown of the impacted canine to apply distally directed extrusive force. **(J)** 6 months of treatment. **(K)** At 1 year of treatment, buccally directed force was applied and a bracket was bonded on the maxillary lateral incisor. **(L–N)** At 1 year 5 months of treatment, mesially directed force was applied on the lingual side and distally directed force was applied on the buccal side to rotate the maxillary right canine distally. For this, a buccal lever arm was inserted on the bracket of the maxillary right canine. This lever arm was activated by pulling the distal end lingually to the main archwire.

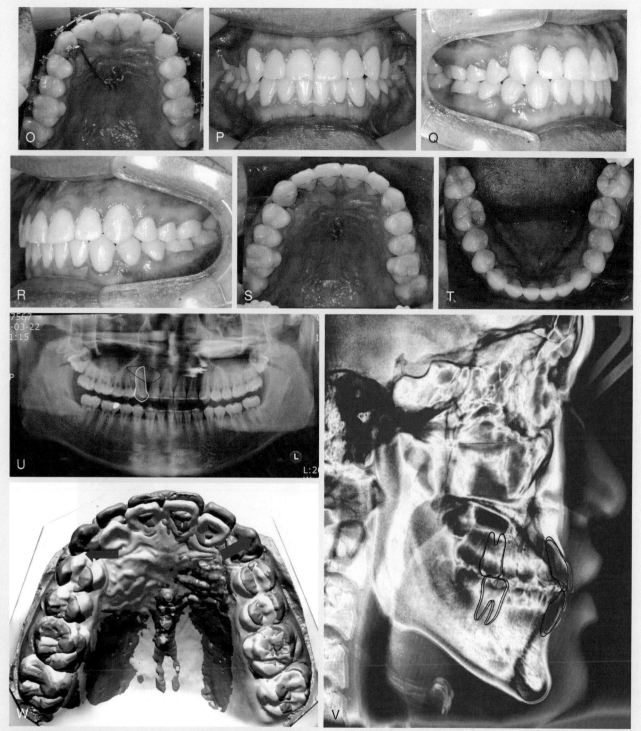

Figure 8.20, cont'd   Traction of impacted canine using LIM plate system. A 25-year-old male was referred from a local clinic for evaluation and treatment of his impacted maxillary right canine. **(O)** At 2 years 1 month of treatment, buccal root torque was applied to the maxillary right canine by inserting a palatal lever spring into the lingual bracket of the maxillary right canine after grinding the end of the lever to be inserted into the .018" slot. **(P–T)** At 2 years 6 months of treatment, debonding was performed. **(U)** Post-treatment panoramic radiograph. **(V)** Superimposition of pre- (blue) and post-treatment (red) cephalograms. Mild flaring of maxillary and mandibular incisors was observed. **(W)**, Superimposition of pre- (white) and post-treatment (blue) digital models. In addition to the flaring of maxillary incisors, expansion of initially constricted maxillary anterior archform was observed.

Vertical and transverse decompensation for orthognathic surgery (Fig. 8.21)

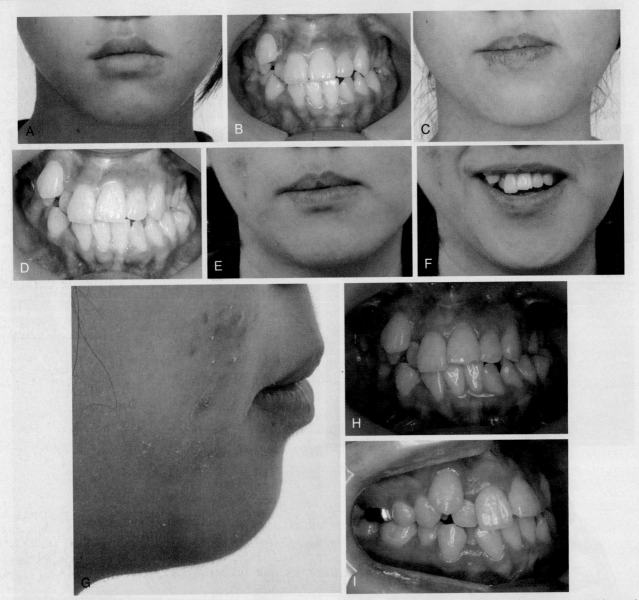

Figure 8.21 Decompensation of vertical and transverse compensation using bracket plate, palatal lever, and buccal mini-implants in a female patient who required combined surgical orthodontic treatment for mandibular asymmetry. **(A and B)** Facial and intraoral photographs taken at 11 years 9 months of age. **(C and D)** Facial and intraoral photographs taken at 14 years 3 months of age. Treatment of facial asymmetry was delayed until completion of facial growth. **(E–G)** Pretreatment facial photographs taken at 18 years 3 months of age. **(H–L)** Pretreatment intraoral photographs.

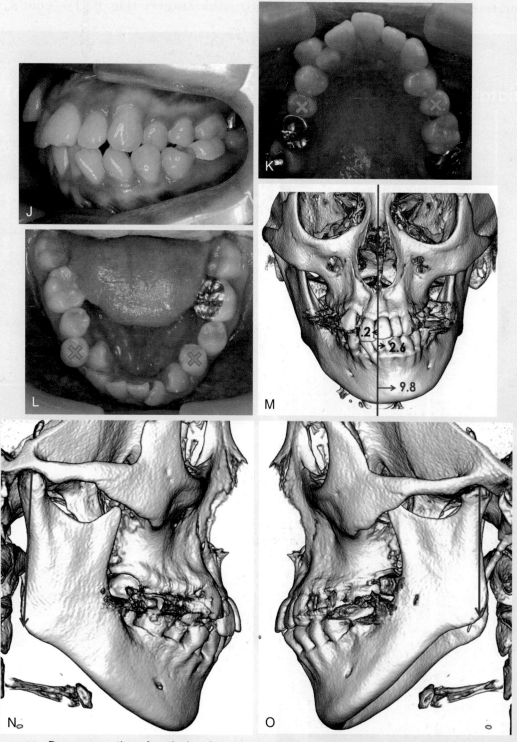

Figure 8.21, cont'd   Decompensation of vertical and transverse compensation using bracket plate, palatal lever, and buccal mini-implants in a female patient who required combined surgical orthodontic treatment for mandibular asymmetry. **(M–O)** Pretreatment cone-beam computed tomography (CBCT) images. Left ramus height was 10 mm shorter than the right ramus height due to previous condylar bone resorption related to degenerative joint disease. Pogonion was deviated 9.8 mm to left. On follow-up observations before orthodontic treatment, further condylar bone resorption was not seen.

Continued

Vertical and transverse decompensation for orthognathic surgery (Fig. 8.21)—cont'd

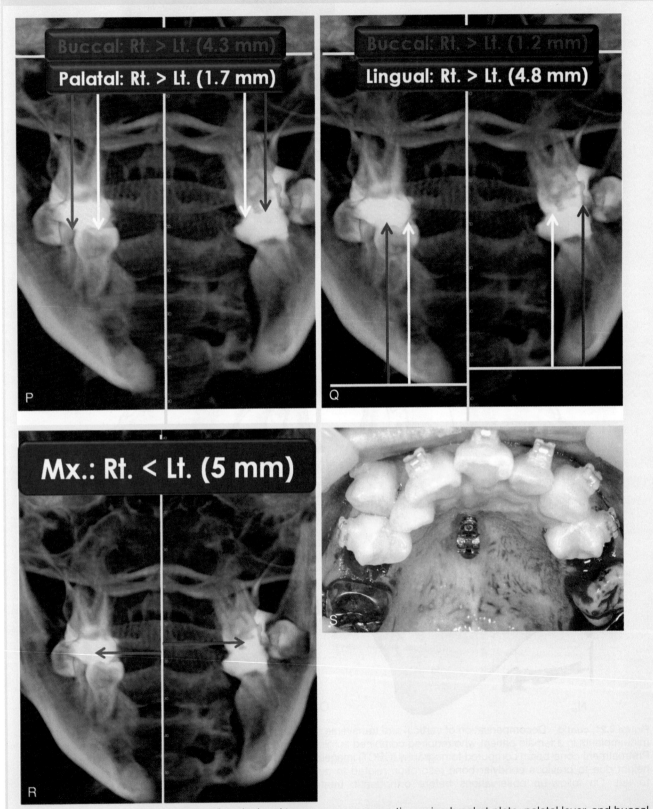

Figure 8.21, cont'd Decompensation of vertical and transverse compensation using bracket plate, palatal lever, and buccal mini-implants in a female patient who required combined surgical orthodontic treatment for mandibular asymmetry. **(P–R)** Coronal clipping view at the anteroposterior level of first molars. Vertical dentoalveolar compensations to shift mandibular to left were noted as an 4.3 mm extrusion of buccal cusp of maxillary right first molar **(P)** and 4.8 mm extrusion of lingual cusp of mandibular right first molar **(Q)**. Transverse dentoalveolar compensation to shift mandibular to the left was noted as 5 mm buccal positioning of the central fossa of the maxillary left first molar relative to the maxillary right first molar **(R)**. **(S)** To resolve crowding, maxillary second premolars which had interproximal caries were extracted and a bracket plate was placed in the mid-palatal suture. In the mandibular arch, first premolars were extracted.

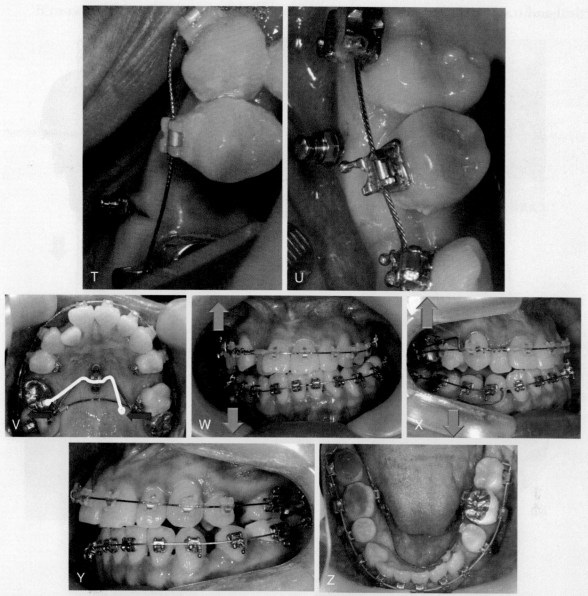

Figure 8.21, cont'd Decompensation of vertical and transverse compensation using bracket plate, palatal lever, and buccal mini-implants in a female patient who required combined surgical orthodontic treatment for mandibular asymmetry. **(T and U)** Buccal mini-implants were placed between maxillary right second premolar and first molar and between mandibular right second premolar and first molar. **(V)** .032" × .032" TMA wire lever was inserted into the bracket plate and activated to move the maxillary molar to the right side. Intrusive force was applied on the right side. **(W–Z)** Rhythmic wires[25] were placed over the buccal mini-implants to intrude the maxillary and mandibular posterior teeth on the right side.

Continued

Vertical and transverse decompensation for orthognathic surgery (Fig. 8.21)—cont'd

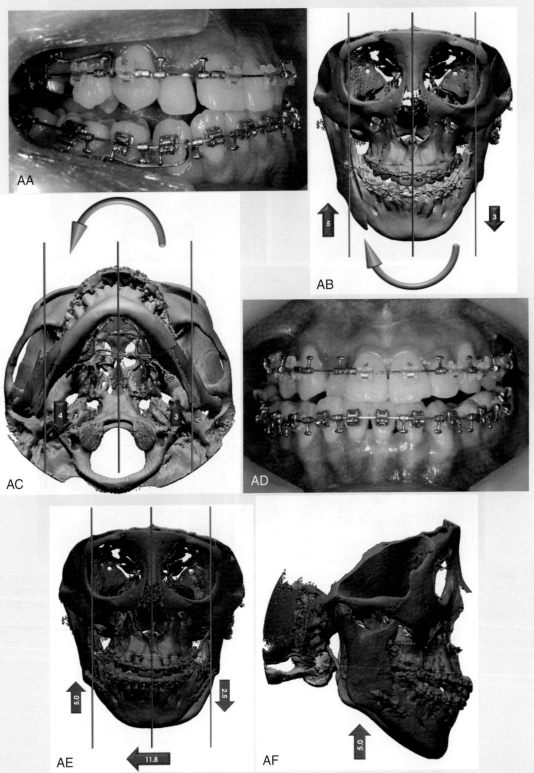

Figure 8.21, cont'd Decompensation of vertical and transverse compensation using bracket plate, palatal lever, and buccal mini-implants in a female patient who required combined surgical orthodontic treatment for mandibular asymmetry. **(AA)** Intraoral photograph before surgery at 11 months of treatment. Posterior open bite was formed on the right side. **(AB** and **AC)** 3D simulation of surgery. In the frontal view, rolling control of the distal segment of the mandible was planned **(AB)**. In the axial view, yawing control of the distal segment of the mandible was planned **(AC)**. Only mandibular surgery was performed using bilateral sagittal split osteotomy and maxillary surgery was not performed. **(AD)** Intraoral photograph two weeks after surgery. **(AE** and **AF)**, Superimposition of presurgery (blue) and two-week-postsurgery (red) cone-beam CT images. Distal segment of mandible was moved similar to the 3D simulation of surgery.

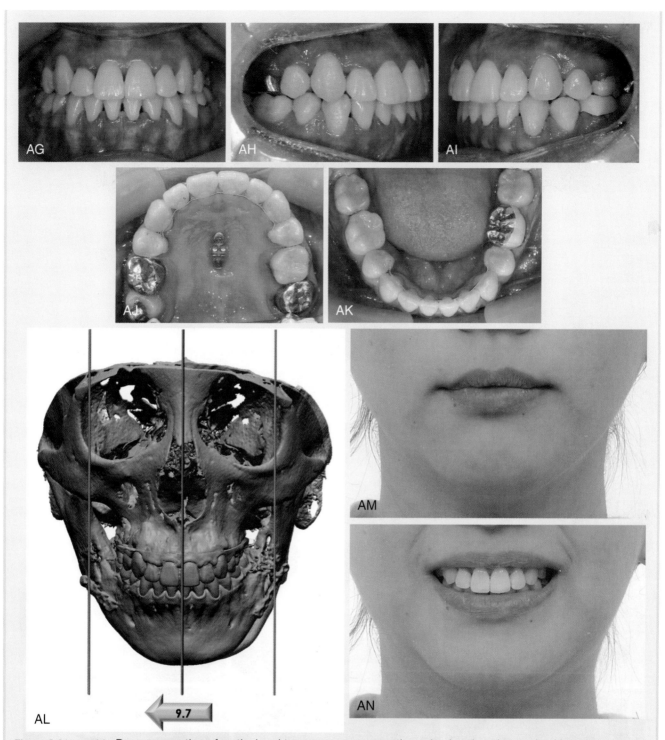

Figure 8.21, cont'd   Decompensation of vertical and transverse compensation using bracket plate, palatal lever, and buccal mini-implants in a female patient who required combined surgical orthodontic treatment for mandibular asymmetry. **(AG–AK)** After 2 years 1 months of treatment, debonding was performed. **(AL)** Post-treatment CBCT image. **(AM–AO)** Post-treatment facial photographs. Mandibular asymmetry was corrected successfully.

Continued

Vertical and transverse decompensation for orthognathic surgery (Fig. 8.21)—cont'd

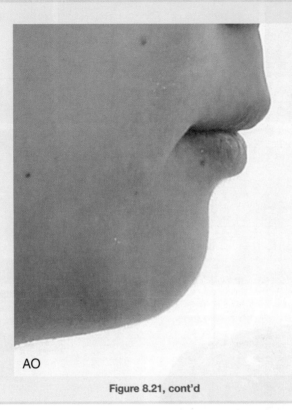

AO

Figure 8.21, cont'd

Protraction of mandibular molars (Fig. 8.22)

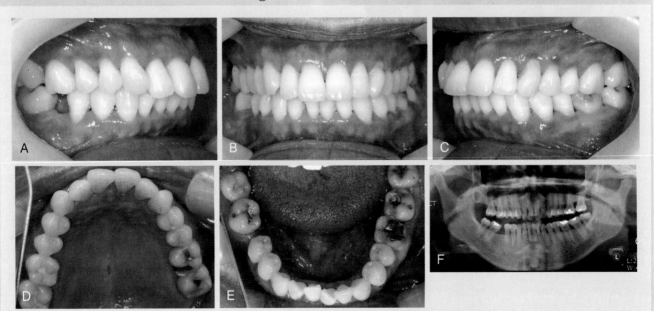

Figure 8.22 Protraction of mandibular molars using LIM plate system. A 33-year-old female patient was referred from the department of prosthodontics for molar uprighting before placement of an implant at the extraction site of mandibular right first molar. Mandibular right first molar was extracted 17 years ago. **(A–E)** Pretreatment intraoral photographs. **(F)** Pretreatment panoramic radiograph. Mesial tipping of mandibular right second and third molars was observed. Full orthodontic treatment was refused and protraction of mandibular right second and third molars was chosen instead of molar uprighting.

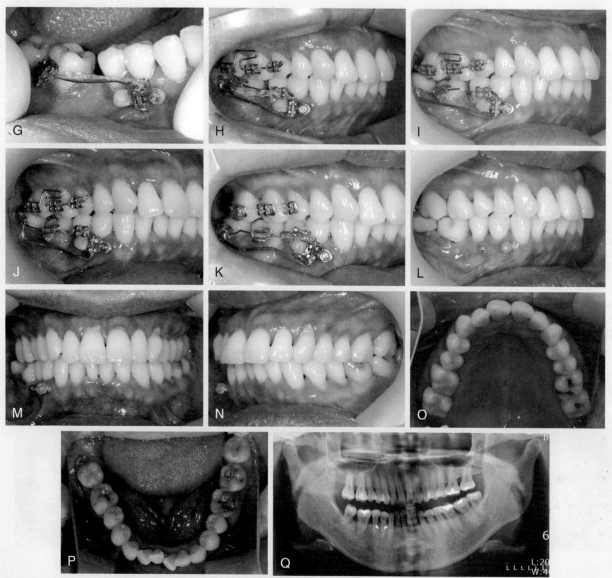

Figure 8.22, cont'd   Protraction of mandibular molars using LIM plate system. A 33-year-old female patient was referred from the department of prosthodontics for molar uprighting before placement of an implant at the extraction site of mandibular right first molar. Mandibular right first molar was extracted 17 years ago. **(G)** Mini-implants were placed between mandibular right canine and first premolar and between first and second premolars. Bracket plate was placed and segment wire connecting the bracket plate and mandibular right second molar was placed. Elastomeric chain was used for sliding protraction of the mandibular right second molar. **(H)** Four months of treatment. To prevent extrusion of the distal part of the mandibular right second molar, .032" × .032" SS lever was placed and intrusive force was applied by pulling the posterior end of the lever toward the distal extension of the wire segment inserted into the bracket bonded on mandibular right second molar. .022" slot bracket was welded to this lever and segment wire connecting this bracket and the mandibular right first molar was used. Elastomeric chain was used for sliding protraction. Brackets were bonded on the maxillary right second premolar and first and second molars, and a segment wire with an L-loop was inserted to intrude the maxillary right first molar. **(I)** One year one month of treatment. Gable bend was formed at centre of the segment wire connecting the bracket on the lever and the bracket on the mandibular right second molar. **(J)** One year six months of treatment. Tube was bonded on the mandibular right third molar and wire segment was inserted from the bracket on the lever to the tube on the third molar. **(K)** One year eleven months of treatment. Finishing wire segment was placed. **(L–P)** After two years and one month of treatment, debonding was performed and a fixed retainer was bonded between the mandibular right second premolar and second molar. **(Q)** Post-treatment panoramic radiograph.

Continued

Protraction of mandibular molars (Fig. 8.22)—cont'd

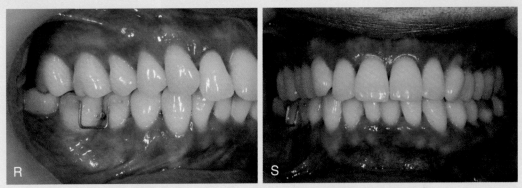

Figure 8.22, cont'd   Protraction of mandibular molars using LIM plate system. A 33-year-old female patient was referred from the department of prosthodontics for molar uprighting before placement of an implant at the extraction site of mandibular right first molar. Mandibular right first molar was extracted 17 years ago. **(R and S)** One year after treatment, occlusion was stable.

CASES USING MINI-IMPLANT PLACED IN THE RETROMOLAR AREA OF THE MANDIBLE

Distalization of mandibular molars (Fig. 8.23)

Figure 8.23   Mandibular molar distalization using mini-implant. A 24-year-old male presented with a chief complaint of anterior crossbite and crowding. **(A–E)** Pretreatment intraoral photographs.

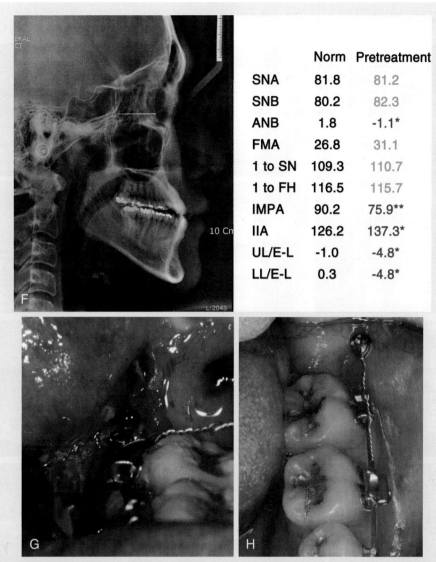

	Norm	Pretreatment
SNA	81.8	81.2
SNB	80.2	82.3
ANB	1.8	-1.1*
FMA	26.8	31.1
1 to SN	109.3	110.7
1 to FH	116.5	115.7
IMPA	90.2	75.9**
IIA	126.2	137.3*
UL/E-L	-1.0	-4.8*
LL/E-L	0.3	-4.8*

Figure 8.23, cont'd   Mandibular molar distalization using mini-implant. A 24-year-old male presented with a chief complaint of anterior crossbite and crowding. **(F)** Pretreatment cephalogram and cephalometric analysis. ANB angle of −1° was observed. Normal inclination of the maxillary incisors and retroclination of the lower incisors were observed. **(G and H)** Orthodontic mini-implants (2.0 mm × 8 mm) were placed at the distobuccal side of the mandibular right and left second molars.

Continued

Distalization of mandibular molars (Fig. 8.23)—cont'd

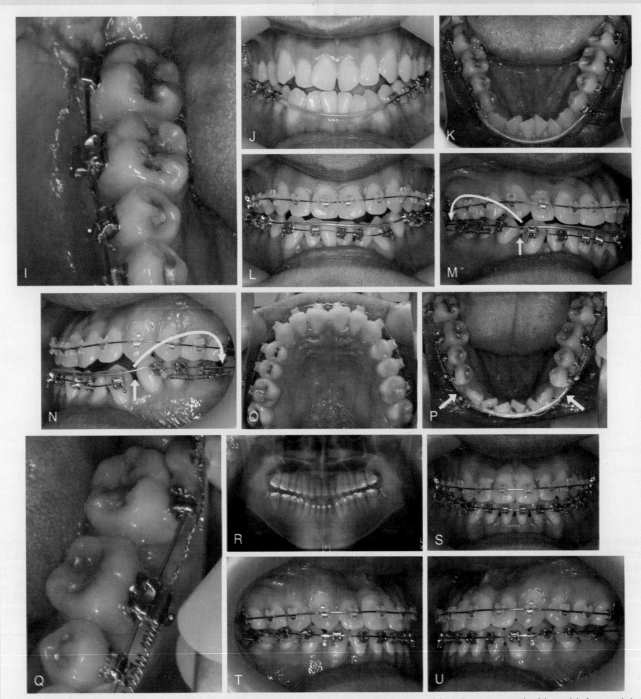

Figure 8.23, cont'd   Mandibular molar distalization using mini-implant. A 24-year-old male presented with a chief complaint of anterior crossbite and crowding. **(I)** One month after placement of right mini-implant, there remained mild soft tissue inflammation around the buried mini-implant and wire extension from the mini-implant head. **(J and K)** Initially, brackets were bonded only on the mandibular posterior teeth. **(L–P)** At eight months of treatment, extrusion of mandibular canines was observed due to counterclockwise rotation of the mandibular occlusal plane caused by the distal force applied to the crown of the mandibular posterior teeth. At this time, brackets were bonded on the mandibular anterior teeth and NiTi anterior segment wire was placed to align these teeth. **(Q)** At 12 months of treatment, mandibular left mini-implant was removed due to the mobility of the mini-implant. **(R)** Panoramic radiograph after removal of left mini-implant. Distal tipping of mandibular second molars was observed. **(S–U)** Fourteen months of treatment.

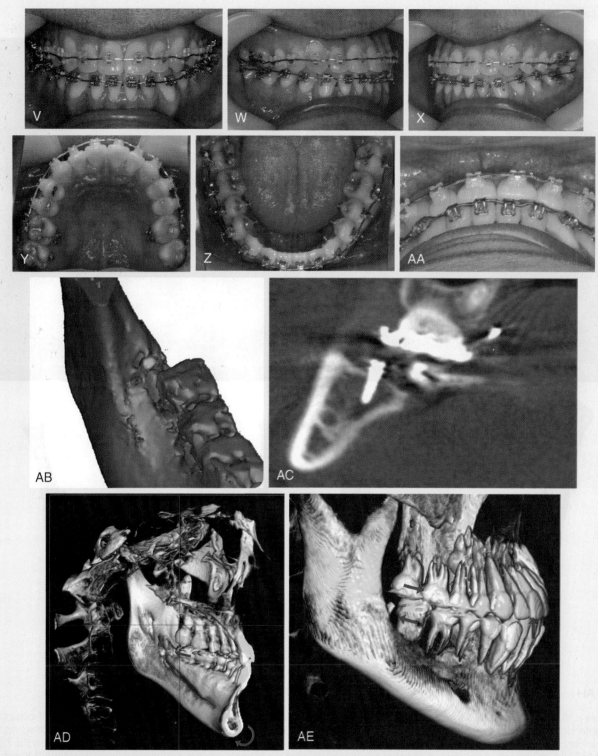

Figure 8.23, cont'd   Mandibular molar distalization using mini-implant. A 24-year-old male presented with a chief complaint of anterior crossbite and crowding. **(V–AA)** At 20 months of treatment, debonding was performed and lingual fixed retainers were delivered. **(AB** and **AC)** Post-treatment CBCT images showed that the mandibular right mini-implant was placed at the buccal border of the retromolar triangle which has low density cortical bone. **(AD** and **AE)** Superimposition of pre- and post-treatment CBCT images based on cranial base. Maxillary teeth were moved forward and the mandible rotated backward.

Continued

Distalization of mandibular molars (Fig. 8.23)—cont'd

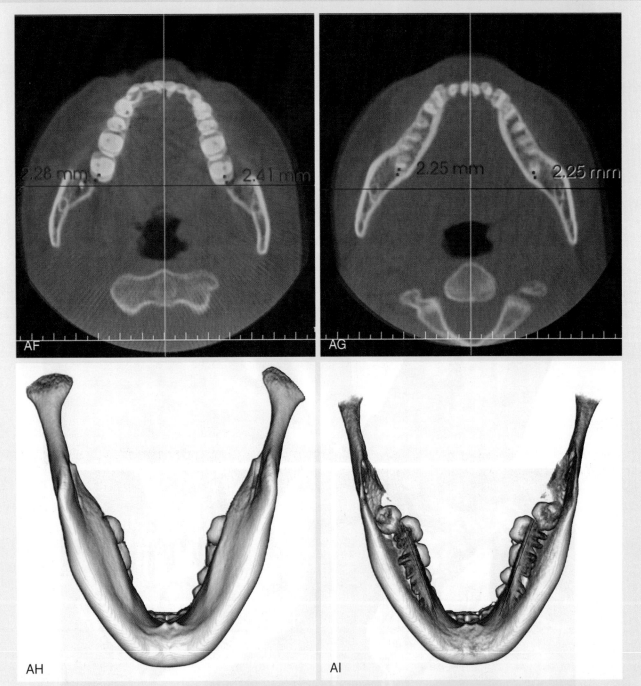

Figure 8.23, cont'd   Mandibular molar distalization using mini-implant. A 24-year-old male presented with a chief complaint of anterior crossbite and crowding. **(AF and AG)** Superimposition of pre- and post-treatment CBCT images based on the mandible. Axial view at the crown level **(AF)** showed that the mandibular second molars were distalized 2.3 mm on the right, and 2.4 mm on the left. Axial view at the root apex showed that the mandibular second molars were distalized 2.3 mm on both sides. Distal root of the mandibular second molars contacted with the lingual cortical bone at the mylohyoid ridge area. **(AH–AK)** mylohyoid ridge observed in the CBCT images. This can hinder distal movement of the mandibular second molar.

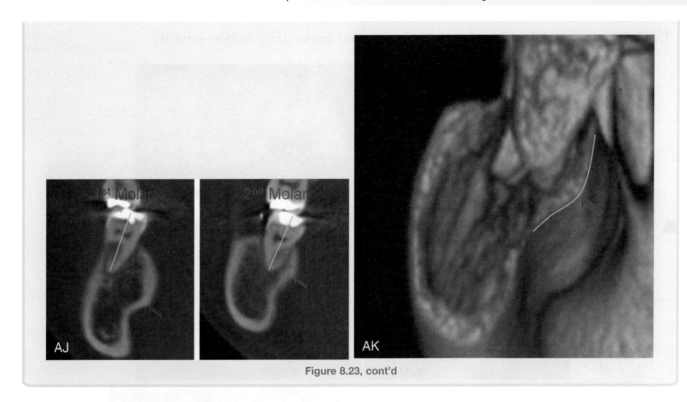

Figure 8.23, cont'd

Uprighting of mesially tipped mandibular second molar (Fig. 8.24)

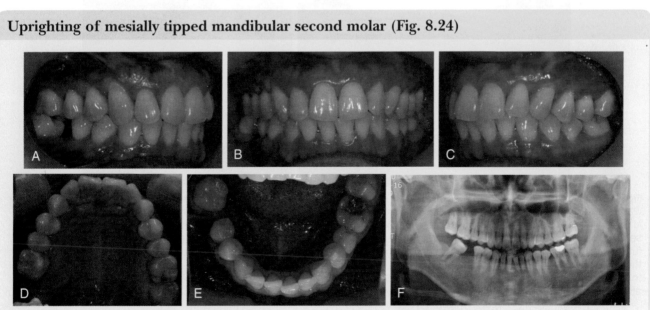

Figure 8.24 Uprighting of mesially tipped mandibular second molar using mini-implant. A 54-year-old male patient was referred for uprighting of mandibular right second molar before placement of prosthodontic implant. **(A–E)** Pretreatment intraoral photographs. **(F)** Pretreatment panoramic radiograph.   *Continued*

Uprighting of mesially tipped mandibular second molar (Fig. 8.24)—cont'd

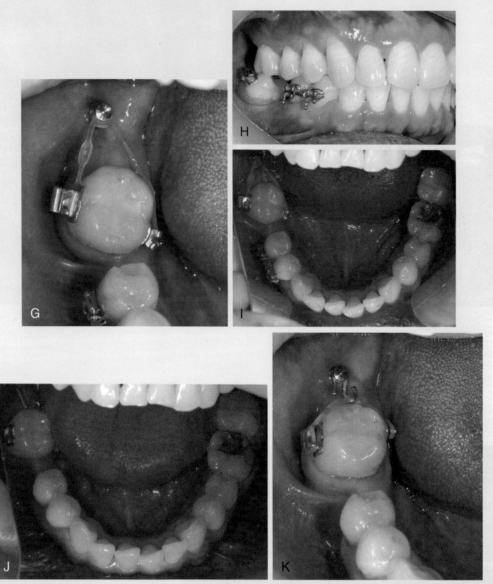

Figure 8.24, cont'd   Uprighting of mesially tipped mandibular second molar using mini-implant. A 54-year-old male patient was referred for uprighting of mandibular right second molar before placement of prosthodontic implant. **(G and H)** Mini-implant was placed at the distobuccal side of the second molar with a distance that is required for distal tipping of the second molar crown. Brackets engaged with full-size SS wire were bonded passively on the mandibular right premolars for future use as anchorage for final positioning of second molar. Elastomeric chains were used buccally and lingually to upright the second molar. **(I)** One month of uprighting. **(J)** Three months of uprighting. Lever was attached to the mini-implant head to apply distal force that passes on the lingual side of the second molar to rotate the tooth mesially. Elastomeric chain was applied only on the lingual side at this time. **(K)** Six months of treatment. Lever was shortened as the second molar uprighted.

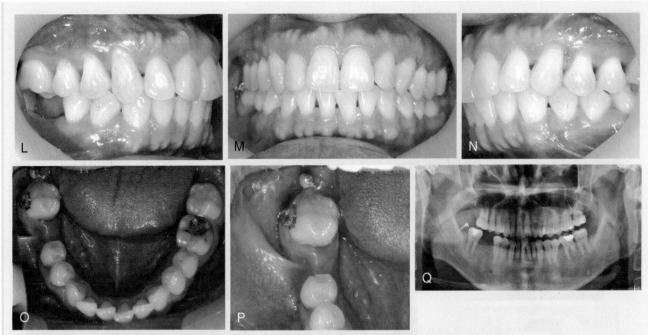

Figure 8.24, cont'd   Uprighting of mesially tipped mandibular second molar using mini-implant. A 54-year-old male patient was referred for uprighting of mandibular right second molar before placement of prosthodontic implant. **(L–P)** After eight months of treatment, debonding was performed. **(Q)** Post-treatment panoramic radiograph.

Uprighting of impacted mandibular molar (Fig. 8.25)

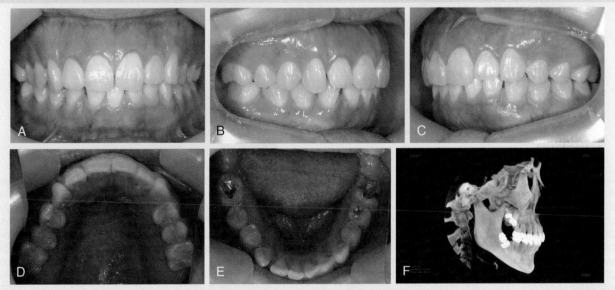

Figure 8.25   Uprighting of impacted mandibular molar using mini-implant. A 16 years 5 months old female patient was referred from a local clinic for impaction of all maxillary and mandibular second molars. **(A–E)** Pretreatment intraoral photographs. **(F–K)** Pretreatment CBCT images showed impaction of all second molars. Mandibular left second molar was impacted horizontally, and mandibular right second molar was blocked by the third molar. Crowns of the maxillary third molars were stuck under the cervical area of the maxillary second molars causing distal tipping of maxillary second molars.

Continued

Uprighting of impacted mandibular molar (Fig. 8.25)—cont'd

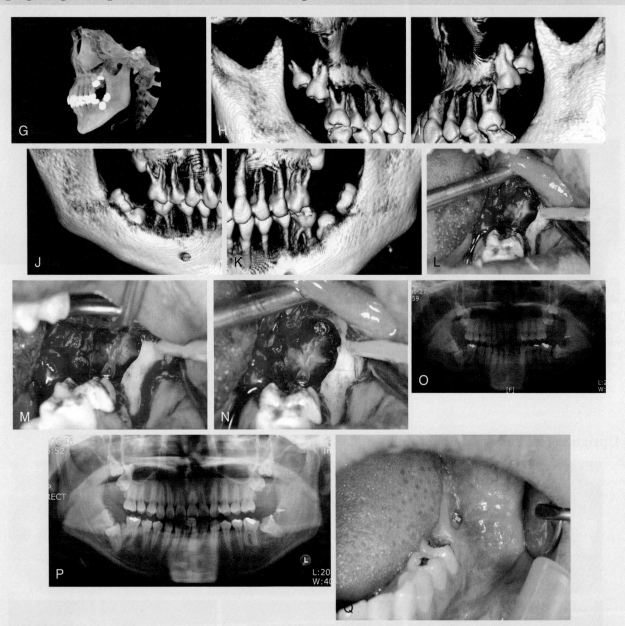

Figure 8.25, cont'd   Uprighting of impacted mandibular molar using mini-implant. A 16 years 5 months old female patient was referred from a local clinic for impaction of all maxillary and mandibular second molars. **(L–N)** Orthodontic mini-implant (2.0 mm × 8 mm) was placed horizontally in the distal wall of the extraction socket of the mandibular third molar. Elastomeric chain was applied between the mini-implant head and the button bonded on the distal surface of the crown of the mandibular second molar. To prevent slippage of the elastomeric chain, 0.3 mm stainless steel ligature wire was tied on the button and mini-implant head. **(O)** Panoramic radiograph taken 1 week after mini-implant placement. **(P)** Panoramic radiographs taken 5 months after mini-implant placement. Mandibular left second molar was uprighted significantly. **(Q)** Intraoral photograph taken 5 months after mini-implant placement. Button bonded on the distal surface of the second molar crown was exposed spontaneously. Elastomeric chain attached to the button is seen as a yellow rubber material around the button.

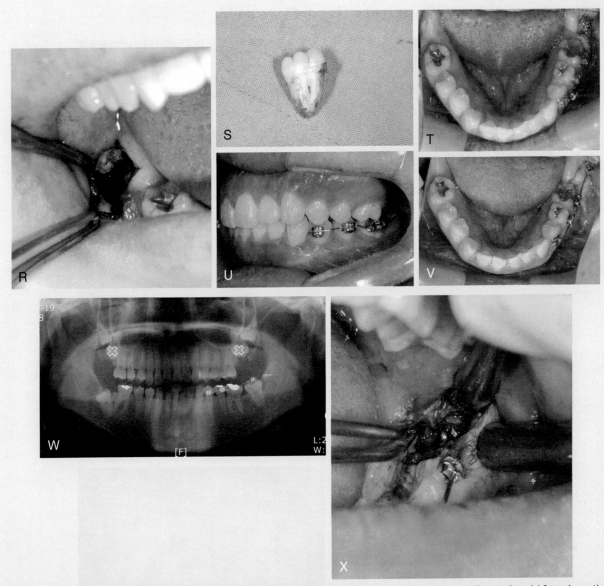

Figure 8.25, cont'd   Uprighting of impacted mandibular molar using mini-implant. A 16 years 5 months old female patient was referred from a local clinic for impaction of all maxillary and mandibular second molars. **(R and S)** Mandibular left third molar was extracted at 5 months of treatment because it was mechanically blocked by the second molar crown. **(T)** At 9 months of treatment, brackets were bonded on the mandibular left posterior teeth and a rigid passive wire segment was inserted on the premolar and first molar brackets. For more uprighting of the mandibular left second molar, an uprighting spring made of titanium molybdenum alloy wire was inserted into the second molar bracket and hooked between the first and second premolars. **(U and V)** At 1 year 5 months of treatment, a continuous wire segment was inserted from 1st premolar to second molar bracket. **(W)** There was no spontaneous eruption of the maxillary second molars. Extraction of the maxillary second molars was then planned in order to allow the eruption of the maxillary third molars into the second molar position. **(X and Y)** At 1 year 7 months of treatment, mini-implant placed in the extraction socket of mandibular left third molar was removed.

Continued

Uprighting of impacted mandibular molar (Fig. 8.25)—cont'd

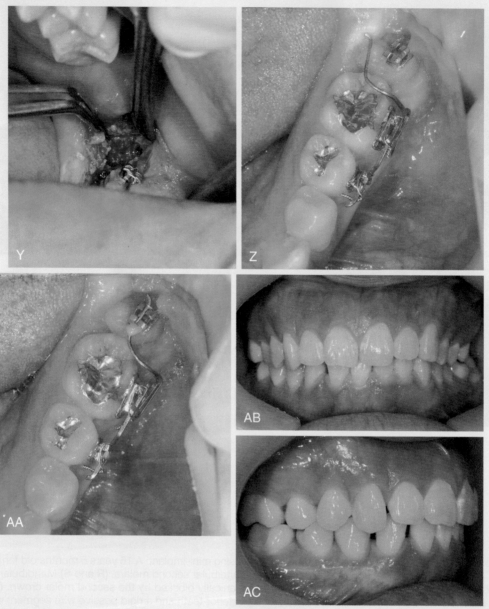

Figure 8.25, cont'd   Uprighting of impacted mandibular molar using mini-implant. A 16 years 5 months old female patient was referred from a local clinic for impaction of all maxillary and mandibular second molars. **(Z and AA)** L-loop was bent between first and second molars to apply lingual force with buccal crown torque to the second molar. AA shows passive configuration of wire before insertion into second molar bracket. **(AB–AG)** Debonding was performed at 2 years 5 months of treatment. Wire segment was bonded on the mandibular left first and second molars to prevent extrusion of mandibular second molar.

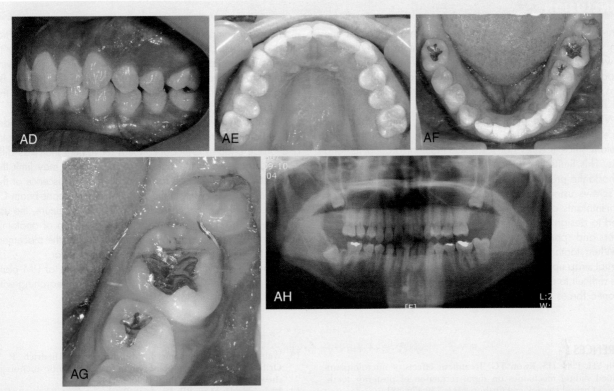

Figure 8.25, cont'd Uprighting of impacted mandibular molar using mini-implant. A 16 years 5 months old female patient was referred from a local clinic for impaction of all maxillary and mandibular second molars. **(AH)** Post-treatment panoramic radiograph. Mesial movement and eruption of maxillary third molars was observed. Mandibular right third molar also erupted maintaining its distal tipping. Further observation is required to evaluate the need of orthodontic traction of unerupted third molars.

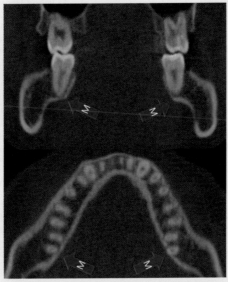

Figure 8.26 Anatomic limit for mandibular molar distalization. Mylohyoid ridge (arrow) extends superior and posterior from the lower part of the symphysis of the mandible. If the apex of the distal root of mandibular second molar contacts mylohyoid ridge (arrow), distal movement of mandibular second molar is almost impossible. Also, intrusion of the mandibular molars can be hindered by the mylohyoid ridge.

CONCLUSION

Mini-implants placed in the buccal interdental alveolar bone can be used for anchorage reinforcement in many cases. However, there are patients whose interdental alveolar bone is too narrow and thin to place a mini-implant. In these situations, mini-implants can be placed in the mid-palate or anterior region of palate successfully.

When a single mini-implant is used, the orthodontic force should be made to pass through the head of the mini-implant since it does not resist the moment around its long axis. This limits the design of force system needed to solve orthodontic problems. Therefore, splinting two mini-implants or screws using plate is necessary in some cases. Splinted mini-implants or bone plate can resist moment and can be used to design complex force systems by connecting various levers and springs.

When tooth movement is required only for a few teeth, partial strap up can be used. But in the partial strap up cases, it is difficult to maintain arch form continuity because the orthodontic forces applied at the bracket level inevitably cause moments inducing unwanted tooth movements. In the partial strap up cases, LIM plate system can be used effectively to prevent unwanted tooth movements by connecting the wire segment to the bracket of the LIM plate system (Fig. 8.22). By using this, orthodontic brackets can be applied only on the teeth to be moved.

When using skeletal anchorage, orthodontist should consider the anatomical limits of tooth movement. Although the skeletal anchorage enables orthodontic tooth movement that was difficult or impossible in the past, anatomical limits may limit the tooth movement or induce root resorption or dehiscence of the alveolar bone. To evaluate the anatomical limit, cone-beam CT can be helpful in some cases (Fig. 8.26). In the future, the use of cone-beam CT images both for the evaluation of anatomic limits and also for the fabrication of the stent for the placement of skeletal anchorage would become more popular.

The video showing the placement procedure of LIM plate system can be viewed at the youTube.com by searching with the keyword of 'Lim plate system'.

REFERENCES

1. Oh YH, Park HS, Kwon TG. Treatment effects of microimplant-aided sliding mechanics on distal retraction of posterior teeth. Am J Orthod Dentofacial Orthop 2011; 139:470–481.
2. Yamada K, Kuroda S, Deguchi T, Takano-Yamamoto T, Yamashiro T. Distal movement of maxillary molars using miniscrew anchorage in the buccal interradicular region. Angle Orthod 2009; 79:78–84.
3. Sharma P, Valiathan A, Sivakumar A. Success rate of microimplants in a university orthodontic clinic. ISRN Surg 2011; 2011. 982671.
4. Jung YR, Kim SC, Kang KH, Cho JH, Lee EH, Chang NY et al. Placement angle effects on the success rate of orthodontic microimplants and other factors with cone-beam computed tomography. Am J Orthod Dentofacial Orthop 2013; 143:173–181.
5. Dalessandri D, Salgarello S, Dalessandri M, Lazzaroni E, Piancino M, Paganelli C et al. Determinants for success rates of temporary anchorage devices in orthodontics: a meta-analysis (n > 50). Eur J Orthod 2013.
6. Buchter A, Wiechmann D, Koerdt S, Wiesmann HP, Piffko J, Meyer U. Load-related implant reaction of mini-implants used for orthodontic anchorage. Clin Oral Implants Res 2005; 16:473–479.
7. Buchter A, Wiechmann D, Gaertner C, Hendrik M, Vogeler M, Wiesmann HP et al. Load-related bone modelling at the interface of orthodontic micro-implants. Clin Oral Implants Res 2006; 17:714–722.
8. Kadioglu O, Buyukyilmaz T, Zachrisson BU, Maino BG. Contact damage to root surfaces of premolars touching miniscrews during orthodontic treatment. Am J Orthod Dentofacial Orthop 2008; 134:353–360.
9. Cho UH, Yu W, Kyung HM. Root contact during drilling for micro-implant placement. Affect of surgery site and operator expertise. Angle Orthod 2010; 80:130–136.
10. Shinohara A, Motoyoshi M, Uchida Y, Shimizu N. Root proximity and inclination of orthodontic mini-implants after placement: cone-beam computed tomography evaluation. Am J Orthod Dentofacial Orthop 2013; 144:50–56.
11. Umemori M, Sugawara J, Mitani H, Nagasaka H, Kawamura H. Skeletal anchorage system for open-bite correction. Am J Orthod Dentofacial Orthop 1999; 115:166–174.
12. De Clerck H, Geerinckx V, Siciliano S. The Zygoma Anchorage System. J Clin Orthod 2002; 36:455–459.
13. Wehrbein H, Glatzmaier J, Mundwiller U, Diedrich P. The Orthosystem—a new implant system for orthodontic anchorage in the palate. J Orofac Orthop 1996; 57:142–153.
14. Wehrbein H, Merz BR, Diedrich P, Glatzmaier J. The use of palatal implants for orthodontic anchorage. Design and clinical application of the orthosystem. Clin Oral Implants Res 1996; 7:410–416.
15. Crismani AG, Celar AG, Burstone CJ, Bernhart TG, Bantleon HP, Mittlboeck M. Sagittal and vertical load-deflection and permanent deformation of transpalatal arches connected with palatal implants: an in vitro study. Am J Orthod Dentofacial Orthop 2007; 131: 742–752.
16. Wehrbein H, Feifel H, Diedrich P. Palatal implant anchorage reinforcement of posterior teeth: A prospective study. Am J Orthod Dentofacial Orthop 1999; 116:678–686.
17. Chung KR, Kook YA, Kim SH, Mo SS, Jung JA. Class II malocclusion treated by combining a lingual retractor and a palatal plate. Am J Orthod Dentofacial Orthop 2008; 133:112–123.
18. Kook YA, Lee DH, Kim SH, Chung KR. Design improvements in the modified C-palatal plate for molar distalization. J Clin Orthod 2013; 47:241–248; quiz 267–248.
19. Wilmes B, Drescher D. A miniscrew system with interchangeable abutments. J Clin Orthod 2008; 42:574–580; quiz 595.
20. Wilmes B, Nienkemper M, Ludwig B, Kau CH, Pauls A, Drescher D. Esthetic Class II treatment with the Beneslider and aligners. J Clin Orthod 2012; 46:390–398; quiz 437.
21. Burstone CJ. Precision lingual arches. Active applications. J Clin Orthod 1989; 23:101–109.
22. Kim YJ, Lim SH, Gang SN. Comparison of cephalometric measurements and cone-beam computed tomography-based measurements of palatal bone thickness. Am J Orthod Dentofacial Orthop 2014; 145:165–72.
23. Kim SJ, Lim SH. Anatomic study of the incisive canal in relation to midpalatal placement of mini-implant. The Korean Journal of Orthodontics 2009; 39:146–158.
24. Burstone CJ. Welding of TMA wire. Clinical applications. J Clin Orthod 1987;21:609–615.
25. Kang YG, Nam JH, Park YG. Use of rhythmic wire system with mini-screws to correct occlusal-plane canting. Am J Orthod Dentofacial Orthop 2010; 137:540–547.

Lingual Orthodontics 9

Toshiaki Hiro and Fernando de la Iglesia

An improvement in one's physical appearance, as is common with orthodontic treatment, can positively affect social and interpersonal interactions. With an increasing number of grown-ups opting for orthodontic treatment, adult patients form a significant segment of practice, making almost up to 40% of certain orthodontic practices. These adults have special aesthetic demands regarding their orthodontic appliance visibility, which prompted the idea of placing brackets on the lingual side, with a resultant introduction of lingual orthodontic treatment methodology.

Traditionally, banding was used to place various orthodontic attachments on teeth. Current development of lingual orthodontics began in early 1970s, when it became apparent that bonding of brackets was a viable clinical procedure and that 'aesthetic' plastic brackets were a compromise. Dr Craven Kurz developed a true lingual appliance, in which he bonded plastic Fischer edgewise brackets to the lingual aspect of the anterior teeth and metal brackets to the lingual aspect of the posterior dentition, for many of his aesthetically conscious adult patients. A product development team of Ormco—orthodontic product manufacturing company in California, USA—developed many prototypes of edgewise lingual appliance. The turning point in the early stages of lingual appliance development was the addition of an 'anterior flat bite plane' as an integral part of the maxillary brackets. This converted the shearing force produced by the lower incisors to compressive force, which was believed to facilitate the anterior intrusion and decreased bond failure.

In the early 1970s, when lingual orthodontics debuted sensationally,[1,2] the number of lingual cases increased exponentially in the United States. However, this rapid increase declined within a few years.[3,4] The reason for this decline is not only due to the ceramic brackets which debuted at the same time but also due to the fact that most of the lingual cases could not finish with satisfactory results, as most orthodontists started lingual treatments without understanding the peculiarities of lingual orthodontics.

Some patient-related problems, like tissue irritation, speech difficulties, gingival impingement and occlusal interferences, and certain operator-related problems, like appliance control, appliance placement and bonding, wire placement, ligation and attaching auxiliaries, were associated with lingual appliance system. However, a continued research in this field over the last few years has led to several improvements in the original lingual appliance and to a variety of new lingual appliance systems. The current lingual appliances are much more refined to address the above-mentioned problems and offer great promise in clinical practice. The development of newer appliances, invention of superelastic wires, such as thermoactive wires and improvements in laboratory procedures[5–12] changed the lingual orthodontic practice, making it easier and more comfortable for the patients. Current lingual orthodontic practice is completely different from the lingual orthodontic practice, 30 years ago.

This chapter deals with certain key features of lingual treatment, efficient bonding procedure and various lingual appliance systems with clinical case presentations.

KEY DIAGNOSTIC AND TREATMENT PLANNING CONSIDERATIONS

It is certainly true that lingual orthodontic appliances in their current forms have helped orthodontic professionals to provide services to a large segment of population that would not have otherwise sought orthodontic treatment. However, every patient seeking lingual orthodontic treatment should be comprehensively examined, and potential difficulties, if any, should be identified to establish appropriate treatment strategy. Patient examination, diagnosis and treatment planning are carried out in a manner similar to established standards; however, certain factors that are specific to lingual treatment mechanics must be considered in diagnosis and treatment planning process.

Patient selection

Some practitioners of lingual orthodontic therapy are quite particular about the selection of specific malocclusion patients for lingual treatment. Authors believe that all cases can be successfully treated with lingual appliance therapy; however, certain morphological characteristics of malocclusion pose challenges, and therefore, limitations to this approach.

- Patients with short clinical crowns do not provide sufficient space for bonding the brackets and tubes, and it is difficult to avoid gingival impingement.
- In patients with dolichofacial patterns, it is critical to take appropriate measures to prevent extrusion of molars when using brackets with bite plane.
- Oral hygiene is another important area in lingual appliance therapy. Its proper assessment should be done prior to the initiation of treatment to make sure that the treatment proceeds smoothly and as planned.
- Juvenile or early teen patients are different from adult patients in several aspects.[13] They are abundant in saliva and the wet condition may cause failure of bonding. Broken brackets or wires are more frequent than

with adult patients, cooperation is consistently poor than adults, gingivoplasty is often required because of insufficient crown height, growth must be managed, etc. The management of such patients was presented at the 2nd World Society of Lingual Orthodontics (WSLO) meeting in Seoul, Korea, 2007.

BRACKET POSITIONING, LABORATORY SETUP AND BONDING PROCEDURE

Bracket positioning

It has been universally recognized that precise bracket placement holds the key to success of the lingual treatment. Considering the difficulty in gaining access to the lingual surfaces of maxillary and mandibular teeth, indirect bonding technique remains the only viable option to control bracket placement. This makes the laboratory setup and indirect bonding procedure a standard protocol in lingual orthodontics.

The most important aspect of bracket placement in lingual orthodontics is that the required tip, torque, in–out and rotational corrections are built into the bonded brackets through the resin beneath the bracket bases. There is no predetermined bracket placement prescription in lingual technique. An accurate bracket positioning on laboratory setup models and precise transfer of the same during bonding procedure are critical steps involved in successful lingual treatment.

More than 30 years have passed since lingual orthodontics appeared.[1,2] During the last 20 years, lingual orthodontics has taken very important revolutionary steps. The current lingual orthodontic practice is quite different from the lingual orthodontic practice, 30 years ago. One of the most dramatic changes is the evolution of the bonding procedures.[5,6,8–12] The indirect bonding technique is pivotal for success in lingual orthodontics. The only indirect bonding technique in the 1980s was silicone tray system made with torque angulation reference guide (TARG) or customized lingual appliance set-up service (CLASS).[8] Some clinicians are still using silicone trays; however, it has a lot of associated problems, such as bonding inaccuracy, bonding failure and increased cost.

In the early 1990s, authors introduced an epoch-making laboratory-indirect bonding system and published it in 1998[8] as the resin core indirect bonding system (RCIBS). Since RCIBS has made a great impact in the lingual orthodontic world, the users did not name it RCIBS but the 'Hiro system'. Currently, the Hiro system is

CASE 1

The patient was a 12-year 9-month-old male. At first examination, the authors did not expect that such a young boy would request for lingual treatment. Molars were Angle Class II on both sides, and the upper incisors were flared out (Fig. 9.1A1–D). After the upper bicuspids were extracted, the treatment began with lower arch (Fig. 9.1E1–H5). Extraction spaces were closed with sliding

mechanics, followed by detailing of dentition. The treatment term was 21 months, large overjet and deep overbite were overcorrected (Fig. 9.1I1–J5). Maxillary and mandibular growth was observed during the treatment. Headgear was not used (Fig. 9.1K). Panoramic radiograph showed a good root paralleling, and dental radiographs showed that root resorption was not observed (Fig. 9.1L–M2).

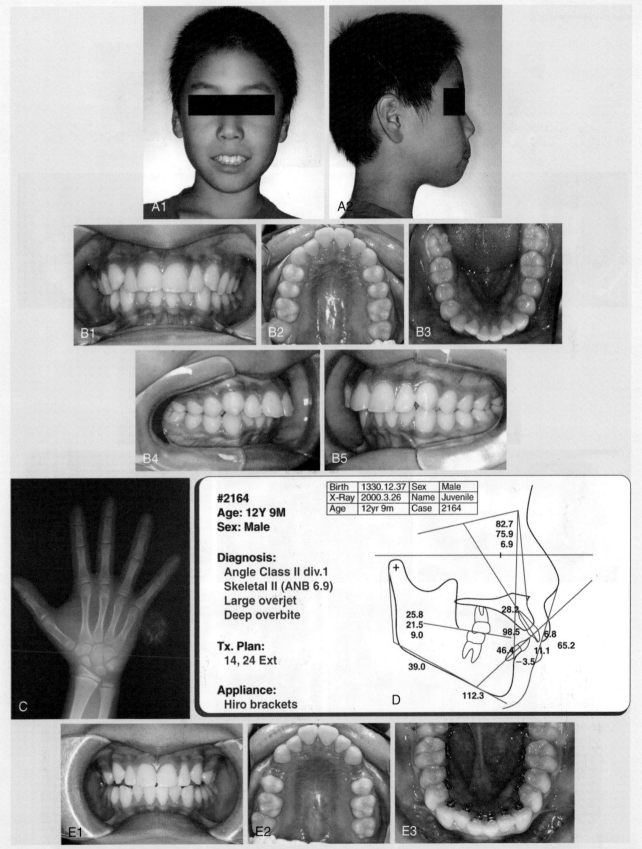

#2164
Age: 12Y 9M
Sex: Male

Diagnosis:
  Angle Class II div.1
  Skeletal II (ANB 6.9)
  Large overjet
  Deep overbite

Tx. Plan:
  14, 24 Ext

Appliance:
  Hiro brackets

Birth	1330.12.37	Sex	Male
X-Ray	2000.3.26	Name	Juvenile
Age	12yr 9m	Case	2164

82.7
75.9
6.9

28.2

25.8
21.5
9.0

98.5

6.8
65.2

46.4
11.1
−3.5

39.0

112.3

Figure 9.1 (**A1** and **A2**) A 12-year 9-month-old male patient. He and his father requested lingual treatment. (**B1–B5**) Pretreatment intraoral pictures. Upper incisors were protruded. Molar relations were almost full Class II. (**C**) Pretreatment hand-wrist X-ray. Sesamoid bone was not appeared yet. It is about stage 3. (**D**) Pretreatment cephalometric tracing, diagnosis and treatment plan. He was skeletal Class II, and maxillary growth control was required. However, he did not accept it. (**E1–E5**) Upper bicuspids were extracted, and brackets were bonded on lower bicuspids. Initial wire was 012NiTi.

Continued

CASE 1—cont'd

Figure 9.1, cont'd (**F1–F5**) Four months into the treatment. Upper brackets were bonded. The archwires were 016 thermoactive in both arches. (**G1–G5**) Eleven months into the treatment. Space closure was done with sliding mechanics. Archwires were 1725 Beta III/0175 square titanium-molybdenum alloy (TMA). (**H1–H5**) Sixteen months into the treatment. Finishing and detailing were done with 1725 Beta III/0175 square TMA.

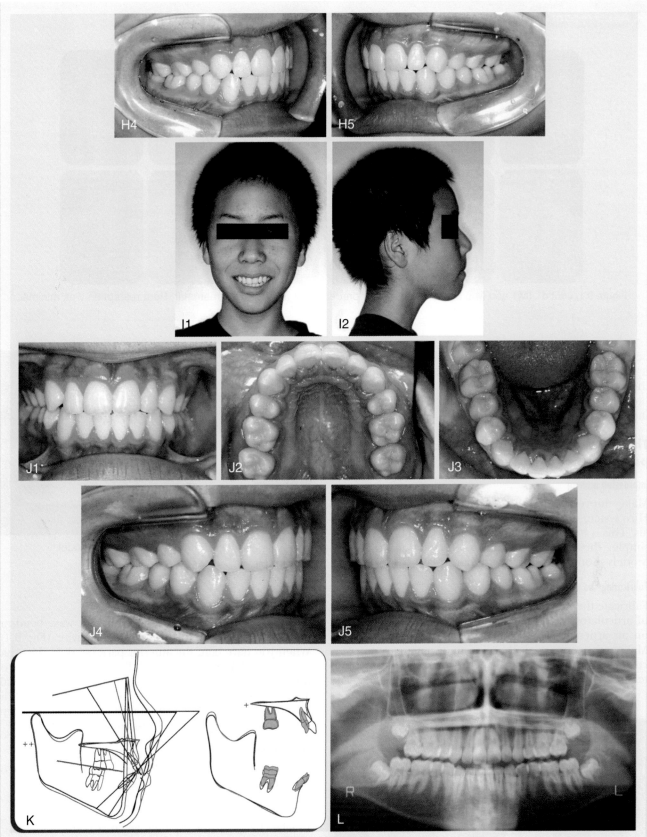

Figure 9.1, cont'd (**I1** and **I2**) Post-treatment facial pictures showing pleasing smile. However, profile was not improved because of lack of maxillary growth control. (**J1–J5**) Post-treatment intraoral pictures showing an excellent occlusion. (**K**) Cephalometric superimpositions show the growth of maxilla and mandible. Anchorage loss was minimal despite not using any additional anchorage. (**L**) Post-treatment panoramic X-ray shows good root paralleling. Lower third molars are not extracted yet.

Continued

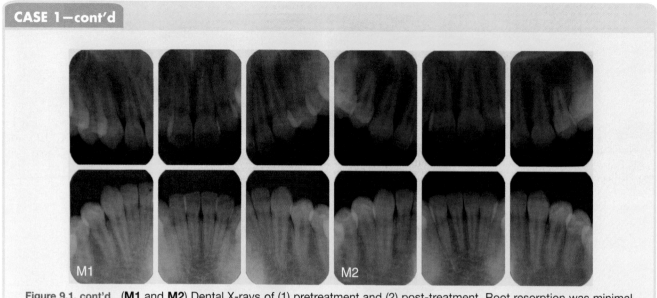

Figure 9.1, cont'd (**M1** and **M2**) Dental X-rays of (1) pretreatment and (2) post-treatment. Root resorption was minimal.

becoming a widely used indirect bonding system because it has improved upon a lot of difficulties associated with the other indirect bonding systems, providing accurate bonding with minimum bonding failure. It allows rebonding and is affordable.

The laboratory and indirect bonding procedure of Hiro system

Impression making

Make impression of the patients' teeth with alginate. Hiro system does not require silicone impression materials. This is because the laboratory work of Hiro system is simple; therefore, the chances of error are reduced. Models should be poured with hard plaster (Fig. 9.2).

Fabricating the setup

Fabricate the setup using articulators (Fig. 9.3). Any kind of articulator is suitable since the purpose of mounting on an articulator is to make the laboratory work easy. Making the setup as ideal occlusion or making some over correction is dependent on the orthodontist's treatment technique. Dr Hiro always uses ideal setup in his practice.

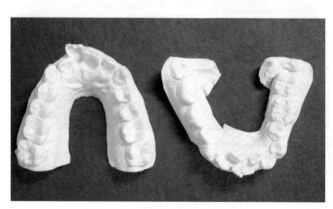

Figure 9.2 Hard plaster models.

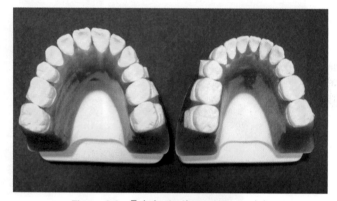

Figure 9.3 Fabricate the setup model.

Prepare the ideal archwire

Once the setup has been fabricated with wax, bend an ideal archwire using full-size rectangular wire (Fig. 9.4). When you have bent the anterior part, bend the bicuspid insets. Not all bonding bases will fit to the tooth surface of the dental cast, but this is fine (Fig. 9.5). Do not make small adjusting bends in the archwire and keep it as smooth as possible. If you make small adjusting bends in this step, they should be continued throughout the treatment.

Mesiodistal position

Mesiodistal position of brackets is normally the middle of the teeth for each tooth.

Bracket height

Bracket height in bicuspid-molar area is normally lower (gingival) than the centre of the crown height (Fig. 9.6). Sometimes gingivoplasty might be necessary for second molars or upper canines in order to place the brackets in ideal position. Do not place the brackets higher than the functional cusps. In the upper anterior part, brackets must be placed close to their gingival margin. This positioning

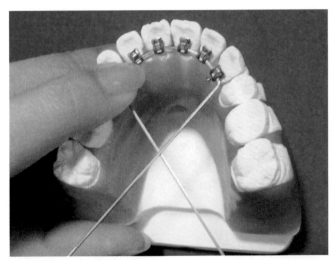

Figure 9.4 Bend an ideal archwire using full-size rectangular wire.

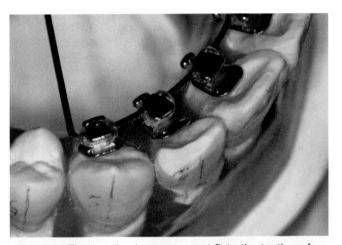

Figure 9.5 The bonding bases may not fit to the tooth surface of the dental cast, but this is fine. Do not make small adjusting bends in the archwire; keep it as smooth as possible.

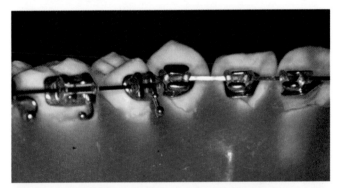

Figure 9.6 Bracket height in bicuspid-molar area is normally gingival than the centre of crown height.

will help the patient's speech and avoid interference to antagonistic teeth. In the lower anterior part, brackets must be positioned at almost the centre of the crown height. To achieve this bracket position, some cases may require vertical steps between canines and first bicuspids. Remember that if this vertical bend is made in the

laboratory archwire, you must bend the archwires for the patient in the same way.

Crimp surgical hooks

When the ideal arch is completed and the brackets positioned (Fig. 9.7), remove the archwire from the setup and crimp three surgical hooks on the wire (Fig. 9.8). One of the hooks is crimped between both the central incisors (Fig. 9.9). Another two hooks are crimped between the first and the second molars on both the sides (Fig. 9.10). Afterwards, the surgical hooks are bent lingually (Fig. 9.11).

Stick dowel pins

Next, heat three dowel pins and stick them in the wax base, just under the surgical hooks (Figs 9.12–9.14).

Fabricate the attachments

Once the dowel pins are fixed in the wax, the next step is to fabricate the attachments with liquid–powder acrylic resin. Use gutta-percha at the two points of the archwire to hold it temporarily. Next, using brush on technique, cover the top of the surgical hooks and the dowel pins with the resin and connect them with each

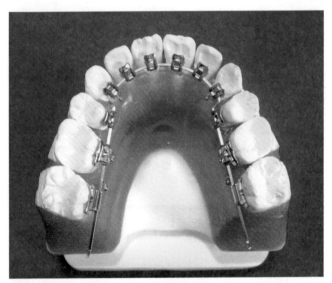

Figure 9.7 Completed ideal arch with brackets.

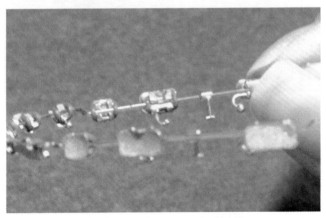

Figure 9.8 Crimped surgical hooks.

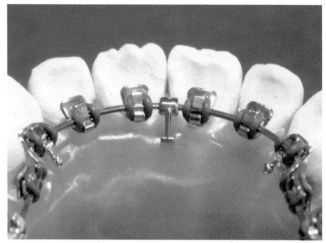

Figure 9.9 One of the hooks is crimped between the central incisors.

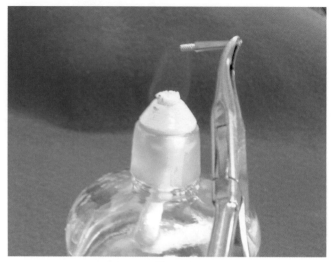

Figure 9.12 Heat dowel pins.

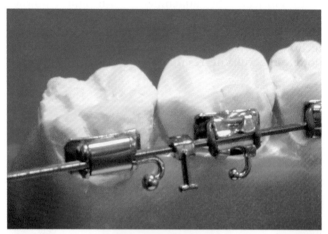

Figure 9.10 Another two hooks are crimped between the first and the second molars on both the sides.

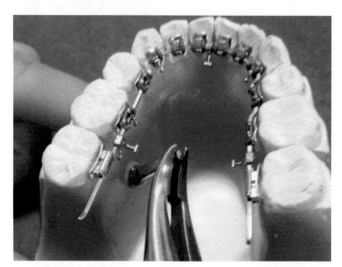

Figure 9.13 Stick dowel pins under the surgical hooks.

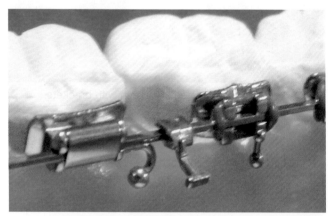

Figure 9.11 Bend the surgical hooks lingually.

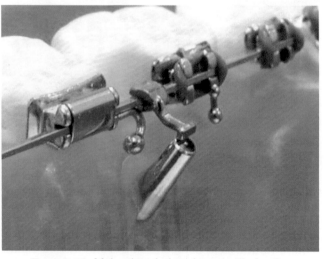

other (Figs 9.15 and 9.16). They work as attachments so that you can replace the archwire exactly in the same position. Therefore, you can reproduce new bracket positions and rebond them anytime in case the patient's brackets break off or are lost. After the resins are cured, remove the gutta-percha and clean the model and the archwire.

Figure 9.14 Make dowel pins closer to the hooks.

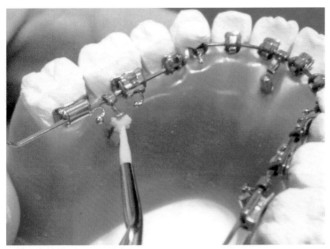

Figure 9.15 Cover the top of the surgical hooks and the dowel pins with the acrylic resin and connect them with each other.

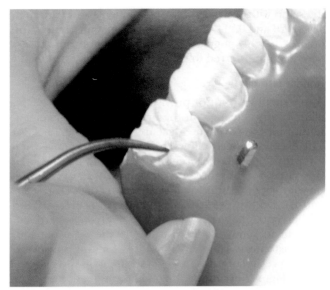

Figure 9.17 Block out the small grooves with wax.

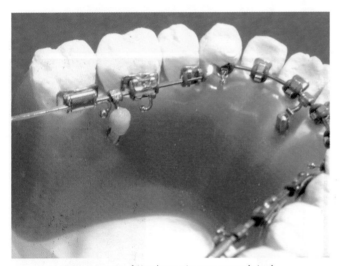

Figure 9.16 Attachments are completed.

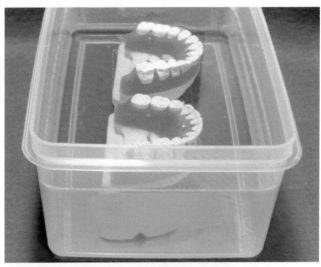

Figure 9.18 Soap the casts.

Prepare the models

Block out deep and small grooves with wax (Fig. 9.17). This prevents imperfect fit of cores when they are placed on the patient's teeth.

Soap the setup model

Put the setup models into a soapy liquid. After 10 min of dipping, polish them with cotton in the water (Figs 9.18 and 9.19). The purpose of soaping is to replace the application of separating medium. The authors had tried all kinds of separating media and found that this is the best way for the future laboratory steps and that the frequency of broken brackets during the treatment is minimum. Do not use Vaseline as separating medium because it causes dislodgement of brackets from the teeth.

Complete the bracket prescription

The next step is to transfer all the information of the setup to the brackets. Apply the light-cure composite resin (Transbond® 3M) on all of the bracket bases, set the archwire on

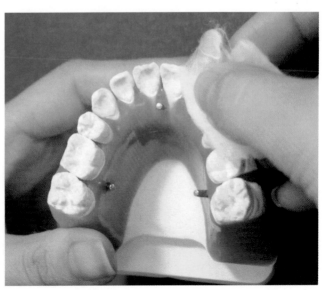

Figure 9.19 Polish them with cotton in the water.

the setup with the help of the attachments and cure them (Figs 9.20 and 9.21). Now, all the information of the setup, bracket height, angulation, in–out, rotation and torque have been transferred to the brackets.[14]

Fabricate resin cores

Apply small amount of provisional dental resin (having elaticity after curing) on the brackets, paying special attention not to cover the ideal archwire (Figs 9.22–9.24). The elastic property allows the clinician to remove them even through the undercut areas, such as tie-wings. Do the same for all the brackets and cure. Use liquid–powder acrylic resins to fabricate resin cores (Fig. 9.25A and B). Do not use composite materials, such as Band-lok, as core materials because they are too hard and difficult to remove.[15] Before the acrylic resin hardens, put elastomeric rings on the cores for the purpose of holding resin cores when we bond them on the patient's teeth (Fig. 9.26A and B). If you make a small hole at the top of lingual cusps of each core, excess adhesive will come out from the hole when you bond them on the patient's teeth.

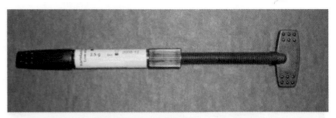

Figure 9.22 Provisional dental resin having elastic property after curing.

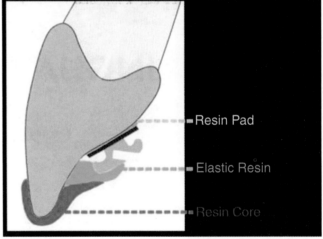

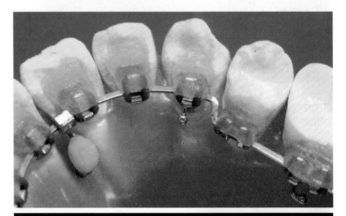

Figure 9.23 Apply provisional resin exhibiting elastic property after curing.

Resin Pad

Elastic Resin

Resin Core

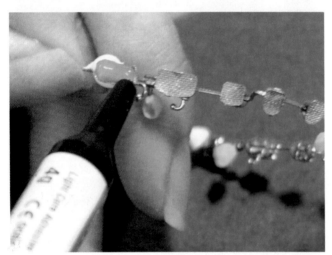

Figure 9.20 Apply light-cure composite resin on the brackets' bases.

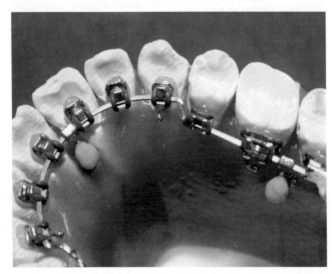

Figure 9.21 Position the ideal arch on the setup model.

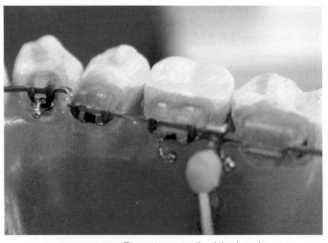

Figure 9.24 Do not cover the ideal arch.

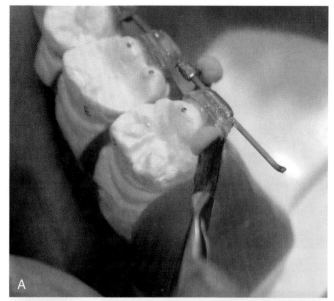

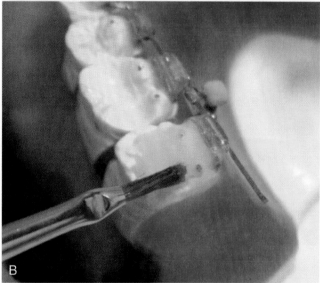

Figure 9.25   (**A** and **B**) Use of liquid–powder acrylic resin to fabricate resin cores.

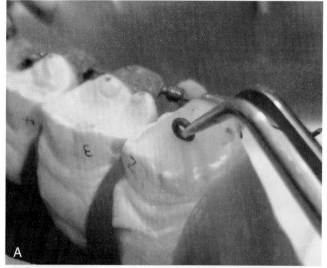

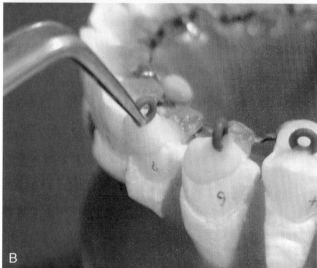

Figure 9.26   (**A** and **B**) Elastomeric ring positioning.

Finalizing the resin cores

After writing down the tooth number on each core, re-move all the cores–brackets–archwires as a unit and grind off the excess resin (Figs 9.27 and 9.28). Cut the elastomeric ligatures with a heated instrument and sepa-rate the brackets from the ideal arch (Fig. 9.29). Now, all of the brackets are ready to bond (Figs 9.30–9.32).

The bonding procedure

Etch the patient's teeth with phosphoric acid, rinse with water and then dry. Apply a thin primer on the etched surface. Hold the elastomeric ring with a bracket holder and apply a very small amount of adhesive on the bonding surface of the brackets (Transbond®). Seat the brackets on the teeth and cure them one by one. After all the teeth are cured, remove the resin core and Fermit® with scalers. Since Fermit has elasticity, its removal is quite easy.

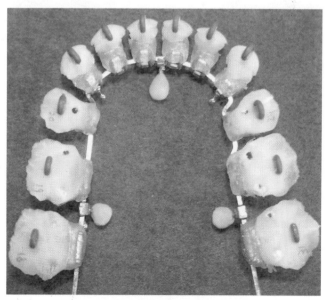

Figure 9.27   Completed resin cores.

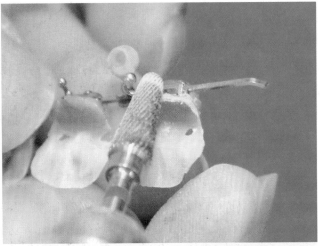

Figure 9.28   Grind off the excess resins.

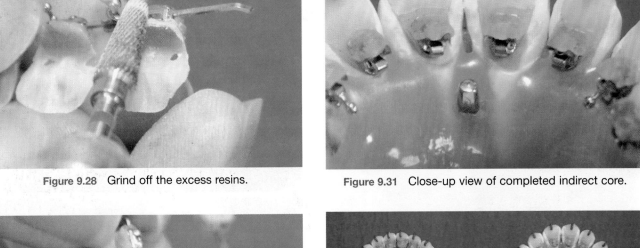

Figure 9.31   Close-up view of completed indirect core.

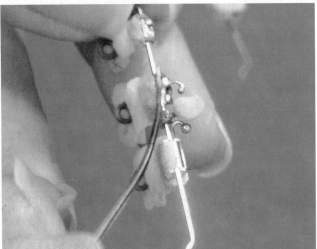

Figure 9.29   Cut the elastic ligatures with heated instruments.

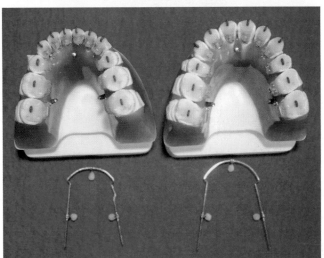

Figure 9.32   Brackets and ideal arches.

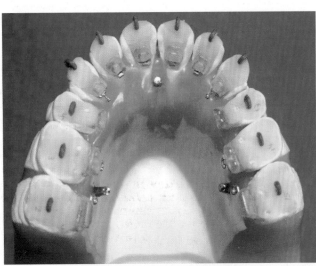

Figure 9.30   All the brackets are completed.

Bracket rebonding

The original Hiro system, published in 1998, did not facilitate rebonding; however, with the most recent Hiro system, it is easy to do so in a few minutes. Put a new bracket on the ideal arch that was explained in the Section, 'Prepare the ideal archwire', and replace it on the setup with the attachments (Figs 9.33–9.37). Next, repeat the steps explained in the Sections, 'Complete the bracket prescription', 'Fabricate resin cores' and 'Finalizing the resin cores'. It takes less than 5 minutes to complete a new bracket for rebonding (Fig. 9.37).

Currently, many types of indirect bonding techniques are used in orthodontic practice.[5–12] In lingual orthodontics, it is well known that brackets must be preadjusted with TARG, CLASS or some electric devices, and afterwards, silicone tray indirect bonding system may be used. However, these laboratory procedures are quite complex and require experience to use them. In spite of meticulous fabrication, the silicone trays do not always fit the patients' teeth, making lingual treatment difficult.[4,16]

The problems associated with silicone indirect bonding technique are as follows:

1. Since they are flexible, deformation and uncertain adhesion often occur. Therefore, brackets are often adhered inaccurately. Inaccurate bonding needs complex wire bending in order to compensate for faulty bracket positions. This makes lingual treatment difficult.

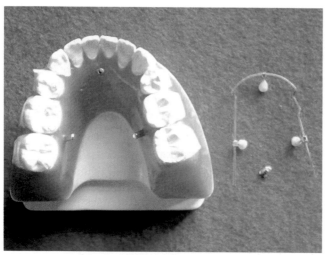

Figure 9.33   Setup and archwire.

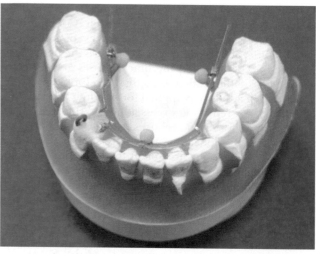

Figure 9.36   Completed new bracket for rebonding.

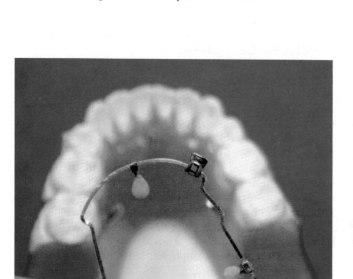

Figure 9.34   Put a new bracket on the wire.

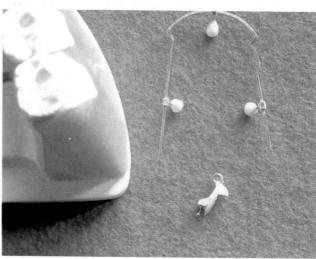

Figure 9.37   Ready for rebonding.

2. A lot of adhesive spreads to gingiva. It is very hard to clean them up perfectly and is also uncomfortable for the patient; if it is incomplete, it causes gingival inflammation.

3. Silicone trays do not fit the patient's teeth in case of minor tooth movements. Therefore, extraction, separation, expansion, etc. must be avoided until bonding is finished. The reason why the Hiro system made such a great impact in lingual orthodontics was that it solved numerous difficulties associated with bonding techniques.

The advantages of Hiro system as compared with other indirect bonding techniques

1. The laboratory procedures are quite simple, and special tools or equipments are not necessary for Hiro system.

2. Simplified laboratory procedures reduce the laboratory costs and errors.

3. Small and rigid individual hard trays provide quite accurate bonding in a short time. Silicone indirect bonding trays are flexible; therefore, bracket placement is affected by the pressure applied to the tray even though outer shells are prepared.

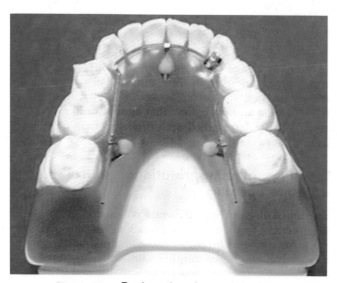

Figure 9.35   Replace the wire on the setup.

4. Individual trays provide good handling, and it takes less than 10 minutes for bonding one arch. Compared to silicone tray indirect bonding, the excess of adhesive is quite little, almost none. This is because the bonding is done one by one, and the bracket bases are perfectly adapted to the patient's teeth; therefore, very little amount of adhesive is applied for bonding. There is no necessity for removing excess adhesive, this makes the chair time shorter and reduces patient's discomfort.

5. Trays are individual, having no relation to adjacent teeth. Therefore, any treatment that may change teeth arrangement, such as extractions, separations, expansion or distalization can be done between the period from making impression to bonding brackets. They are contraindicated in silicone tray indirect bonding system.

6. In cases of severe crowding, we can improve the crowding with temporarily adhered brackets, and afterwards we can bond the real one. This is easier to manage than with other lingual indirect bonding procedures.

7. In case of lost or broken brackets, we can refabricate them immediately at the chairside, anytime, easily and involving less cost.

8. Hiro system does not have any commercial relationship with any company; hence it is not necessary to pay royalties to anyone.

The Hiro system does not require any special tools or equipments. It is easy to make, provides accurate bonding with less cost and any kind of brackets can be used. It is pivotal for lingual orthodontics.

ARCHWIRES USED IN LINGUAL THERAPY

Orthodontic management of malocclusions with lingual appliances requires different archwire configurations and certain modifications of the conventional mechanotherapy used with labial appliances. When the brackets are placed on the lingual instead of the labial, the interbracket distances in the anterior region of the arches are decreased considerably. The decreased interbracket distance associated with lingual appliances makes a wire approximately three times as stiff as when used with labial appliances for first- and second-order bends and approximately one-and-half times as stiff for third-order bends.[17] Also, the stresses produced by the lingual appliances are slightly higher, as the archwire between the anchor units is lesser in lingual than in labial, thus producing greater forces on equal activation.

To overcome these problems inherent with the lingual system, it is appropriate to select a wire of low stiffness and good resilience. The clinician should consider the wire stiffness as the first criterion in the selection of a particular wire, as it determines the force and deflection in the ideal working range. The initial tooth alignment and final detailing of tooth positions are usually considered to pose a great challenge to the orthodontist. This may be partially as a result of using too stiff archwires that do not compensate for the decreased lingual interbracket distance in the anterior dental arches.

Archwire shape

The effect of variations in labiolingual tooth dimensions is significant enough on the lingual aspect to require nearly routine first-order bends distal to the cuspids and mesial to the molars. It has been found that the attempts to eliminate these bends have resulted in an unacceptably high bracket profile.[18]

Kinya Fujita[19,20] in 1979 introduced the concept of 'mushroom-shaped archwire' in conjunction with the lingual appliance. This design is smoother than just incorporating the compensatory offsets. These offsets should be sharp enough to reduce the chance of binding in the archwire slot.

Typical lingual archwire configuration

- *Cuspid-bicuspid offset:* A horizontal bend placed between cuspid and bicuspid. The precise amount of the offset is determined by the differences in the facial-lingual thickness of the cuspids and bicuspids. These bends may vary on the right and left sides.
- *Molar offset:* A lingual offset is often required mesial to the first molar due to the broader buccolingual dimension of the molars.

ANCHORAGE CONTROL

In lingual technique, extraction spaces are usually closed by en masse retraction of anterior teeth. This approach prevents opening of spaces mesial to cuspids, respecting patient's aesthetic concern; however, it taxes the anchorage. The clinician should consider anchorage in both sagittal and vertical planes for efficient and effective mechanics.

The mechanical advantage inherent with the lingual system facilitates more tooth movement with lesser demand on posterior anchorage in lingual than in labial appliance technique. However, in certain clinical situations with higher anchorage demands, several methods of anchorage control, like transpalatal arches, combination of various elastics, microimplants, etc., can be used to reinforce the anchorage.

TREATMENT SEQUENCE

In a broader sense, the lingual mechanics generally consists of the following four primary phases of treatment.[21]

1. Levelling, aligning, rotational control and bite opening
2. Torque control
3. Consolidation and retraction
4. Finishing and detailing

These phases of treatment are usually characterized by a progressive increase in wire stiffness. Various clinicians have suggested various archwires in lingual mechanics. However, the authors believe that there should not be any typical or predetermined archwire sequencing, rather it should be case-specific.

Levelling, aligning, rotational control and bite opening

The initial phase of lingual therapy is aimed at levelling and alignment of teeth, eliminating rotations, gaining adequate space for rotation correction and additional bracket placement, obtaining initial torque control when required, etc. The goal of initial treatment phase is to initiate tooth movement with light continuous forces and provide adequate time for patient adaption. Considering the reduced inter-bracket distance, it is appropriate to use resilient archwires and get them fully seated into the bracket slot for better alignment and wire progression. The commonly used initial wires may be 0.012 NiTi or 0.016 thermoactive NiTi wires.

Archwire ligation

Conventional steel ligation techniques used on the facial brackets are not as effective on the lingual brackets. This is because the lingual bracket slot is highly torqued in relation to its base. For the ligation method to be effective, the force of ligation must pull the archwire in a direction parallel to the bracket slot. Inadequate archwire engagement into the bracket slot interferes with the ability of the archwire to correct rotations and achieve proper tooth alignment and with archwire progression. The authors have explained in the later part of the chapter the reason why the double over-tie was used in lingual and why they had designed their original bracket system.

Retraction or consolidation mechanics

The lingual appliance mechanics for retraction and arch consolidation follows conventional appliance procedures, using sliding mechanics, closing loop arches or combinations. Buccal segments should be levelled and aligned prior to retraction mechanics. Retraction of the entire anterior segment, following initial alignment, should be performed on a rectangular wire with a relatively high stiffness factor.

Torque control

Following retraction, any additional arch consolidation, torque control and arch levelling can be accomplished with appropriate archwires.

Finishing and detailing

This is a final step in lingual technique and the last opportunity for the clinician to fine-tune tooth positions and achieve good occlusion. Desired relationships, maximum intercuspation and levelled marginal ridges should be achieved. It is important to make sure that the maxillary and mandibular midlines and archforms are coordinated. In extraction cases, the roots of the adjacent teeth at the extraction site should be parallel, and the closure of extraction spaces should be maintained.

VARIOUS LINGUAL APPLIANCE SYSTEMS

Kurz appliance

Currently, lingual orthodontics is expanding in European and Asian countries, but it is not as popular in the United States. However, it was Cravin Kurz,[22] an orthodontist from California, who made one of the biggest accomplishments in the history of lingual orthodontics. He invented the 'Kurz Lingual Appliance'. So far, as of 2009, it had undergone seven times modifications and improvements from the first prototype.[3] Although it causes some hindrances, such as speech problems, tongue irritations, need for double over-tie, etc., the Kurz appliance has been practiced for many years around the world. The authors have used this appliance extensively, with more than 300 cases treated with the Kurz appliance.

The seventh-generation Kurz lingual appliance has the following features:

- The maxillary anterior inclined plane is now heart-shaped with hooks.
- All hooks have a greater access for ligation.
- Premolar brackets were widened mesiodistally and the hooks were shortened. The increased width of the bicuspid brackets allows better rotational control.
- The molar tube is now available with either a hinge cap or a terminal sheath.
- The bonding base of the bracket is well contoured to approximate the lingual morphology of each individual tooth.
- The brackets have been redesigned with smooth exterior surface and have a low profile.

CASE 2

The case of a 24-year-old female treated with the Kurz appliance is presented. The patient suffered from anterior crowding of both arches and a protruded upper left lateral incisor. The molar relation was a full Class II on either side; severe crowding and a deep overbite were observed (Fig. 9.38A1–B5). Figure 9.38C shows the head plate, diagnosis and treatment plan. The patient's treatment began with the extraction of the upper bicuspids. Considering the molar relations and the arch length discrepancy, it seemed that this would be a surgical case. Had the authors treated her with a labial appliance, the patient would have required surgery; however, the patient was treated without surgery. This exemplifies that the treatment planning in lingual orthodontics is different from that in labial orthodontics.[4,23]

When the brackets were bonded on the upper arch, the sandwich technique (resin buildup on molars) was used (Fig. 9.38D1–D5). Generally, composite materials, such as Bandlok, are applied on the functional cusps of lower molars; however, the authors used a liquid–powder acrylic resin on the occlusal surface of the upper molars. This is because the acrylic resin gradually wears down as the treatment progresses, and the resin is very easy to remove with Band Slitting Pliers.

Since this case was treated in 1998, the upper first molars were banded; headgear and transpalatal bar were used, but if the authors were to treat this case now, microimplants would be used instead of the headgear and the transpalatal bar (Fig. 9.38E1–E5). The extraction spaces were closed with sliding mechanics and detailing was followed with Beta III wires (Fig. 8.38F1–G5). The patient's treatment was finished within 23 months of the treatment term with excellent results (Fig. 9.38H1–I5). The superimpositions show the uprighting of lower molars (Fig. 9.38J). Panoramic radiographs showed a near-perfect paralleling of the roots, and the dental radiographs showed that the root resorption was minimal (Fig. 9.38K–L2).

Continued

CASE 2—cont'd

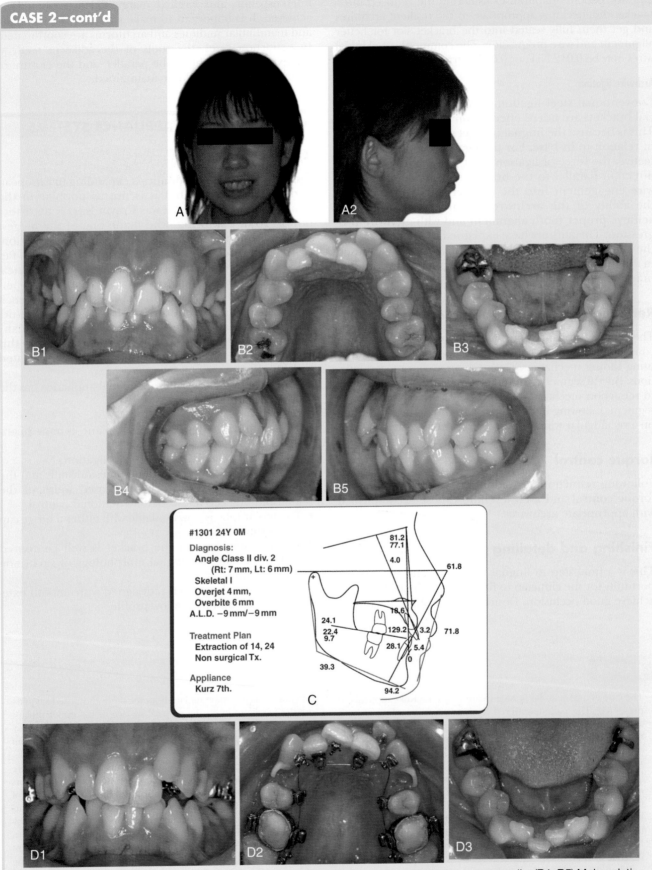

Figure 9.38   **(A1 and A2)** A 24-year-old female patient showing protruding, crowded incisors upon smile. **(B1–B5)** Molar relation was full Class II on both sides with severe crowding and deep overbite. **(C)** ANB showed skeletal Class I, and the profile was good. Mandibular plane was normal. **(D1–D5)** After bicuspid extractions, brackets were bonded on the upper arch. Because of severe crowding, some brackets could not be bonded. Labial brackets and hooks were bonded temporarily.

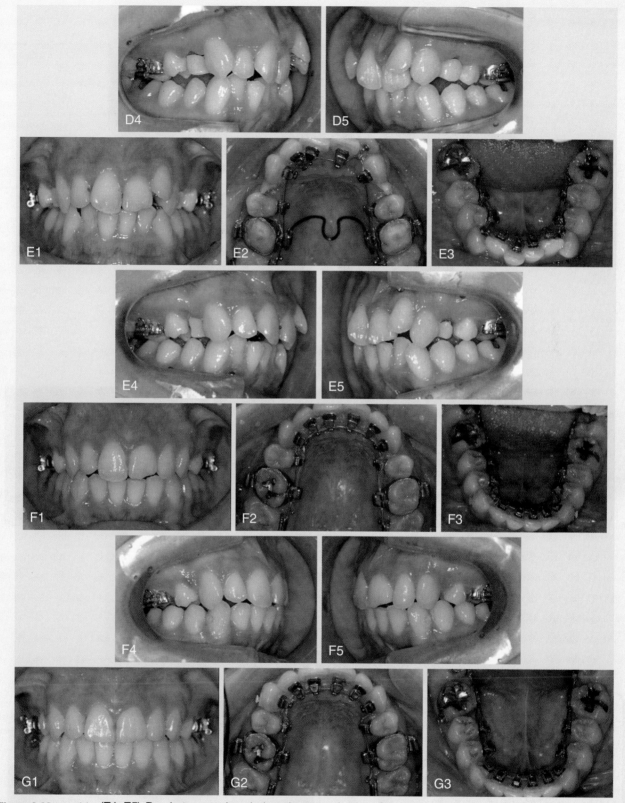

Figure 9.38, cont'd **(E1–E5)** Brackets were bonded on lower arch also. Since this case was treated in 1998, upper first molars were bonded; headgear and transpalatal arch were used. **(F1–F5)** Twelve months into the treatment, levelling and space closure were almost finished. The archwires were 1725 TMA/018 TMA. **(G1–G5)** Finishing and detailing stage after 17 months into the treatment. The fractured 21 was reshaped.

Continued

CASE 2—cont'd

Figure 9.38, cont'd   (H1 and H2) Post-treatment facial pictures. Pleasing smile was achieved in 23 months of treatment. (I1–I5) Post-treatment intraoral pictures. (J) Cephalometric superimpositions show upright lower molars. (K) Post-treatment panoramic X-ray shows good root paralleling.

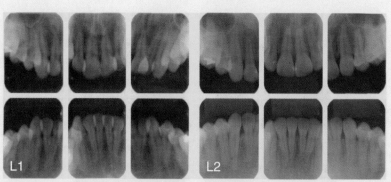

Figure 9.38, cont'd (**L1** and **L2**) Dental X-rays of (1) pretreatment and (2) post-treatment. Root resorption was minimum.

Creekmore system

The Creekmore appliance[24] has some unique points in comparison with the Kurz appliance.

The lingual bracket system by Creekmore—conceal bracket system—had the slot opening occlusally rather than lingually. This approach made the archwire insertion, seating and removal easier than in case of lingually opening slots. These brackets were designed around the Unitwin bracket 'centred slot' concept. This provided the advantages of both single and twin brackets by allowing maximum interbracket distance for optimal expression of tip and torque while offering twin tie-wings for rotational control. The bracket slot was 0.016" horizontally and 0.022" vertically with built-in T hooks in canine and lateral incisor brackets for intramaxillary and intermaxillary elastics. The first 1 mm of molar tube opened occlusally, providing direct guidance for insertion of the archwire; while the anterior brackets had a Y configuration with a single tie-wing projecting gingivally and twin tie-wings projecting occlusally, hence making the archwire ligation easier. This lingual appliance configuration provided positive control for each of the tip, torque and rotation functions while optimizing interbracket distance to provide maximum mechanical advantage. Personally, the authors support this appliance; however, one faces some difficulty in molar width control because of its reduced slot size.

Lingual straight wire appliance

So far as the authors have investigated, the first attempts to develop the Lingual Straight Wire Appliance (LSWA) were begun in the early 1980s by Hee-Moon Kyung, Korea.[25] Later, Takemoto and Scuzzo also started developing an LSWA.[26] The authors were associated with Takemoto and Scuzzo's LSWA development and presented their cases in 2002 ESLO meeting in Berlin.[27] At that time, Ormco did not assist the project; therefore, the first prototype did not have any bonding bases. Then the authors purchased readymade bonding bases, soldered the bracket bodies and the bonding bases by hand, one by one, and began the treatments (Fig. 9.40).

The lingual straight wire brackets are smaller mesiodistally. The bracket slot is horizontal, but the insertion of the wire is from the opposite direction in the anteroposterior plane. This reverse slot direction ensures that the archwire is fully seated in the bracket slot, and the torque control is improved. This appliance system allows the use of preformed archwires with few additional bends, which substantially reduces chair time and allows the use of simple sliding mechanics.

CASE 3

A 20-year-old female patient had severe crowding in both the arches (Fig. 9.39A1–B5). Figure 9.39C shows the diagnosis and treatment plan. This case was treated as a non-extraction case, but if she would have been treated with the labial appliance, four of the bicuspids would have been extracted. Brackets were bonded on both arches with the Hiro system. Hooks were bonded on 23, 32, 34 and 41 because of severe crowding (Fig. 9.39D1–D5). After 4 months of levelling, those temporarily adhered hooks were removed and the brackets were bonded with the Hiro system (Fig. 9.39E1–E5). Since the Creekmore appliance has a vertical slot, some of the teeth were vertically double over-tied in order to get wire engagement (Fig. 9.39F1–F5). The treatment was finished within 22 months (Fig. 9.39G1–H5). In spite of the severe crowding pretreatment, the upper and lower incisors were bodily moved, and they did not flare out (Fig. 9.39I). Panoramic radiographs show good root paralleling, and the dental radiographs show that no root resorption was observed (Fig. 9.39J–K2).

Continued

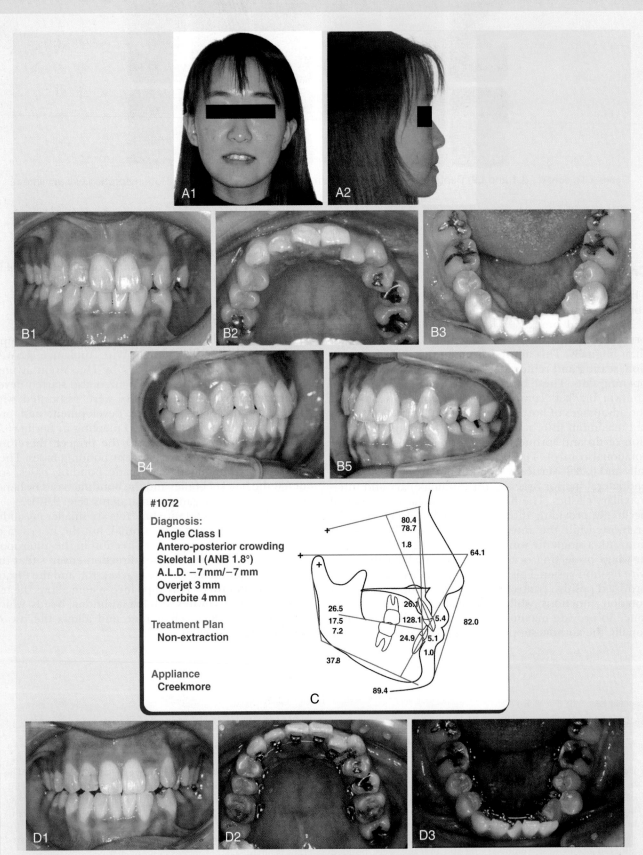

Figure 9.39 (**A1** and **A2**) A 20-year-old female patient. (**B1–B5**) Molars were Class I with severe crowding in both arches. (**C**) She had a good profile. Mandibular plane was normal. (**D1–D5**) The treatment was started with Creekmore brackets. Hooks and labial brackets were bonded on 13, 23, 32, 34 and 41 because of severe crowding. The archwires were 0.012 NiTi in both the arches.

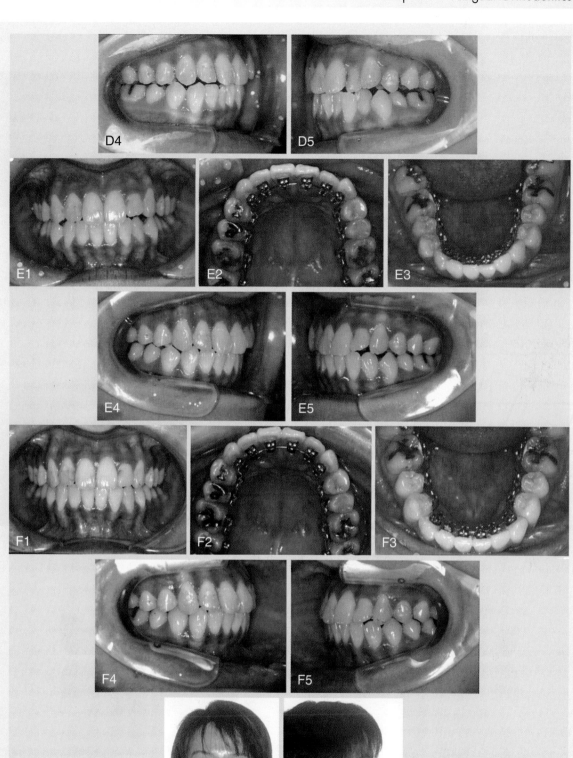

Figure 9.39, cont'd **(E1–E5)** Five months into the treatment. Provisionally adhered brackets and hooks were removed, and new brackets were bonded indirectly. The archwires were 0.016 SS and 0.014 NiTi wires. **(F1–F5)** Finishing and detailing stage after 16 months into the treatment. The archwires were 0.016 SS and 0.014 SS. **(G1 and G2)** Post-treatment facial pictures exhibiting good smile and profile.

Continued

Figure 9.39 (H1–H5) Post-treatment intraoral pictures showing an excellent result. (I) Cephalometric superimpositions show the uprighted lower molars and slightly labially moved incisors. (J) Post-treatment panoramic X-ray shows good root paralleling. (K1 and K2) Dental X-rays of (1) pretreatment and (2) post-treatment. Root resorption was not observed.

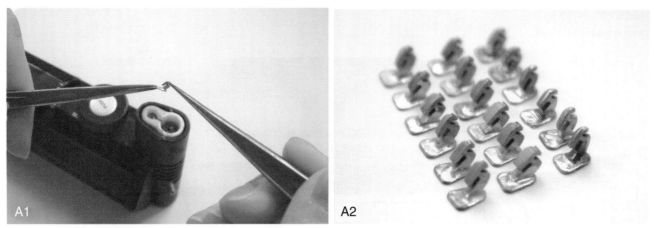

Figure 9.40 (**A1** and **A2**) Soldering bracket body on the bonding bases by hand (1); in total, more than 50 brackets were done one by one. Original bulky and high profile bracket bodies were shortened before soldering.

CASE 4

A 39-year-old female patient exhibited protruded incisors and an incomplete lip seal (Fig. 9.41A1–B5). The cephalometric analysis showed that the upper and lower incisors were extremely protruded with an interincisal angle of 92° (Fig. 9.41C). After four bicuspids were extracted, a headgear was worn and the brackets were bonded on the lower teeth (Fig. 9.41D1–D5). Space closure was done by loop mechanics after levelling (Fig. 9.41E1–F5). Since this case was treated in 1997, the authors used headgear and loop mechanics; however, if they were to treat the patient now,

microimplant anchorage and sliding mechanics would have been used. During the finishing stage, tiny spaces were closed with elastic chains and the treatment was finished (Fig. 9.41G1–G5). Quite an excellent result was obtained within 26 months of treatment (Fig. 9.41H1–I5). The excessively protruded incisors were retracted, the profile was dramatically improved and 92° interincisal angle became 137° (Fig. 9.41J). Panoramic radiograph shows good root paralleling with a slight root resorption (Fig. 9.41K–L2).

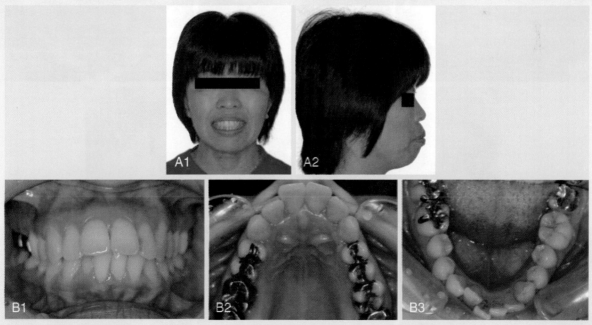

Figure 9.41 (**A1** and **A2**) A 39-year-old female patient had an extremely protruded profile. (**B1–B5**) Intraorally, upper and lower incisors were extremely protruded and lower incisors were crowded. Molars were Class I on both the sides.

Continued

CASE 4—cont'd

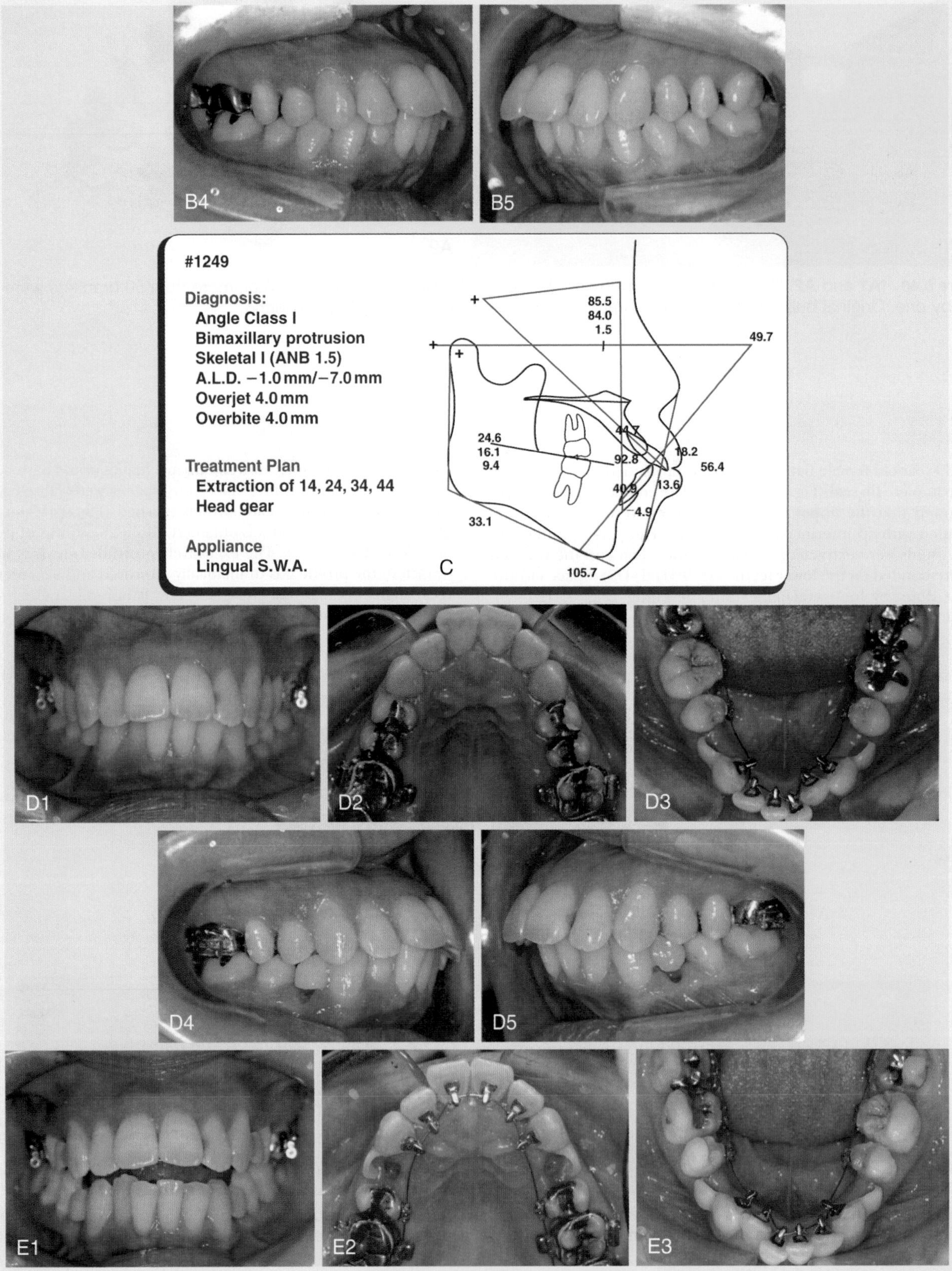

B4
B5
#1249
Diagnosis:
Angle Class I
Bimaxillary protrusion
Skeletal I (ANB 1.5)
A.L.D. −1.0 mm/−7.0 mm
Overjet 4.0 mm
Overbite 4.0 mm
Treatment Plan
Extraction of 14, 24, 34, 44
Head gear
Appliance
Lingual S.W.A.
C
85.5
84.0
1.5
49.7
24.6
16.1
9.4
44.7
92.8
18.2
56.4
40.9
13.6
4.9
33.1
105.7
D1
D2
D3
D4
D5
E1
E2
E3

Figure 9.41, cont'd **(C)** Pretreatment head plate, diagnosis and treatment plan. (**D1–D5**) Upper first molars were bonded for headgear. Brackets were bonded on lower first molars. (**E1–E5**) One month later, brackets were bonded on upper also. Archwires were 0.016 NiTi and 0.014 NiTi.

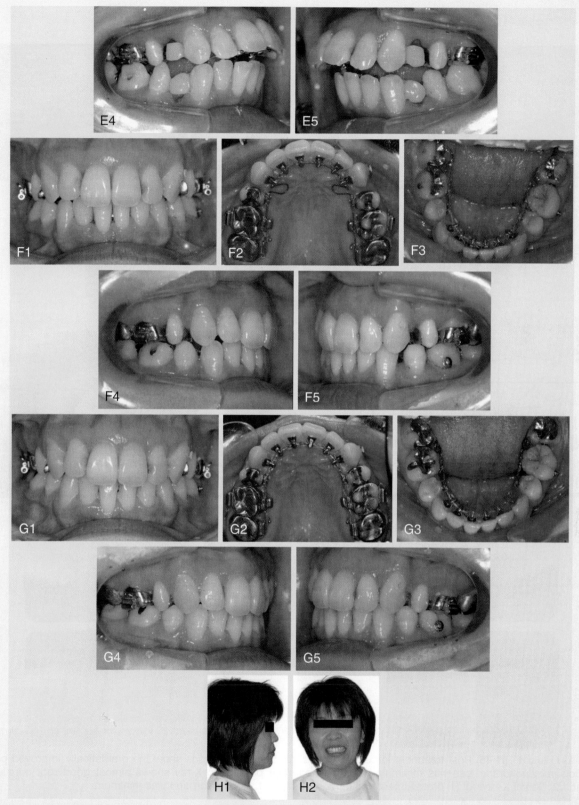

Figure 9.41, cont'd (**F1–F5**) Sixteen months into the treatment. Space closure was done with loop mechanics. Archwires were 1725 Beta III in both the arches. (**G1–G5**) Twenty-five months into the treatment. Finishing and detailing with 1725 Beta III. Elastic chains were worn *from second molar to second molar* to tighten contacts. (**H1** and **H2**) Post-treatment facial pictures. Original protruded incisors were well retracted and profile was dramatically improved.

Continued

CASE 4—cont'd

Figure 9.41, cont'd **(I1–I5)** Post-treatment intraoral pictures. **(J)** Superimpositions show the dramatically improved profile and incisors. Anchorage loss was minimum. **(K)** Post-treatment panoramic X-ray shows almost good root paralleling. **(L1** and **L2)** Dental X-rays of (1) pretreatment and (2) post-treatment. Root resorption was minimum.

Experimentally made 45° torque twin brackets

In 1994, the authors developed 45° torque twin brackets. At that time, the Kurz appliance was widely used around the world, but the authors were not satisfied with it.

Therefore, they experimentally made new brackets[4] in order to improve the six difficulties associated with Kurz appliance. These were introduced at the first International Lingual Orthodontic Congress in Tokyo, Japan, 1999 and at the Korean Society of Lingual Orthodontic Meeting in Seoul, Korea, 1999.

Double over-tie

The well-known reason why the Kurz appliance requires the double over-tie[18] is because of the relationship between the wings and the slot direction. Figure 9.42 shows the lateral view of the Kurz appliance. Yellow rectangle shows the archwire and red circles show the ligature wires. Note the angle between both the tie-wings and the bracket slot. It is very small, almost 20° as opposed to the ideal right angle. Therefore, if it were conventionally tied, the archwire would not be seated to the bottom of the bracket slot. The conventional tie does not push the archwire in the direction of the bracket slot. In order to seat the archwire to the bottom of the bracket slot, the double over-tie must be used (Fig. 9.43). The authors made a hypothesis that if the angle between the tie-wings and the slot is less than 45°, the conventional ties are able to seat the archwire into the bracket slot. This is a very important point and we must keep it in our mind because some brackets that are currently being marketed have almost the same feature as Kurz appliance. Check the brackets laterally and observe the angle between the slot direction and the tie-wings. If more than 45°, double over-ties must be used even though they are newly designed.

Speech difficulties

Authors often experienced patients complaining about speech problems, and many patients quit their treatment just a week after the Kurz appliance was bonded because of the size and bulk of the appliance, especially in the upper anterior region. For better pronunciation, the authors made the brackets smaller and thinner (Fig. 9.44A1).

Tongue irritation

Big and bulky appliance also causes tongue irritations. The Kurz appliances are very thick, especially in the bicuspids area. The authors made their appliance thinner,

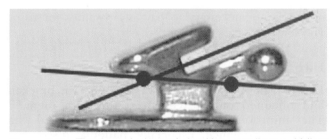

Figure 9.42 The lateral view of the Kurz appliance. Yellow rectangle shows the archwire, and red circles show the ligature wires. Note the angle between both the tie-wings and the bracket slot. It is very small, almost 20° as opposed to the ideal right angle.

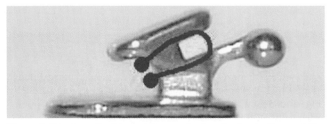

Figure 9.43 In order to seat the archwires to the bottom of the bracket slot, the double over-tie must be used.

and the tongue irritation was dramatically reduced (Fig. 9.44A2).

Bracket interference

The disadvantages of big and bulky appliances are not only the pronunciation problems and tongue irritation but also the large bite planes of Kurz appliance interfering with antagonistic teeth or adjacent teeth, making finishing difficult (Fig. 9.45). The authors made their brackets smaller and without bite planes. Small brackets have distinct advantage, especially in crowding cases (Fig. 9.46).

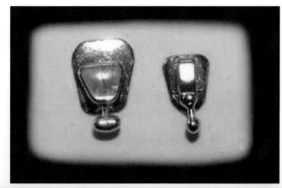

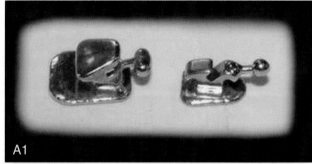

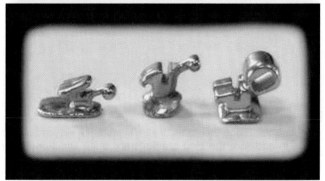

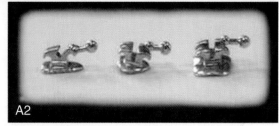

Figure 9.44 **(A1)** Comparison of Kurz appliance (left) and Hiro brackets (right). **(A2)** Comparison of Kurz appliance (above) and Hiro brackets (below).

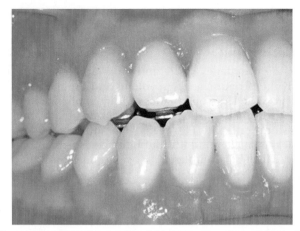

Figure 9.45   Bite planes often interfere with antagonistic teeth.

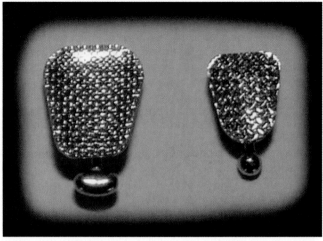

Figure 9.47   The comparison of the bonding mesh of Kurz (left) and Hiro brackets (right). Kurz's mesh is much too fine. Hiro brackets used rougher mesh for better retention, and therefore, frequency of bond failures was decreased.

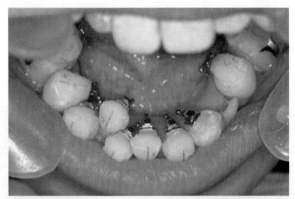

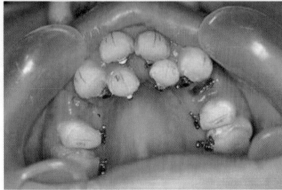

Figure 9.46   Since the cores of Hiro system are very small and thin; in addition, the Hiro brackets are quite small and they can be bonded on such a severely crowded case.

Brackets being broken off

The authors often experienced the Kurz appliance brackets breaking off from the teeth. Whenever it happened, adhesive remained on the teeth and nothing on the bonding bases. This indicates there are some difficulties in the bonding meshes. In fact, one hundred meshes are used for the Kurz appliance, and it is much too fine. Therefore, the authors made the bonding mesh rough and the frequency of broken brackets decreased (Fig. 9.47).

Cost

Reducing costs is quite important not only for the orthodontist but also for the patients because increased costs push up the treatment fees. The authors provide Hiro brackets at cheaper cost than any other brackets, and it is not necessary to pay any royalties for using Hiro system.

Hiro brackets

In 1994, the authors made 45° torque twin brackets and obtained quite excellent results with them.[4,28] They improved all the six difficulties associated with the Kurz appliance. Especially, patients' discomfort and pronunciation difficulties[29] were dramatically improved. Therefore, the authors evolved them to be smaller and thinner in 1999. Compared with the Kurz appliance, these Hiro brackets that were introduced at the 6th ESLO meeting in Barcelona were quite small and thin (Fig. 9.44).

CASE 5

The patient, a 26-year-old female, visited the authors' clinic complaining about anterior crowding and protrusive profile. Molar relation was Class I on both the sides and severe crowding was observed in both the arches (Fig. 9.48A1–C). After four bicuspids were extracted, the treatment was initiated (Fig. 9.48D1–G5).

Quite an excellent result was obtained in 24 months of treatment (Fig. 9.48I1–J). Panoramic radiographs show good root paralleling, and dental radiographs do not show any root resorption (Fig. 9.48K–L2).

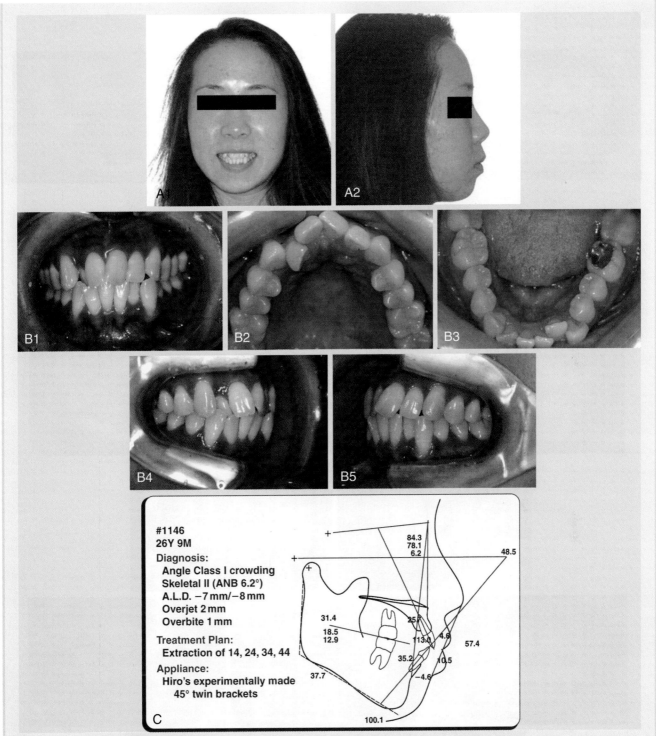

#1146
26Y 9M
Diagnosis:
  Angle Class I crowding
  Skeletal II (ANB 6.2°)
  A.L.D. −7 mm/−8 mm
  Overjet 2 mm
  Overbite 1 mm

Treatment Plan:
  Extraction of 14, 24, 34, 44

Appliance:
  Hiro's experimentally made
    45° twin brackets

Figure 9.48 (**A1** and **A2**) A 26-year-old female patient had a bimaxillary protruded profile. (**B1–B5**) Pretreatment intraoral pictures. Molars were Class I and severe crowding was observed in both the arches. (**C**) Cephalometric tracing and diagnosis. Four bicuspids were extracted to improve the profile and crowding.

Continued

CASE 5—cont'd

Figure 9.48, cont'd (**D1–D5**) Brackets were bonded, and initial archwires were 0.012 NiTi in both the arches. Labial brackets were used for the bicuspids and molars. (**E1–E5**) Six months into the treatment. Archwires were 0.014 SS in both the arches, and canines were slightly retracted. (**F1–F5**) Ten months into the treatment. Archwires were 0.014 SS/1622 TMA.

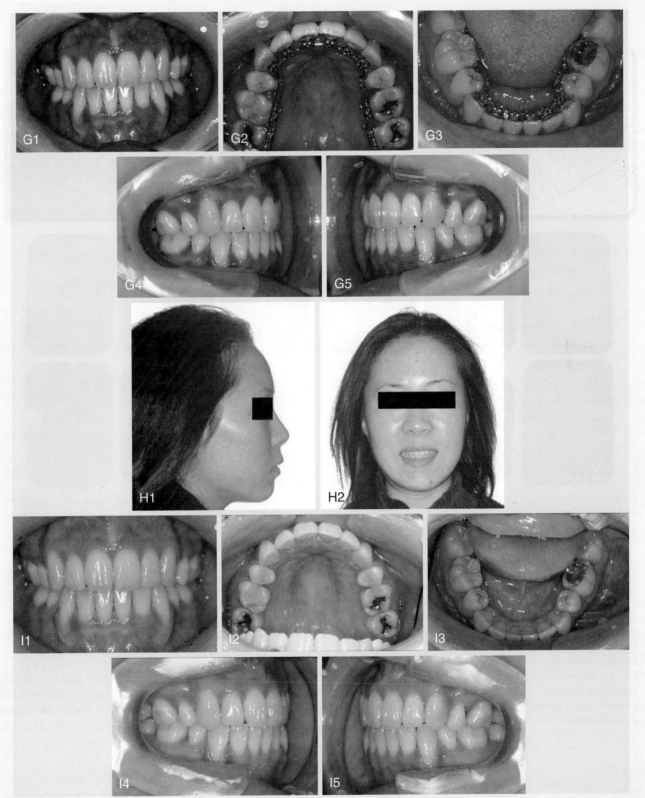

Figure 9.48, cont'd   **(G1–G5)** Twenty months into the treatment. Finishing and detailing of dentition done. (**H1** and **H2**) Post-treatment facial pictures. Protruded profile was improved. (**I1–I5**) Post-treatment intraoral pictures. The treatment term was 24 months, and quite an excellent result was obtained with experimentally made twin brackets.

Continued

CASE 5—cont'd

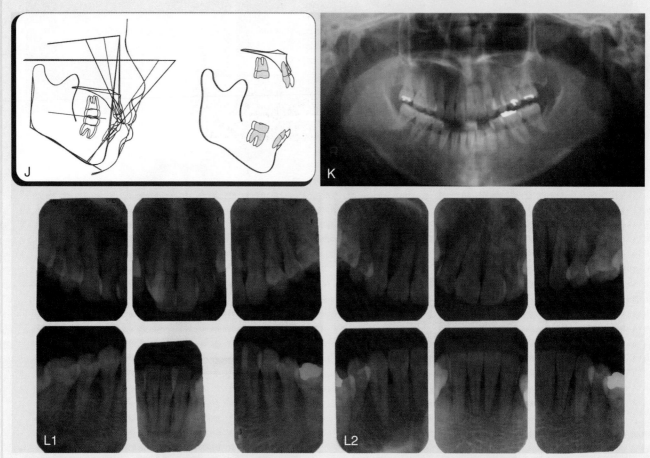

Figure 9.48, cont'd **(J)** Pretreatment and post-treatment cephalometric superimpositions. Incisors were well retracted and the profile was improved. Additional anchorage was not used. **(K)** Post-treatment panoramic X-ray shows good root paralleling. **(L1 and L2)** Dental X-rays of **(1)** pretreatment and **(2)** post-treatment. Root resorption was minimum.

Hiro lingual bracket system offers some critical technical improvements and has the following features:

- Anatomical design that reduces bracket debonding
- Curved wings to secure ligature retention
- Double premolar wings for easier derotation
- Hooks on canine and molar facilitate the use of intermaxillary elastics
- Bracket body is gingivally displaced to reduce occlusal interference

- Optimal slot depth for maximum torque control
- Low-profile bracket design
- All these features contribute to more comfort, less friction and lingual irritation and proper speech.

Since Hiro brackets greatly improved patient comfort and pronunciation, the authors introduced them on his website in 2002 and at the ESLO meeting in Barcelona in 2004.

CASE 6

A 19-year-old female patient demonstrated maxillary protrusion and anterior crowding. On intraoral examination, the molar relations were found to be Angle Class II on both sides and the maxillary incisors were protruded (Fig. 9.49A1–C). At the initial stage of treatment, cross-elastics were used for the correction of scissors bite of the right second molars (Fig. 9.49D1–D5). Space closure was done with sliding mechanics, and the treatment was finished within 16 months (Fig. 9.49E1–H5). Regularly, correction of deep overbite is done not by upper incisor intrusion but by lower incisor intrusion[30,31] (Fig. 9.49I). Panoramic radiograph shows good root paralleling. Impacted mandibular third molars were extracted during the treatment. No root resorption was observed (Fig. 9.49J–K2).

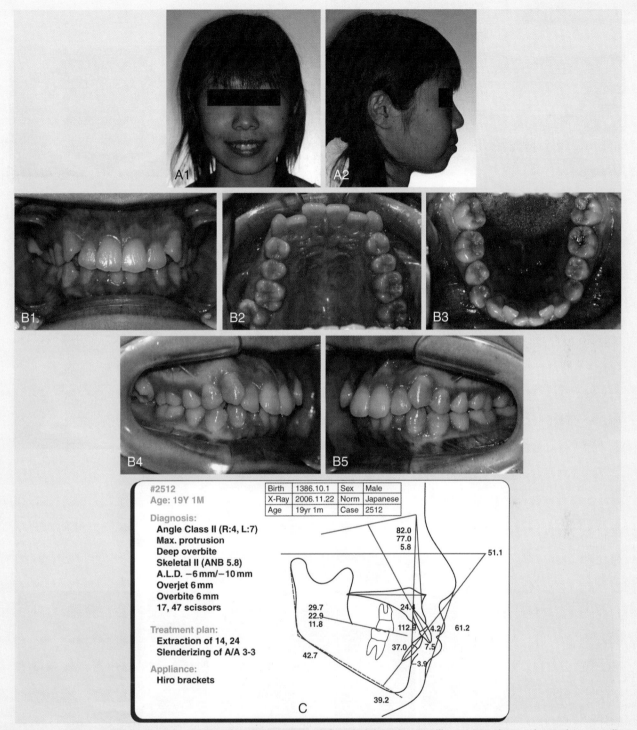

#2512
Age: 19Y 1M

Birth	1386.10.1	Sex	Male
X-Ray	2006.11.22	Norm	Japanese
Age	19yr 1m	Case	2512

Diagnosis:
 Angle Class II (R:4, L:7)
 Max. protrusion
 Deep overbite
 Skeletal II (ANB 5.8)
 A.L.D. −6 mm/−10 mm
 Overjet 6 mm
 Overbite 6 mm
 17, 47 scissors

Treatment plan:
 Extraction of 14, 24
 Slenderizing of A/A 3-3

Appliance:
 Hiro brackets

82.0
77.0
5.8
51.1
29.7
22.9
11.8
24.4
112.9
4.2
61.2
37.0
7.5
42.7
−3.9
39.2

C

Figure 9.49 (**A1** and **A2**) A 19-year-old female patient. Her chief complaint was maxillary protrusion and anterior crowding. (**B1–B5**) Pretreatment intraoral pictures. Anterior teeth were protruded and crowded. (**C**) Pretreatment cephalometric tracing, diagnosis and treatment plan.

Continued

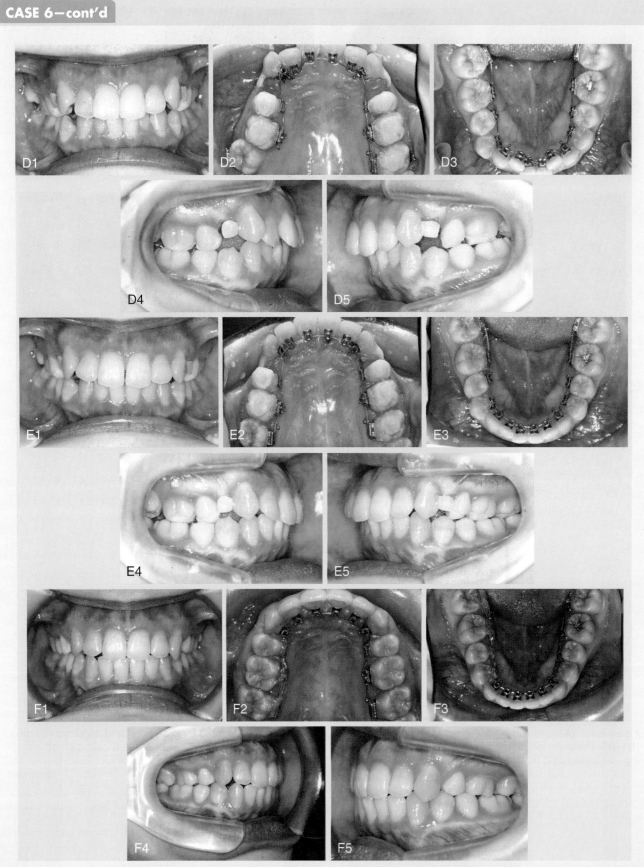

Figure 9.49, cont'd   **(D1–D5)** Upper bicuspids were extracted and the treatment was started. Archwires were 0.016 NiTi in both the arches. **(E1–E5)** Two months into the treatment. Crowding of upper and lower incisors was almost relieved. Archwires were 016 Beta III/ 0175 square TMA. **(F1–F5)** Twelve months into the treatment. Space closing was already completed. The archwires were 0175 square TMA.

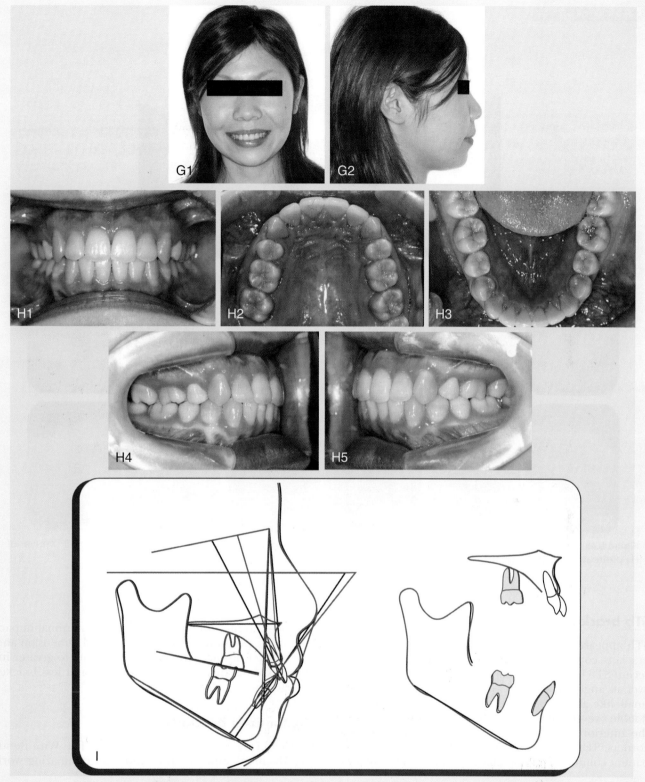

Figure 9.49, cont'd (**G1** and **G2**) Post-treatment facial pictures. A beautiful smile and nice profile were obtained. (**H1–H5**) Post-treatment intraoral pictures. Original protruded upper incisors were well retracted. An excellent result was obtained within 16 months of treatment term. (**I**) Superimpositions show intrusion of upper incisors.

Continued

CASE 6—cont'd

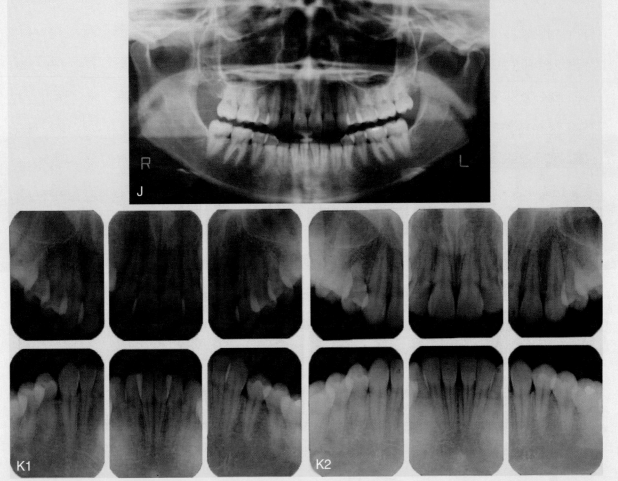

Figure 9.49, cont'd **(J)** Post-treatment panoramic X-ray shows good root paralleling. **(K1** and **K2)** Dental X-rays of (1) pretreatment and (2) post-treatment. Root resorption was none.

STb bracket system

STb appeared few years after the introduction of Hiro brackets, copying all concepts of Hiro brackets. The most recent STb has quite similar looks to Hiro brackets; however, its angle between tie-wings and bracket slot is quite small like Kurz appliance (Fig. 9.42). Therefore, the double over-tie must be used for STb in order to control the anterior teeth. With their reduced size and rounded corners, STb brackets are designed to provide maximum patient comfort. This appliance system has a low-bracket profile—1.5 mm total thickness—and a minimal impact on tongue position and speech. Reduced dimension and low bracket profile significantly contribute to greater interbracket distance for reduced forces and less bracket interference.

Customized brackets

In 1998, Dirk Wiechmann introduced 'The Wire Bending Machine'. Since then he did a lot of amazing work

CASE 7

A 28-year-old female patient treated with STb bracket system is shown in Figure 9.50. Her chief complaints were anterior crowding and convex profile (Fig. 9.50A1–B5). Cephalometric analysis shows bimaxillary protrusion and high angle (Fig. 9.50C). After four bicuspids were extracted, treatment was started with STb and an excellent result was obtained (Fig. 9.50D1–J). The treatment term was 28 months because it took a long time to control the anterior torque. Panoramic radiograph shows good root paralleling, and dental radiograph shows that root resorption was not observed (Fig. 9.50K–L2).

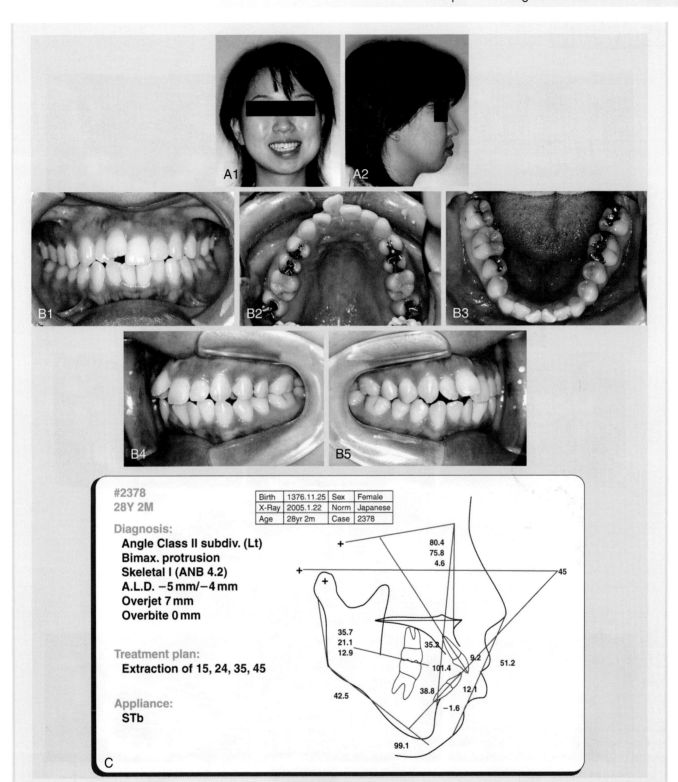

Figure 9.50 **(A1** and **A2)** A 28-year-old female patient visited the authors' office complaining about anterior crowding and convex profile. **(B1–B5)** Pretreatment intraoral pictures. The maxillary right central incisor was excessively protruded and molar relation was Class II on left side. **(C)** Pretreatment cephalometric tracing, diagnosis and treatment plan. Upper and lower incisors were flared out.

Continued

CASE 7—cont'd

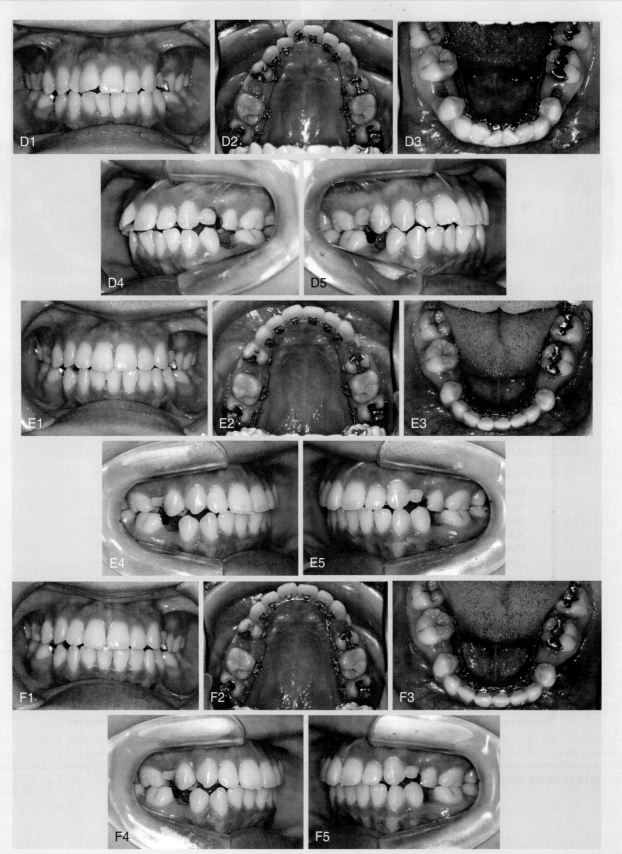

Figure 9.50, cont'd (**D1–D5**) Brackets were bonded on upper and lower. Initial wires were 012 NiTi in both the arches. (**E1–E5**) Levelling was achieved in 5 months. Archwires were 0175 square TMA/014 NiTi. (**F1–F5**) Six months into the treatment, space closing with elastic chains. Both archwires were 1725 Beta III.

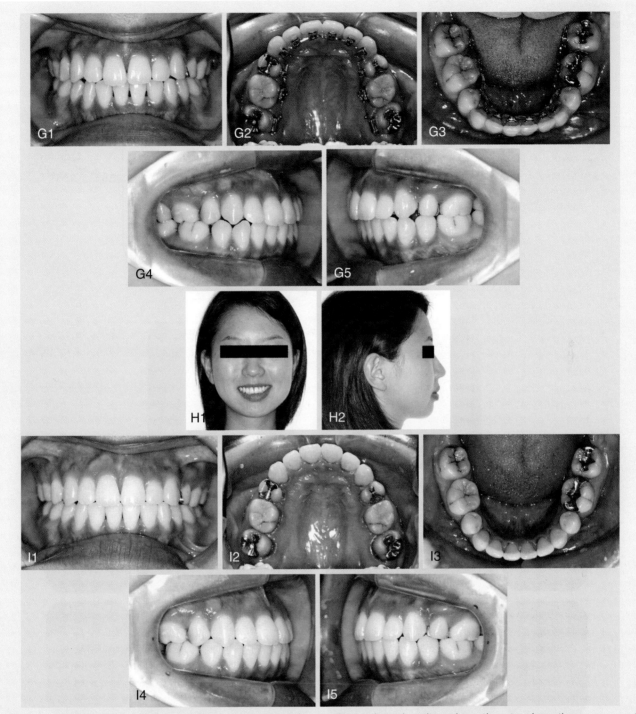

Figure 9.50, cont'd **(G1–G5)** Twenty-three months into the treatment. It took quite a long time to close the space, and then spent many months to control anterior torque. **(H1 and H2)** Facial pictures showing pleasing smile after treatment. **(I1–I5)** Post-treatment intraoral pictures. It took 28 months to finish the treatment but an excellent occlusion was obtained.

Continued

CASE 7—cont'd

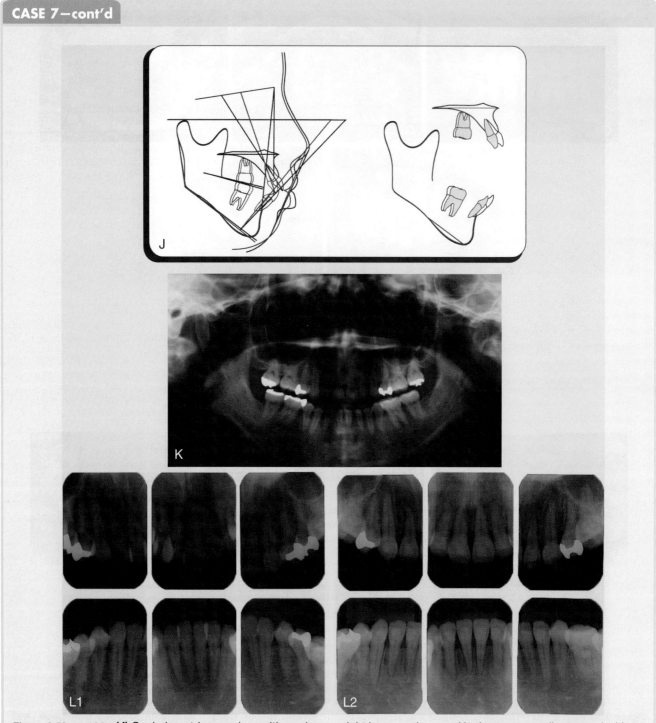

Figure 9.50, cont'd **(J)** Cephalometric superimpositions show upright lower molars, and incisors were well retracted without any additional anchorage. **(K)** Post-treatment panoramic X-ray. 44 and 46 should have uprighted but could not do so because the treatment was already extended. **(L1** and **L2)** Dental X-rays of (1) pretreatment and (2) post-treatment. Root resorption was very less.

and finally achieved a great innovation, computerized custom-casted appliance for individual teeth, 'Incognito'. Currently, he holds Incognito courses around the world. The authors also took his course and ordered a few cases. Checking the setups with internet, the authors received a package just a month after the initial contact (Fig. 9.51A1 and A2).

Customized bracket system for individual patient was introduced to solve some crucial problems associated with prefabricated mass-produced lingual brackets using CAD/CAM technology. Both the processes involved fabrication of brackets and optimal positioning of brackets customized to individual patient and are fused into a single process. This is later followed by precise archwire bending using a robot.

INCOGNITO

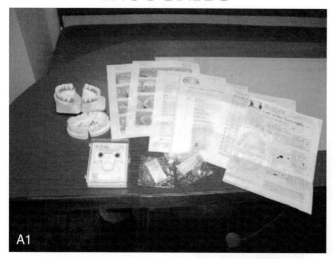

A1

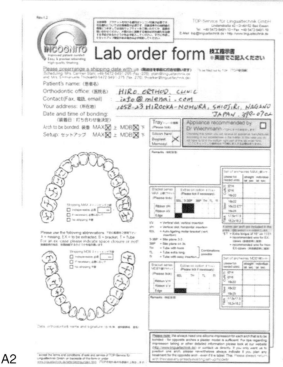

A2

Figure 9.51 (A1) The package from Bad Essen enclosed the setup, three sets of archwires, the order form, a packing list, workers list, material list and the Incognito brackets with silicone trays. Everything was perfectly cleaned and packed with desiccants. Authors had never experienced such an impressive work. **(A2)** The order form of Incognito. The client can select the kind of indirect bonding trays, the direction of the slot and the direction of wires from Ribbon VH, Ribbon VV and EW. Also, we can order some extras, autoligating molar brackets, bite plane for 3 × 3 or just canines, tube with hooks and easy insertion tubes. We can order archwires as we want.

This appliance system involves a customized target setup made of each malocclusion cast, and it is then scanned under a 3D scanner. The scanned data is fed into a software program that designs the dimensions of the base pad that will be adapting to the lingual surface. The bracket bodies with vertical slots are designed on computer. Wax analogues are produced using rapid prototyping machine. These analogues are then cast in a high gold content alloy. Due to precise base design, these brackets can be directly or indirectly bonded.

BIOMECHANICS AND CASE SELECTION

The article of LSWA[26] written by Takemoto and Scuzzo is well known around the world. The authors had assisted their work, submitted the article 'The Six Keys to Success in Lingual Orthodontics'[4] for the future users of LSWA and also presented successful results[28] with LSWA. However, they quit their trial for the LSWA and developed a very different concept bracket, STb. There are three major reasons why they changed their direction. First, the prototype of LSWA had a very high profile; hence patients suffered excessive speech problem and tongue irritation. Second, contrary to the labial appliances,[32] the treatment with lingual SWA was rather difficult than that with lingual non-SWA because of its high profile. This is because the archwires of LSWA are distant from the teeth; therefore, very small adjustments of the archwires induce quite a large movement of the teeth.[4] Third, the high profile brackets make the interbracket distance shorter,[33] which is against the ideals of orthodontics. The authors had introduced the successful results of LSWA by putting some modifications, such as cutting the bracket bodies shorter to make the slot closer to the teeth and reshaping the sharp-edged bracket body round.

As the authors indicated in their article, comprehensive understanding of force systems[34] of lingual orthodontics is pivotal to obtain successful results, especially in LSWA. This is because high-profile brackets accentuate the teeth movement. For example, anterior segment tips lingually if the orthodontist does not manage the anterior torque during the space closure; as a result, vertical bowing effect occurs.[35–37] Another example is that the terminal molars move lingually during space closure; as a result, horizontal bowing effect occurs.

These effects are observed in both loop mechanics and sliding mechanics. Most lingual orthodontists explain that these are peculiarities of lingual orthodontics; however, the authors have a different opinion. That is, the same situations are occurring in labial treatment. Here is an example. In space closing stage of labial treatment, if the clinician applies elastomeric chain on the terminal molars of maxilla, they move buccally. Then if the archwire is not adjusted, buccal overjet will be increased in that area. Simultaneously, the upper incisors will tip lingually and extrude and then the overbite becomes deep. These are the same phenomena as the bowing effect of lingual treatment, but they are less remarkable in labial treatment.

So, how can we prevent them? The answer is simple. They can be prevented by putting the αβ, gable bends between the anterior segment and the posterior segment, as we usually do for labial treatment.[38] Another example is the difficult anchorage control, that is, the posterior segments do not lose their anchorage. Generally, it is explained as due to the cortical bone anchorage; however, the authors have a different opinion. The torque control of anterior segment has quite an important role for the success of the treatment. Regrettably, some brackets that are currently being marketed have difficulty in controlling the anterior torque. The bracket selection is as important as understanding the force system.

These issues will help the case selection for beginners.[39] Some experts say that beginners of lingual orthodontics

CASE 8

The patient shown in Figure 9.52 is a 20-year-old female and had an anterior crossbite. The molars were severe Class III on both the sides (Fig. 9.52A1–B5). She had severe skeletal Class III; however, the authors started her treatment without extraction or surgery (Fig. 9.52C1–F5). An excellent result was obtained with

22 months of treatment. Even though she was treated without surgery, the original concave profile was improved. Lower molars were uprighted and mandible showed slight backward rotation (Fig. 9.52G1–K2).

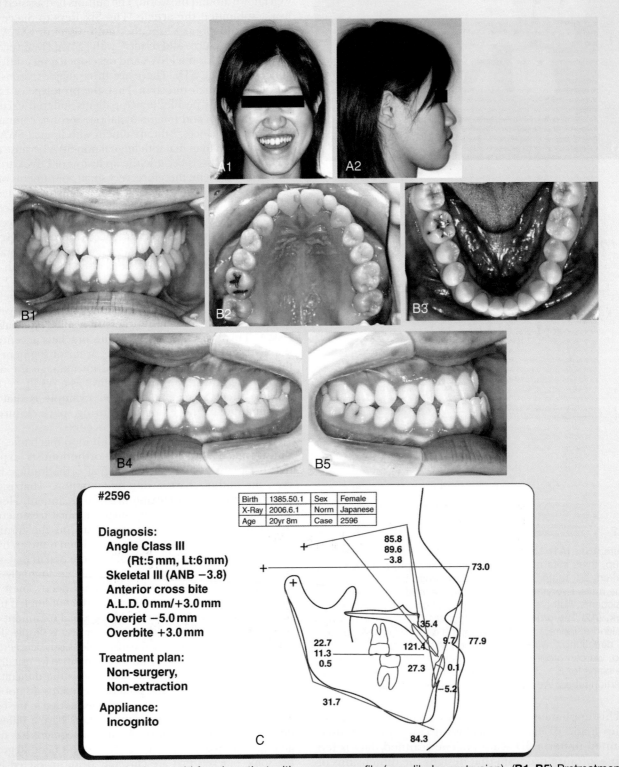

#2596

Birth	1385.50.1	Sex	Female
X-Ray	2006.6.1	Norm	Japanese
Age	20yr 8m	Case	2596

Diagnosis:
  Angle Class III
      (Rt:5 mm, Lt:6 mm)
  Skeletal III (ANB −3.8)
  Anterior cross bite
  A.L.D. 0 mm/+3.0 mm
  Overjet −5.0 mm
  Overbite +3.0 mm

Treatment plan:
  Non-surgery,
  Non-extraction

Appliance:
  Incognito

85.8
89.6
−3.8

73.0

35.4

22.7
11.3
0.5

121.4

9.7   77.9

27.3   0.1

−5.2

31.7

84.3

C

Figure 9.52 (**A1** and **A2**) A 20-year-old female patient with concave profile (mandibular protrusion). (**B1–B5**) Pretreatment intraoral pictures. Molar relation was full Class III and anterior crossbite. (**C**) Pretreatment cephalometric tracing, diagnosis and treatment plan. The authors started her treatment without extraction and surgery.

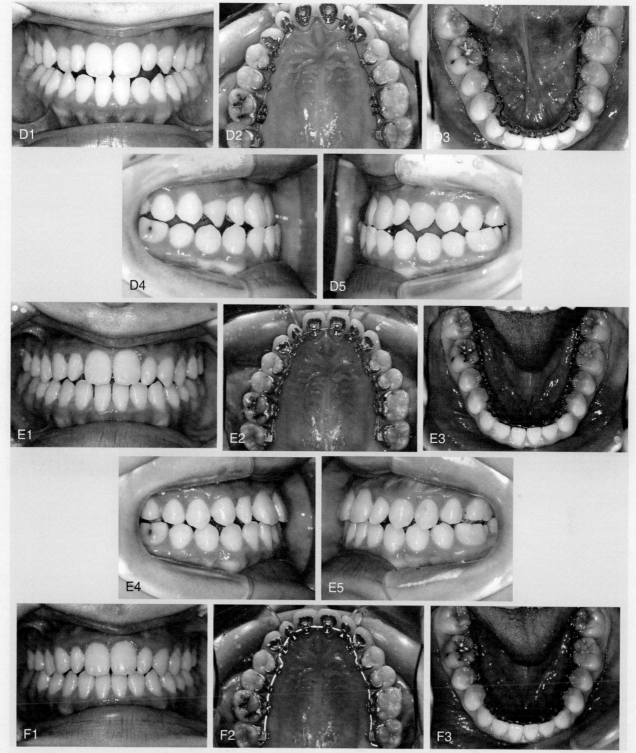

Figure 9.52, cont'd (**D1–D5**) The appliance was bonded on maxillary and mandibular arches. The initial wire was 012 NiTi/1622 super elastic. (**E1–E5**) Six months into the treatment. Class III elastics were worn all day long, and the anterior crossbite was improved. The archwires were 1622 super elastic for both the arches. (**F1–F5**) Twelve months into the treatment, Class III elastics were continued.

Continued

Figure 9.52, cont'd **(G1** and **G2)** Post-treatment facial pictures with pleasing smile   achieved without surgery and extraction. **(H1–H5)** Post-treatment intraoral pictures showing good occlusion. The treatment term was 22 months. **(I)** Cephalometric superimpositions show upright lower molars and incisors. Backward rotation of mandible was observed.

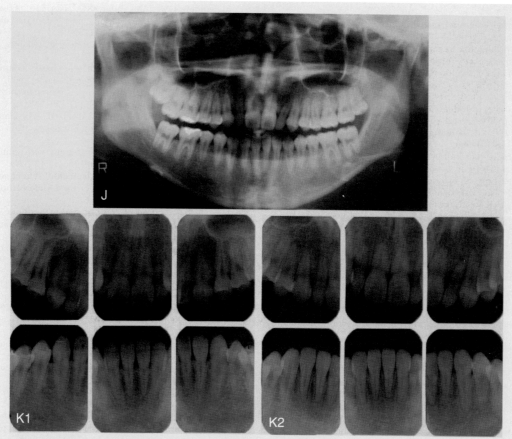

Figure 9.52, cont'd **(J)** Post-treatment panoramic X-ray shows good root paralleling. **(K1** and **K2)** Dental X-rays of (1) pretreatment and (2) post-treatment. Root resorption was not significant.

should start from Class II division 2 cases; however, after reviewing the force systems, it has been pointed out that it is not correct. The Class II division 2 cases have deep overbites with lingually inclined upper incisors and are the most difficult cases to treat, requiring perfect control of anterior torque and enough experience. We must remember that when we intrude the anterior teeth in lingual treatment, they tip lingually. Original lingually inclined incisors will have further lingual tipping by intrusion force.

Considering the force mechanics, Class II division 1 cases with large overjet appear to be difficult cases, but actually they are easier than Class II division 2 cases. The authors recommend that the orthodontists who are thinking to start lingual orthodontics should start from Class I non-extraction cases. Next, treat Class II division 1 upper bicuspid extraction cases. Some experts recommend that when treating minor crowding cases, we should bond the brackets directly, and it is not necessary to make setup or indirect cores; however, the authors strongly oppose this opinion. In order to keep the treatment simple and obtain excellent results, we must not ignore the precise bracket positioning, laboratory setup and efficient and effective bonding procedure.

CONCLUSION

Almost 20 years have passed since the authors started lingual orthodontics. Currently, they do not select the cases for lingual; in their practices, they belive in the philosophy 'All the cases that can be treated with Labial Orthodontics can be treated with Lingual Orthodontics'. This is what they always explain to their patients, and the selection of appliance is 100% done by patients.

The most important factor in achieving excellent results in lingual treatment is to address the following issues.

1. *Bracket placement:* The quality of laboratory work plays quite an important role.
2. *The performance of brackets:* The thinness and the shape of the bracket are important for better comfort and pronunciation of the patients. Suitable wires for every situation—there is no routine wire sequence and ideal archform. Just as in labial treatment, we must make decisions and carry them out for every visit.
3. *Mastering the force system and diagnosis of lingual:* When compared with the lingual practice 20 years ago, current lingual practice is totally different. We can obtain as excellent results as labial orthodontics, and sometimes better than labial orthodontics, without any troubles.

The authors always remember Dr Harry Daugherty's words— '3Hs'. They are 'Hands', 'Head' and 'Heart'.

REFERENCES

1. Fujita K. Orthodontic appliance (Multiple Lingual Orthodontic Appliance), Japan patent, 55–48814, Field; 1976.
2. Fujita K. New orthodontic treatment with lingual bracket mushroom arch wire appliance. Am J Orthod 1982; 82(2):120–140.
3. Mori Y., et al. Lingual orthodontics – Dr. Gorman technique, chap. 1. Tokyo: Ishiyaku; 1996. p. 1–27.
4. Hiro T. Preparation for the new generation of lingual orthodontics – Six keys to success with lingual straight wire appliance. J Lingual Orthod 2002; 2:29–47.
5. Aquirre MJ. Indirect bonding for lingual orthodontics. J Clin Orthod 1984; 18:565–569.
6. Kyung HM. Individual indirect bonding technique (IIBT) using set-up model. J Kor Dent Assoc 1989; 27:73–82.
7. Mori Y, et al. Lingual orthodontics – Dr. Gorman technique, chap. 4. Tokyo: Ishiyaku; 1996. p. 71–110.
8. Hiro T, Takemoto K. Resin core indirect bonding system – improvement of lingual orthodontic treatment. Orthod Waves 1998; 57:83–91.
9. Huge S. The customized lingual appliance set-up service system in lingual orthodontics. Ontario: BC Decker; 1998. p. 163–173.
10. Kim TW, Bae Gi – Sun, Cho J. New indirect bonding method for lingual orthodontics. J Clin Orthod 2000; 34:348–350.
11. Koyata H. Esthetic orthodontics – basic technique of lingual orthodontics, chap. 11. Tokyo: Quintessence; 2003. p. 80–92.
12. Matsuno I, Okuda S, Nodera Y. The hybrid core system for indirect bonding. J Clin Orthod 2003; 37(3):160–161.
13. Breece GL, Nieberg LG. Motivation for adult orthodontic treatment. J Clin Orthod 1986; 20:166–171.
14. Kyung HM, Kim BC, Sung HJ. The effect of resin base thickness on shear bonding strength in lingual tooth surface. J Lingual Orthod 2002; 2(1):15–21.
15. Scuzzo G, Takemoto K. Invisible orthodontics, chap. 4. Germany: Quintessence; 2003. p. 39–45.
16. Hiro T, Iglesia F, Andreu P. Indirect bonding technique in lingual orthodontics: the HIRO system. Prog. Orthod 2008; 9(2):34–45.
17. Kirk IM. Relative wire stiffness due to lingual vs labial inter-bracket distance. Am J Orthod Dentofac Orthop 1987; 92(1):24–32.
18. Smith JR, Gorman JC, Kurz C et al. Keys to success in lingual therapy – Part-2. J Clin Orthod 1986; 20(5):330–340.
19. Kinya F. New orthodontic treatment with lingual bracket mushroom archwire appliance. Am J Orthod 1979; 76(6):657.
20. Kinya F. Multilingual-bracket and mushroom archwire technique. A clinical report. Am J Orthod Dentofac Orthop 1982; 82(2):120–140.
21. Alexander CM, Alexander RG, Gorman JC et al. Lingual orthodontics: a status report: part 5-Lingual mechanotherapy. J Clin Orthod 1983; 17(2):99–115.
22. Kurz C. Lingual orthodontic course syllabus. Ormco Corp: Orange, CA, USA; 1989.
23. Koyata H. Esthetic orthodontics — basic technique of lingual orthodontics, chap. 1. Tokyo: Quintessence; 2003. p. 8–14.
24. Creekmore T. Lingual orthodontics its renaissance. Am J Orthod Dentfacial Orthopedics 1989; 96(2):120–137.
25. Kyung HM, Park HS, Bae SM et al. The lingual plain-wire system with microimplant anchorage. J Clin Orthod 2004; 38(7):388–395.
26. Takemoto K, Scuzzo G. The straight wire concept in lingual orthodontics. J Clin Orthod 2001; 35(1):46–52.
27. Hiro T. Fallberichte zur Lingualtechnik-Therapie mit lingualen Straight-Wire Apparaturen. Inf Orthod Kieferorthop 2003; 35:249–258.
28. Hiro T. Presentation of eight lingual orthodontic cases submitted for the European Board of Orthodontists examination. J Int Orthod 2008; 1:53–132.
29. Koyata H. Esthetic orthodontics—basic technique of lingual orthodontics, chap. 13. Tokyo: Quintessence; 2003. p. 104–5.
30. Koyata H. Esthetic orthodontics—basic technique of lingual orthodontics, chap. 15. Tokyo: Quintessence; 2003. p. 1110–1132.
31. Bennett RK. A study of deep overbite correction with lingual orthodontics, Master's thesis. Loma Linda Univ. 1988.
32. Andrews LF. JCO interviews on the straight wire appliance. J Clin Orthod 1990; 24:493–508.
33. Koyata H. Esthetic orthodontics—basic technique of lingual orthodontics, chap. 5. Tokyo: Quintessence; 2003. p. 20–23.
34. Koyata H. Esthetic orthodontics—basic technique of lingual orthodontics, chap. 8. Tokyo: Quintessence; 2003. p. 44–60.
35. Smith JR, Gorman JC, Kurz C et al. Key to success in Lingual therapy Part 1. J Clin Orthod 1986; 20(4):252–262.
36. Garland-Parker L. The complete Lingual Orthodontic training manual. 3rd edn. Professional Orthodontic Consulting; 1994.
37. Echarri P. Sagittal and vertical control in lingual orthodontics. J Lingual Orthod 2002; 2:48–56.
38. Mulligan TF. Common sense mechanics, Phoenix. CMS: Arizona, USA; 1982.
39. Mori Y, et al. Lingual orthodontics—Dr. Gorman technique, chap. 2. Tokyo: Ishiyaku; 1996. p. 29–33.

Management of Cleft Lip and Cleft Palate Patients

10

Pradip R Shetye, Hitesh Kapadia and Barry H Grayson

The management of patients with cleft lip and cleft palate requires prolonged orthodontic treatment and an interdisciplinary approach in providing these patients with optimal aesthetics, function and stability. This chapter describes current concepts and principles in the treatment of patients with cleft lip and palate. Orthodontic or orthopaedic management in infancy, in early mixed dentition, in early permanent dentition and after the completion of facial growth will be discussed. The focus of this chapter will be on the interdisciplinary approach to treatment planning and treatment sequencing.

Cleft lip and palate are the most frequently occurring congenital anomalies. Depending on the extent of the cleft defect, patients may have complex problems dealing with facial appearance, feeding, airway, hearing and speech. Patients with cleft lip and palate are ideally treated in a multidisciplinary team setting involving specialities from the following disciplines: paediatrics, plastic and reconstructive surgery, orthodontics, genetics, social work, nursing, ENT, speech therapy, maxillofacial surgery, paediatric dentistry, prosthetic dentistry and psychology. The orthodontic treatment of patients with clefts is extensive, initiating at birth and continuing into adulthood until the completion of craniofacial skeletal growth. The role of the orthodontist in timing and sequence of treatment is important in terms of overall team management. The goal for complete rehabilitation of patients with clefts is to maximize treatment outcome with minimal intervention. This chapter presents current orthodontic treatment concepts for the management of patients with clefts.

ROLE OF THE ORTHODONTIST

In a patient with cleft lip and palate, the malocclusion can be related to soft tissue, skeletal or dental defects. Some cleft orthodontic problems are directly related to the cleft deformity itself, such as discontinuity of the alveolar process and missing or malformed teeth. Some aspects of the malocclusion are secondary to the surgical intervention performed to repair the lip, nose, alveolar and palatal defects. The malocclusion may exist in all the three planes of space: anteroposterior, transverse and vertical. The malocclusion may reflect the severity of the initial cleft deformity and the growth response to the primary surgery. As malocclusion in patients with clefts is often a growth-related problem, the effect of the cleft deformity and primary surgery will be observed throughout the growth of the child until skeletal maturity. The orthodontist must make critical decisions for orthodontic intervention at the appropriate time and prioritize treatment goals for each intervention. For the purpose of organization, the orthodontic treatment of patients with clefts will be presented in four distinct treatment phases: infancy, primary dentition, mixed dentition and permanent dentition.

INFANCY

Presurgical infant orthopaedics has been used in the treatment of cleft lip and palate patients for centuries. The early techniques were focused on elastic retraction of the protruding premaxilla followed by stabilization after surgical repair. There still exists a debate on the long-term benefits of presurgical infant orthopaedics, and abundant literature has been published presenting various sides of this story.

The modern school of presurgical orthopaedic treatment in cleft lip and palate was started by McNeil in 1950. Burstone further developed and popularized McNeil's technique. In 1975, Georgiad and Latham introduced a pin-retained active appliance to simultaneously retract the premaxilla and expand the posterior segments over a period of several days. Hotz in 1987 described the use of a passive orthopaedic plate to slowly align the cleft segments. In 1993, Grayson et al[1] described a new technique, nasoalveolar moulding (NAM), to presurgically mold the alveolus, lip and nose in infants born with cleft lip and palate. The NAM appliance consists of an intraoral moulding plate with nasal stents to mold the alveolar ridge and nasal cartilage concurrently. The objective of presurgical NAM is to reduce the severity of the original cleft and nasal and alveolar deformities and thereby enable the surgeon to achieve a better primary repair of the lip and nose. The NAM technique has been shown to significantly improve the surgical outcome of primary repair in cleft lip and palate patients compared with other techniques of presurgical orthopaedics.

Impression technique, appliance fabrication and design

The initial impression of the infant with cleft lip and palate is obtained within the first week of birth using a heavy body silicone impression material. The impression must be taken in a clinical setting that is prepared to handle an airway emergency and in the presence of a surgeon. The moulding plate is made of hard, clear, self-cure acrylic that is 2–3 mm in thickness to provide structural integrity and to permit adjustments during the process of moulding. A retention button is fabricated and positioned anteriorly at an angle of approximately 40° to the plate (Fig. 10.1A–D). The nasal stent is not fabricated at this time. Instead, its construction is delayed until the cleft of the alveolus is reduced to approximately 5–6 mm in width.

Appliance insertion and taping

The appliance is then secured extraorally to the cheeks and bilaterally by surgical tapes that have orthodontic elastic bands at one end. The use of skin barrier tapes on the cheeks, like Duoderm or Tegaderm is advocated to reduce irritation on the cheeks. The horizontal surgical tapes are one-quarter inch (0.25") in width and approximately 3–4" in length. The elastic on the surgical tape is actively engaged on the retention button of the moulding plate, and the tape is secured to the cheeks (Fig. 10.2). Parents are instructed to keep the plate in the mouth full time and to remove it for daily cleaning. The infant may require time to adjust to feeding with the NAM appliance in the first few days.

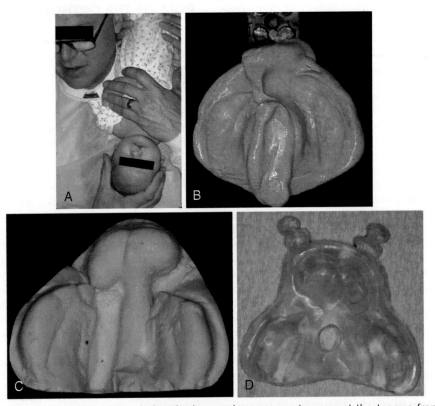

Figure 10.1 **(A)** Infant held in inverted position during the impression process to prevent the tongue from falling back and to allow fluids to drain out. **(B)** Impression of a unilateral cleft patient using custom tray and heavy body silicone impression material. **(C)** Plaster stone working model of a bilateral cleft patient for appliance fabrication. **(D)** Bilateral nasoalveolar moulding plate with retention buttons fabricated using self-cure acrylic resin.

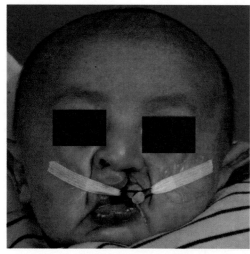

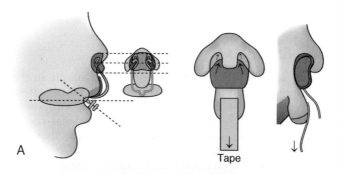

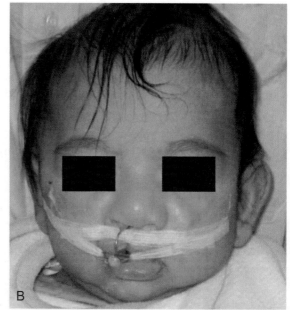

Figure 10.2 Unilateral cleft baby with NAM plate showing the retention arm positioned approximately 40° down from horizontal to achieve proper activation and to prevent unseating of the appliance from the palate. Note that there is no nasal stent placed for the first few weeks of treatment.

Appliance adjustments and nasal stent fabrication

The baby is seen weekly to make adjustments to the moulding plate to bring the alveolar segments together. These adjustments are made by selectively removing the hard acrylic and adding soft denture base material to the moulding plate. No more than 1 mm of modification of the moulding plate should be made at one visit. The nasal stent component of the NAM appliance is incorporated when the width of the alveolar gap is reduced to approximately 5 mm. The stent is made of 0.36" round stainless steel wire and takes the shape of a 'swan neck'. The intranasal hard acrylic component is shaped into a bilobed form that resembles a kidney, and a layer of soft denture liner is added to the hard acrylic for comfort. The upper lobe enters the nose and gently projects forward the dome, and the lower lobe of the stent lifts the nostril apex and defines the top of the columella (Fig. 10.3A–C).

Nonsurgical columella lengthening in bilateral cleft lip and palate

In bilateral cases, the attention is focused on nonsurgical lengthening of the columella by manipulation of the nasal stent. To achieve this objective, a horizontal band of denture material is added to join the left and right lower lobes of the nasal stent, spanning the base of the columella (Fig. 10.3A). This band sits at the nasolabial junction and defines this angle. Tape is adhered to the prolabium, and it applies a downward force to stretch the columella tissues. This tape contains elastics that are engaged to the retention buttons. The downward pull on the prolabium and columella provides a counter force to the upward force that is applied to the nasal tip by the stent. Taping downward on the prolabium helps to lengthen the columella and vertically lengthens the often small prolabium. The

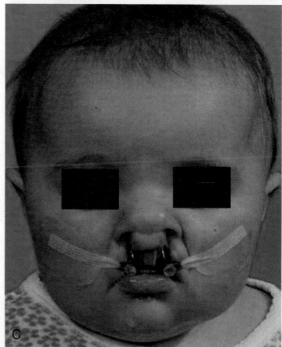

Figure 10.3 **(A)** Figure showing the design of the nasal stent and the position of the nasal stent in the nostril. **(B)** Unilateral NAM plate with nasal stent showing lip taping. **(C)** The bilateral NAM plate in position showing the tape adhered to the prolabium and stretched to the plate and attached to the plate.

horizontal lip tape is added after prolabium tape is in place.

Benefits of NAM

There are several benefits of the NAM technique in the treatment of cleft lip and palate deformity. Proper alignment of the alveolus, lip and nose helps the surgeon to achieve a better and more predictable surgical result. Long-term studies of NAM therapy indicate that the change in nasal shape is stable.[2] There is less scar tissue as the surgical correction is less invasive. The improved quality of primary surgical repair reduces the number of surgical revisions, oronasal fistulas and secondary nasal and labial deformities (Fig. 10.4).

If the alveolar segments are in the correct position and a gingivoperiosteoplasty is performed, the resulting bone bridge across the former cleft site improves the conditions for eruption of the permanent teeth and provides

them with better periodontal support. Studies have also demonstrated that 60% of the patients who underwent NAM and gingivoperiosteoplasty did not require secondary bone grafting.[3] The remaining 40% who did need bone grafts showed more bone remaining in the graft site compared with patients who have had no gingivoperiosteoplasty.[4] Fewer surgeries also result in substantial cost savings for families, insurance companies and government medical programmes. Studies have demonstrated that midfacial growth in the sagittal and vertical plane was not affected by gingivoperiosteoplasty.[5]

Since the introduction of NAM, there have been significant differences in the outcome of primary surgical cleft repair. With proper training and clinical skills, NAM has been demonstrated to provide tangible benefits to the patients, as well as to the surgeons performing the primary repair.

ORTHODONTIC/ORTHOPAEDIC TREATMENT IN THE PRIMARY DENTITION

Cleft lip and palate have an impact on multiple developmental and functional processes. As a result, the orthodontist must keep in mind the overall needs of the patient. At our institution, the orthodontic goals during the primary dentition stage of development are focused on the acquisition of normal speech function, which is managed by the speech therapist/pathologist and the surgeon. Once it is determined that a child has established proper speech function, the orthodontist can proceed with treatment.

The primary dentition is typically erupted by 3 years of age. Though it may not be readily apparent at this stage, the deleterious consequences of the clefting process on nasomaxillary growth become increasingly evident as the child grows. This is manifested as constriction of the maxillary arch transversely and anteroposteriorly. Dentally, an anterior crossbite with accompanying unilateral or bilateral posterior crossbites is observed. The decision whether to correct a crossbite at this stage is driven by the presence or absence of a functional mandibular shift. If it is caused by incisal or occlusal interference, selective enameloplasty or adjunctive orthodontics may be used to eliminate the centric relation (CR)–centric occlusion (CO) shift. If a functional occlusal interference occurs secondary to transverse constriction, the maxilla may be widened with the use of fixed or removable orthodontic expansion appliances. Since correction of a sagittal discrepancy tends to recur as the child grows, only the most severe maxillary retrognathia should be treated in this time period.

Another important component of care for a patient during this time period includes routine follow-up with a paediatric dentist. It is important that the paediatric dentist be made aware that every effort must be made to restore rather than extract a tooth. Though only a primary tooth, it may be used as anchorage for various appliances (i.e. palatal expander and protraction headgear [PHG]) during the mixed dentition phase. Regular 4–6-month visits to the paediatric dentist have the added benefit of exposing the children at an early age to a dentist's office, enabling them to feel comfortable when orthodontic care is required.

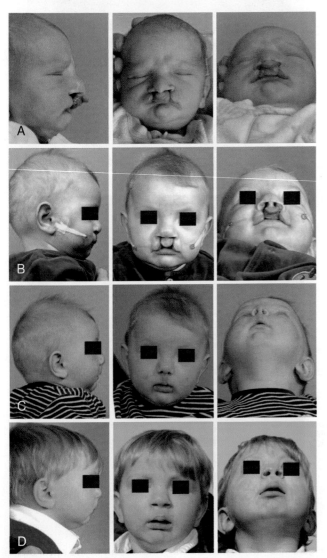

Figure 10.4 A bilateral complete cleft lip and palate infant treated with NAM therapy. **(A)** Prenasoalveolar moulding therapy. **(B)** Postnasoalveolar moulding therapy; note the nonsurgical columella elongation. **(C)** Postsurgical photograph. **(D)** 1-year follow-up.

MIXED DENTITION

The transition from primary dentition to mixed dentition commences at 6 years of age with the eruption of the first permanent tooth and continues until all the primary teeth are exfoliated at approximately 12 years of age. It is during this time that the child's psychosocial needs are brought to the forefront: as the child begins school, feelings of self-awareness and regard for appearance are heightened. This is also the time during which orthodontic treatment begins in earnest. As a result, the formulation of an appropriate treatment plan becomes paramount. The process begins with the collection of a set of diagnostic records, which includes intraoral and extraoral medical photographs, study models, orthopantomogram (panoramic radiograph), lateral cephalogram and periapical radiograph(s) of the cleft site(s). The advent of cone beam computed tomography enables a three-dimensional view of the cleft site defect and enhanced resolution of adjacent structures.

The treatment objectives for a child as he or she enters mixed dentition are directed toward resolution of problems, as they develop in the three planes of space: anteroposterior, vertical and transverse. Equally important during this time is the assessment and management of the alveolar bone at the cleft site, as well as missing, malformed or supernumerary teeth.

Intermediate secondary alveolar bone graft

Intermediate secondary, or delayed, alveolar bone grafting is defined as a graft that is placed between 6 and 15 years of age.[6] The timing of the graft is primarily dependent on the status of the maxillary lateral incisor, if present, or the maxillary canine. If the lateral incisor is present, it is preferred to perform the alveolar bone graft prior to its eruption. On the other hand, if the lateral incisor is absent, a bone graft should be performed before the eruption of the maxillary canine, when its root is half to two-thirds formed (Fig. 10.5A–F). The principal benefits of alveolar bone grafting are: (1) to provide sufficient bone for the eruption of either the maxillary lateral incisor or the canine, (2) to provide adequate bone and soft tissue coverage around teeth adjacent to the cleft site, (3) closure of oronasal fistulae to prevent nasal air escape and fluid or food leakage, (4) to provide additional support and elevation to nasal structures, (5) to restore the alveolar ridge in the area of the cleft, thereby allowing orthodontic tooth movement and future placement of a dental implants and (6) to stabilize premaxillary segments in patients with bilateral clefts (Fig. 10.5).[6]

Discrepancies in maxillary archform or transverse width should be improved prior to the secondary alveolar bone graft. It is important that the surgeon and orthodontist must work in concert to determine the anatomical limits of presurgical maxillary expansion. This is imperative, as over-expansion may create an oronasal fistula or a defect that is beyond the limits of surgical closure. Presurgical expansion in our unit is most commonly accomplished through the use of an occlusally bonded acrylic fan expander or a conventional Haas rapid palatal expander.

The deciduous teeth that are found along the cleft margin help to conserve or maintain bone volume along the facing alveolar walls. However, teeth that are present along the margin of the alveolar cleft may prevent adequate soft tissue closure at the time of the bone graft surgery. If a tooth requires extraction, it should be performed 3 weeks prior to the bone graft in order to allow adequate time for gingival healing and not enough time for loss of bone height along the cleft margins. If the intent is to maintain the tooth, it may be retracted away from the cleft margin prior to surgery.

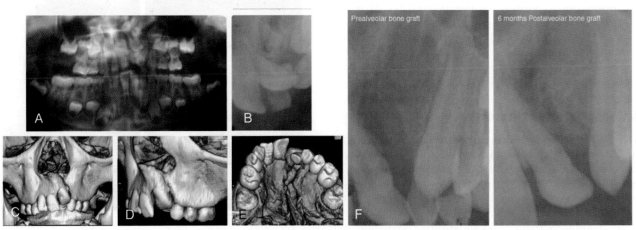

Figure 10.5 **(A)** Panoramic radiograph of a patient with left cleft lip and palate. The panoramic radiograph fails to show conclusively the extent of the cleft defect. **(B)** The periapical radiograph shows a definitive need for an alveolar bone. However, the spatial orientation of the unerupted permanent teeth and their proximity to the cleft defect are not clear. **(C–E)** Cone beam computed tomography images showing the alveolar cleft defect on the lateral wall of the maxillary left central incisor. In addition, the severity of the cleft defect, as well as the three-dimensional arrangement of the teeth in the surrounding area, can also be observed from such an image. **(F)** Periapical radiograph of prealveolar and postalveolar bone graft sites. Note the large alveolar defect on the lateral wall of the maxillary left central incisor. The postalveolar bone graft periapical radiograph shows good fill-in of the alveolar cleft, 6 months postiliac bone graft.

In order to provide the most stable environment for integration of the alveolar bone graft and maintenance of palatal expansion, we routinely place an occlusally bonded acrylic splint at the time of surgery. The splint serves to immobilize the alveolar segments, as well as prevent relapse of presurgical maxillary expansion. The splint remains in place for 8 weeks postsurgery. During this time, the patient consumes nutritionally rich and balanced liquids for the first week and soft foods for the remaining time while in the splint. In addition, a chlorhexidine antiseptic rinse is used twice daily, starting the night before surgery and continuing for 8 weeks until splint removal.

Bilateral cleft lip and palate: Premaxillary position

The management of a bilateral cleft lip and palate patient may pose a unique challenge with respect to the position of the premaxilla prior to bilateral alveolar bone grafts. The ideal position of the premaxillary segment is between the lateral alveolar segments and in occlusion with the mandibular dentition. However, it is frequently observed that the premaxilla may be ectopically positioned vertically and anteroposteriorly. This may also be complicated by medial collapse of the lateral alveolar segments. Presurgical expansion (fan expansion) may be used to improve the transverse relationship between the premaxilla and the lateral segments. In less severe cases, the premaxilla may be intruded using conventional intrusion mechanics or with the aid of temporary anchorage devices. In severe cases, the vertically descended premaxilla may be repositioned intraoperatively, to the level of the occlusal plane, at the time of bilateral alveolar bone grafts. The anteroposterior position of the premaxilla may also be corrected at the time of the bone graft, with the intent to leave it as protrusive as possible, while allowing for adequate soft tissue coverage. Similar to the unilateral bone graft, a bonded occlusal splint is used to stabilize the postsurgical position of the premaxilla. However, the premaxillary teeth are not bonded to the splint so that they are not stressed upon splint removal. Instead, the teeth that are found on the premaxilla receive bonded orthodontic brackets that are secured to the splint by stainless steel ligature wires.

Anteroposterior discrepancy

A child with cleft lip and palate often shows a concave facial profile, which characteristically worsens with maturation and growth of the mandible. An anterior crossbite of skeletal aetiology, as determined by a lateral cephalometric analysis, can be corrected in the mixed dentition for both aesthetic and functional reasons. If allowed to persist, an anterior crossbite may contribute to hypereruption of the maxillary and mandibular anterior teeth, displacement of the premaxilla and a CR–CO mandibular shift. This malocclusion may also result in errors in speech articulation. We routinely use PHG therapy for the correction of mild mid-face retrusion. The protraction facemask is used in conjunction with a bonded appliance with full occlusal coverage to optimize the orthopaedic response, while minimizing anterior dental tipping. Transverse discrepancies may also be addressed simultaneously with an expansion screw built into the PHG appliance (Figs 10.6–10.8). The appliance is generally used for 6 months. PHG may need to be repeated as facial concavity may return with normal mandibular growth. Vertical hypoplasia of the maxilla often accompanies the sagittal discrepancy. Both PHG and distraction osteogenesis can address the vertical hypoplasia of the maxilla. In the mandibular arch, a lingual arch that passively rests on the cingulae of the mandibular anterior teeth can effectively prevent their supraeruption and development of an excessive curve of Spee.

Transverse discrepancy

Maxillary constriction should also be corrected during the mixed dentition stage. Our preferred appliance is the bonded acrylic splint with full occlusal coverage. This allows for equal distribution of force across all teeth, thereby minimizing effects on dental position and maximizing skeletal and alveolar expansion. In the patient with bilateral cleft lip and palate, a fan expander is usually indicated as there is often greater constriction in the anterior region than in the posterior maxillary dental arch. Similar to the conventional expander, the fan expander is an occlusally bonded appliance with palatal tissue coverage (Fig. 10.9). Once expansion is complete, it is essential to maintain it by either a removable retainer or a fixed transpalatal archwire with soldered lingual extensions along the palatal aspect of the buccal segments (Fig. 10.10).

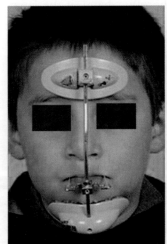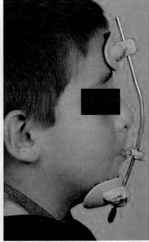

Figure 10.6 Frontal and lateral views of protraction headgear (PHG) appliance. The PHG appliance consists of the extraoral device and the intraoral acrylic appliance that is bonded to the incisal and occlusal surfaces of all teeth in the maxillary arch. The direction of force applied to the maxilla is approximately 25° from the maxillary occlusal plane, and the magnitude of force is 800 g. The appliance is worn for 12–14 h per day.

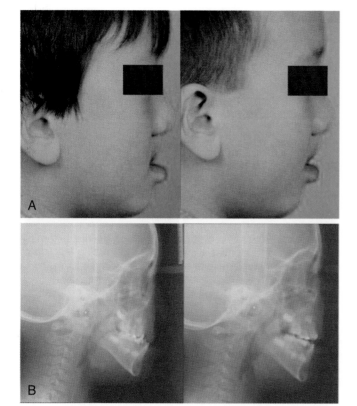

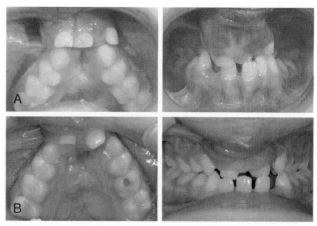

Figure 10.9 (A) Occlusal and frontal views of a patient with bilateral cleft lip and palate who underwent rapid maxillary expansion with a bonded acrylic fan expander. **(B)** Following transverse expansion, patient had bilateral alveolar bone grafts and premaxillary repositioning.

Figure 10.7 (A) Pre-PHG and post-PHG lateral photos following 6 months of PHG therapy. Note the improvement in mid-face projection and facial convexity. **(B)** Pre-PHG and post-PHG lateral cephalograms of the patient shown in Figure 10.7A. They show clearly an improvement in maxillary and mandibular relationships.

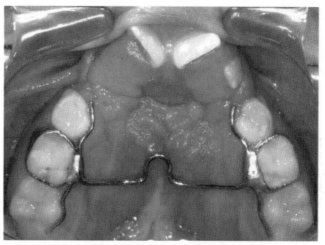

Figure 10.10 Once maxillary expansion is complete, a transpalatal arch is used to maintain the transverse dimension. Here, the transpalatal arch is soldered to bands on the maxillary right and on the left primary second molars. A 0.036" stainless steel wire is also soldered to the palatal surface of the bands and extends anteriorly and posteriorly to maintain expansion in the buccal segments.

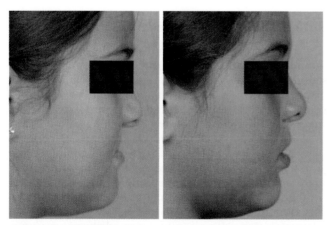

Figure 10.8 Pre-PHG and post-PHG lateral photos following 6 months of PHG therapy. Note the improvement in mid-face projection and facial convexity.

PERMANENT DENTITION

This is an important developmental stage in which the orthodontist makes critical decisions as part of the multidisciplinary team that is treating patients with cleft lip and palate. Lateral cephalometric growth studies have shown that the maxilla in treated patients with cleft lip and palate shows variable degrees of maxillary hypoplasia. The reasons for abnormal facial morphology in treated cleft patients may involve either intrinsic skeletal and soft tissue deficiencies or iatrogenic factors introduced by treatment or a combination of both. At birth, cleft lip and palate deformities vary greatly in severity. In some patients, there is adequate tissue volume, and the cleft segments have failed to fuse together. In others, there may be varying amounts of missing tissue (bone, soft tissue and teeth) associated with non-fusion of the cleft segments. Both groups of patients may respond differently to surgical treatment.

Clinically, patients with clefts may present with a concave profile, mid-face deficiency and Class III skeletal pattern. The maxilla may be also deficient in transverse and vertical planes contributing to posterior skeletal crossbite and reduced mid-face height. Dentally, there may be lingually inclined incisors and constricted maxillary posterior arch width causing anterior or posterior crossbite. The extent of abnormal mid-face growth may vary from mild to severe. The severity distribution of abnormal mid-facial growth is concentrated in the centre of the bell curve, whereas patients with good growth and severe growth disturbances are dispersed on either side of the curve.[7] Depending on the severity of the malocclusion presented by the cleft patient, the management can be categorized into the following three types. In the first category, the patients have no skeletal discrepancy, and orthodontic correction is limited to tooth movement only. In the second category, the patients have a mild skeletal discrepancy and will benefit from camouflaging the malocclusion by orthodontic tooth movement alone. In the last category, the patients have moderate to severe skeletal deformity, and optimal results can only be obtained by combined surgical and orthodontic intervention. It is important to establish as early as possible, if the patient will be treated with orthodontics alone or with orthodontics in conjunction with surgery. The direction of orthodontic tooth movement to camouflage a very mild mid-face deficiency is opposite to that of tooth movement required to prepare a patient for mid-face advancement surgery.

Patients with no skeletal deformity

If a patient with cleft in permanent dentition presents with no skeletal deformity (anteroposterior, transverse or vertical), then the management of the dental malocclusion does not differ very much from that of the noncleft patient. Patients with isolated clefts of the lip and alveolus or clefts of the soft palate may fall into this group and will benefit from fixed orthodontic treatment alone. The dental malocclusion may be limited to mild dental anterior or posterior crossbites, rotated and malposed teeth and missing lateral incisor in the cleft area. Mild anterior crossbites can be corrected with an advancing archwire and posterior crossbite with an archwire expansion or with a removable quad helix.

There are two options available for the management of the missing lateral incisor, either maintenance of the space for a dental implant or movement of the canine into the lateral incisor space, recontouring it to resemble a lateral incisor. If the decision is made to maintain space for a dental implant, then optimal space must be made available for the implant to replace the missing lateral incisor. During active orthodontic treatment, this space can be maintained with the use of a pontic tooth that contains a bracket and is ligated to the orthodontic archwire. At the conclusion of treatment, a cosmetic removable prosthesis should be fabricated to maintain the space. Once craniofacial skeletal growth is complete, a single tooth implant can be placed (Fig. 10.11).

If canine substitution is planned for replacement of the missing lateral incisor, then several canine crown modifications are needed to achieve optimal aesthetics.

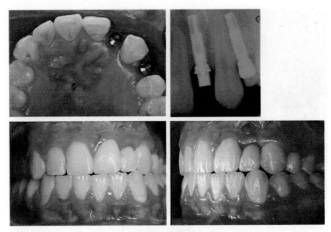

Figure 10.11 Series of a cleft patient with no skeletal deformity treated with orthodontics alone. Here, the missing left lateral incisor and left first bicuspid were replaced with implants.

The permanent canine will need recontouring on incisal, labial, mesial, distal and lingual surfaces. Recontouring can be done progressively during active orthodontic treatment. When bonding this tooth, a lateral incisor bracket will be placed more gingivally in order to bring its gingival margin down to the level of the adjacent central incisor. The first bicuspid will then take the canine position and will also need reshaping to resemble a permanent canine. The second bicuspid and first and second molars are moved mesially. The patient's orthodontic treatment is completed with a Class II occlusal relationship on the side of the missing lateral incisor. With successful aesthetic bonding, excellent results can be achieved with this option (Fig. 10.12).

Patients with mild skeletal discrepancy

In patients presenting with mild skeletal discrepancy and minimal aesthetic concern, orthodontic dental compensation may be recommended. A thorough clinical exam, growth status and stature, hand-wrist films and serial cephalometric assessments need to be performed before suggesting this option. However, the patient and the family should be cautioned that the outcome can be compromised, if the patient outgrows the dental compensation and ultimately may need extended orthodontic treatment to remove the compensations and prepare for orthognathic surgery. Proclination of the maxillary incisors and lingual inclination of the lower incisor can adequately camouflage a mild skeletal discrepancy. Sometimes, extractions in mandibular arch will be necessary to achieve a satisfactory result.

Patients with moderate to severe skeletal discrepancy

Patients presenting with moderate to severe skeletal discrepancy have an opportunity to achieve the best aesthetic and functional results through a combination of orthodontic treatment that is carefully coordinated with orthognathic surgery. Depending on the severity of the skeletal discrepancy, the patient may require only maxillary

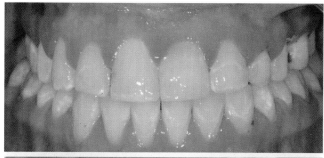

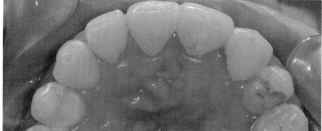

Figure 10.12 Frontal and occlusal photographs of a left unilateral cleft patient with missing left lateral incisor treated by canine substitution.

advancement or a combination of maxillary advancement and mandibular setback (Figs 10.13 and 10.14). If the surgical or orthodontic option is elected, then timing of the orthodontic and surgical treatments becomes critical.

Under normal conditions, it is recommended to remove all dental compensations and to align the teeth in an optimal position relative to the skeletal base and alveolar processes. The orthodontist will plan the coordination of maxillary and mandibular arch widths by hand articulating progress dental study models into the predicted postsurgical occlusion. Once the presurgical orthodontic treatment goals are achieved (coordinated maxillomandibular arch width, compatibility of occlusal plans, satisfactory intercuspation), the appliance may be debonded and removable retainers are placed until craniofacial skeletal growth is complete. This assessment is made by observation of the closing sutures in the hand-wrist radiographs, by measurements of mandibular body length in serial lateral cephalograms and by measurements of change in stature or height. The patient is placed on fixed orthodontic appliances for a short pre-surgical orthodontic treatment phase, prior to orthognathic surgery. The combined surgical and orthodontic treatment goals are planned in close coordination with the surgeon. After surgical correction is completed, a 12-month post-surgical

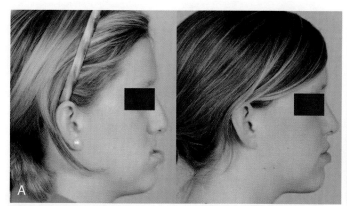

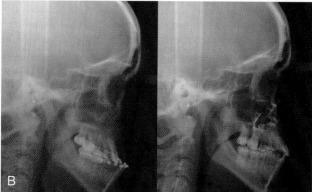

Figure 10.13 Unilateral cleft patient treated with Le Fort I maxillary advancement. **(A)** Presurgical and postsurgical lateral profile photographs showing improvement after maxillary advancement. **(B)** Presurgical and postsurgical lateral cephalograms.

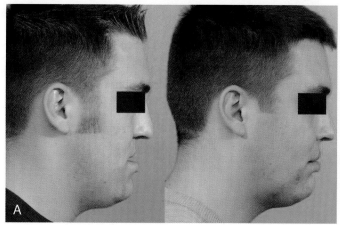

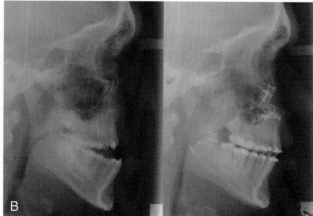

Figure 10.14 Bilateral cleft patient treated with two-jaw surgery. **(A)** Presurgical and postsurgical lateral profile photographs showing significant improvement after Le Fort I maxillary advancement and bilateral sagittal split osteotomy. **(B)** Presurgical and postsurgical lateral cephalograms.

orthodontic phase of treatment begins. The objectives of postsurgical orthodontics are to balance the forces of skeletal relapse with intermaxillary elastics, to observe skeletal stability of the surgical correction and to detail the postsurgical occlusion.

Sometimes, a maxillomandibular skeletal discrepancy is severe, and due to psychosocial reasons, early surgery during the mixed or permanent dentition is indicated. However, the patients and their family must be cautioned that the patient may outgrow the surgical orthodontic correction and may need another corrective surgery upon the completion of skeletal growth. In these cases, distraction osteogenesis may be considered to be an alternative. The advantages of distraction osteogenesis in a growing patient with cleft lip and palate include generation of new bone at the site of the osteotomy, large advancement without the need for a bone graft and gradual stretching of the scarred soft tissue. Since distraction osteogenesis and mid-face advancement are performed at the rate of 1 mm per day, changes in velopharyngeal competency can be monitored during the advancement. For the skeletally mature cleft patient who shows severe maxillary deficiency, advancement of the mid-face with distraction osteogenesis is also a good treatment option (Figs 10.15 and 10.16).

Distraction in the cleft patient can be achieved with external or internal distraction devices. Depending on the surgeon's preference and clinical presentation of deformity, either approach may be used to achieve the desired result. The internal distraction devices are more acceptable to the patient; however, they offer some clinical limitations. The external devices can be adjusted to change the vector of skeletal correction during the active phase of distraction, while the internal device cannot be adjusted in this way. After the Le Fort I osteotomy and a latency period of 5–6 days, the distraction device is activated at the rate of 1 mm per day until the desired advancement is achieved. Interarch elastics may be used during the active phase of distraction osteogenesis, to guide the maxilla to its optimal position and the teeth to optimal occlusion. On completion of the advancement, there is an 8-week period of bone consolidation where the distraction devices serve as skeletal fixation appliances. Following this period of bone healing, the distraction devices are removed and postdistraction orthodontics is initiated. The objective of postdistraction orthodontics is to retain the position of the advanced mid-facial skeleton and to fine-tune the occlusion.

The successful management of a patient with cleft lip and palate requires careful coordination of all members of the cleft palate team. Perhaps the most important members of this team are the patients and their family. We are indebted to the many extraordinary patients and families who have collaborated with our cleft palate team to achieve lifelong functional and aesthetic solutions to their problems.

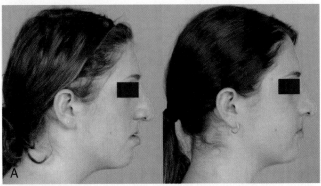

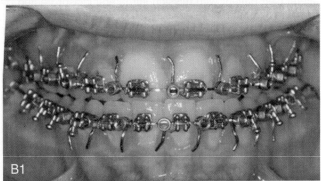

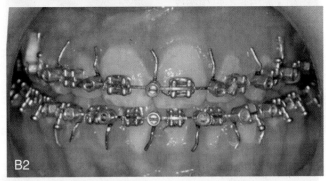

Figure 10.15 Patient treated with Le Fort I mid-face advancement through an internal distraction osteogenesis device. **(A)** Presurgical and postsurgical lateral profile photographs showing significant improvement. (**B1** and **B2**) Presurgical and postsurgical intraoral photographs.

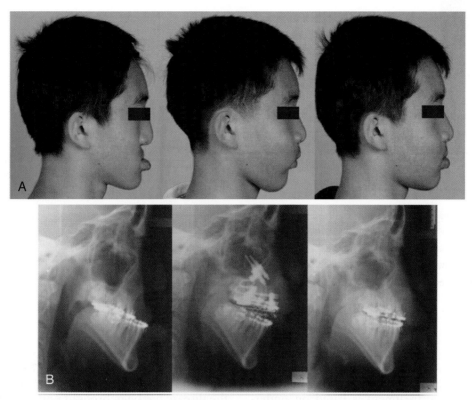

Figure 10.16 Patient treated with Le Fort I mid-face advancement with an internal distraction osteogenesis device. **(A)** Predistraction, distraction and postdistraction lateral profile photographs. **(B)** Lateral cephalograms.

CONCLUSION

Cleft lip and palate are the most frequently occurring congenital anomalies. Such patients often present with a malocclusion that may exist in all the three planes of space: anteroposterior, transverse and vertical. The management of patients with cleft lip and cleft palate requires prolonged orthodontic treatment and an interdisciplinary approach to treatment planning and treatment sequencing. This chapter has provided an insight into orthodontic or orthopaedic management in infancy, in early mixed dentition, in early permanent dentition and after the completion of facial growth, for optimal aesthetics, function and stability. A careful coordination of all members of the cleft palate team remains the key to successful management of a patient with cleft lip and palate.

REFERENCES

1. Grayson BH, Cutting C, Wood R. Preoperative columella lengthening in bilateral cleft lip and palate. Plast Reconstr Surg 1993; 92(7):1422–1423.
2. Maull DJ, Grayson BH, Cutting CB, et al. Long-term effects of nasoalveolar moulding on three-dimensional nasal shape in unilateral clefts. Cleft Palate Craniofac J 1999; 36(5):391–397.
3. Cutting C, Grayson B, Brecht L, et al. Presurgical columellar elongation and primary retrograde nasal reconstruction in one-stage bilateral cleft lip and nose repair. Plast Reconstr Surg 1998; 101(3):630–639.
4. Pfeifer TM, Grayson BH, Cutting CB. Nasoalveolar moulding and gingivoperiosteoplasty versus alveolar bone graft: an outcome analysis of costs in the treatment of unilateral cleft alveolus. Cleft Palate Craniofac J 2002; 39(1):26–29.
5. Lee CT, Grayson BH, Cutting CB, et al. Prepubertal mid-face growth in unilateral cleft lip and palate following alveolar moulding and gingivoperiosteoplasty. Cleft Palate Craniofac J 2004; 41(4): 375–380.
6. Losee J, Kirschner R. Comprehensive cleft care. 1st ed. McGraw-Hill: New York, United States; 2008.
7. Ross RB. Treatment variables affecting facial growth in complete unilateral cleft lip and palate. Cleft Palate J 1987; 24(1):5–77.

11 Treatment of Periodontally Compromised Patients

A Bakr M Rabie, Yanqi Yang and Ricky WK Wong

Orthodontic tooth movement in periodontally involved patients constitutes a problem distinct from routine orthodontics. Orthodontic treatment is based on understanding the relationship between the orthodontic tooth movement and the different biologic processes that will take place. This chapter deals with the understanding of the health and status of the supporting structures of the teeth, the need for altered orthodontic mechanics, defining treatment goals, treatment planning and sequencing, treatment outcome and retention and stability considerations. It will also describe the role of periodontist and prosthodontist as a part of an interdisciplinary approach in the management of periodontally compromised patients.

Patients with advanced periodontal disease may experience tooth migration involving single or multiple teeth. The most common symptoms may include tipping and extrusion of one or several incisors and development of single or multiple diastemas of the anterior teeth.[1] Correction of these problems demands advanced techniques and an understanding of the biologic situation present in those patients.[2]

Periodontal disease is not a continuous and steadily progressive degenerative process.[3] Instead, it is characterized by episodes of acute attack on some but usually not all areas of the mouth, followed by quiescent periods. It is obviously important to identify high-risk patients and high-risk sites. At present, persistent bleeding on probing is the best indicator of active and presumably progressive disease. New diagnostic procedures to evaluate subgingival plaque and crevicular fluids for the presence of indicator bacteria, enzymes or other chemical mediators show promise and are likely to be clinically useful in the near future. There appear to be at least three risk groups in the population: those with rapid progression (approximately 10%), those with moderate progression (the great majority, approximately 80%) and those with no progression despite the presence of gingival inflammation (approximately 10%).[4]

There is no contraindication to treating adults who have had periodontal disease and bone loss, as long as the disease has been brought under control. Progression of untreated periodontal breakdown must be anticipated; however, the periodontal situation must receive major attention in planning and executing orthodontic treatment for all adults.[5]

The aims of this chapter are to illustrate and discuss, by means of case reports, the inter-relationship of orthodontics, periodontics and prosthetic dentistry to fulfil the needs of periodontally involved patients and to highlight the benefits of the team approach.

MINIMAL PERIODONTAL INVOLVEMENT

Any patient undergoing orthodontic treatment must take extra care to clean the teeth, but this is even more important in adult orthodontics. Bacterial plaque is the main aetiologic factor in periodontal breakdown, and plaque-induced gingivitis is the first step in the disease process.[5] Orthodontic appliances simultaneously make maintenance of oral hygiene more difficult and more important. In children and adolescents, even if gingivitis develops in response to the presence of orthodontic appliances, it almost never extends into periodontitis. This cannot be taken for granted in adults, no matter how good their initial periodontal condition is.[6]

A periodontal evaluation in an adult orthodontic patient must include an assessment of the level and the condition of the attached gingiva—the part of the gingiva that is tightly bound to the underlying bone. Earlier animal experiments suggested that the thickness of the gingiva, rather than its surface qualities, could be the key factor that influences the occurrence of recession.[7] Proclination of incisors in some patients may be followed by thinning of the alveolar bone, leading to thinning of the attached gingiva. These patients are at higher risk for gingival recession and loss of attachment. The risk is greatest when irregular teeth are aligned by expanding the dental arch. Lower incisors in patients with a prominent chin and compensation in the form of lingual tipping of these teeth are at particular risk of recession, and thin gingival tissue probably is the reason. For adult orthodontic patients, it is much better to prevent gingival recession than to try to correct it later. Once recession begins, it can progress rapidly, especially, if there is little or no keratinized attached gingiva and the attachment is only alveolar mucosa.[5] Therefore, the gingival condition must receive major attention when planning the orthodontic treatment.

For the cases with abnormal gingival margins and gingival height, innovative orthodontic concepts should be used to enhance biologic structure, as well as the aesthetics of the supporting tissues. In many situations, orthodontic treatment can achieve results that could not be attained by restorations and other mean of cosmetic dentistry, especially when dealing with gingival margins and gingival height.[8] In the following case report, orthodontic intervention was used to move the gingival margin of a maxillary canine incisally by almost 9 mm to mimic a lateral incisor. Increasing the thickness of the labial plate of bone of the canine and subsequently increasing the thickness of the attached gingiva before extrusion prevented gingival recession at a later stage. A step-by-step approach to achieving these treatment objectives is described.

In Case 1, the attached gingiva was very thin because of the canine prominence, and the gingival margin was 9 mm higher than that of the adjacent teeth (Fig. 11.1). The width of the attached gingiva was 2 mm, considerably

CASE 1

A healthy 34-year-old Indian woman complained about a long tooth and crowding (Fig. 11.1). Her maxillary left lateral incisor had been extracted previously, and the canine was moved into place with a removable appliance. The dentist tried to substitute the canine for the lateral incisor, but the clinical crown was too long to create an acceptable aesthetic result. Furthermore, the gingival height and a bony depression caused by the canine eminence were also major concerns for her. The patient had a straight lateral profile with a Class I malocclusion. Her incisors were Class III with an overjet of 0.5 mm and a minimal overbite of 1.5 mm. The first premolars were positioned in buccal crossbite. Severe crowding of 12 mm was present in the mandibular arch. Both the maxillary right canine and the maxillary left lateral incisor were missing. Her mandibular dental midline deviated to the right by 0.5 mm, but the maxillary dental midline coincided with the facial midline (Figs 11.1 and 11.2). The orthopantomogram revealed bony defects in the areas of the missing teeth (Fig. 11.3).

TREATMENT OBJECTIVES

The dentobasal objectives were to normalize overjet and overbite and eliminate the crossbite. The dentoalveolar objectives were to extrude the maxillary left canine to mimic a lateral incisor, to level the gingival height at the maxillary left lateral site, to eliminate and improve the bony depression at the mesial of the maxillary left canine, to correct the midline, to align the teeth and to coordinate the archforms.

TREATMENT PLAN

In the mandibular arch, the treatment option included extracting the right and left first premolars and using a fixed appliance to level and align the teeth; maximum anchorage would be needed. In the maxillary arch, a fixed appliance would be used to level and align the teeth. Special consideration for the maxillary left canine would be needed: (1) a fixed appliance would be used to torque the root palatally followed by extrusion and alignment, (2) the root would be moved mesially to reduce the bony depression and (3) the maxillary left canine would substitute for the lateral incisor.

TREATMENT PROGRESS

The patient's oral hygiene was monitored regularly throughout treatment. She was referred for extraction of the mandibular right and left first premolars as planned. Initially, only the mandibular

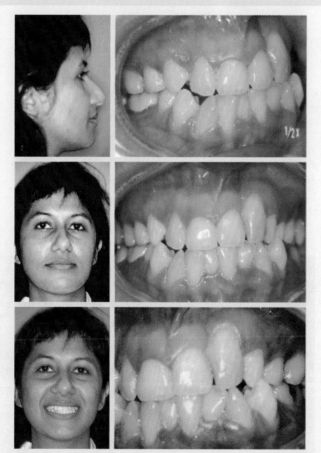

Figure 11.1 Pretreatment photos of a 34-year-old Indian woman with maxillary left canine replacing missing lateral incisor. Profile photo shows straight lateral facial profile. Intraoral photos show high gingival margin of maxillary left canine with composite buildup to mimic lateral incisor and bony depression on mesial of tooth. (Figs 11.1–11.8, Reproduced with permission from Chay SH, Rabie AB. Am J Orthod Dentofacial Orthop 2002; 122:95–102).

Continued

CASE 1—cont'd

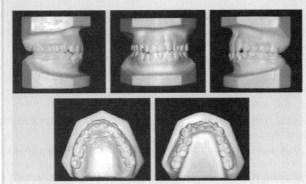

Figure 11.2   Pretreatment study models.

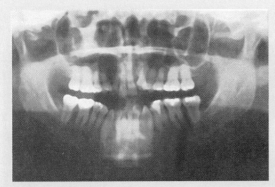

Figure 11.3   Pretreatment panoramic radiograph showing bony defects at areas of missing maxillary right canine and maxillary left lateral incisor.

arch was banded and bonded, bypassing the anterior teeth to avoid their proclination. A 0.022" slot preadjusted system and triple tube bands in the maxillary arch and double tube bands in the mandibular arch were used. After initial levelling and aligning with a 0.016" NiTi wire, a segmental 0.017" × 0.025" titanium molybdenum alloy (TMA) wire with closing loops was used to retract the canines into the extraction spaces.

Spontaneous alignment of the mandibular anterior teeth could be seen as space was created during distal movement of the canines. After 3 months, the mandibular incisors and the maxillary dentition were bonded. The bracket on the maxillary left canine was tilted distally to help upright the root. Levelling and aligning were carried out with an auxiliary 0.016" NiTi wire placed from the auxiliary tube on the band of the maxillary right molar to the bracket on the maxillary left canine to the auxiliary tube on maxillary left molar (Fig. 11.4A). The auxiliary wire was then switched to a 0.017" × 0.025" TMA wire with palatal root torque to move the roots palatally to increase the thickness of the labial plate of bone before the extrusion (Fig. 11.4B).

Extrusion of the maxillary left canine was carried out with 0.016" stainless steel archwire with two boot loops (butterfly loop; Fig. 11.4C). This loop design is versatile and flexible. Height adjustment of the tooth was easily performed, and activation was simple with no fear of running out of space. As extrusion proceeded, the composite restoration was gradually removed from the incisal tip of the canine. After sufficient extrusion (Fig. 11.4D), the bracket was repositioned properly (Fig. 11.4E) and further alignment was carried out. Meanwhile, the mandibular extraction spaces were closed with closing loops by using a 0.017" × 0.025" TMA wire with lingual root torque on the incisors.

Both the maxillary and mandibular archwires were changed progressively with 0.019" × 0.025" TMA wire for optimal torque control. Finishing and detailing were completed with 0.017" × 0.025" TMA wires. Buccal root torque was increased on teeth numbers 14 and 24 to mimic the prominence of canines. An artistic bend was added to the wire at tooth number 41 to close the open gingival embrasure on the distal. A composite restoration was placed on the mesioincisal angle of the maxillary left canine to mimic a lateral incisor (Fig. 11.4F).

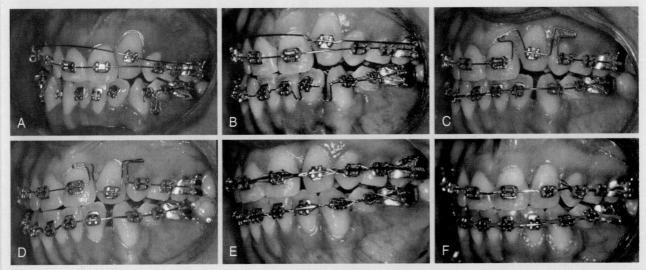

Figure 11.4   **(A)** Distally tipped bracket on maxillary left canine and auxiliary 0.016" NiTi wire to level and align it. **(B)** Palatal root torque to maxillary left canine using auxiliary 0.017" × 0.025" TMA archwire. **(C)** Extrusion of maxillary left canine with 0.016" stainless steel archwire with two boot loops (butterfly loop); composite buildup gradually removed from incisal tip. **(D)** Maxillary left canine extruded. Note the closed boot loops, now passive. **(E)** Bracket on maxillary left canine repositioned. **(F)** Composite buildup on mesioincisal angle of maxillary left canine to mimic lateral incisor.

TREATMENT RESULTS

After 28 months of active treatment, the patient was debonded (Figs 11.5 and 11.6), and a mandibular fixed retainer and a maxillary modified Hawley retainer were inserted. All treatment objectives were achieved, and the patient's aesthetic demands were accomplished. The height of the gingival margin of the maxillary left canine was corrected and is nearly at the same level as the contralateral incisor. The clinical crown length of the maxillary left canine was greatly reduced with extrusion and aesthetic dental procedure to mimic a lateral incisor (Fig. 11.7). The bony depression on the mesial of the maxillary left canine was reduced substantially, as the root was moved mesially (Fig. 11.8). The overbite and overjet were improved, and the crossbite and the midlines were corrected. The Class I molar relationship was maintained.

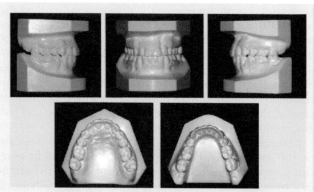

Figure 11.6   Post-treatment study models.

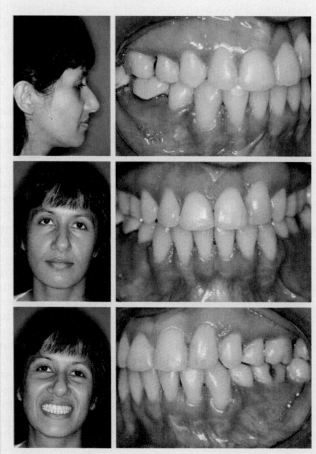

Figure 11.5   Post-treatment photos, after 28 months of orthodontic treatment.

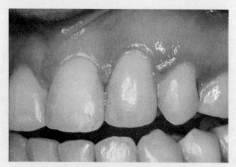

Figure 11.7   Note gingival level and composite buildup of maxillary left canine to mimic lateral incisor.

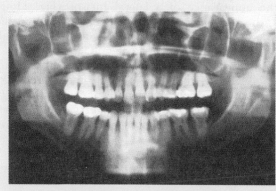

Figure 11.8   Post-treatment panoramic radiograph. Note the reduction of bony defects at the sites of missing maxillary right canine and maxillary left lateral incisor.

less than that of the adjacent teeth. The width of the attached gingiva is measured as the amount of keratinized gingiva between the depth of periodontal probing and the beginning of the alveolar mucosa.[9] Therefore, in planning the treatment for this patient, protective measures were taken to increase the thickness of the labial plate of bone and subsequently the thickness of the attached gingiva before extruding the canine.

Determining the sequence of this patient's orthodontic treatment was based on understanding the relationship between the orthodontic tooth movement and the different biologic processes that would take place. The first step in the orthodontic treatment was palatal root torque of the maxillary left canine. As the root moved palatally, the periodontal ligament (PDL) was stretched on the labial surface, leading to bone deposition at the crest of the alveolus.[9] The increase in the thickness of the labial plate of bone produced an increase in the thickness of the attached gingiva.[10,11] It is believed that for some adult patients, gingival grafting before orthodontic treatment prevents gingival recession. Increasing the thickness rather than the width of the attached gingiva probably produces this protective effect. Increasing the thickness of the labial plate of bone through palatal root torque could also increase the thickness of the attached gingiva and therefore, could also prevent gingival recession. Increasing the thickness of the labial plate of bone may render a healthier attachment around the tooth and ensure that both the bone and the gingiva follow the tooth during extrusion.

The application of palatal torque was made possible on the second visit, before levelling and alignment were completed. The rectangular wire was placed in the auxiliary tubes of the first molars, bypassing all teeth until it was tied to the bracket of the maxillary left canine (Fig. 11.4B). Four months later, the attached gingiva looked healthier (Fig. 11.4C), and the prominence of the root was less apparent. The width of the attached gingiva increased as the palatal root torque was improved. This was the indication to begin gradual extrusion of the maxillary canine. As the canine was extruded, the gingiva followed (Fig. 11.4D). The composite restoration on the incisal edge was removed gradually to provide enough space for the extrusion. After the extrusion was completed, a lateral incisor bracket was placed on the maxillary left canine in an ideal position, and the root was moved mesially to reduce the bony depression. Because the root of the maxillary left canine was moved palatally, it was safe to move the root mesially. This movement was accomplished with a gable bend in the wire, and the mesial of the tooth was extruded and the distal intruded (Fig. 11.4E). The patient was then referred to a dentist to restore the maxillary left canine with composite to simulate the appearance of a lateral incisor (Fig. 11.4F). Again, the sequence of treatment ensured a successful result because the root of the canine was tipped mesially only after the root was moved palatally.

Therefore, if the attached gingiva appears thin and vulnerable and there is a chance of gingival recession with orthodontic tooth movement, increasing the thickness of bone through orthodontic intervention may be a way to create healthier attached gingiva before tooth movement.

MODERATE PERIODONTAL INVOLVEMENT

Before orthodontic treatment is attempted for patients who have pre-existing periodontal problems, dental and periodontal disease must be brought under control. In situations where tooth movement is indicated as an adjunct to periodontal therapy, vigorous preparation of root surfaces and gingival tissues should precede placement of the orthodontic appliance.[12] Deep pockets must be eliminated before orthodontic treatment is initiated so as to prevent apical displacement of plaque that could establish progressive periodontal lesions.[13] Results of a longitudinal study of adults with reduced gingival height and a healthy periodontium showed that orthodontic treatment did not result in significant further loss of attachment.[14] This finding depended on the prerequisite that periodontal treatment was provided to arrest active disease before orthodontic treatment was begun.

Furthermore, these patients received monthly reinforcement of plaque removal and also received subgingival debridement at 3-month intervals during orthodontic treatment to maintain healthy gingival tissues.[14]

Disease control also requires endodontic treatment of any pulpally involved teeth. There is no contraindication to the orthodontic movement of an endodontically treated tooth, so root canal therapy before orthodontics will cause no problems. Attempting to move a pulpally involved tooth, however, is likely to cause a flare-up of the periapical condition.[5]

The relationship between periodontal disease and malocclusion has been a controversial subject. Tooth malpositioning has been recognized as both an aetiologic factor contributing to periodontal destruction and a result of chronic destructive periodontal disease.[15] Malposed or rotated teeth may be predisposed to more rapid breakdown of the periodontium when the roots are too close to one another, resulting in a thin interproximal septum.[16] Klassman and Zucker[17] reported that correction of these malposed teeth may be therapeutic or prophylactic. At the present time, there have been no significant studies that confirm a definite relationship between malocclusion and periodontal disease.[18,19] On the contrary, the consensus of the majority of studies is that there is no relation between various types of malocclusion and periodontal diseases.[15,19] In a study of 188 persons with periodontal disease, no relationship was found between periodontal disease and Angle's classification, overbite, overjet, open bite, rotation or inclination of the mandibular incisor. Grewe et al[20] reported that plaque retention based on oral hygiene habits may be the major factor in periodontal disease, while irregularities of tooth position may play another minor complicating role. The only exceptions to this appear to be extremely severe overbite, in which there is direct impingement of the teeth on the soft tissues, and localized crossbite with traumatic occlusion, which results in destructive effects on the periodontal supporting structure. Gingival recession and mobility affecting isolated mandibular incisors are not uncommon in association with lingually positioned incisors.[21] In such cases, the risk of accelerated loss of attachment appears likely.[21] Because traumatic occlusion may have been a predisposing factor for the gingival recession and tooth mobility, elimination of traumatic occlusion becomes a major objective of the treatment planning.

On the one hand, traumatic occlusion may contribute to destructive periodontal disease, but on the other hand, advanced periodontal disease with the loss of periodontal supporting structure can cause migration, extrusion, flaring and loss of teeth.[12,22] This is because a secondary occlusal trauma may further complicate an already difficult problem. The most common symptoms may include tipping and extrusion of one or several incisors and development of single or multiple diastemas of the anterior teeth.[1] Correction of these problems demands advanced techniques and an understanding of the biologic situation present in those patients.[2] Melsen et al[12,13] concluded that intrusion of incisors in adult patients with marginal bone loss offers a beneficial effect on the periodontal condition at the clinical and radiographic levels.

It has been proposed that orthodontic treatment may be used to attain more favourable bone levels and contours around periodontally involved teeth.[15,23] Kessler[15] proposed that changes in osseous topography could be accomplished by moving teeth into an area of the arch that has a greater volume of bone and by repositioning periodontally involved anterior teeth. This type of orthodontic treatment is considered adjunctive orthodontic treatment.[5] By definition, it is the tooth movement carried out to facilitate other dental procedures necessary to control disease and restore function.[24]

During the treatment planning for this adjunctive orthodontic treatment, special biomechanical considerations were emphasized. The design of the appliance used depended on the number of teeth to be moved, the availability of anchorage and the desired direction and amount of crown or tooth movement. At the same time, orthodontic goals and mechanics must be modified to keep orthodontic forces to an absolute minimum.[6,25] This is necessary when a bone has been lost because the PDL area decreases, and the same force against the crown produces greater pressure in the PDL of a periodontally compromised tooth than in a normally supported one.[26,27] Because the margins of bands can make periodontal maintenance more difficult, it is usually better to use a fully bonded orthodontic appliance for periodontally involved adults.[5] Self-ligating brackets or steel ligatures also are preferred for periodontally involved patients rather than elastometric rings to retain orthodontic archwires because patients with elastomeric rings have higher levels of microorganisms in gingival plaque.[28]

One potential problem with intrusion in periodontally involved adults is the prospect that a deepening of periodontal pockets might be produced by this treatment. Ideally, of course, intruding a tooth would lead to a reattachment of the periodontal fibres, but there is no basis for expecting this. What seems to happen instead is the formation of a tight epithelial cuff so that the position of the gingiva relative to the crown improves clinically, while periodontal probing depths do not increase. Histologic slides from experimental animals show a relative invagination of the epithelium but with a tight area of contact that cannot be probed.[5] It can be argued that this leaves the patients at risk for rapid periodontal breakdown, if inflammation is allowed to recur. Certainly intrusion should never be attempted without excellent control of inflammation. On the other hand, if good hygiene is maintained, clinical experience has shown that it is possible to maintain teeth that have been treated in this way, and both dental aesthetics and function improve after the intrusion.[12,29] The following case report describes orthodontic intrusion treatment of periodontally involved teeth.

Before orthodontic intrusion was initiated, deep pockets were eliminated to prevent apical displacement of plaque that could have produced periodontal lesions.[13] Once the patient had demonstrated the ability to maintain a high level of oral hygiene, orthodontic treatment was begun. During treatment, the patient received monthly reinforcement of plaque removal and subgingival debridement at 3-month intervals, as recommended by Vanarsdall.[14]

Full-mouth periapical radiographs were taken to allow a thorough assessment of every tooth for orthodontic mechanotherapy. Because the second molars showed more bone loss than the first molars, the first molars were used as anchorage units.

We selected to start treatment in the mandibular arch to create enough overjet for retraction of the flared maxillary incisors. This also allowed us to delay bonding of the periodontally involved maxillary central incisors until absolutely necessary. Once adequate overjet had been attained, lingual root torque was applied to compensate for the moment created during retraction of the maxillary incisors. By moving the roots palatally, we could also improve the labial bone plate. As Kessler[15] noted, favourable changes in osseous topography can be accomplished by moving teeth into an area of the arch with greater bone volume and by repositioning periodontally involved teeth.

The finding of Melsen et al[12,13] that incisor intrusion in adult patients with marginal bone loss has a beneficial periodontal effect was substantiated by the present case, where the post-treatment radiographs showed positive bone remodelling (Fig. 11.11). Melsen et al[30] also reported that a new connective tissue attachment can be formed during the intrusion of periodontally involved teeth, if gingival inflammation is eliminated and root surfaces are adequately scaled. Other researchers, however, have found only pseudo- or hemi-desmosomal attachment rather than a new PDL attachment.[31,32]

A given force applied to the crown of a periodontally compromised tooth produces greater pressure on the PDL than it would on a normally supported tooth because of the diminished PDL area.[26,27] In this case, the long span of the initial 2×2 maxillary appliance, followed by the 2×4 appliance (Fig. 11.10D), allowed us to keep the orthodontic forces to less than 20 g per incisor.

Once the overjet and overbite had been almost normalized, the aesthetic dentist was consulted about the composite buildup of the maxillary central incisors and the space available for prosthetic replacement of the missing mandibular incisor. This prosthesis also served as an orthodontic fixed retainer and a periodontal splint for the adjacent teeth. Because bonded bridges, especially those with multiple abutments, are known for bond failures, we decided to perforate the framework, as originally described by Rochette[33] with a periodontal splint and later by Howe and Denehy with a bridge. The perforation makes it easy to rebond by removing the cement through the holes, without having to remove the whole prosthesis (Fig. 11.12).

A completely passive retainer should be used to ensure stability of the orthodontically moved teeth between the impression taking and the cementation of the prosthesis. The retainer is removed for the impression, which is taken with an elastometric material, and replaced in exactly the same position while the prosthesis is being constructed.

Case 2 shows that intrusion is a reliable therapeutic method for orthodontic treatment of periodontally involved patients. A multidisciplinary approach can better serve the needs of periodontally involved patients with malposed teeth.

CASE 2

A 55-year-old woman presented with the chief complaint of incisor spacing and protrusion and consequent speech difficulties. The mandibular left central incisor had been extracted at an earlier age. She had a history of severe periodontal disease that had been treated over a 5-month period with deep scaling and root planing, followed by regular periodontal maintenance. Clinical examination revealed generalized gingival recession with 3-mm pockets, no bleeding on probing and incisor mobility limited to Grade 2. The patient displayed a full profile with potentially competent lips. She had a Class I buccal occlusion with proclined, spaced and elongated incisors, 10 mm of spacing in the maxillary arch and 9 mm of spacing in the mandibular arch (Fig. 11.9). The orthopantomogram showed generalized horizontal bone loss, particularly in the incisor regions, and furcation involvement of the mandibular molars.

TREATMENT PLAN

The treatment plan called for the following:

1. Intrusion and retraction of the mandibular incisors and then the maxillary incisors with torque control
2. Reinforcement of anchorage with a mandibular lingual holding arch and a transpalatal arch
3. Redistribution of space, according to the recommendation of the aesthetic dentist, to allow prosthetic replacement of the missing mandibular incisor
4. Maintenance of periodontal health by home care, under the supervision of a specialist

5. Finishing and detailing
6. Retention with a maxillary fixed lingual retainer and a mandibular Rochette-bonded bridge

TREATMENT MECHANICS AND PROCESS

The mandibular lingual holding arch was cemented to the first molars and placed gingivally enough to permit retraction of the mandibular incisors. A full 0.022" preadjusted edgewise appliance was bonded to the mandibular arch, and a 0.016" × 0.022" TMA archwire with anterior closing loops was inserted and activated slightly (Fig. 11.10A). After the mandibular incisors had been retracted and adequate overjet achieved (Fig. 11.10B), treatment was begun in the maxillary arch with cementation of the transpalatal arch and bonding of the central incisors only. A 0.017" × 0.025" TMA archwire with bilateral closing loops and an intrusion bend was used to simultaneously retract and intrude the maxillary central incisors (Fig. 11.10C). The activation force of the maxillary and mandibular closing loops was kept at a minimum to prevent further periodontal damage during treatment.

The mandibular wire size was progressively increased to 0.017" × 0.025", and lingual root torque was applied to the incisors. Once significant intrusion of the maxillary central incisors had been achieved, the lateral incisors were incorporated in the archwire for alignment (Fig. 11.10D). Maxillary closing loops were reactivated for retraction and intrusion, and elastic chain was added for incisor retraction. Six months into

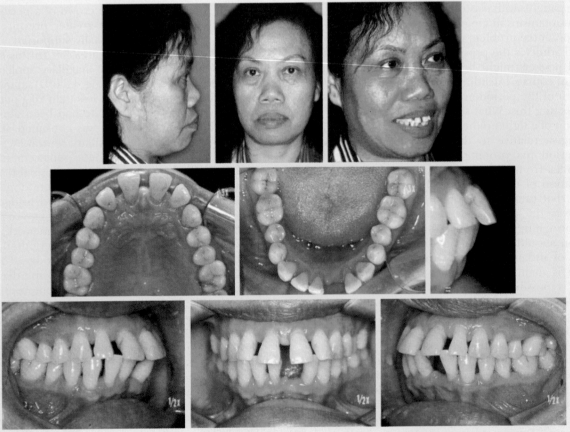

Figure 11.9 A 55-year-old woman with Class I malocclusion, excessive overjet and flared, spaced and elongated incisors before treatment. (Figs 11.9–11.12, Reproduced with permission from Sam K, et al. J Clin Orthod 2001; 35:325–330).

treatment, 6 mm of space was available for prosthetic replacement of the missing mandibular incisor (Fig. 11.10E). Residual maxillary spaces were closed by adding composite resin to the distal of the central incisors.

After another month of treatment, the orthodontic appliances were removed. A multistranded 0.018" wire was bonded lingually for maxillary retention. The mandibular resin-bonded bridge served not only as a prosthetic replacement but also as a fixed retainer.

TREATMENT RESULTS

After orthodontic treatment, the patient showed an improvement in lip competence. The dental midlines were coincident with the facial midline; both archforms had improved, and the good buccal occlusion was preserved. The incisal relationship was normalized with proper overjet and overbite. Intrusion of the incisors was evident both clinically and radiographically, and the periodontal condition had improved (Fig. 11.11). The maxillary and mandibular spaces were eliminated by the orthodontic retraction, prosthetic replacement of the missing incisor and composite restoration of the maxillary central incisors (Fig. 11.12). Because of the improvement in aesthetics and speech, the patient reported a higher level of self-confidence and self-esteem and was generally happier and more cheerful.

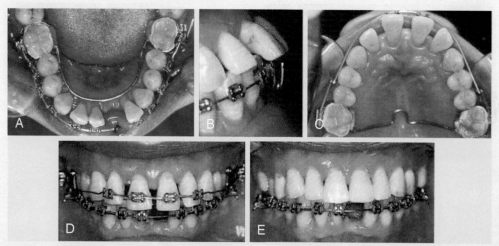

Figure 11.10 (A) Lingual holding arch for anchorage and 0.016" × 0.022" TMA archwire with compensating bends in buccal segment. (B) Overjet after mandibular incisor retraction. (C) Transpalatal arch for anchorage and 0.017" × 0.025" TMA archwire for maxillary intrusion and space closure. (D) Maxillary lateral incisors incorporated into retraction archwire after significant intrusion of central incisors. (E) Residual space distributed distal to maxillary central incisors, which were then built up distally with composite resin.

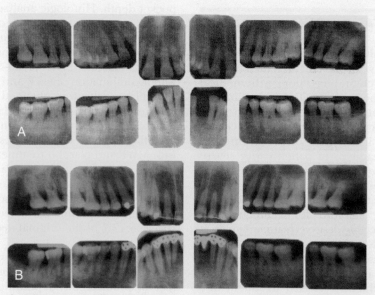

Figure 11.11 (A) Periapical radiographs before treatment, showing reduced periodontal support. (B) Radiographs after treatment, showing improved periodontal condition after orthodontic intrusion.

Continued

CASE 2—cont'd

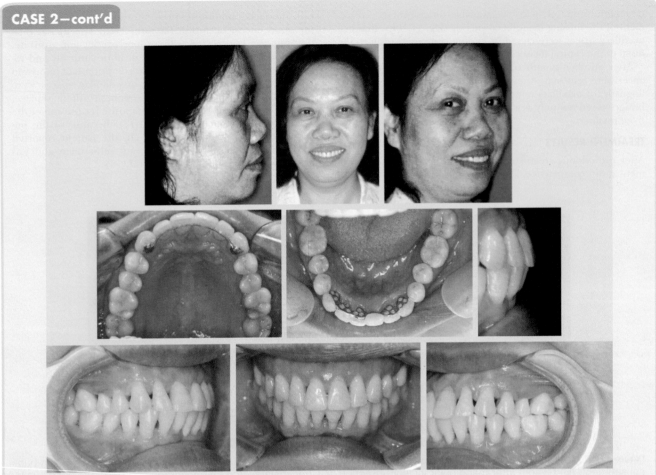

Figure 11.12   Patient after 7 months of orthodontic treatment and placement of resin-bonded prosthesis. Buccal occlusal relationship has been preserved; midlines are coincident, and patient has normal overjet and overbite.

SEVERE PERIODONTAL INVOLVEMENT

The management of adult orthodontic patients with severe bone loss continues to present a challenge. The outpouring of new research findings, along with medical and technological advances, necessitates constant re-examination of out treatment philosophies and techniques. We can integrate current thoughts and successful clinical techniques used in the field of periodontology into our orthodontic treatment of patients with severe bone loss to regenerate lost periodontal structures.

A task force of periodontitis[34] examined clinical and experimental outcomes for the treatment of intrabony defects and researched the literature for techniques that would achieve most predictable desired treatment goals. It was concluded that guided tissue regeneration (GTR), GTR combined with the use of demineralized bone matrix (DBM), and DBM alone are the most predictable regenerative procedures for achieving selected treatment outcomes.[34,35] These findings were later echoed by several researchers[36] who established a large body of clinical evidence that clearly indicated periodontal bone grafts consistently led to better bone fill of the defect than the nongrafted controls. In addition to gain in bone levels, there was improvement in attachment levels and reduction in probing pocket depth. Histologic analyses of cementum regeneration in experimental animals conclusively demonstrated that regenerative treatment with bone grafting leads to some degree of regenerated bone, cementum and PDL.[37,38] A mean attachment gain of 2.6–3.0 mm has been reported with a combination of GTR and DBM.[35,39]

Similar results were obtained experimentally and clinically using Emdogain (Biora, Malmo, Sweden), an enamel matrix derivative.[40–42] Emdogain was used as an adjunct to modified-Widman flap (MWF) surgery and was compared with MWF and placebo treatments. A 36-month follow-up showed a 2.2-mm attachment gain in the Emdogain group and a 66% bone gain in the defect.[40] Histologic assessment of the effect of Emdogain on periodontal regeneration in one human experimental defect showed new cementum covering 73% of the original defect and 65% bone height regain.[41]

General factors, such as the morphology of the defect, plaque control and patient compliance, can directly affect the predictability of periodontal regeneration. Defect selection is critical to achieving a successful outcome; deep and narrow defects showed the most predictable positive response to regenerative procedures.[34] Orthodontic intrusion can change a horizontal bony defect into a deep and narrow defect that is more favourable for regeneration of the periodontium through grafting

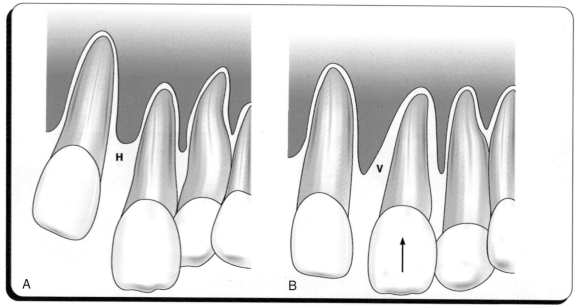

Figure 11.13 (A) Severe bone loss, spacing and extrusion of incisors. Horizontal bony defect (H) around the maxillary left central incisor. **(B)** Orthodontic intrusion changes the topography of the defect into a vertical (V), deep and narrow defect. (Figs 11.13–11.15, Reproduced with permission from Rabie ABM, Boisson M. World J Orthod 2001; 2:142–153).

procedures (Fig. 11.13). Therefore, the field of orthodontics should consider the combined regenerative and periodontal surgical treatments an invaluable addition to the armamentarium available for the orthodontic treatment of adult patients with severe loss of periodontal tissues.[43] Similarly, the field of periodontics should recognize the importance of orthodontic intervention in achieving results unattainable with periodontal treatment alone.[43]

The following two cases will illustrate the interplay among periodontics, orthodontics and bone induction.

In case 3 (Fig. 11.14), the defect was deep with a vertical bony wall, making it a prime candidate for combined surgical and bone induction procedures. This type of defect most likely has a high chance of periodontal tissue regeneration because the bony wall and periosteum are a good source of mesenchymal cells that can be acted upon by bone morphogenetic proteins and other cytokines present in the DBM and induce their differentiation into osteoblasts.[45]

Since this vertical bony wall provides a good source of resident mesenchymal cells, orthodontic intrusion could favourably change a horizontal bony defect into a bony defect with a vertical wall. Figure 11.13 shows the transformation of a horizontal bony defect into a vertical defect by orthodontic intrusion. Furthermore, orthodontic intrusion could contribute to the process of periodontal tissue regeneration by enhancing the circulation of new blood supply into the defect site.

The changes in blood circulation in teeth and supporting structures incident to experimental tooth movement were reported by Vandevska-Radunovic et al.[46] Fluorescent microspheres were used to quantify the effect of orthodontic forces on blood flow in the PDL, pulp and alveolar bone in a fluorescent microscope. The results showed that the blood flow was significantly lower in the PDL on the first day. However, a steady significant increase in the blood flow was observed in the PDL and alveolar bone on the third and seventh day. It was concluded that tooth movement initiates a generalized blood flow response in the PDL, pulp and alveolar bone. Therefore, orthodontic intrusion of such extruded teeth should lead to a generalized increase in blood flow into the defect area.

Tissue regeneration and bone healing are biologic events that are strictly dependent on the rapid ingrowth of new capillary blood vessels, a process termed *angiogenesis*.[47] These blood vessels provide a good source of mesenchymal cells that can differentiate into useful cells, such as osteoblasts and fibroblasts, during regeneration of the periodontal structures. In the presence of DBM, these mesenchymal cells differentiate into bone-making cells and induce new bone formation.[45] Furthermore, a close correlation between ingrowth of new blood vessels and new bone formation induced by DBM has been reported.[48] Therefore, orthodontic intrusion could benefit periodontal tissue regeneration using combined surgery and DBM by providing a vertical bony defect and an increase in blood flow into the defect and by increasing the population of mesenchymal cells that could, in the presence of osteoinductive factor, differentiate into cells capable of regenerating the periodontal structures.

Case 4 (Fig. 11.15) demonstrated the vital role of orthodontic intrusion in providing a suitable environment for periodontal tissue regeneration using bone-inductive matrices. It is important to understand that we are emphasizing a treatment philosophy rather than a recommendation of DBM, Emdogain or other bone-inductive proteins. The team approach is essential in designing a treatment plan that allows the orthodontist to favourably change the topography of a given defect, since defect shape is considered a critical factor in the success of the regeneration process.[34] Periodontal surgery and bone induction should be included as integral parts of orthodontic treatment options for adult patients with severe loss of periodontal structures.

CASE 3

This adult patient (Fig. 11.14) suffered from a deep vertical bony defect on the mesial root of the mandibular right first molar (Fig. 11.14A and B). Periodontal therapy included an MWF combined with bone induction using DBM and GTR. The pretreatment intraoral photograph (Fig. 11.14C) shows the bony defect at the mesial root of the first molar; bifurcation involvement is also evident. Combined periodontal surgery and bone induction using DBM and GTR (Fig. 11.14D) before orthodontic therapy resulted in a considerable gain in bone height, as demonstrated radiographically (Fig. 11.14F–H).

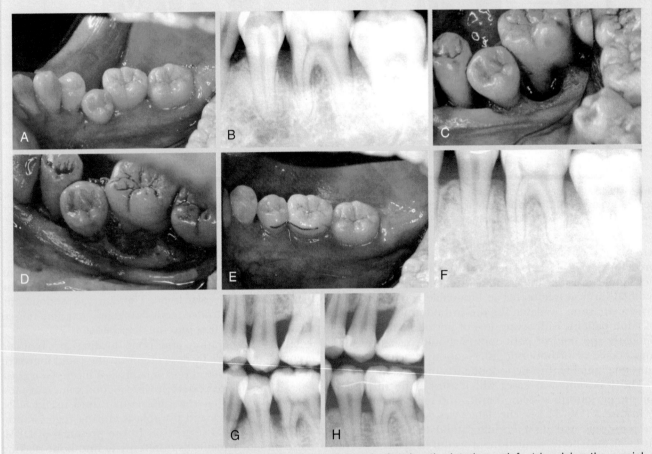

Figure 11.14   (A) Pretreatment intraoral view. **(B)** Periapical radiograph showing the intrabony defect involving the mesial root of the mandibular right first molar. **(C)** Surgical flap showing the extent of the defect. **(D)** DBM packed into the defect. **(E)** Post-treatment intraoral view **(F)** Post-treatment radiograph showing bone regeneration in the bifurcation area and around the mesial root. **(G and H)** Post-treatment radiographs showing considerable regain of lost bone.

CASE 4

The patient was a 35-year-old Chinese woman with spaced and extruded maxillary incisors (Fig. 11.15A–D). Periapical radiographs of the maxillary left central incisor showed horizontal bone loss with bone covering the apical one-third of the mesial aspect of the root (Fig. 11.15G). A team including the orthodontist, the periodontist and the prosthodontist judiciously planned the combined treatment.

TREATMENT PLAN

1. Periodontal treatment, including scaling and root planing, before orthodontic intrusion
2. Adjunctive orthodontic intrusion with a simple fixed appliance to intrude and align the maxillary left central incisor and to create a vertical defect
3. Periodontal surgery, packing DBM around the maxillary left central incisor to regenerate bone into the vertical defect

4. Composite buildups on mandibular incisors to close mandibular spaces
5. Endosseous dental implants in the edentulous areas
6. Retention using a maxillary fixed lingual retainer

TREATMENT PROCESS

The treatment was performed as planned. After the initial periodontal therapy was completed and oral hygiene was monitored for a few months, the orthodontic treatment started by bonding a maxillary simple fixed appliance. The maxillary right second premolar, the maxillary left first molar and the maxillary left incisors were bonded with a 0.022" slot preadjusted edgewise appliance. A 0.016" stainless steel archwire with an intrusion bend was used to intrude the maxillary left central incisor (Fig. 11.15E and F). The 2 × 1 simple fixed appliance used to intrude the maxillary left central incisor provided a long inter-bracket distance that ensured light force.

Melsen et al [12] suggested that when a bone has been lost and the PDL area has decreased, the same force against the crown produces greater pressure in the PDL of a periodontally compromised tooth than in a normally supported one. In addition, the centre of resistance becomes more apical with bone loss.[44] The centre of resistance is defined as the midpoint of the root embedded in bone. Therefore, the absolute magnitude of force used to move teeth must be reduced when periodontal support has been lost.[44]

The intrusion bend would place the wire at the gingival margin before tying the wire into the bracket of the maxillary left central incisor (Fig. 11.15E and F). Intrusion was completed within 3–4 months, and the remaining incisors were bonded, levelled and aligned. A 0.017" × 0.025" TMA rectangular wire was placed, and palatal root torque was applied on the maxillary left central incisor to increase the thickness of the labial plate of bone. Also, a gable bend was added to move the root mesially; this increased the amount of bone distal to the root (Fig. 11.15H and I). The reasons to intrude the maxillary left central incisor were fourfold: (1) alignment of the tooth would improve aesthetics, (2) embedding more root into the bone would increase the root-to-crown ratio, (3) the horizontal bone defect around the tooth would change into a vertical bone defect and (4) increased blood flow into the defect would enhance the regenerative response during osteoregeneration.

At this stage of treatment, the patient was readied for periodontal structure regeneration by packing DBM into the vertical defect. A flap was raised and root planing was carefully performed, and DBM was packed into the defect site (Fig. 11.15I and J). The teeth were retained with rectangular wire, the same as used earlier, for 3 months (Fig. 11.15H). Radiographic examination at the time of surgery showed a deep and narrow defect (Fig. 11.15H). Three months later, new bone formation had taken place, as demonstrated by the bone fill into the defect area (Fig. 11.15K). Radiographic analysis also showed slight blunting of the apex with intrusion of the maxillary left central incisor. Radiographs (Fig. 11.15L) taken 2 years after completion of treatment showed the stability of the treatment results (Fig. 11.15M-P).

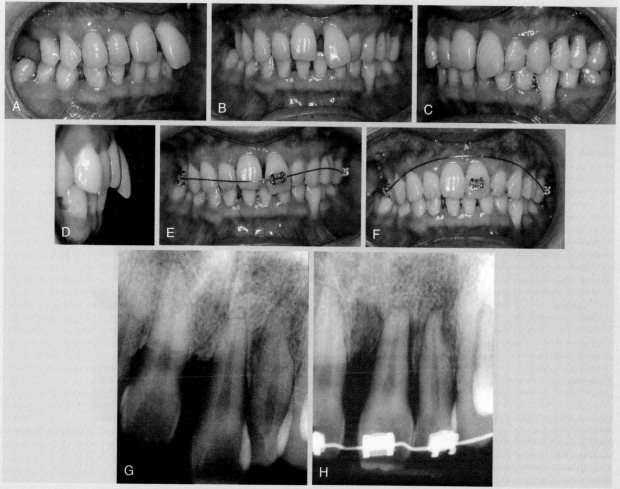

Figure 11.15 **(A–D)** Intraoral views showing extruded and spaced incisors. Mucogingival lesion noticed at the mandibular left first premolar was treated during the follow-up period. **(E)** Intraoral view showing a 2 × 1 appliance to intrude the maxillary left central incisor. **(F)** Successful intrusion after 3 months of using a 0.016" stainless steel archwire with an intrusion bend. Note that the wire rests at the gingival margin when not engaged in the bracket. **(G)** Pretreatment radiograph of the maxillary left central incisor, showing bone loss. Bone is covering only one-third of the root on the mesial side. **(H)** Radiograph of the maxillary left central incisor at the end of intrusion. The defect topography has changed from a horizontal defect to a narrow and deep defect. Note the gable bend in the wire that moved the root of the maxillary left central incisor mesially. Note also the root blunting of the tooth.

Continued

CASE 4—cont'd

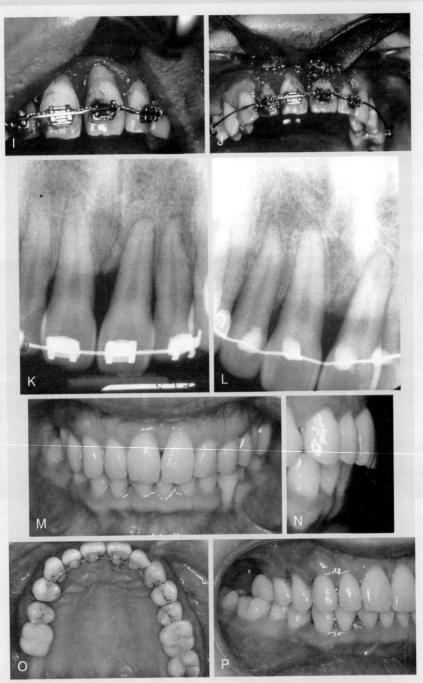

Figure 11.15, cont'd (I) The defect after intrusion of the maxillary left central incisor. **(J)** Surgical packing of DBM in the defect. **(K)** Radiograph at 3 months postgrafting. Note the regain of bone into the defect area. **(L)** One year postretention radiograph, i.e. 15 months after DBM grafting, showing stability of the regained bone. **(M–O)** Intraoral views at 2-year post-treatment. The mandibular left first premolar needs to be treated with a mucogingival procedure. **(P)** An endosseous implant was placed in the maxillary right first molar region.

Results of Cases 3 and 4 clearly demonstrated that combining orthodontic treatment with periodontal surgery and bone induction is a promising approach. However, the reader might question the safety of DBM and the fate of DBM particle. Demineralized bone matrices have been used safely in the field of dentistry for the past 20 years.[49–51] The fate of DBM particles and effects of the residual particles within grafted human intrabony

defects were reported by Reynolds and Bowers in a series of articles.[52–54] Their study examined 12 healthy volunteers with two or more premolars, canines or incisors demonstrating advanced periodontal disease; the teeth had been recommended for extraction. The treatment included periodontal surgery and bone induction using DBM. At 6 months, the teeth were removed en bloc for histologic analysis to examine the fate of DBM particles and to compare the amount of new attachment apparatus formation, including component tissues, in relation to the presence or absence of DBM particles. Analysis of histologic sections revealed that 72% of the grafted defects exhibited residual DBM particles. These particles were amalgamated within the new viable bone. This result supported the experimental findings showing DBM particles iterated and amalgamated within the newly formed bone.[55] Defects harbouring residual graft particles exhibited significantly greater amount of new attachment apparatus formation (1.74 versus 0.23 mm), including new bone (2.33 versus 0.23 mm), cementum (1.74 versus 0.23 mm) and associated PDL, than those found in sites without evident grafted DBM. The presence or absence of DBM particles within a grafted site was directly related to the degree of inflammation within the defect area. The histologic level of inflammatory cell infiltrate was more extensive in specimens lacking the DBM particles than in defects harbouring them.

Case 4 demonstrated the successful outcome of orthodontic intrusion as an adjunct to periodontal therapy. However, several factors influence the feasibility of such an approach. The availability of good anchorage units and the condition of the supporting structures of the anchor units should be taken into account.

In conclusion, combined bone induction, periodontal surgery and orthodontics should be added to the armamentarium available to the orthodontist for the management of orthodontic patients with severe bone loss.

FINISHING AND RETENTION

Positioners are rarely indicated as finishing devices for patients with moderate to severe periodontal bone loss. These patients should be brought to their final orthodontic relationship with archwires and then stabilized with immediately placed retainers before eventual detailing of occlusal relationships by equilibration.[5]

Fixed and permanent retainers are highly recommended to be delivered to patients with periodontal bone loss. Resin-bonded bridge can serve not only as prosthetic replacement but also as an orthodontic retainer and a periodontal splint for the adjacent teeth.

Oral hygiene maintenance is life-long task, and regular review of the periodontal condition should be carried out.

CONCLUSION

- Orthodontic tooth movement in periodontally involved patients constitutes a problem distinct from routine orthodontics.
- Any patient undergoing orthodontic treatment must take extra care to clean the teeth, especially for adult patients.
- A periodontal evaluation in an adult orthodontic patient must include an assessment of the level and the condition of the attached gingiva. So the gingival condition must receive major attention when planning the orthodontic treatment.
- If the attached gingiva appears thin and vulnerable and there is a chance of gingival recession with orthodontic tooth movement, increasing the thickness of bone through orthodontic intervention may be a way to create healthier attached gingiva before tooth movement. Before orthodontic treatment is attempted for patients who have pre-existing periodontal problems, dental and periodontal diseases must be brought under control. These patients received monthly reinforcement of plaque removal and also received subgingival debridement at 3-month intervals during orthodontic treatment to maintain healthy gingival tissues.
- Because traumatic occlusion may have been a predisposing factor for the gingival recession and tooth mobility elimination of traumatic occlusion becomes a major objective of the treatment planning.
- During the treatment planning for this adjunctive orthodontic treatment, special biomechanical considerations were

emphasized. The design of the appliance used depended on the number of teeth to be moved, the availability of anchorage and the desired direction and amount of crown or tooth movement. At the same time, orthodontic goals and mechanics must be modified to keep orthodontic forces to an absolute minimum.
- If good hygiene is maintained, intrusion of incisors in adult patients with marginal bone loss offers a beneficial effect on the periodontal condition at clinical and radiographic levels.
- Orthodontic intrusion can change a horizontal bony defect into a deep and narrow defect that is more favourable for regeneration of the periodontium through grafting procedures.
- Combined bone induction, periodontal surgery and orthodontics should be added to the armamentarium available to the orthodontist for the management of orthodontic patients with severe bone loss.
- Judicious interdisciplinary treatment planning should involve team approach, i.e. orthodontics, periodontics, prosthetic dentistry and bone induction.
- Fixed and permanent retainers are highly recommended to be delivered to patients with periodontal boneloss. Oral hygiene maintenance is life-long task, and regular review of the periodontal condition should be carried out.

REFERENCES

1. Eliasson LA, Hugoson A, Kurol J, et al. The effects of orthodontic treatment on periodontal tissues in patients with reduced periodontal support. Eur J Orthod 1982; 4:1–9.
2. Williams S, Melsen B, Agerbaek N, et al. The orthodontic treatment of malocclusion in patients with previous periodontal disease. Br J Orthod 1982; 9:178–184.
3. Brown LJ, Brunelle JA, Kingman A. Periodontal status in the United States, 1988–1991: prevalence, extent, and demographic variation. J Dent Res 1996; 75:672–683.
4. Albandar JM. Epidemiology and risk factors of periodontal diseases. Dent Clin North Am 2005; 49:517–532, v–vi.
5. Proffit WR. Special considerations in treatment for adults. In: Proffit WR, Fields Jr HW, Sarver DM, eds. Contemporary orthodontics, chap. 18. 4th edn. St Louis: Mosby; 2007. 635–685.
6. Boyd RL, Leggott PJ, Quinn RS, et al. Periodontal implications of orthodontic treatment in adults with reduced or normal periodontal tissues versus those of adolescents. Am J Orthod Dentofacial Orthop 1989; 96:191–198.

7. Wennström JL, Lindhe J, Sinclair F, et al. Some periodontal tissue reactions to orthodontic tooth movement in monkeys. J Clin Periodontol 1987; 14:121–129.

8. Chay SH, Rabie AB. Repositioning of the gingival margin by extrusion. Am J Orthod Dentofacial Orthop 2002; 122:95–102.

9. Lindhe J, Karring T. Anatomy of the periodontium. In: Lindhe J, Karring T, Lang NP, eds. Clinical periodontology and implant dentistry. Copenhagen: Munksgaard; 1997. 23.

10. Boyd RL. Mucogingival considerations and their relationship to orthodontics. J Periodontol 1978; 49:67–76.

11. Hall WB. The current status of mucogingival problems and their therapy. J Periodontol 1981; 52:569–575.

12. Melsen B, Agerbaek N, Markenstam G. Intrusion of incisors in adult patients with marginal bone loss. Am J Orthod Dentofacial Orthop 1989; 96:232–241.

13. Melsen B. Tissue reaction following application of extrusive and intrusive forces to teeth in adult monkeys. Am J Orthod 1986; 89:469–475.

14. Vanarsdall RL. Orthodontics and periodontal therapy. Periodontol 2000. 1995; 9:132–149.

15. Kessler M. Interrelationships between orthodontics and periodontics. Am J Orthod 1976; 70:154–172.

16. Stenvik A, Mjör IA. Pulp and dentine reactions to experimental tooth intrusion. A histologic study of the initial changes. Am J Orthod 1970; 57:370–385.

17. Klassman B, Zucker HW. Treatment of aperiodontal defect resulting from improper tooth alignment and local factors. J Periodontol 1969; 40:401–403.

18. Ericsson I, Thilander B. Orthodontic relapse in dentitions with reduced periodontal support: an experimental study in dogs. Eur J Orthod 1980; 2:51–57.

19. Artun J, Urbye KS. The effect of orthodontic treatment on periodontal bone support in patients with advanced loss of marginal periodontium. Am J Orthod Dentofacial Orthop 1988; 93:143–148.

20. Grewe JM, Chadha JM, Hagan D, et al. Oral hygiene and occlusal disharmony in Mexican-American children. J Periodontal Res 1969; 4:189–192.

21. Shaw WC. Risk-benefit appraisal in orthodontics. In: Shaw WC, ed. Orthodontics and occlusal management. 1st edn. Cambridge: Oxford; 1993. 134–155.

22. Wagenberg BD, Eskow RN, Langer B. Orthodontic procedures that improve the periodontal prognosis. J Am Dent Assoc 1980; 100:370–373.

23. Musich DR. Assessment and description of the treatment needs of adult patients evaluated for orthodontic therapy. II. Characteristics of the dual provider group. Int J Adult Orthodon Orthognath Surg 1986; 1:101–117.

24. Rabie AB, Deng YM, Jin LJ. Adjunctive orthodontic treatment of periodontally involved teeth: case reports. Quintessence Int 1998; 29:13–19.

25. Thilander B. The role of the orthodontist in the multidisciplinary approach to periodontal therapy. Int Dent J 1986; 36:12–17.

26. Kusy RP, Tulloch JF. Analysis of moment/force ratios in the mechanics of tooth movement. Am J Orthod Dentofacial Orthop 1986; 90:127–131.

27. Miller BH. Orthodontics for the adult patient. Part2–The orthodontic role in periodontal, occlusal and restorative problems. Br Dent J 1980; 148:128–132.

28. Forsberg CM, Brattström V, Malmberg E, et al. Ligature wires and elastomeric rings: two methods of ligation, and their association with microbial colonization of Streptococcus mutans and lactobacilli. Eur J Orthod 1991; 13:416–420.

29. Sam K, Rabie AB, King NM. Orthodontic intrusion of periodontally involved teeth. J Clin Orthod 2001; 35:325–330.

30. Melsen B, Agerbaek N, Eriksen J, et al. New attachment through periodontal treatment and orthodontic intrusion. Am J Orthod Dentofacial Orthop 1988; 94:104–116.

31. Polson A, Caton J, Polson AP, et al. Periodontal response after tooth movement into intrabony defects. J Periodontol 1984; 55:197–202.

32. Ericsson I, Thilander B, Lindhe J, et al. The effect of orthodontic tilting movements on the periodontal tissues of infected and non-infected dentitions in dogs. J Clin Periodontol 1977; 4:278–293.

33. Rochette AL. Attachment of a splint to enamel of lower anterior teeth. J Prosthet Dent 1973; 30:418–423.

34. Cortellini P, Bowers GM. Periodontal regeneration of intrabony defects: an evidence-based treatment approach. Int J Periodontics Restorative Dent 1995; 15:128–145.

35. Blank BS, Levy AR. Combined treatment of a large periodontal defect using GTR and DFDBA. Int J Periodontics Restorative Dent 1999;19:481–487.

36. Rosenberg E, Rose LF. Biologic and clinical considerations for auto grafts and allografts in periodontal regeneration therapy. Dent Clin North Am 1998; 42:467–490.

37. Kim CK, Cho KS, Choi SH, et al. Periodontal repair in dogs: effect of allogenic freeze-dried demineralized bone matrix implants on alveolar bone and cementum regeneration. J Periodontol 1998; 69:26–33.

38. Caplanis N, Lee MB, Zimmerman GJ, et al. Effect of allogeneic freeze-dried demineralized bone matrix on regeneration of alveolar bone and periodontal attachment in dogs. J Clin Periodontol 1998; 25:801–806.

39. Kassolis JD, Bowers GM. Supracrestal bone regeneration: a pilot study. Int J Periodontics Restorative Dent 1999; 19:131–139.

40. Heijl L, Heden G, Svärdström G, et al. Enamel matrix derivative (EMDOGAIN) in the treatment of intrabony periodontal defects. J Clin Periodontol 1997; 24:705–714.

41. Heijl L. Periodontal regeneration with enamel matrix derivative in one human experimental defect. A case report. J Clin Periodontol 1997; 24:693–696.

42. Heden G, Wennström J, Lindhe J. Periodontal tissue alterations following Emdogain treatment of periodontal sites with angular bone defects. A series of case reports. J Clin Periodontol 1999; 26:855–860.

43. Rabie ABM, Boisson M. Management of patients with severe bone loss: Bone induction and orthodontics. World J Orthod 2001; 2:142–153.

44. Geramy A. Alveo lar bone resorption and the center of resistance modification (3-D analysis by means of the finite element method). Am J Orthod Dentofacial Orthop 2000; 117:399–405.

45. Rabie AB, Dan Z, Samman N. Ultra-structural identification of cells involved in the healing of intramembranous and endochondral bones. Int J Oral Maxillofac Surg 1996; 25:383–388.

46. Vandevska-Radunovic V, Kristiansen AB, Heyeraas KJ, et al. Changes in blood circulation in teeth and supporting tissues incident to experimental tooth movement. Eur J Orthod 1994; 16:361–369.

47. Polverini PJ. The pathophysiology of angiogenesis. Crit Rev Oral Biol Med 1995; 6:230–247.

48. Rabie AB. Vascular endothelial growth pattern during demineralized bone matrix induced osteogenesis. Connect Tissue Res 1997; 36:337–345.

49. Rabie AB, Chay SH. Clinical applications of composite intramembranous bone grafts. Am J Orthod Dentofacial Orthop 2000; 117: 375–383.

50. Rabie AM, Comfort MB. Composite bone grafts inalveolar ridge augmentation for implants. In: Rabie ABM, Urist MR, eds. Bone formation and repair. Amsterdam: Elsevier Science BV; 1997. 47–58.

51. Mulliken JB, Glowacki J. Induced osteogenesis for repair and construction in the craniofacial region. Plast Reconstr Surg 1980; 65:553–560.

52. Reynolds MA, Bowers GM. Fate of demineralized freeze-dried bone allografts in human intrabony defects. J Periodontol 1996; 67:150–157.

53. Bowers GM, Chadroff B, Carnevale R, et al. Histologic evaluation of new attachment apparatus formation in humans. Part I. J Periodontol 1989; 60:664–674.

54. Bowers GM, Chadroff B, Carnevale R, et al. Histologic evaluation of new attachment apparatus formation in humans. Part III. J Periodontol 1989; 60:683–693.

55. Rabie AB, Lie Ken Jie RK. Integration of endochondral bone grafts in the presence of demineralized bone matrix. Int J Oral Maxillofac Surg 1996; 25:311–318.

Interdisciplinary Orthodontics

12

Ashok Karad and Ratnadeep Patil

Orthodontic treatment of adults has been the fastest growing area in orthodontics in recent years. Many orthodontic practices today include 45% of patients as adults. This is probably because of an increased awareness of malocclusion and functional benefits of orthodontic treatment. In addition to aesthetics, recent advances in orthodontic materials, aesthetically pleasing and biomechanically sound appliances, and interdisciplinary treatment philosophy have all played an important role in making orthodontic treatment popular in adult population. This chapter presents the philosophy and treatment approach needed to bring together a diverse group of professionals into a cohesive team to provide treatment strategies for adult patient. It explains existing and new orthodontic, periodontic, surgical and restorative techniques that provide the best possible solution to complex dentofacial problems.

In clinical practice, orthodontic treatment of adults may be somewhat different from that of most adolescents.[1] Adult patients are usually motivated for improved oral hygiene, and they are cooperative. Compared with adolescents, adults are more likely to have dentitions that have undergone some degree of mutilation over a period of time. In addition to the malaligned teeth and jaws, adult orthodontic patients may have other problems that demand some alterations in treatment strategy. These include excessive tooth wear, missing teeth, restored teeth, periodontally compromised teeth, endodontically involved teeth, etc., which make the treatment more challenging. In such clinical situations, orthodontist needs to coordinate treatment with other specialist or multiple specialists in order to optimize the treatment results.[2,3]

This involvement of various specialists, like orthodontist, prosthodontist, periodontist and endodontist, should be maintained with active communication among themselves throughout treatment, from the diagnosis and treatment planning stages through to the completion of active treatment and into the retention phase. In adult patients having periodontally compromised dentition with significant bone and attachment loss, conventional approach to orthodontic tooth movement does not produce the desired results, as this may lead to increased tipping of teeth.[4] Therefore, in such clinical situations, entirely different biomechanical strategies are required for efficient and desired tooth movement.[5] Absence of growth potential in adults as opposed to growing patients is another factor that influences the orthodontic treatment strategy to resolve adult malocclusions.

INTERDISCIPLINARY PHILOSOPHY

An interdisciplinary dentofacial therapy is the effective and efficient utilization of the expertise and skills in the various disciplines of dentistry.[6] Its key is the combination of diagnostic, treatment planning and therapeutic procedures with extensive communication among the team members. An interdisciplinary approach to the management of complex dentofacial problems produces consistent optimal results. By providing solutions to variety of problems, an interdisciplinary treatment simplifies and idealizes the treatment plan that improves the overall treatment prognosis and enhances the treatment results.

Diagnostic and treatment planning process

Establishing proper diagnosis is the most important step to formulate the treatment plan and to prevent any complications and confusion in the final treatment. The goal of the diagnostic process in an interdisciplinary treatment is to produce a comprehensive but concise list of patient's problems and to synthesize the various treatment options into a plan that gives maximum benefit to the patient. In diagnosis and treatment planning, the orthodontist should

1. recognize the various elements of malocclusion and characteristics of dentofacial deformity,
2. have comprehensive knowledge of different disciplines of dentistry to generate the pertinent data other than orthodontics,
3. define the nature of the problem and
4. design a treatment strategy based on the specific needs and desires of the patient.

During the process of diagnosis, while assessing complex dentofacial problems, orthodontists should not focus only on specializedareas ignoring the patient's main concern. The basic tenet of establishing diagnosis is the development of a comprehensive but concise database of useful information that can be derived from: (a) patient's history, (b) clinical examination and (c) analysis of diagnostic records (study models, full-mouth radiographs and facial and intraoral photographs; Fig. 12.1).

This database is then well structured and organized in such a way that it gives a systematic description of the patient's problems that can be easily referred to during the treatment planning process. This leads to a development of a problem list. While arranging the database of a complex dentofacial problem in a systematic manner, if the problem list becomes very extensive, it is advisable to classify the problem list into various areas, like orthodontic problem list, restorative problem list and periodontal problem list (Fig. 12.2).

Defining treatment goals

Since the problem list of the complex dentofacial abnormalities is multifaceted and involves multiple disciplines of dentistry, it is extremely important to address the patient's main concern, i.e. chief complaint, whether the patient is seeking treatment for functional or aesthetic improvement or both, while formulating the treatment

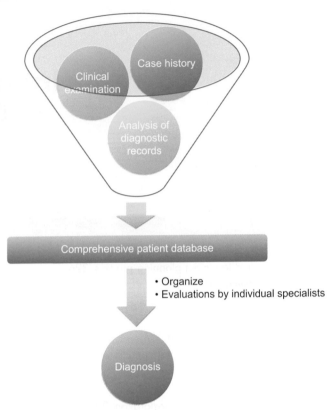

Figure 12.1 Diagnostic process.

plan. The treatment planning process in an interdisciplinary therapy involves finding a solution to each individual problem that leads to the formulation of a definitive treatment plan.[7] The key here is to follow a logical sequence to develop an interdisciplinary problem list, which can be synthesized to establish a final treatment plan. The entire process of treatment planning is focused on arriving at an unbiased treatment plan that promotes optimal overall treatment results. This may involve a compromise of individual concerns of different members of an interdisciplinary team, like prosthodontist, periodontist and orthodontist, according to their relative importance to the overall treatment.[8] A well-structured and organized list of problems makes sure that all areas have been evaluated in the diagnostic phase and also serves as a valuable reference tool during the course of treatment. All specialists involved in formulating the treatment plan for the patients should provide possible solutions to individual problems based on their own areas of expertise, and no problem should be treated as less important. These problems are then prioritized in order of importance, related to one another, and overall effects are carefully studied to establish alternate tentative treatment plans. Provisional treatment plans are then compared with respect to their overall effects, and the plan that enhances the treatment and provides maximum benefit to the patient, considering the patient's chief complaint, is then regarded as final and definitive treatment plan.

Orthodontists should be able to visualize or foresee the final treatment outcome before implementing the definitive treatment plan. This requires that the treatment goals are clearly defined, which set the direction to the proposed treatment plan. In an adult patient with

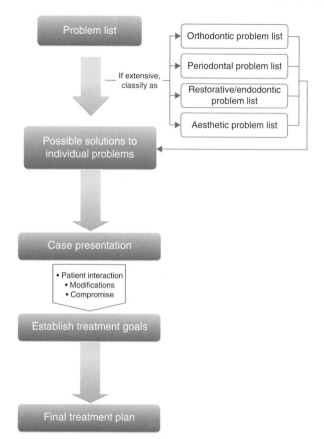

Figure 12.2 Development of a final treatment plan.

restorative and periodontal treatment needs, it should be remembered that the established treatment objectives are realistic, as opposed to idealistic treatment objectives in nonrestored adolescent patient. Economics also plays an important role in the patient's selection of treatment plan. If the treatment goals are not economically viable, the patient may not even proceed with the restorative or periodontal treatment after orthodontic therapy. Therefore, in interdisciplinary treatment, the ideal treatment plan would be the plan that addresses maximum number of highest priority problems including the chief complaint and optimizes the treatment results with maximum benefit to the patient and with less risk involved.

Case presentation

Once the potential risks and benefits to the patient and all other factors that contribute to the optimal treatment plan have been openly and honestly discussed among the team members, it is time to schedule an appointment for case presentation. This is the most critical element of interdisciplinary therapy, as the outcome of this meeting determines whether the patient is willing to accept the proposed treatment plan or not. This meeting is aimed at making patient fully aware of his or her existing problems and possible solutions by presenting the detailed diagnostic findings, the alternative treatment plans with potential risks and benefits and the cost involved. This should be done thoroughly by using actual diagnostic records and visual aids and presentation of similar cases with pretreatment and post-treatment photographs. This

definitely helps to establish the patient's trust and confidence in the treatment providers and enhances the patient's perceived value of therapy.[7] Ideally, the multispecialist consultation with the patient is very effective; however, it may not be realistic, if it is not a group practice setup. The goal of this meeting is to make patient fully aware of his or her dentofacial problems and needs by presenting the detailed diagnostic findings and the proposed tentative treatment plans to help the patient to decide on what is important to him or her. Since the interdisciplinary treatment involves services from multiple specialists, it is important for the patient to understand the financial matters, which should be best handled by individual team members. After the patient has accepted the proposed treatment plan, it should be fine-tuned based on the outcome of the case presentation with the patient. This should be followed by a detailed outline of treatment sequence, listing the various specialists involved and making them responsible for their respective areas.

Treatment sequencing

After the finalization of a definitive treatment plan, it is an important step in interdisciplinary therapy to establish the sequence of treatment. All specialists involved in providing services should meet and discuss the definitive treatment plan before it is implemented. During this meeting, it is essential that the team members understand their responsibilities and are fully aware of the planned sequence of therapy. This should be recorded, and a copy should be given to each of the team member and to the patient.[7,9] This helps to make sure that the proposed plan is proceeding properly, any team specialist can review the sequence at any stage of treatment and the patient is aware of the direction and the stage of treatment completion. The treatment planning process almost always follows the same events; however, the sequence of treatment varies significantly from patient to patient based on the treatment priority. Here, the main goal is to organize the sequence of various treatment procedures into a logical order so that each intervention performed by one of the specialists from the interdisciplinary team facilitates the next in order[10] (Fig. 12.3). Figure 12.4 illustrates a 14-point treatment protocol for interdisciplinary cases.

PERIODONTALLY COMPROMISED PATIENT

One of the most important aspects of orthodontic treatment while treating adult population is the proper assessment of their periodontal health. This should be done before the placement of fixed orthodontic appliances in order to avoid adverse iatrogenic effects on the periodontium. Adequate maintenance of dental and periodontal health is an integral part of the treatment performed by every specialist who is a part of the interdisciplinary team. Many adult patients who are the candidates for restorative treatment often have abnormal tooth positions. This compromises their ability to adequately clean their dentitions and maintain the oral hygiene, leading to periodontal breakdown. Orthodontic tooth movement plays

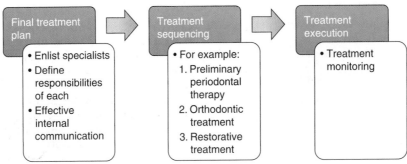

Figure 12.3   Treatment execution.

- Case history
- Clinical examination
- Full-mouth radiographic survey, panoramic radiograph
- Study models
- Extraoral photographs
- Intraoral photographs
- Evaluations by individual specialists involved
- Preliminary problem list
- Diagnosis
- Treatment plan
- Treatment sequencing
- Execution of treatment
- Treatment progress assessment
- Continued maintenance

Figure 12.4   A 14-point interdisciplinary treatment protocol.

an important role in improving the prognosis of periodontally compromised teeth.

Tooth position and periodontal condition

There are several studies that show pathogenic correlation between tooth position in the dental arch and periodontal condition (Fig. 12.5). An ectopically positioned tooth or a tooth that is labially placed is often associated with soft tissue breakdown, which is expressed clinically as gingival recession. Such teeth, when moved orthodontically into areas of better bone support, have been shown to partially gain attachment[11–13] (Fig. 12.6).

Irregularity of teeth is a predisposing factor to plaque accumulation and also results in unfavourable topography of gingiva and interradicular bone. The pathologic levels of microorganisms are significantly higher in the crowded dentition than in the well-aligned teeth.[14] Orthodontic correction of crowded dentition improves the topography of interdental gingiva and bone by establishing normal contact points, which in turn facilitates to adequately maintain the oral hygiene. It has been shown that the alveolar bone height is significantly reduced in regions of severe malocclusion (8 mm of overjet) as compared to the regions of normal occlusion.[15]

Preliminary periodontal therapy

Periodontal disease control, prior to the initiation of orthodontic treatment, contributes significantly to the success of treatment. It is extremely important to control periodontal inflammation, as the orthodontic treatment in presence of this inflammation can lead to rapid bone loss.[16,17] Gingival bleeding on gentle probing is the most reliable indicator of clinically significant gingivitis.[18] Excessive pocket probing depth should also be reduced with the preliminary periodontal therapy. A thorough scaling, root planing and sub-gingival curettage are often performed to keep the gingival tissues free from clinical signs of inflammation prior to and also during therapy (Fig. 12.7I and J). Since the orthodontic treatment itself can often improve the topography of alveolar bone, more extensive periodontal procedures, like flap and osseous surgery, are contraindicated as a part of preliminary periodontal therapy.[19] However, after the initial periodontal therapy, if signs of active periodontal disease or severe pocket probing depths of 5–6 mm or more are still present, flap surgical procedure may be required.[20] The presence of significant bone loss and furcation involvement are also the indications for scaling and root planing with periodontal flap surgery. As far as possible, soft tissue periodontal surgical procedures should be scheduled after orthodontic treatment, since these procedures will allow periodontal fibres to get reorganized to the new tooth positions, thereby preventing the relapse.[21]

In addition to establishing the normal health of the periodontium, the goal of the preliminary periodontal therapy is to generate some useful diagnostic information to develop an optimal definitive treatment plan. This

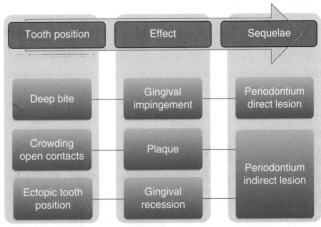

Figure 12.5   Influence of tooth position on periodontal health.

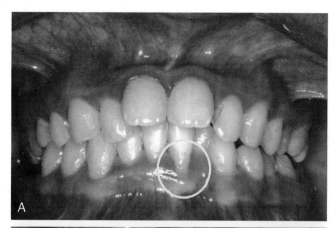

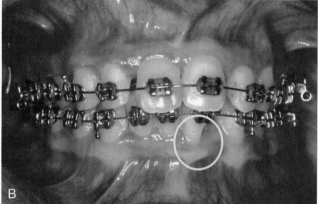

Figure 12.6 Tooth position and periodontal condition. **(A)** Labially positioned mandibular left central incisor associated with soft tissue breakdown. **(B)** Orthodontic positioning of teeth into areas of better bone support shows partial attachment gain.

information includes the response of the tissues to the initial periodontal therapy, the level of patient compliance, the prognosis of periodontally involved teeth, etc. It is focused at nonsurgically controlling the clinical signs and symptoms of inflammation and reducing the pocket probing depth to facilitate orthodontic therapy and later possible bony or soft tissue enhancements. If the patient requires periodontal osseous surgery, it would be appropriate to complete the orthodontic treatment first, establish a stable occlusion, evaluate the periodontal health after 6 months and then decide on definitive periodontal procedures.

After the preliminary periodontal therapy, supportive periodontal treatment that consists of periodontal and dental maintenance is necessary for the success of definitive therapy.[22] During the interdisciplinary therapy, it is the responsibility of every specialist involved in the team to monitor the dental and periodontal status at each visit. It is of utmost importance to make sure that the supportive periodontal treatment is strictly instituted during active orthodontic therapy. This is because orthodontic fixed appliances often cause mechanical irritation to the soft tissues and interfere with oral hygiene and with the potential for occlusal trauma due to tooth movement. To prevent caries and periodontal damage, effective and efficient oral hygiene measures should be reinforced during orthodontic therapy.[23,24]

A typical oral hygiene maintenance protocol during the supportive periodontal treatment should include the use of effective toothbrushing with proper technique, the use of chlorhexidine mouth rinse, the use of fluoride and, above all, the use of plaque-control instructions. It is advisable to recommend the rotary electric toothbrushes since they are more effective in reducing plaque accumulations than manual toothbrushes during orthodontic treatment.[25] Accumulation of plaque around the brackets and behind the archwire frequently leads to decalcified enamel white lesions that can be reduced by the prescribed use of fluoride.[26] The use of chlorhexidine mouth wash can significantly control the periodontal inflammation.[27] While the periodontal control program is being strictly adhered to, the entire dentition should be monitored and evaluated both clinically and radiographically for caries, decalcification, root resorption and endodontic involvement of teeth during orthodontic treatment.

Endodontic treatment

Adult patients undergoing interdisciplinary treatment often present with teeth with pulpal or periapical infections, which may require either endodontic treatment or extraction at some stage during the course of treatment. After thorough scaling and polishing of teeth, all carious lesions should be excavated and restored (Fig. 12.7K). However, the deep carious lesions that may be a threat to the pulp should be thoroughly excavated and restored with a temporary sedative filling material. It is important to initiate endodontic treatment of teeth with symptomatic and asymptomatic necrotic pulps in order to control and resolve active pulpal pathology and assess the initial prognosis of the affected teeth.[28,29] If the infected tooth cannot be restored and maintained due to its extensive involvement, its extraction should be considered prior to the orthodontic appliance placement. The decision to extract a tooth and its timing should be discussed among the members of the interdisciplinary team, as it affects the treatment plan. As a general rule, it works better for the orthodontist to maintain as many teeth in the dental arch as possible for adequate anchorage.

Implants for anchorage and restoration

Dental implants have become an integral part of modern dental practice. They provide single unit or multiple unit restorations with optimal aesthetics.[30,31] There are different types of implant systems available to provide optimal anchorage for tooth movement. In case of a severely periodontally compromised patient, it would be appropriate to assess the periodontal response to preliminary periodontal therapy. With positive tissue response and satisfactory patient compliance, the next phase of interdisciplinary treatment can be initiated. If an adult patient undergoing interdisciplinary therapy has a single or several dental units missing and requires a definitive restorative treatment at a later stage, restorative implants can be placed at a predetermined location, which can be used initially for orthodontic anchorage and later for restorations.[32]

While selecting the dental implants, those having an attachment through fibro-osseous integration, like blades

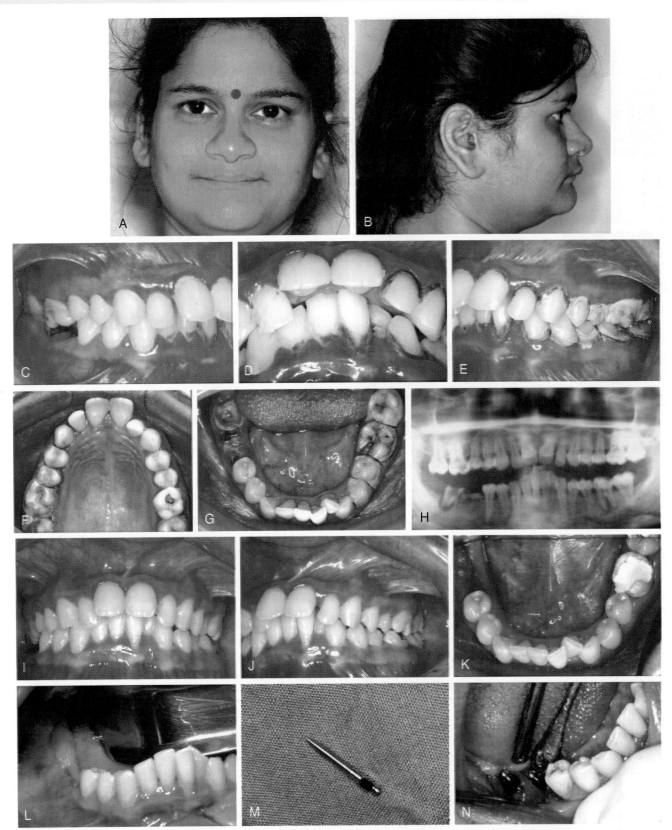

Figure 12.7 **(A** and **B)** Pretreatment facial features. Straight profile, acute nasolabial angle, deep mentolabial groove, prominent chin, poor vermilion show and decreased lower facial height. **(C–G)** Pretreatment intraoral features. Maxillary anterior proclination with spacing, mandibular incisor supraeruption and crowding, periodontitis (severely periodontally compromised dentition), incisor mobility, mutilated teeth and deep overbite (traumatic). **(H)** Pretreatment radiograph. **(I** and **J)** Preliminary periodontal therapy involving thorough scaling and subgingival curettage shows improved tissue response. **(K)** Endodontic treatment of periapically infected teeth. **(L–N)** Placement of implants in the region of mandibular right first and second molars.

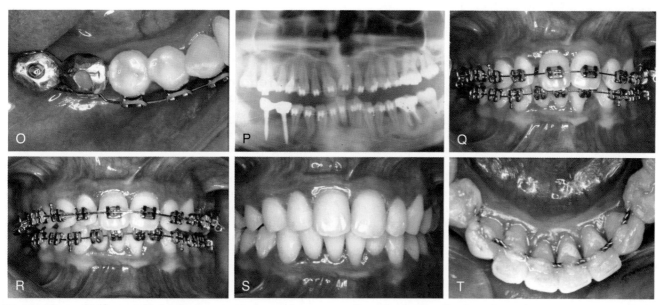

Figure 12.7, cont'd (O and **P)** Implant-supported metal crowns with orthodontic attachments and compensatory archwire configuration. **(Q)** Orthodontic treatment to move teeth into areas of better bone support and to correct occlusal problems. **(R)** Orthodontic treatment progress showing partial attachment gain in the region of mandibular left central incisor, overall improvement in occlusal condition and improvement in the angulation of teeth. **(S)** Post-treatment occlusion. **(T)** Bonded flexible spiral wire mandibular retainer.

and subperiosteal implants, are known to have less stability and success rate due to tissue breakdown around the implant.[33] On the other hand, osseointegrated implant systems have a very long-term success rate.[34] Apart from the type of the implant, it is important to determine the appropriate time for the implant placement. They can be placed either prior to the orthodontic appliance placement or after the orthodontic treatment. If the intended use of the implant is also to provide adequate anchorage for orthodontic tooth movement, it should be placed before the commencement of orthodontic treatment. After the placement of osseointegrated implants, they should be allowed to integrate with the adjacent bone for a period of 4–6 months prior to loading or application of orthodontic forces. However, the recent research shows more rapid development of bone on the implant surface when implants are loaded with static or continuous load in the same direction[35,36] and much less bone development on the implant surface when they are subjected to dynamic load (not continuous and different directions).[36] Therefore, based on these research findings, it is clear that since orthodontic forces are continuous, and if the biomechanics involved is such that the reciprocal force applied to the anchor implants is in the same direction, they can be loaded immediately. Another type of implants known as *transitional implants*, which are available in the form of screws, offer the similar advantage of immediate loading (Fig. 12.7M and N). These implants will then receive a tooth-shaped plastic or metal provisional restoration, which will allow the placement of orthodontic attachments (Fig. 12.7O). The timing of implant placement varies according to each patient's individual requirements. If patient requires periodontal surgery, the implant placement procedure can be timed at the same time in order to save time and avoid additional surgical procedure, provided the results of periodontal surgery are predictable, and it is not expected to generate some useful diagnostic information to develop optimal definitive treatment plan. Osseointegrated implants can be placed in extraction sockets immediately after extraction, which saves time, shortens treatment time and helps in prevention of alveolar bone resorption.[37]

Orthodontic treatment

Before beginning orthodontic tooth movement, patient's periodontal health, status of endodontically treated teeth and implants placed for both anchorage and future restorations should be thoroughly evaluated (Fig. 12.7Q and R). This is critical because orthodontic tooth movement, if carried out in the presence of inflammation, leads to further loss of attachment and crestal bone loss. However, research and clinical studies have shown that orthodontic tooth movement of periodontally involved dentition, performed in the absence of periodontal inflammation, improves the prognosis of the case.[19,38] When planning a tooth movement by orthodontic appliances, it is essential for the orthodontist to understand the existing periodontal status of patient and its impact on orthodontic biomechanics.

- Periodontally involved teeth with pre-existing attachment loss incident to periodontal disease offer decreased anchorage value. Therefore, it is difficult to control undesirable side effects.
- The centre of resistance of a tooth is more apical in the periodontally compromised teeth, requiring a different set of force systems to determine the type of tooth movement.
- Such patients require the delivery of ultralight orthodontic forces for a tooth movement without any side effects due to reduced alveolar bone support.

Pathologic tooth migration

Flared maxillary and mandibular incisors incidentto advanced periodontitis is a common finding in adults. Incisors suffer from periodontal attachment loss and lead to apical shifting of the centre of resistance, thereby altering the biomechanics of the periodontal anchorage. In such clinical situation, occlusal forces and abnormal forces from lip to tongue due to dentomuscular imbalance significantly contribute to the progression of incisor flaring (Fig. 12.7C–F). Preliminary periodontal therapy to control inflammation induces tissue shrinkage leading to the development of dark triangular spaces. Therefore, in adult population, progressive incisor flaring with its elongation and dark triangular spaces considerably contribute to the impairment of dentofacial aesthetics. The altered interincisal relationship encourages further overeruption of incisors and often the development of traumatic gingival lesions in more severe cases (Fig. 12.7D).

The goal of orthodontic treatment is to establish normal incisal relationship for optimal aesthetics, function, stability and longevity of dentition. Ultralight, continuous force to bring about various orthodontic tooth movements like extrusion, intrusion, tipping and translation has been the key to success in dealing with adult population. The combination of intrusive and retrusive movements helps to reduce dark interdental triangles and shift them apically. The intrusion of anterior teeth during levelling of the occlusal plane to correct deep overbite should be done with great caution, as the force is concentrated at the apex.

Restorative treatment

If the interdisciplinary treatment of a periodontally compromised patient also involves restorative treatment, orthodontic treatment should be focused at positioning teeth to facilitate restorative phase of treatment. Final fixed restorations are rarely placed prior to orthodontic treatment. Orthodontic treatment improves the root position for health of the supporting tissues and optimally positions teeth to facilitate proper placement of margins of restorations. The treatment goals established at the beginning of treatment should be monitored during the entire course of treatment, and the dentition should be assessed from the point of patient's restorative needs. This exercise should be done in consultation with a restorative dentist during the finishing stage of orthodontic treatment, preferably 6 months prior to the appliance removal. After the completion of active orthodontic tooth movement, provisional restorations can be given to prepare the teeth to withstand the stresses of final restorations without any iatrogenic interference.

ORTHO-RESTORATIVE INTERRELATIONSHIP

An adult orthodontic patient is frequently characterized by various degrees of edentulousness and various stages of periodontal pathology. Ideal orthodontic treatment goals for growing patients may not always be necessary or realistic to achieve in adult population.

Therefore, quite often, compromised treatment goals can be developed to achieve optimal interdisciplinary treatment results.

Space regaining: Molar uprighting and distalization

The loss of a permanent tooth, if not restored at an early stage, leads to a number of occlusal problems that are challenging to correct orthodontically and restore prosthetically. Such cases can be managed either by space closure or by space gaining depending on careful evaluation of the clinical situation. Following the loss of first permanent molars, the decision to achieve adequate space closure is taken considering the number of factors: the presence of third molar, the eruptive stage of the bicuspids and second molars, overjet and overbite relationship and presence of crowding or spacing.[39]

If space closure is not a treatment option, the mesially tipped molar is carefully uprighted and, if required, distalized to gain adequate space for the pontic (Fig. 12.8). The mesially tipped molars are often associated with periodontal involvement and angular bone loss on the mesial aspect (Fig. 12.8D). Studies have shown the pocket depth reduction after these teeth are optimally uprighted.[40] This improvement in the periodontal health is usually the result of the levelling of the cementoenamel junction and subsequent eversion of the apical portion of the soft tissue defect.[40] If the uprighted first molar needs subsequent distalization to reopen adequate restorative space, it may be necessary to remove the third molar. If the second molar is compromised, it may be desirable to keep the third molar. It is advantageous to optimally position teeth adjacent to the restorative space to facilitate restorative treatment. It is extremely important to decide on the type of restorations before the initiation of orthodontic therapy, as specific restorations require different types of tooth positioning.

Tooth positioning for proper restoration

Adult patients are likely to have dentitions that have undergone some degree of mutilation over a period of time, which may require some alterations in treatment strategy. The management of such patients requires interdisciplinary treatment often involving periodontal therapy, operative dentistry, orthodontics, restorative dentistry, surgery, etc. An effective communication among different disciplines should allow the formulation of treatment goals for optimal results with acceptable degree of compromise and long-term prognosis. Prerestorative orthodontic therapy involves proper positioning of teeth in order to achieve parallelism of abutment teeth, coordination of upper and lower archforms, proper distribution of teeth and spaces, redirection of occlusal forces and improved crown-to-root ratio (Fig. 12.9).

Orthodontic positioning of teeth in the orthodontic-restorative patient may not always ensure complete interdigitation of teeth and Class I molar relationship as against the goals for adolescent patient. Before the initiation of orthodontic treatment, it is important to decide on the type of restoration, as different types of restorations

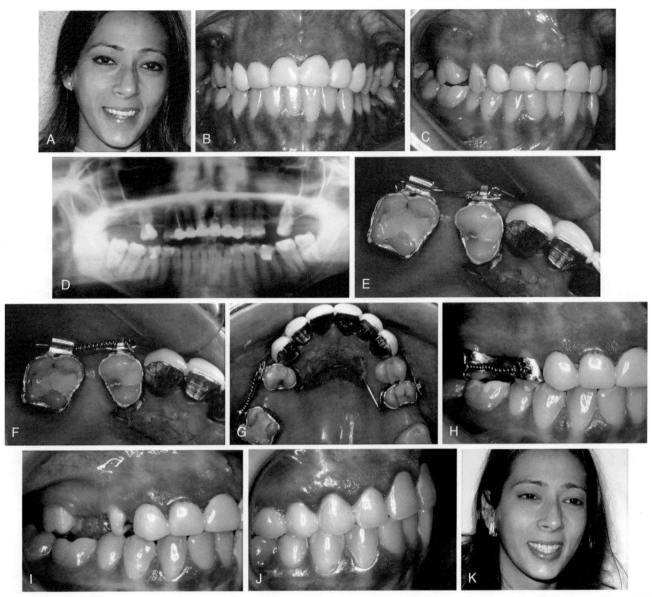

Figure 12.8 (**A** and **B**) Pretreatment unpleasant smile due to unaesthetic anterior restoration. (**C**) Missing maxillary right second bicuspid leading to mesial drifting of first molar and inadequate pontic space for the restoration. (**D**) Angular bony defect on the mesial aspect of maxillary right first molar. (**E** and **F**) Derotation and distalization of maxillary right first molar to gain optimal space for the pontic. (**G** and **H**) Maxillary right first molar distalized to a super Class I relationship, anchorage units maintained in their original positions. (**I**) Distalizing appliance removed and teeth prepared for the restoration. (**J** and **K**) Final restoration in place, post-treatment pleasing smile as a result of new anterior aesthetic restoration.

require different tooth positioning. The main goal is to position teeth to facilitate restorative treatment. A typical orthodontic-restorative situation involves patient with mutilated dentition with the attrition of teeth, often with aesthetically and functionally compromised old restorations. Such patients quite often exhibit collapsed maxillary and mandibular arches in vertical, sagittal and transverse planes. Frequently, both upper and lower incisors are upright or retroclined with a lack of proper incisor guidance and vertical stop, promoting their supra-eruption that leads to deep bite. Interproximal decay and faulty restorations with the break in continuity of dental arch lead to drifting of the adjacent teeth. Over a period of time, there is significant amount of sagittal discrepancy, loss of vertical dimension and decreased arch width

(Fig. 12.9B–F). Such teeth often exhibit the roots that are not parallel to one another with uneven interradicular spaces. In such cases, the prerestorative orthodontic treatment is aimed at proper positioning of teeth that establishes normal interincisal relationship with proper anterior guidance, well-coordinated upper and lower archforms and parallelism of roots for proper distribution of occlusal forces. This forms a good foundation for a long-term and predictable restoration, both aesthetically and functionally. The key element in managing such patients with interdisciplinary treatment is to have an effective communication between orthodontist and prosthodontist. During the finishing stage of orthodontic treatment, orthodontist should fine-tune the tooth positions based on the information received from the

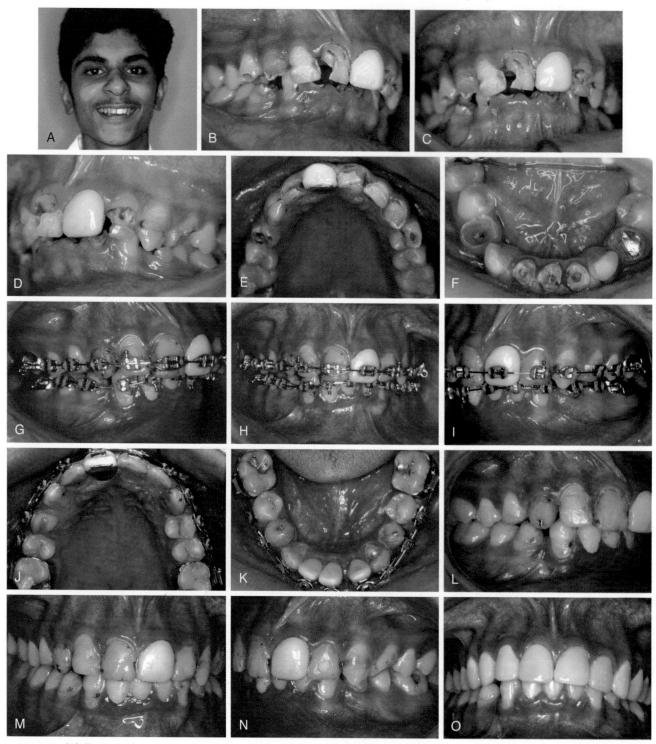

Figure 12.9 **(A)** Pretreatment extraoral features show impaired dentofacial aesthetics, and the smile reveals unaesthetic (lack of proportion, symmetry and shade of displayed teeth) anterior restorations. **(B–D)** Pretreatment intraoral photographs show severely mutilated dentition, unaesthetic restorations, badly decayed and broken teeth, deep overbite and poor periodontal condition. **(E and F)** Contracted and collapsed maxillary and mandibular arches. Uneven root spacing and old endodontic restorations. **(G–K)** Orthodontic treatment to achieve bite opening, coordinated archforms, root parallelism and proper interincisal relationship. Note the transitional restorations and tooth buildups to receive orthodontic attachments. **(L–N)** Post-treatment occlusal condition. Proper angulation of teeth, bite opening, progressive buccal root torque on maxillary posterior teeth and clinically evident normal root eminences.

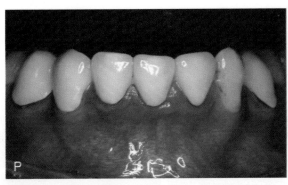
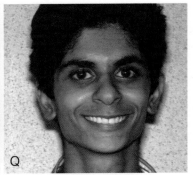

Figure 12.9, cont'd (**O** and **P**) Post-treatment photographs show final restorations in place. (**Q**) Pleasing smile.

restorative dentist to facilitate restorative therapy. The removal of orthodontic appliances should be well planned and coordinated with the prosthodontist so that the provisional restorations following the tooth preparation can be given immediately in order to avoid any untoward movement of teeth.

Gaining distal abutment tooth

Missing dental units in the distal part of dental arch is a frequent finding in a periodontally compromised patient. The only restorative option in such clinical situations is either a partial denture or an implant-supported prosthesis. Another treatment approach is to distalize the second bicuspid in a distal edentulous area and in a favourable position to be used as a distal bridge abutment. This has proved to be a prognostically favourable alternative to an implant placement.[41,42] The distal abutment can also be gained by sagittal orthodontic tooth movement of hemisected molar roots or by alignment of impacted third molars. Quite often, impacted third molars with well-formed roots are also a frequent finding in such clinical situations. These teeth can be surgically exposed and moved vertically with forced eruption in a favourable position to serve as a distal abutment tooth (Fig. 12.10). They should be stabilized in their new positions to allow reorganization of periodontal fibres. In a retrospective long-term study,[43] 32 distalized premolars to serve as posterior abutment teeth for fixed restorations were evaluated, with a mean distalizing distance of 9 mm and an investigation period of 14 years. The results showed that none of the premolar abutments was lost and all of them retained their vitality. The periodontal parameters, like probing depth, sulcus bleeding and attachment level, showed no significant detrimental effects.

MANAGEMENT OF CONGENITALLY MISSING MAXILLARY LATERAL INCISORS

The management of patients with congenitally missing maxillary lateral incisors is challenging for both orthodontist and restorative dentist. Such patients exhibit the presence of anterior spacing, diastema between the central incisors and compromised lateral incisor space due to the mesial drifting of the canines and the posterior segment. The maxillary midline shift and tooth-size discrepancy are also common clinical findings. Since these abnormalities are present in the aesthetic zone, the management of such cases raises several important treatment planning concerns. There are two basic treatment options, which include the following:

1. Missing lateral incisor space closure: In this approach, the missing lateral incisor space is closed by the mesial movement of cuspids and the protraction of the entire buccal segment. The case is often finished in a Class II molar relationship. The canine and first bicuspid are then reshaped to achieve maximum aesthetic result.
2. Opening of missing lateral incisor space: The missing lateral incisor space can be opened optimally to restore with either a tooth-supported restoration or a single-tooth implant.

Restoration of missing lateral incisor with implant

If a single-tooth implant is the treatment option to replace the maxillary lateral incisor (Fig. 12.11), it is critical to evaluate the smile line and gingival contour. The implant site should be carefully studied to ascertain the height and width of available bone, the root position of adjacent teeth, the form of adjacent teeth, the local gingival thickness and architecture, etc. One of the most important factors to be considered here is to determine the amount of space required for the restoration. This should be followed by gaining adequate space by carefully planning the orthodontic tooth movement based on the occlusal abnormalities.

There are many methods for determining the optimal space required to restore the appropriate width of lateral incisor. The contralateral lateral incisor, if it is not malformed or peg-shaped, can be used to establish the appropriate width of missing lateral incisor.[44] Another method is the golden proportion. Since the maxillary teeth are positioned along an arc, each tooth should be 61.8% wider than the distal tooth.[45] Bolton analysis can be used for determining the proper space for missing or malformed teeth.[46,47] The construction of diagnostic wax-up is the most predictable method to determine the appropriate space for the missing maxillary lateral incisors. In this method, after arranging the anterior and posterior teeth in their ideal functional and aesthetic relationships, the residual space is used for the restoration of a lateral incisor.[44,48]

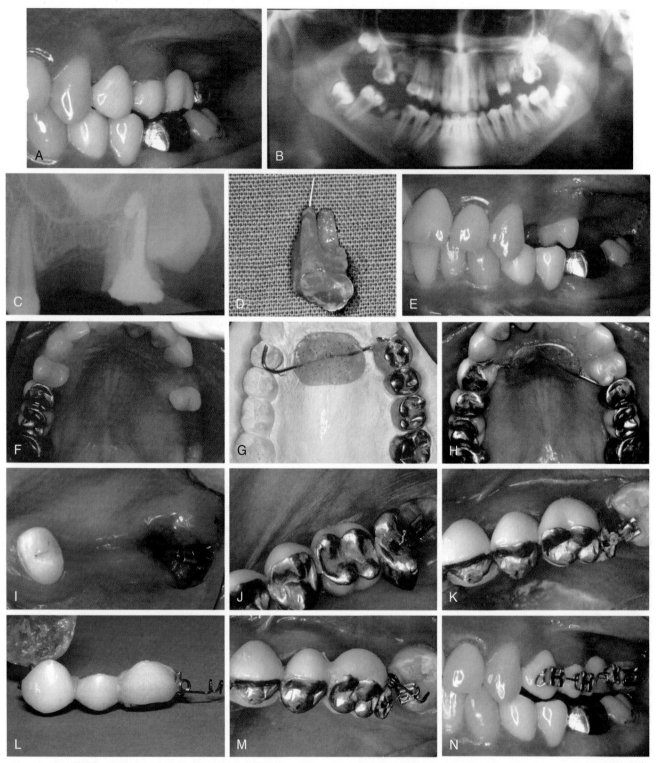

Figure 12.10 **(A)** Pretreatment intraoral photographs showing multiple restorations. Patient's only concern was pain in connection with maxillary left second molar. **(B)** Pretreatment radiograph. **(C)** Intraoral periapical X-ray showing endodontically treated maxillary left second molar. **(D)** Second molar extraction was considered since it was infected; extracted second molar shows overextended endodontic restoration. **(E and F)** Extraction of maxillary left second molar resulted in a long edentulous span with no distal abutment tooth. Pretreatment radiograph **(B)** shows unerupted maxillary left third molar, and the treatment plan involved the surgical exposure and forced eruption of this tooth to get it in the second molar region to serve it as a distal abutment tooth. **(G and H)** The existing bridge is to be used as an orthodontic appliance, and a large palatal button and an occlusal rest on the right first bicuspid to reinforce the anchorage. **(I)** Surgically exposed third molar with bonded attachment. **(J)** The distal half of the second molar metal crown of the bridge was cut, and the whole assembly was bonded in place. A hole created on occlusal aspect of the remaining portion of the second molar crown received the ligature wire from the third molar attachment to guide the occlusal and mesial movement of third molar. **(K)** As the third molar moved in a mesial and occlusal direction, the metal crown was progressively cut to allow this movement. **(L and M)** Later, a spring was designed and embedded in a distal aspect of the bridge to move the third molar occlusally.

Chapter 12 — Interdisciplinary Orthodontics   337

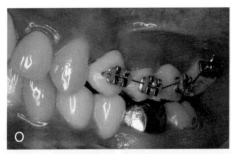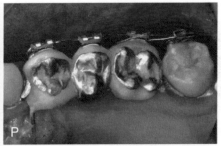

Figure 12.10, cont'd (N and **O)** Brackets were bonded to the crowns, and the molar tube was bonded to the buccal surface of the third molar to receive segmental archwire. **(P)** Third molar position was fine-tuned, followed by the stabilization period of 4 months.

Optimal implant space

Once the optimal space has been gained with appropriate treatment mechanics, acrylic tooth of proper size and colour shade can be bracketed and attached to the archwire for aesthetic purpose (Fig. 12.11J). If the space gained for the lateral incisor is in excess, the bracketed acrylic tooth can be used as a template, which will help determining the residual space closure. Clinical evaluation of the edentulous space and radiographic evaluation of the root position of the adjacent teeth should precede appliance removal.

Adequate space gained for the restoration of the normal width of missing lateral incisor based on aesthetics and occlusion will determine the appropriate size of the implant to be placed. When selecting the size of the implant, it is important to have 1.5–2.0 mm space between the coronal diameter of the implant and the adjacent teeth for the development and maintenance of the papillae.[49] After the evaluation of coronal space, it is important to radiographically evaluate the interradicular space. The roots of the adjacent teeth should be parallel to slightly divergent with adequate space between the roots for implant placement (Fig. 12.11P and Q). The final implant restoration is significantly influenced by the position and angulation of implant placement. For proper placement of an implant, the minimum space between the adjacent teeth roots is usually 5 mm, providing enough room for small diameter implant placement, leaving approximately 0.75 mm of space for the bone between the implant and the adjacent roots.[50]

It is a common observation that when an orthodontist is opening up the space for missing lateral incisor, as the force is applied on the crowns of the central and canine teeth, the roots get tipped into the lateral incisor region. This leads to an adequate crown space, but the space between the adjacent roots gets reduced, making it impossible for the surgeon to place an implant. It is equally important to take sufficient care to make sure that there is adequate interocclusal space for the implant restoration. It is, therefore, critical to establish optimal intracoronal and interradicular spaces, evaluated clinically and radiographically, respectively, for proper implant placement and long-term predictable restoration.

It is best to place an implant during the finishing stage of orthodontic treatment, which allows finer manipulation of space, maintenance of space and sufficient time for osseointegration by the time appliances are removed. However, if the implant placement procedure is planned after the removal of orthodontic appliances, the gained space should be maintained during the retention phase.

Implant site development

One of the prerequisites for placing an implant and a subsequent good soft tissue integration for more aesthetic implant restoration is to have an excellent alveolar ridge. It is a common clinical observation that unrestored edentulous areas typically exhibit compromised bone levels due to alveolar bone atrophy. Research studies have shown that if maxillary anterior teeth are extracted, the alveolar ridge will narrow by 34% over period of 5 years.[51] However, these findings related to the alveolar resorptive change do not hold true in cases where the edentulous span has been created by orthodontic tooth movement. Another study that evaluated the long-term width of the alveolar ridge after the required space was created for missing maxillary lateral incisors in adolescent orthodontic patients revealed that the amount of bone loss as result of resorptive changes was less than 1% over a period of 4 years.[44] Orthodontic implant site development is a process involving the root movement that creates adequate alveolar ridge width through stretching of the periodontal ligament fibres prior to the implant placement. This can be accomplished in any part of the alveolar ridge. In addition to the compromised alveolar ridge width, vertical bony defect at the site of implant placement can be influenced by controlled vertical root movement to generate osteoblastic activity before implant placement (Fig. 12.11D, K, M and P). The goal is to create an ideal implant site by establishing adequate alveolar ridge width and height for a predictable and more aesthetic implant restoration.

AESTHETICS

Aesthetics forms an integral part of any orthodontic treatment plan. The objectives of orthodontic treatment are to achieve good occlusal result, to improve the health of the supporting structures and to achieve optimal dentofacial aesthetics. However, traditionally, orthodontic treatment was focused more on the achievement of occlusal objectives—both static and dynamic—with less emphasis on improving the periodontal health and the aesthetic appearance of teeth. Today, increased awareness of aesthetics and resulting patient expectations have challenged the orthodontic profession to look at other

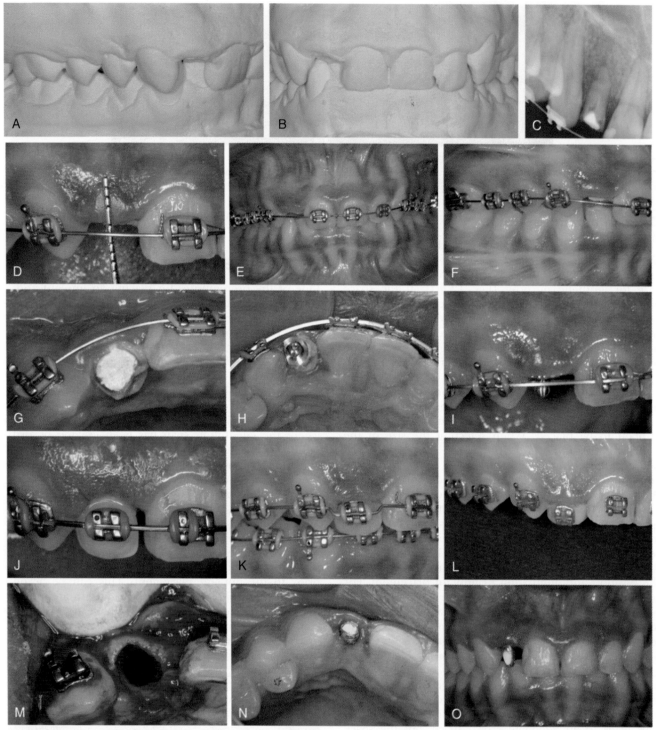

Figure 12.11 (**A** and **B**) Pretreatment models showing deep overbite. (**C**) Intraoral periapical radiograph showing the presence of maxillary right lateral incisor root piece, note good interproximal bone levels. (**D**) Pocket depth of 5 mm in the lateral incisor region indicating facial bone loss. (**E** and **F**) Orthodontic treatment to gain adequate space for implant placement in the maxillary right lateral incisor region, implant site development and to improve deep overbite. (**G**) Endodontic treatment done. (**H** and **I**) Temporary post placed. (**J**) Orthodontic bracket attached to temporary crown. (**K**) Controlled vertical eruption of maxillary right lateral incisor root in progress. (**L**) Extrusion completed. (**M**) Lateral incisor root piece extracted, note the presence of adequate bony socket walls. (**N** and **O**) Implant placed and abutment loaded. Note the ideal facial gingival contour and level.

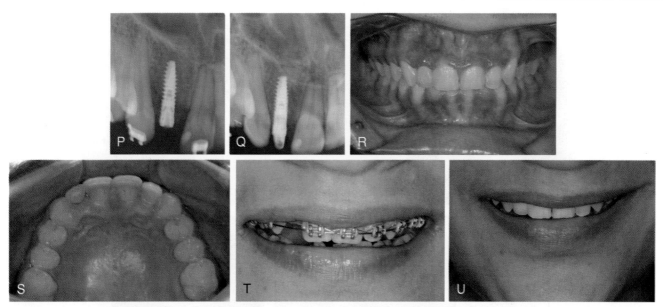

Figure 12.11, cont'd (**P** and **Q**) Intraoral periapical radiographs after implant placement and after abutment loading. (**R** and **S**) Maxillary right lateral incisor implant restoration. (**T** and **U**) Smile before and after restoration of maxillary right lateral incisor.

parameters contributing to optimal aesthetics in a more organized and systematic manner. Therefore, treatment planning process must incorporate clearly defined aesthetic objectives and development of a definite plan without compromising structural balance and functional efficiency. In this approach, the orthodontists should be able to use various clinical procedures from other disciplines of dentistry and integrate them with orthodontic treatment to maximize aesthetics.

Excessive gingival display ('gummy' smile)

The proper amount of gingival exposure during smile is essential for optimal aesthetics. In a normal situation, when the patient smiles, the lip is raised to the level of the gingival margins of the maxillary central incisors showing approximately 1–2 mm of gingiva.[52] However, an excessive gingival display upon smile appears to be highly unaesthetic (Fig. 12.12). Though the clinicians consider the gummy smile to be unaesthetic, most patients do so only in more extreme cases. Before any treatment is instituted, it is important to establish differential diagnosis of excessive gingival display.

There are many factors that contribute to the development of the problem:

1. *Role of growth:* Disproportionate vertical overdevelopment of the maxilla, especially in patients with increased facial height.
2. *Role of the upper lip:* Shorter upper lip contributes to the excessive gingival display.
3. *Eruption process:* Supraeruption of the maxillary teeth.
4. *Periodontal contribution:* Delayed apical migration of the gingival margins over the anterior teeth.

The gummy smile as a result of the overgrowth of the maxilla, leading to the overeruption of all teeth, requires orthosurgical approach to superiorly position the entire maxilla. Quite often, the problem is seen in patients with deep overbite due to supraeruption of maxillary incisors. As the teeth overerupt, there is a concomitant coronal movement of the gingival margins, resulting into an excessive display of the gums. This clinical situation is managed by orthodontic intrusion of supraerupted teeth, which in turn will position the gingival margins more apically. For optimal aesthetics, the gingival margins of the central incisors should be positioned apical to the lateral incisor gingival margins. Prior to orthodontic intrusion, it is important to evaluate the presence of excessive gingival tissue that needs to be excised. This is done by probing the gingival sulci to determine the sulcular depth, the normal being 1 mm.

The gummy smile can also be caused by delayed apical migration of the gingival margin over the maxillary anterior teeth.[53] During childhood and adolescence, the gingival margin tends to migrate apically as the teeth erupt to reach to its normal adult position. This adult position of the free gingival margin is usually 1-mm coronal to the cementoenamel junction.[54,55] If the patient has thick and fibrotic gingival tissues, the apical migration of the gingival margins towards the cementoenamel junction is delayed, resulting in excessive gingival display upon smile. To determine the depth of the sulcus and its location with respect to the cementoenamel junction, it is advisable to probe the gingival sulci of the maxillary anterior teeth. If the gingival tissues are not inflamed, the sulcular depth is more than normal, and the cementoenamel junction is located at the depth of the sulcus; aesthetic gingival surgery can be performed to position the gingival margin apically.

The relationship between the crest of the alveolar bone and the cementoenamel junction determines the type of the gingival surgery to be performed. In adults, the distance between the alveolar crest and the cementoenamel junction is approximately 2 mm.[54] If the alveolar crest and the cementoenamel junction relationship are normal, which is determined by pushing the periodontal probe from the bottom of the gingival sulcus through the epithelial attachment and connective tissue to the bone

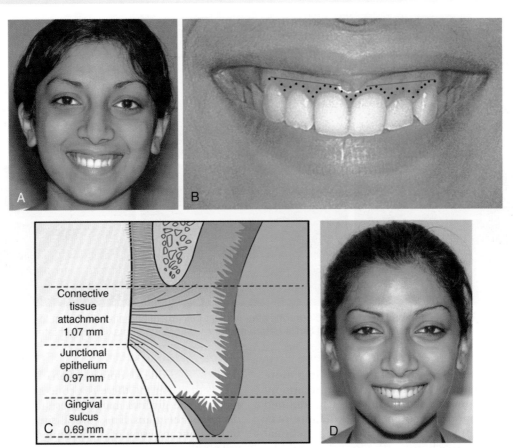

Figure 12.12 **(A)** Excessive gingival display upon smile. **(B)** Projected ideal gingival margin location while maintaining the gingival architecture. **(C)** Biologic width and its components comprising mean gingival sulcus depth of 0.69 mm, junctional epithelium measuring 0.97 mm and mean supra-alveolar connective tissue attachment of 1.07 mm. Total attachment of 2.04 mm is essential for the preservation of periodontal health. **(D)** Post-treatment smile shows reduced gingival display following aesthetic gingival surgery. Note the relapse of gingival tissue position in the left lateral incisor region due to violation of biologic width. Combining this surgical procedure with bone recontouring along with gingival recontouring would have ideally elicited a better tissue response in this region.

level, excisional gingival surgery would be the treatment of choice. However, if the distance between the alveolar crest and the cementoenamel junction is less than normal, an apically positioned flap with recontouring of the crestal bone is recommended.[56] These surgical procedures position the gingival margins apically and expose the complete crown length of the anterior teeth, with a resultant reduction in gingival display upon smile (Fig. 12.12).

These aesthetic gingival surgical procedures can be performed after the removal of orthodontic appliances, if the incisal edges are at the same level and unworn, indicative of the cementoenamel junctions being at the same height.[53] However, if the cementoenamel junctions are at different levels, determined by the presence of worn incisal edges, the gingival surgery should be performed before the removal of orthodontic appliances.[57] This will help the clinician to correct the vertical gingival margin discrepancy with the forced eruption and incisal equilibration of the longer tooth.

Gingival architecture and teeth remodelling

Colour, contour and health of the gingival tissues provide the framework and backdrop for the aesthetic smile.

Even if the case is well finished with orthodontic treatment, the gingival discrepancy either in the form of loss of papilla or in the form of asymmetrical pattern displayed upon smile leads to a poor result.[58] While evaluating the aesthetics related to gingival architecture, it is important to consider two key factors:

1. Gingival levels
2. Gingival margin contour or gingival zenith

It should be remembered that establishing a normal gingival architecture, either with orthodontic tooth movement or with surgical intervention, is purely a cosmetic procedure. Therefore, it is necessary to evaluate the relationship between the gingival margin of the maxillary anterior teeth and the patient's lip line upon smile. If the patient does not display gingival margins while smiling, it does not require correction. However, if the gingival discrepancy is apparent, measures should be taken to establish ideal gingival form for optimal aesthetics.

Ideally, the free gingival margins of the maxillary central incisors and the cuspids are positioned at the same level. The lateral incisor gingival margins are coronal to that of the centrals and the cuspids. The gingival papillary tip should be halfway between the incisal edge and the labial gingival height of contour over the centre of each anterior tooth. The contour of the margins of gingiva should mimic the cementoenamel junctions. The most apical point of the labial gingival contour, called the *gingival zenith*, is located just distal of the long axis of the central incisors and cuspids, whereas the gingival zenith for the lateral incisors coincides with their long axis.[59] In other words, the height of the gum line across the face of the tooth should be centred on the lateral incisors and positioned in the distal one-third of the face of the tooth for the centrals and canines. This gives the gingiva a semicircular appearance for the lateral incisors and an elliptical appearance for the central incisors and the cuspids.

During the process of eruption, the whole periodontal apparatus is carried with the erupting tooth. When there is asymmetric eruption of the teeth, it will also result in discrepancies in heights of the underlying crestal bone. This, in turn, results into asymmetries in gingival heights from one side of the arch to the other (Fig. 12.13B). This type of a clinical situation can be managed orthodontically by intrusion or extrusion of teeth.

In a clinical situation where missing maxillary lateral incisor space has been closed by mesialization of the posterior segment, the cuspid and the first bicuspid can be remodelled and shaped to simulate the lateral incisor and the cuspid, respectively, (Fig. 12.13F–I). This procedure should be supported by the establishment of normal gingival architecture.

UNSTABLE OCCLUSION

Occlusal consideration during all dental procedures is a critical factor in determining the longevity of the treatment and patient satisfaction. Occlusion is of fundamental importance in clinical dentistry, as all restorations placed in the mouth can have a profound effect on it. It involves not only the static relationship of teeth but also their functional inter-relationship and all the components of the masticatory system. The muscles of mastication, the neural feedback pathways, the temporomandibular joints and the shape of the occluding surfaces of the teeth influence the positions and movements of the mandible. The way in which teeth meet and move over each other must be understood so that any restoration placed in a mouth will be part of a harmoniously functioning occlusion.[60] Improperly adjusted restorations can predispose to occlusal and neuromuscular disparity resulting in detrimental effects on the stomatagnathic system (Fig. 12.14).

Temporomandibular dysfunction (TMD) is a collective term embracing a number of clinical problems that involve the masticatory musculature, the temporomandibular joint (TMJ) and associated structures, including the teeth. TMD has been identified as a major cause of non-dental pain in the orofacial region and is considered to be a subclassification of musculoskeletal disorders.[61] TMD signs and symptoms may occur before, during and after orthodontic treatment. Therefore, an attentive orthodontist should always identify and document findings of the TMJ and related structures. Since it is a multifactorial and complex phenomenon, Orthodontists

should, therefore, be familiar with the key features of temporomandibular disorders and be prepared to play an important role in managing these patients, especially in the areas of occlusion, temporomandibular joint and muscle function. The key to understanding temporomandibular joint disorders (TMDs) is the differential diagnosis of joint (internal derangement) as against muscle pathology (myofacial pain) or combination of the two. The location of the pain helps in diagnosis. The pain in TMDs is centred immediately in front of the tragus of the ear and projects to the ear, temple, cheek and along the mandible.

Management of pain before rehabilitation procedures can pose a formidable challenge to the clinician. Certain non-invasive procedures offer symptomatic relief to pain, however, complete elimination of these symptoms is feasible by appropriate and sequential elimination of causative factors. Diagnosing the contributing factor is imperative before initiation of irreversible treatment modalities. It is important to decide whether to reorganize the occlusion or to conform with the patient's existing intercuspal position (ICP).

Reorganizing the occlusion is not something that needs to be undertaken for many patients, as it involves deliberately changing or reconstructing the pattern of occlusal contacts.[62] The occlusal modification can be achieved by variety of methods, like selective grinding, restorative procedures, orthodontics and surgery.

Achieve a reproducible mandibular position

Orthopaedic instability of the temporomandibular joint may lead to parafunctional activities of the mandible, causing trauma to either the teeth, muscles or the joint itself. A stable and repeatable mandibular position is important as a functional goal of orthodontic treatment. Achieving optimal functional occlusion requires a careful consideration of mainly three areas of functional occlusion: centric relation, anterior guidance, and stability of posterior tooth arrangement. Orthodontics is the least invasive and most favourable, yet necessitating the requirement of precision during accomplishment of finishing phase. Good orthodontics can produce a reliable and stable occlusion. However, comprehension of prerequisite to permanently modify the occlusal scheme should be supported by evidence of trauma occurring as a result of occlusion.

Establish proper vertical dimension

It is critical to determine the vertical height at which the occlusion will be reorganized. In case of incisor attrition, the amount of space required to restore the incisor height will determine the new vertical dimension. However, in a mutilated partial dentition, an increase in vertical dimension may be required to level the occlusal plane. In clinical situations, where posterior teeth have lost height due to occlusal wear, or faulty restorations, resulting in overclosure of the mandible, the vertical dimension of occlusion may be increased by couple of millimetres. To test the patient's response to increased vertical dimension prior to definitive restorations, a stabilization splint may be used. As an alternative approach to splint therapy, composite build-ups of posterior teeth may be done, and sequentially adjusted

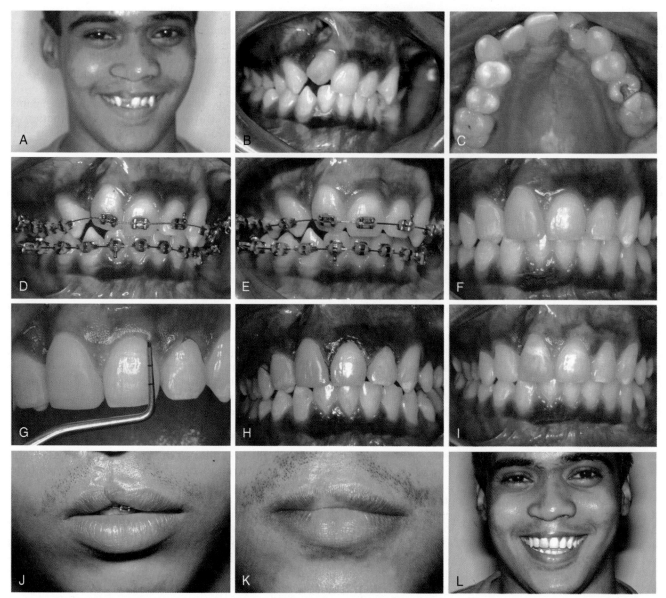

Figure 12.13 **(A)** Pretreatment extraoral features showing impaired dentofacial aesthetics and unpleasant smile due to dental asymmetry, lack of dental proportions, repaired cleft lip and nasal deformity. **(B** and **C)** Intraoral condition reveals repaired alveolar cleft between 11 and 13, apically positioned maxillary right central incisor, mesially drifted maxillary right canine, crowding of anterior teeth and palatally placed and malformed maxillary right lateral incisor. **(D** and **E)** Treatment plan included combination of ortho-restorative procedure and plastic surgery procedure. Orthodontic treatment for alignment of teeth and for improving occlusal relationships. **(F–I)** Aesthetic finishing procedures. Correction of gingival height discrepancies by forced eruption of 11 and crown lengthening of 21, 22, composite buildup of 11 and remodelling and reshaping of maxillary right cuspid and first bicuspid to look like lateral incisor and cuspid. **(J)** Residual upper lip deformity due to postsurgical scar tissue causing uneven interlabial gap. **(K)** Residual upper lip correction by plastic surgical procedure. **(L)** Post-treatment pleasant smile. Rhinoplasty will be planned at a later stage.

to a new comfortable position (Fig.12.14 H). Cores or provisional restorations may also be used for this purpose (Fig.12.14 O). This is then followed by strategically building the posterior definitive restorations to the new established dimension.

Achieving stability in intercuspal position (ICP)

When the mandible is brought into closure in the musculoskeletal stable position (CR), the posterior teeth contact evenly and simultaneously. All contacts occur between centric cusp tips and flat surfaces, directing occlusal forces through the long axes of the teeth.

During anterior excursion, the anterior teeth contact and the posterior teeth disclude. During the lateral mandibular excursive movements, cuspids are in the best position to provide the main gliding inclines, with no interferences on the balancing side. In the upright head position (alert feeding position), the posterior tooth contacts are more prominent than the anterior tooth contacts.

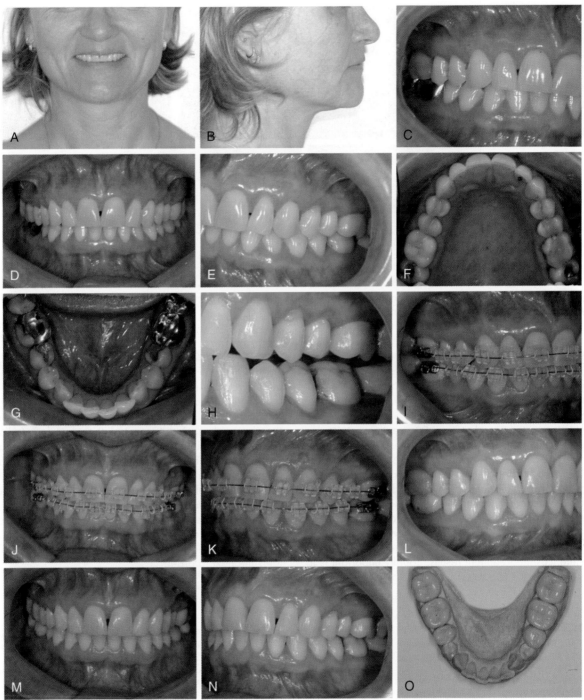

Figure 12.14 Orthorestorative treatment in unstable occlusion. A 45-year-old female patient reported with a chief complaint of pain around the dentofacial region, including the shoulders, neck and lower jaw. Inability to comfortably chew food was also a prime concern. (**A** and **B**) Pretreatment extraoral photographs. (**C–G**) Pretreatment intraoral photographs demonstrate healthy teeth and gingiva, and old posterior restorations. However, instability in occlusion existed. Lingually displaced mandibular canines, attrition of mandibular incisors, absence of canine-guided occlusion, with significant prematurities between teeth, were causing the mandible to deflect from its stable centric position. Musculoskeletal disparity was leading to bruxism, causing attrition of teeth. Therapeutic measures to diminish prematurities of teeth and restore lost tooth structure thereby reducing deleterious effects resulting from parafunctional mandibular activities were aimed for. Reduction of symptomatic pain upon use of a deprogrammer assured the necessity to modify the occlusal scheme to repeatable CR, to attain musculoskeletal stability. (**H**) The deprogrammer was replaced with composite build-ups of posterior teeth. (**I- K**) Establishment of proper anterior guidance, and maximum intercuspation to coincide with stable CR were accomplished with orthodontics. Posterior occlusal composites during orthodontic treatment allowed adjustment of vertical dimensions. Definitive height adjustments of restorations were done with intent of acquiring stable centric stops, to counter elimination of mandibular slide. (**L–N**) Post-orthodontic treatment occlusion. (**O**) Provisional posterior crowns prior to final restorations.

Continued

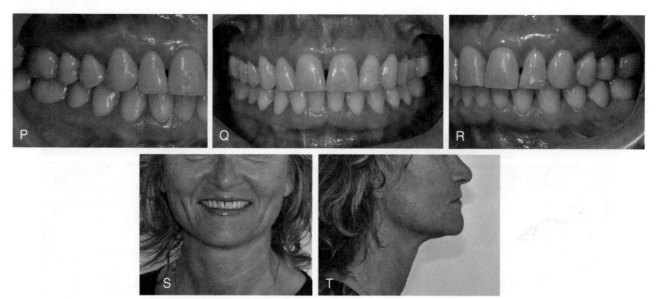

Figure 12.14, cont'd (P–R) Post-treatment occlusion. The posterior teeth were restored with all ceramic crowns as a definitive prosthesis. **(S** and **T)** Post-treatment extraoral photographs.

CONCLUSION

An interdisciplinary orthodontic therapy presents the philosophy and treatment approach that involves a group of professionals from different disciplines of dentistry into a cohesive team. It is aimed at providing treatment strategies for adult patients having multiple problems by effectively and efficiently utilizing expertise and skills of these specialists. This treatment approach is characterized by the combined diagnostic, treatment planning and therapeutic procedures with extensive communication among the treatment providers. The goal is to simplify and idealize the treatment plan by providing solutions to a variety of clinical situations, which improves the overall treatment prognosis and enhances the treatment results. Equally important is to generate some useful clinical diagnostic information from a specific treatment procedure to develop an optimal final treatment plan. For example, the preliminary periodontal therapy implemented to control the periodontal disease prior to the initiation of orthodontic treatment provides a useful information like the tissue response to the initial periodontal therapy, the level of patient compliance and the prognosis of periodontally involved teeth. The key to the management of complex dentofacial problems is to organize the sequence of various treatment procedures into a logical order so that each intervention performed by one of the specialists from the interdisciplinary team facilitates the next in order.

REFERENCES

1. Levitt HL. Modification of appliance design for the adult mutilated dentition. Int J Adult Orthod Orthognath Surg 1988; 3:9–21.
2. Musich DR. Assessment and description of the treatment needs of adult patients evaluated for Orthodontic therapy: II. Characteristics of the dual provider group. Int J Adult Ortho d Orthognath Surg 1986; 1:101–117.
3. Musich DR. Assessment and description of the treatment needs of adult patients evaluated for orthodontic therapy: III. Characteristics of the multiple provider group. Int J Adult Orthod Orthognath Surg 1986; 1:251–274.
4. Alexander RG, Sinclair PM, Goates LJ. Differential diagnosis and treatment planning for the adult nonsurgical orthodontic patient. Am J Orthod 1986; 89:95–112.
5. Lindauer SJ, Rebellato J. Bio mechanical considerations for orthodontic treatment of adults. DCNA Adult Orthodon I 1996; 40(4):811–836.
6. Roblee RD. Interdisciplinary dentofacial therapy. In: Roblee RD, ed. Interdisciplinary dentofacial therapy – a comprehensive approach to optimal patient care. Quintessence publishing: Printed in Singapore; 1994. 17–43.
7. Roblee RD. Treatment planning: phase II of IDT. In: Roblee RD, ed. Interdisciplinary Dentofacial therapy – a comprehensive approach to optimal patient care. Quintessence publishing: Printed in Singapore; 1994. 77–99.
8. Proffit WR, Fields HW. Orthodontic treatment planning:from problem list to final plan. In: Proffit WR, ed. Contemporary orthodontics. 2nd edn. St Louis: Mosby; 1992. 186–224.
9. Kokich V, Spear F. Guidelines for managing the orthodontic–restorative patient. Semin Orthod 1997; 3:3–20.
10. Spear FM, Kokich VG, Mathews DP. Interdisciplinary management of a patient with a skeletal deformity. Adv Esthetic interdiscip dentistry 2005; 1(2):12–18.
11. Boyd RL. Mucogingival considerations and their relationship to orthodontics. J Periodontol 1978; 49:67–76.
12. Geiger AM. Mucogingival problems and the movement of mandibular incisors. Am J Orthod 1980; 78:511–527.
13. Engelking G, Zachrisson BU. Effects of incisor repositioningon the monkey periodontium after expansion through the cortical plate. Am J Orthod 1982; 83:23–32.
14. Baldinger J, Chung C-H, Vanarsdall R. The presence of periopathogenic organisms in crowded versus aligned teeth in the anterior adult dentition, Thesis, Philadelphia, June 1998, University of Pennsylvania.
15. Bjornaas T, Rygh P, Boe OE. Severe overjet and overbite reduced alveolar bone height in 19-year old men. Am J Orthod Dentofac Orthop 1994; 106:139.
16. Ericsson I, Thilander B. Orthodontic forces and recurrence of periodontal disease. Am J Orthod 1978; 71:41–50.
17. Ericsson I, Thilander B, Lindhe J, et al. The effect of Orthodontic tilting movements in the periodontal tissue of infected and

non-infected dentitions in dogs. J Clin Periodontol 1977; 4: 278–293.

18. Greenstein G, Canton J, Polson AM. Histologic characteristics associated with bleeding after probing and visual signs of inflammation. J Periodontol 1981; 52:420–425.

19. Brown IS. The effect of orthodontic therapy on certain types of periodontal defects. J Periodontol 1973; 44:742–756.

20. Caffesse RG, Sweeney PL, Smith BA. Scaling and root planing with and without periodontal flap surgery. J Clin Periodontol 1986; 13:205–210.

21. Crum RE, Anderson GF. The effect of gingival fiber surgery on the retention of rotated teeth. Am J Orthod 1974; 65:626–637.

22. Wilson TG. Supportive periodontal treatment for patients with inflammatory periodontal diseases. In: Wilson TG, Korman KS, Newman MG, eds. Advances in periodontics. Chicago: Quintessence publishing; 1992. 195–204.

23. Zachrisson BB. Cause and prevention of injuries to teeth and supporting structures during orthodontic treatment. Am J Orthod 1976; 69:285–300.

24. Yeung SC, Howell S, Fahey P. Oral hygiene programs for orthodontic patients. Am J Orthod 1989; 96:208–213.

25. Boyd RL, Murray P, Robertson PB. Effect of rotary electric toothbrush on periodontal status during orthodontic treatment. Am J Orthod Dentofac Orthop 1989; 96:342–347.

26. Geiger AM, Gorelick L, Gwinnett AJ, et al. Reducing white spot lesions in orthodontic populations with fluoride rinsing. Am J Orthod Dentofac Orthop 1992; 101:403–407.

27. Brightman LJ, Terezhalmy GT, Greenwell H, et al. The effects of a 0.12% chlorhexidine gulconate mouth rinse on orthodontic patients aged 11 through 17 with established gingivitis. Am J Orthod Dentofac Orthop 1991; 100:324–329.

28. Goering AC, Neaverth EJ. Case selection and treatment planning. In: Cohen S, Burns RC, eds. Pathways of the pulp. 5th edn. St Louis: Mosby; 1991. 48–60.

29. Glickman GN, Schwartz SF. Preparation for treatment. In: Cohen S, Burns RC, eds. Pathways of the pulp. 5th edn. St Louis: Mosby; 1991. 61–93.

30. Spitzer D, Kastenbaum F, Wagenberg B. Achieving ideal esthetic in osseointegrated prosthetics. Part II: the single unit. Int J Periodont Rest Dent 1992; 12:501–507.

31. Kasterbaum F. Achieving ideal esthetic in osseointegrated prosthesis. Part I: multiple units. Int J Periodont Rest Dent 1992; 12:153–159.

32. Kokich V. Comprehensive management of implant anchorage in the multidisciplinary patient. In: Hiiguchi K, ed. Orthodontic application of osseointegrated implants. Chicago: Quintessence publishing; 2000. 21–32.

33. Smithloff M, Fritz ME. The use of blade implants in a selected population of partially edentulous adults: a ten-year report. J Periodontol 1982; 53:413–418.

34. Adell R, Lekholm U, Rockler B, et al. A15-year study of osseointegrated implants in the treatment of the edentulous jaw. Int J Oral Surg 1981; 10:387–416.

35. Piatelli A, Corigliano M, Scarano A, et al. Immediate loading of titanium plasma – sprayed implants: an histologic analysis in monkeys. J Periodontol 1998; 69:321–327.

36. Duyck J, Rønold HJ, Van Oosterwyck H, et al. The influence of static and dynamic loading on marginal bone reactions around osseointegrated implants: an animal experimental study. Clin Oral Implants Res 2001; 12:207–218.

37. Lazzara R. Implant placement into extraction sites: Surgical and restorative advantages. Int J Periodont Res Dent 1989; 9(5):332–343.

38. Geraci TF. Orthodontic movements of teeth into artificially produced infrabony defects in the rhesus monkey: a histological report. J Periodontol 1973; 44:116.

39. Moyers RE. Handbook of orthodontics. 4th edn. Chicago: Year Book Medical Publishers; 1988.

40. Brown S. The effects of orthodontic therapy on certain types of periodontal defects: I. Clinical findings. J Periodont 1973; 44:742–756.

41. Diedrich P, Erpenstein H. Die Distalisierung endständiger Prämolaren zur vermeidung von freiendsätteln. Dtsch Zahnärztl Z 1984; 39:644–649.

42. Vanarsdall RL. Correction of periodontal problems through orthodontic treatment. In: Hos E, Baldauf A, Diernberger R, et al., eds. Orthodontics and periodontics. Chicago: Quintessence publishing; 1985; 127–167.

43. Diedrich P, Fuhrmann RAW, Wehrbein H, et al. Distal movement of premolars to provide posterior abutments for missing molars. Am J Orthod Dentofac Orthop 1996; 109:355–360.

44. Spear F, Mathews D, Kokich VG. Interdisciplinary management of single-tooth implants. Semin Orthod 1997; 3:45–72.

45. Lombard RE. The principles of visual perception and their clinical application to denture esthetic. J Prosthet Dent 1973; 29: 358–382.

46. Freeman JE, Maskeroni AJ, Lorton I. Frequency of Bolton tooth-size discrepancies among orthodontic patients. Am J Orthod Dentofacial Orthop 1996; 110:24–27.

47. Bolton WA. Disharmony in tooth size and its relation to the analysis and treatment of malocclusion. Angle Orthod 1958; 28:113–130.

48. McNeil RW, Joondeph DR. Congenitally absent maxillary lateral incisors: treatment planning considerations. Angle Orthod 1973; 43:24–29.

49. Saadun AP, LeGall M, Touati B. Current trends in implantology: Part II – treatment planning and tissue regeneration. Pract Periodontics Aesthet Dent 2004; 16:707–714.

50. Kinzer GA, Kokich VO. Managing congenitally missing lateral incisors. Part III: single-tooth implants. J Esthet Restor Dent 2005; 17:202–210.

51. Carlsson GE, Bergman B, Hedegard B. Changes in contour in the upper alveolar process under immediate dentures: A longitudinal clinical and x-ray cephalometric study covering 5 years. Acta Odont Scand 1967; 25(1):45–75.

52. Vig R, Brundo G. The kinetics of anterior tooth display. J Prosthet Dent 1978; 39:502–504.

53. Vincent KG. Esthetic: the orthodontic–periodontic restorative connection. Semin Orthod 1996; 2:21–30.

54. Garguilo A, Wenz F, Orban B. Dimensions and relation at the dentogingival junction in humans. J Periodontol 1961; 32:261–267.

55. Maynard J, Wilson R. Physiologic dimension of the periodontium fundamental to successful restorative dentistry. J Periodontol 1979; 50:170–174.

56. Prichard J. Gingivectomy, gingivoplasty, and osseous surgery. J Periodontol 1961; 32:257–262.

57. Kokich VG. Anterior dental esthetic: an orthodontic perspective. I. Crown length. J Esthet Dent 1993; 5:19–23.

58. Karad A. Excellence in finishing: current concepts, goals and mechanics. J Ind Orthod Soc 2006; 39:126–138.

59. Rufenacht CR. Fundamentals of esthetic. Chicago: Quintessence publishing; 1990:124–127.

60. McCullock AJ. Making Occlusion Work: I.Terminology, Occlusal Assessment and Recording. Dent Update 2003; 30: 150–157.

61. McNeill C. Management of temporomandibular disorders: concepts and controversies. J Prosthet Dent 1991;77:510–522.

62. Robert Wassell, Amar Naru, Jimmy Steele, Francis Nohl. Reorganizing the occlusion. In: Applied occlusion, Prosthodontics-5, Ed. Nairn H F Wilson. Quintessence Publishing Co. Ltd., London. 2008: 31–48.

Functional Occlusion Goals in Orthodontics

Kazumi Ikeda

More than 100 years have elapsed since modern orthodontics gathered momentum under the leadership of Edward H Angle.[1] Has his theory that good function and facial aesthetics would automatically follow, if the patient bites into Class I ever been validated?[2] Angle's concept is still widely accepted as truth without ever having been questioned. Is it true that function improves automatically, if the teeth are aligned within the dental arches with the molars in Angle Class I?[3] Is there a body of evidence in the literature demonstrating that orthodontic treatment based on the Angle philosophy will always result in functional improvement?[4,5] The teeth will certainly be straighter and aesthetically more pleasing with treatment, but we must pay closer attention to functional aspects of occlusion and question ourselves, if function has really been enhanced and maintained as a result of treatment. While there have been remarkable advancements in orthodontic appliances and materials since the days of Edward H Angle, basic principles of orthodontic diagnosis and treatment have remained relatively unchanged. Should mere straightening of all teeth in the mouth automatically lead to the establishment and maintenance of good function? Why are so many patients

seeking retreatment? Something seems to be missing here. In the author's view, it is the awareness of treatment goals in terms of functional occlusion that is lacking in the orthodontist's mind.[6] We have no clearly defined goals with clear-cut criteria as to what needs to be done for each patient we treat. If orthodontic procedures are meant to be therapeutic rather than simply cosmetic, the post-treatment health of the patient's stomatognathic system should be improved with lasting effect.[7,8] Can we really expect long-term stability of the post orthodontic result with traditional methods of diagnosis and treatment? Unfortunately, the answer to this question is negative. Treatment focusing only on the alignment of teeth and improvement of form often fails to attain functional improvement, let alone consistently achieve long-term stability, though one may get lucky every once in a great while. Orthodontists throughout the world are still making diagnoses and treating patients in a manner similar to our predecessors in Angle's days whose orthodontic goal was simply to align teeth. The time has come for us as professionals to seriously reflect upon orthodontic goals for good functional occlusion. If we fail to do so, orthodontics would be left behind without further progress except for the development of new appliances and materials. This chapter describes the concept that will help us improve the function and form of the dentition through goal-directed treatment.

GOALS OF ORTHODONTICS FOR OCCLUSION

The orthodontic treatment goal in terms of function is to create the occlusion that allows the upper and lower teeth to come into maximum intercuspation, while condyles are positioned such that there is minimal strain on the muscles of mastication. At the same time, the position of the teeth should be in harmony with the face, lips, tongue and periodontium (Fig. 13.1).

In a normally developing temporomandibular joint (TMJ), the basic structures comprising the joint—namely the disc, condyle and eminence—are intimately related to one another. By age of about 10 years, the eminence will have sufficient height to disclude the posterior teeth in mandibular movements.[9] The child has a mixed dentition at this age, and it will take a few more years before the permanent dentition is complete from second molar to second molar. In the meantime, the first permanent molars and deciduous molars provide posterior support. Anterior guidance[10] has not yet been established. Lateral movement is guided mostly by the permanent incisors or deciduous canines or by the deciduous molars and first permanent molars in some situations.

As a starting point for orthodontic tooth movement, we should first aim at achieving proper positioning of the condyles in the fossae where there is minimum masticatory muscle activity, followed by the provision of posterior support and proper alignment of the anterior teeth that guide protrusive and lateral movements. When this relationship between the occlusion and the joints is established, the efficiency of the masticatory muscles can be maximized without an increase in muscle tension.[11] The clinical significance of orthodontics thus lies in the establishment of a harmonious relationship between the joints and the occlusion that does not require excessive muscle

tension. Once the harmony has been achieved, orthodontic treatment results will remain stable (Fig. 13.2).

No dentist seems to argue against the importance of optimum condylar position as the basis of functional occlusion,[12–14] yet this fundamental principle of dentistry is not clearly defined and often disregarded in our current clinical practice. Use of traditional orthodontic records for diagnosis does not allow us to determine, if the patient's existing mandibular position is appropriate or not. These records contain no objective data to show discrepancies in the joints. Hand-held models, for example, provide no information on mandibular position and provide no indication about where condyles are positioned in the fossae. The same is true for lateral cephalograms, which is a two-dimensional representation of three-dimensional anatomical structures, such as the joints derived from mere addition of the left and right and divided by two. Then, how can we capture data on mandibular position? Knowing the answer to this question would help to enhance the quality of our clinical practice.

MANDIBULAR POSITION AS A FUNCTIONAL GOAL OF ORTHODONTIC TREATMENT

A stable and repeatable mandibular position is important as a functional goal of orthodontic treatment. Without this functional goal, teeth may appear nice and straight in the mouth, but the tooth alignment thus obtained would not last long and may even do harm to the gnathic system. The following five requirements must be fulfilled to achieve this stable and repeatable mandibular position:

1. Discs are correctly positioned on the condyles (Fig. 13.3).
2. Condyle, disc and eminence are intimately related with close contact.
3. There is no looseness in the collateral ligaments fixing the disc directly to the lateral and medial poles of the condyle, no distention of the joint capsule or no joint effusion.

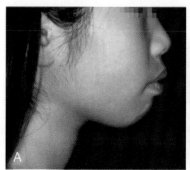
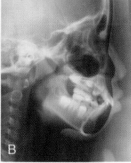
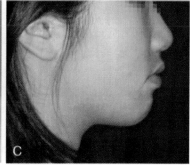
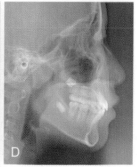

Figure 13.1 (**A** and **B**) Before orthodontic treatment. (**C** and **D**) After orthodontic treatment. Post-treatment facial profile is in harmony with tooth alignment, and perioral muscles are naturally relaxed. Condylar position was stabilized before initiating tooth movement. Careful tooth movement and counterclockwise mandibular growth allowed the chin to come forward without an increase in lower facial height, providing good function and facial harmony, which resulted in relaxed muscles and stable tooth position.

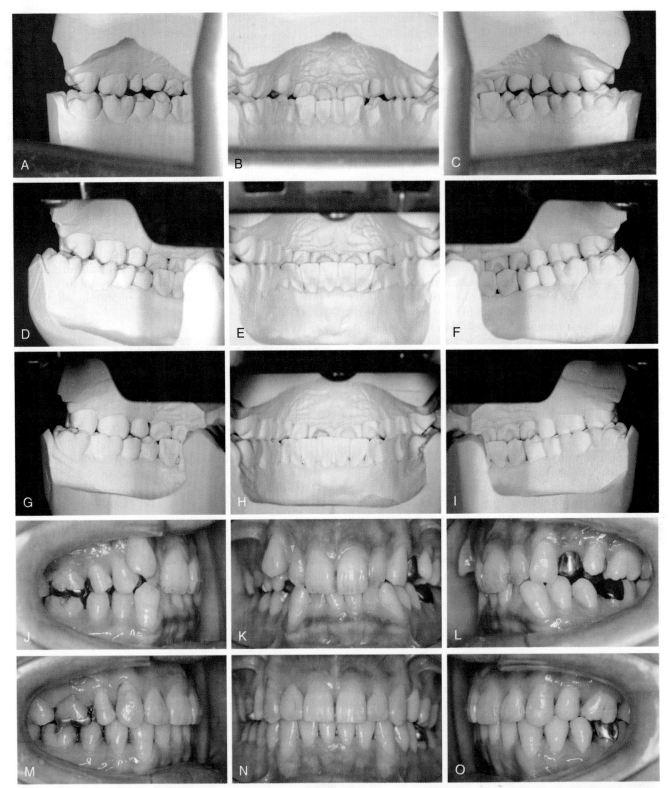

Figure 13.2   15 years out of treatment. Establishment of functional occlusion through maximum intercuspation of posterior teeth, adequate anterior coupling and canine guidance seems to have contributed greatly to the post-treatment stability. (**A–C**) Lingual views of initial mounted models. (**D–F**) Lingual views of post-treatment mounted models. (**G–I**) Occlusion remains stable, 15 years out of treatment. (**J–L**) Pretreatment labial and buccal views. (**M–O**) Post-treatment labial and buccal views.

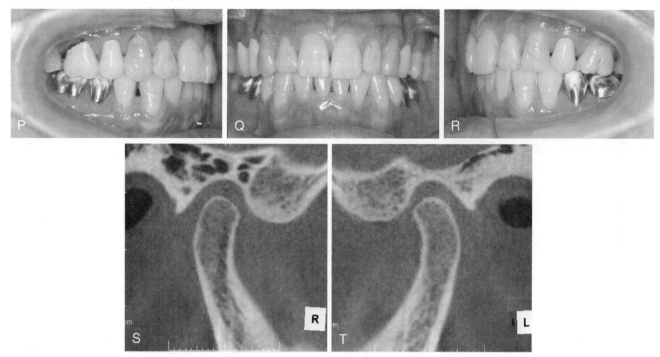

Figure 13.2, cont'd (**P–R**) Labial and buccal views, 15 years after treatment. (**S** and **T**) The cone-beam computed tomography (CBCT) images of the right and left joints, 15 years after treatment, show well-rounded functional articular surfaces, normal position of the condyles relative to the fossae and eminentia and well-preserved bone structures.

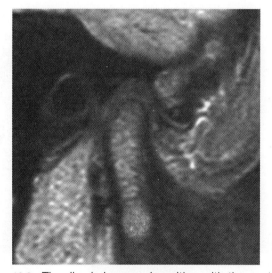

Figure 13.3 The disc is in normal position with the posterior band at 12 O'clock and the intermediate zone interposed intimately between the eminence and condyle.

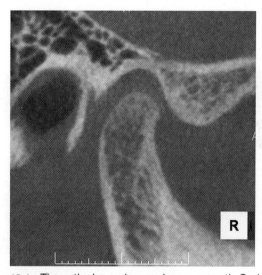

Figure 13.4 The articular eminence has a smooth S-shaped curve. The condyle also has a rounded surface and is in normal position within the fossa.

4. Condyles are seated at the superior most position in relation to the fossae (Fig. 13.4).
5. In the frontal plane, the condyles are centred in the fossae without medial or lateral deviation (Fig. 13.5).

A stable and repeatable mandibular position requires the disc to be optimally placed on the condyle in close contact with the eminence without capsular or ligamentous laxity or excess synovial fluid. When these requirements are met, the condyles are seated against the discs at the most superior-anterior position against

the eminentia, leading to a stable position of the condyles in the fossae.

Condylar position then becomes repeatable with the condyles always returning to the same position. This is illustrated with the MRI images of the movement of the condyle–disc assembly in Figure 13.6. At the start of opening, the condyle is situated against the intermediate zone of the disc at the most superior position in the fossa in close contact with the eminence. Upon opening, the condyle begins to rotate and translate as it goes down the slope of the eminence without losing the close contact with the

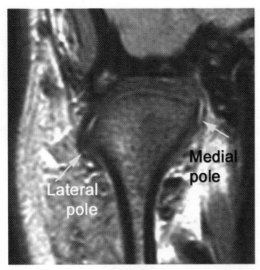

Figure 13.5 This coronal magnetic resonance imaging (MRI) of a right TMJ shows no lateral or medial shift of the disc. The condyle is also centred mediolaterally within the fossa.

eminence via the intermediate zone of the disc. In closing, the condyle follows the identical reciprocal path to return to the starting position. The movement is thus repeatable.

When the teeth close into maximum intercuspation with the condyle and disc seated at the most superior position in the fossa, that is, when there is harmony between the occlusion and the joints—the associated muscles are so relaxed that bite registration becomes very easy. However, this is rarely the case when we examine our orthodontic patients, both adults and children, at their initial visits. It is important to realize that a majority of our patients have varying degrees of disc displacement. These patients naturally have strained masticatory and perioral muscles, necessitating very careful registration of mandibular position at the time of initial examination.

JOINTS FIRST

If we are to establish the harmony between occlusion and joints, which should we look at first when examining our patients, the occlusion or the joints? The answer is 'the joints first'. The status of the joints should be closely examined before intraoral examination of occlusal relationship. Traditionally, orthodontists have attached importance to the way the upper and lower teeth fit together in the mouth and assumed that the joints would adapt to the occlusion. Are the joints always so pliable? With the advent of advanced imaging modalities, such as CBCT and MRI, we are now able to visualize the joint structures more precisely. Accumulating data suggest that the joints may not be so adaptable. Three postorthodontic cases are shown to illustrate this point.

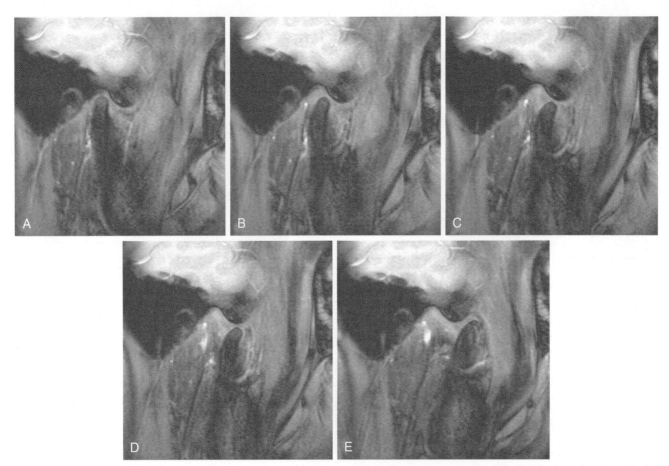

Figure 13.6 **(A–E)** Every cut from this MRI movie of condylar movement from centric occlusion (CO; habitual occlusal position) to maximum opening demonstrates the stable spatial relationship between the condyle and the eminence throughout the movement.

The first case is a male patient treated at the author's office and is out of treatment for 7 years (Fig. 13.7). He was 13 years old at his initial visit, his masticatory muscles were very tight, making bite registration difficult. He was also experiencing frequent headaches. He was, therefore, placed on a stabilization splint (hereinafter referred to *Splint)* in order to stabilize his mandibular position, prior to orthodontic treatment. The direction and amount of tooth movements were determined based on the results of the rediagnosis made in the stabilized mandibular position. The second case is a patient treated elsewhere, 2 years prior to coming to the author's office with parents for consultation because of unstable orthodontic results (Fig. 13.8). The previous orthodontic treatment did some good in that the teeth were well aligned. However, the imaging of the joints revealed hidden discrepancies.

Case 2 had a problem with the position of the condyles in the fossae. The condyles were significantly displaced inferiorly with the loss of intimate relationship between the condyle, disc and eminence. The shape of the condyles had also been greatly altered along with a decrease in size, precluding normal condylar movement. In Case 1, the condyle–disc–eminence relationship has been maintained with optimum condylar morphology and position in the fossae, allowing for normal function.

At the tooth level, Case 1 has adequate coupling of the anterior teeth and good canine guidance for lateral movement. The buccal cusps of the mandibular posterior teeth are either on the marginal ridges or in the central fossae of the upper posterior teeth. In contrast, Case 2 lacks in both anterior guidance for protrusive movement and canine guidance for lateral movement due to inadequate overbite. Case 2 also lacks stable posterior support.

What was the orthodontist's treatment goal for Case 2? Without harmony between the occlusion and the joints, we cannot expect long-term stability of the post orthodontic treatment result. The patient will most likely be subjected to muscle strain, tooth mobility and occlusal wear.

Case 3 is also a post orthodontic patient, 3 years out of treatment (Figs 13.9–13.12). The patient, being a dentist herself, was aware of functional problems with a complaint of muscle fatigue from chewing. Her bite changed within a single day with full-time splint wear. How can we explain the changes? Solely based on what we see in the mouth, we cannot explain this phenomenon. Even if we could relate the intraoral changes to changes in condylar position, there is

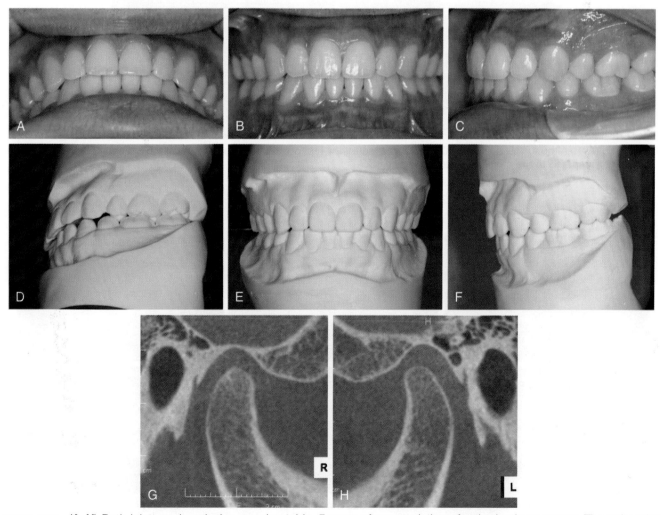

Figure 13.7 **(A–H)** Both joints and occlusion remain stable, 7 years after completion of orthodontic treatment. The trabecular bone of the articular structures exhibits a functional pattern outlined with uninterrupted cortication.

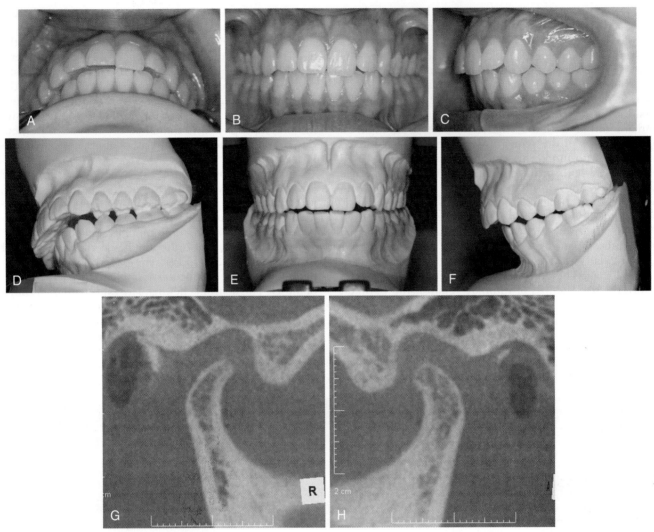

Figure 13.8 (**A–H**) Although teeth are still aligned, 2 years after the first orthodontic treatment, unstable bite and poor joint health are evident compared to the case presented in Figure 13.7.

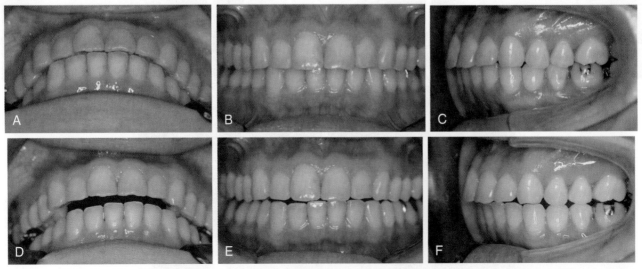

Figure 13.9 (**A–F**) The bite changed after 24 h of splint wear. Since it is inconceivable that the teeth moved with only 1 day of splint use, the bite change can be attributed to changes at the joint level.

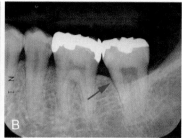

Figure 13.10 (**A** and **B**) Periapical radiograph of the patient's lower left second molar. The PDL space is widened (arrow), indicating increased tooth mobility. Localized gingival recession (arrow) around the same tooth and tooth wear on canine cusp are also evident intraorally.

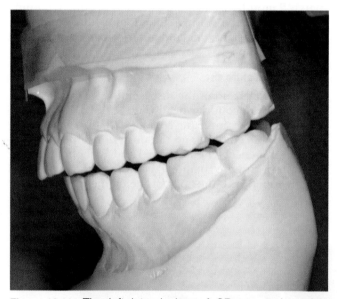

Figure 13.11 The left lateral view of CR-mounted models taken at initial visit reveals a premature contact on the lower left second molar. When performed properly, CR mounting may uncover what cannot be seen intraorally.

no way of knowing in which direction and to what extent the condyles moved in the three planes of space. This case, like Case 2, had well-aligned teeth and could bring the teeth into intercuspation. Both cases would be considered well-treated cases in traditional orthodontics. In reality, however, they had major discrepancies hidden in the joints, were suffering from masticatory fatigue and had adverse effects on the muscles, teeth and periodontium. Their gnathic systems were not functioning in an ideal manner. Figure 13.10 shows a periapical radiograph of the second molar on the lower left side with widened periodontal ligament (PDL) space, indicating occlusal trauma. The tooth also had pathological mobility and gingival recession. The intraoral photograph taken after full-time splint wear reveals a premature contact between the upper and lower second molars on the left side. However, prematurity could not be found in the mouth at her initial visit. Figure 13.11 shows the patient's initial models mounted in centric relation (CR). Her initial CR bite was taken with wax and the models were mounted on an articulator using the CR bite. It was possible to capture the premature contact at the left second molars on the initial CR-mounted models, while the prematurity was completely hidden in the

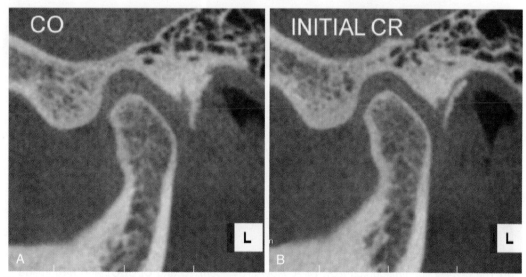

Figure 13.12 (**A** and **B**) The condyle is positioned noticeably more forward and upward in CR bite (**B**) relative to CO bite (**A**), indicating that CR bite allows anterosuperior seating of the condyle.

patient's mouth. This phenomenon is caused by the neuro-muscular protective mechanism. The hidden contact cannot be found during initial examination unless the models are mounted using a CR bite carefully taken while avoiding any tooth contact between the upper and lower teeth.

The recent advent of CBCT allows direct visualization of the CO-CR discrepancies in the joints for this case (Fig. 13.12). These images were taken upon patient consent with her initial CR bite in place, showing that the use of a carefully taken initial CR bite enables us to visualize and even quantify superior-anterior seating of the condyles in the fossae. We can also see CO-CR discrepancies in the joints by comparing CBCT images taken in the two different positions. CBCT images thus demonstrate through the visualization of the joint structures that the use of a properly taken CR bite allows the condyles to seat superiorly and anteriorly in the fossae.

More than 99% of orthodontists seem to make diagnoses and assess postorthodontic results solely based on what they see in the mouth as in Cases 2 and 3. We should not believe what we see in the mouth before confirming the condylar position. The author uses the records shown in Figures 13.11 and 13.12 to make a diagnosis, since his orthodontic goal is to attain harmony of the occlusion with the dictates of the joints, which is different from the traditional orthodontic goal of aligning teeth. To pursue this goal, it is essential to first examine the joints, hence 'the joints first'.

ANATOMY OF THE TEMPOROMANDIBULAR JOINTS

Disc

Structure of the disc

The disc, which mainly consists of dense collagen fibres without any innervation or vascularization, is divided into the anterior band, intermediate zone and posterior band. The intermediate zone, in particular, is a good shock absorber with collagen fibres oriented predominantly in anteroposterior (PA) direction. The disc of a newborn is biplanar in shape with all three sections equal in thickness but soon becomes biconcave, in approximately 2 months, as the joint start to function. According to Hansson,[15] the normal functioning disc's posterior band, intermediate zone and anterior band are 3, 1 and 2 mm in thickness, respectively.

Normal position of the disc

The posterior band of the disc is at the 12 O'clock position relative to condylar head (Fig. 13.13). The intermediate zone is in intimate contact with the articulating surface of the condyle and the posterior slope of the articular eminence. The anterior band is slightly inferior and anterior to the rotational centre of the condyle and slightly superior to the apex of the eminence.

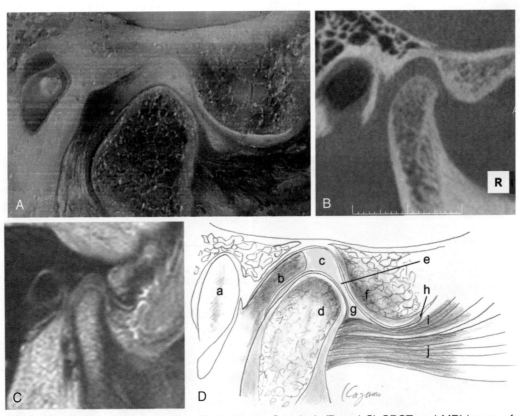

Figure 13.13 **(A)** The cryosection *(Image courtesy: Dr A. Isberg, Sweden)*, **(B** and **C)** CBCT and MRI image of same patient. **(D)** Illustration depicts normal joints: a, auditory canal; b, posterior disc attachment; c, posterior band; d, condylar head of mandible; e, intermediate zone; f, articular eminence; g, anterior band; h, anterior limit of capsular insertion; i, superior head of lateral pterygoid muscle; and j, inferior head of lateral pterygoid muscle.

Roles of the disc

The disc has two main roles. The first role of the disc is to stabilize the condyle in the fossa with the assistance of associated ligaments and muscles. The posterior band of the disc, being at the 12 O'clock position in a normal joint, serves as a good indicator for the most superior position of the condyle during mouth closure. This disc–condyle relationship makes the terminal hinge axis (THA) stable and repeatable. The second role of the disc is to distribute the load applied to the articulating surfaces of the condyle and eminence during mandibular function by interposing between the two structures. The presence of just enough synovial fluid outlining the joint surfaces also serves as a lubricant to allow smooth movement of the condyle. The disc contributes to the maintenance of anatomical configuration of the condyle and eminence by preventing excessive loading to these structures. The position and function of the disc thus have major impact on mandibular structural development in growing children by providing the optimum force on the cartilage at the growing aspect of the bone.

Key factors necessary for stability of the disc

- Harmony between tooth alignment and the joints
- Healthy ligaments and capsules
- Relaxed muscles
- Presence of an appropriate amount of synovial fluid
- An adequate, neither excessive nor insufficient, amount of load

Reversibility

Positive remodelling of the condyle and eminence is routinely observed on CBCT images as mandibular position becomes stabilized even in cases of disc displacement without reduction. These positive morphological changes may be accompanied with improvements in disc position in some patients with early to moderate disc displacement. The amount of synovial fluid is normalized at the same time (Fig. 13.14).

Condyle

Structure of the condyle

The condyle is covered with dense connective tissue similar to periosteum. Underneath this covering is an undifferentiated mesenchymal cell layer. Under this layer, there is a cartilaginous layer with chondrocytes.[16] The cartilage here is called secondary cartilage, which is different in nature from the cartilage in the growth centre of a long bone in that its proliferation depends on the surrounding environment rather than the growth hormones.[17] Its proliferative capacity is retained through adulthood, allowing the condyle to adapt to environmental changes. The bone is formed through ossification of this cartilage. The undifferentiated mesenchymal cell layer remains until an advanced age, although its thickness decreases after the end of growth.[18] It contributes to chondrocyte proliferation, if such a need arises (Fig. 13.15).

Factors causing condylar deformity

- Trauma, such as accidents or major surgical trauma of orthognathic procedures[19] and repetitive minor trauma of bruxism and other parafunctional habits.
- Disc displacement, particularly the displacement without reduction and some degree from early stages of disc displacement.
- Systemic conditions, such as rheumatoid arthritis.

Reversibility

The intact fibrous covering of the condyle permits positive remodelling of the condyle even in adults. The shape of the condyle can be improved when aetiological factors of condylar deformity are removed[20] (Fig. 13.16).

Eminence

Structure of the eminence

The eminence basically has the same structure as the condyle. When the condyle undergoes negative remodelling or resorption in response to a factor causing joint instability, the eminence is also subjected to more or less similar changes. Conversely, when mandibular position is stabilized, positive remodelling is observed in the eminence and in the condyle.

Normal configuration of the eminence

The articular eminence is a convex area of the articulated surface of the temporal bone with a gentle and

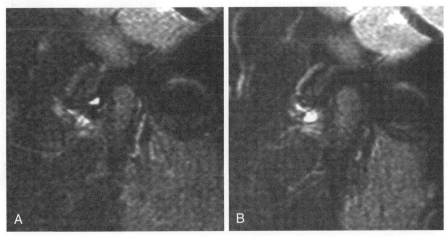

Figure 13.14 (**A** and **B**) The disc was recaptured with stabilization splint therapy in this teenage patient. The T2-weighted MRI illustrates decreased joint effusion (**B**), suggesting close association between disc displacement and joint effusion.

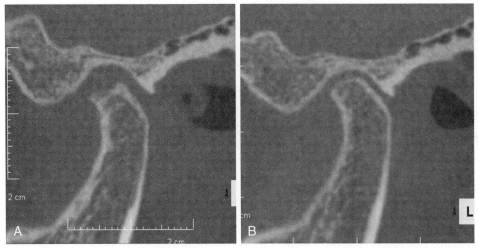

Figure 13.15 **(A)** Splint therapy was initiated in this 69-year-old female patient presenting with pain in the left joint. **(B)** This image shows her joint status, 1 year after 6 months of splint therapy. She has been free of TMJ pain since splint therapy.

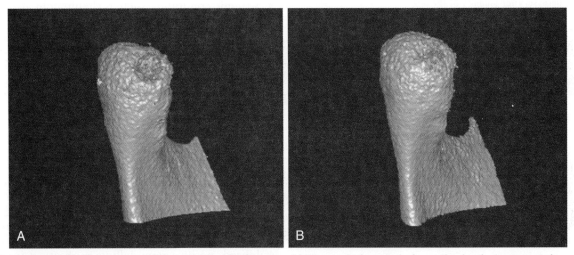

Figure 13.16 **(A and B)** Comparison of the condyle of a 31-year-old woman before and after orthodontic treatment demonstrates positive remodelling or restoration of the major bone defect that was present initially on the posterior surface. Orthodontic mechanics was designed to minimize stress to the joints, so that post-treatment CO-CR discrepancy could be kept to a minimum.

smooth S-shaped curve and a thin cortical outline. The more superior the condyle is positioned in the fossa, the steeper the slope of the eminence becomes. This facilitates the disclusion of the posterior teeth in mandibular movements.

The anterior limit of the joint is determined by the insertion of the capsular attachment (Fig. 13.17).

Factors causing morphological changes of the eminence

- Overloading, e.g. parafunctional habits, such as bruxism
- Disc displacement without reduction
- Systemic condition of rheumatoid arthritis

Reversibility

When appropriately loaded, the eminence will undergo positive remodelling as is the case with the condyle (Fig. 13.18).

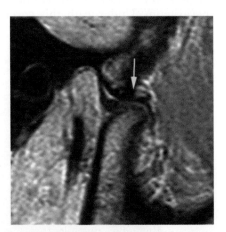

Figure 13.17 MRI of a normal joint at maximum opening. The arrow indicates the insertion of capsular attachment at the anterior limit of condylar movement. Excessive condylar movement beyond this limit is called *hypermobility* or *loose joint*, which is often associated with disc displacement.

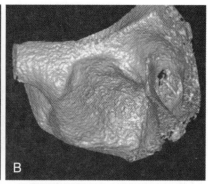

Figure 13.18 (**A** and **B**) Comparison of the articular fossa of a 49-year-old man before (**A**) and after splint therapy (**B**). Positive remodelling of the fossa, eminence and condyle is seen after splint therapy.

OPTIMUM CONDYLAR POSITION

History of optimum condylar position

The concept of concentric condylar position proposed by Weinberg[21] and others was dominant until the 1970s. In the 1980s, Pullinger et al showed variations in condylar position; 50% in the centre and the rest equally divided between anterior and posterior positions with the proportion of anterior position being slightly higher.[22] This concept of variations in condylar position still prevails today. Faced with variations, one would naturally wonder where the optimal position of the condyle is in the fossa. Diagnostic criteria are needed to answer this question. The current concept of condylar position takes only the PA dimension into account and disregards the vertical aspect. In the field of orthodontics, Ricketts[23] produced data on a normal position of the condyle from the measurements made on laminographs in the 1960s. However, his data showed large variations ranging from 1.0 to 4.0 mm (mean of 2.5 mm) for superior space and from 0.5 to 2.5 mm (mean of 1.5 mm) for anterior space. His study sample included not only subjects with normal Class I occlusion but also a few Class II and Class III cases. Another problem was that the orientation of joint sections was not calibrated according to the long axis of condyle.

Optimum condylar position

The next question that may arise is whether individuals with optimum jaw function and intact discs also show variations in condylar position. Again, we need some criteria for optimum condylar position to find an answer to this question.

In conducting a study to identify optimum condylar position, the sample must be carefully selected. The inclusion criterion of having no TMJ symptom alone would not suffice, since MRI studies have found that nearly 30% of asymptomatic individuals have disc displacements.[24,25] Based on this number, it is possible that the so-called 'normal' samples of previous studies on optimum condylar position contained asymptomatic subjects with disc displacement. Since the position of the condyle in the fossa is influenced by disc position, a study conducted in a heterogeneous sample in terms of disc status would naturally show greater variations in condylar position with larger standard deviations (SDs).

The author's group conducted a study on optimum condylar position on a carefully selected sample. Not only the absence of disc displacement but also the shape of the disc was confirmed on MRI images. Subjects with good disc position but hypertrophic or altered disc configuration were excluded. CBCT was used to identify any osseous change in the structures of the TMJ. Mandibular border movements, i.e. lateral, protrusive and opening movements, were recorded to ensure that the subjects had no disharmony in any of these movements. Joint laxity was limited to maximum 1 mm of immediate side shift. Muscle tension was checked on facial photographs and with palpation. CO-CR discrepancies measured at the joint level using condylar position indicator (CPI) had to be 1 mm or less in the sagittal plane and 0.5 mm or less in the transverse plane.[26] The study included 24 joints of 22 subjects in adolescence to early adulthood with a mean age of 18 years who met all these inclusion criteria. Figure 13.19 shows the data obtained from the study.[27]

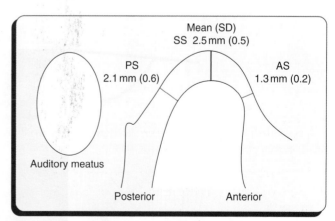

Figure 13.19 Diagram illustrates optimum position of the condyle in the fossa. A few studies have previously evaluated disc position on MRI, and many studies have defined asymptomatic joints as normal joints, leading to wide variations in normal condylar position. A study on a carefully selected sample[27] showed anterosuperior position of the condyles in normal joints with much smaller SDs.

Major study findings:

- No gender difference
- Far smaller SDs than in previously conducted similar studies
- Smallest SD of ±0.2 mm for anterior space, indicating that there is little variation in the amount of space between the condyle and eminence with intimate contact between the two joint structures via the intermediate zone of the disc in the subjects with normal disc position who met all the above-mentioned criteria.

JAW MOVEMENT RECORDINGS

Posselt[28] extensively discusses mandibular movement in his textbook *The Philosophy of Occlusion and Rehabilitation*. The Posselt envelope of mandibular motion recorded at incisor point is well known. Lundeen and Gibbs[29] carried out detailed studies on condylar motion and published their results in 1978. Robert L Lee[30] created fossa boxes that reproduced condylar movements in three dimensions based on these results and developed a simple but clinically useful semi-adjustable articulator by incorporating these fossa boxes to enable the clinician to study the patient's occlusion while reproducing the jaw movements. Lee also devised an instrument to measure CO-CR discrepancies in three planes of space at the level of the joints rather than at the tooth level. Another device that measures mandibular movements at the joint level was developed. With this device, condylar movements, particularly border movements, can be recorded and measured three-dimensionally and transferred to an articulator using the patient's THA, allowing construction of occlusal surfaces in harmony with jaw movement, as well as diagnosis of occlusion and joint function.

Research by Lundeen and Gibbs[31] has shown that chewing movement is more vertically oriented with canine guidance and becomes more horizontal without canine guidance. They have thus demonstrated with objective data that anterior guidance plays an important role in longevity of the teeth and periodontium. What is the significance of recording border movements? It lies in the ability to identify potential disharmony of the occlusion with jaw movements and to minimize destructive effects of parafunction on the gnathic system. If there is no disharmony of the occlusion with condylar movement, the patient would have no chewing problem. If parafunction exists, its damaging effects must be kept to minimum. Bruxing, for example, takes place outside the range of chewing movement or near the border movement paths. Elimination of disharmony between the occlusion and the jaw movement within the envelope of motion would, therefore, minimize adverse effects of bruxing.

Figure 13.20A and B shows the orbit of the axis of rotation (hinge axis) of the mandible in the sagittal plane in a normal individual. The red dot represents the hinge axis. Being at the terminal position, it is called the THA. The movement paths scribed in the sagittal plane by the hinge axis consists of protrusive, mediotrusive and opening paths, which are superimposed on top of one another to form a single line for the first 8 mm or so from THA.[32] From there, the axis moves slightly more inferiorly in mediotrusive movement and goes up a little in opening movement. The axis moves slightly more forward in protrusive movement before reaching the border.

Relaxed muscles and stable mandibular position make the location of THA very easy, while it is difficult to locate THA in an individual with unstable mandibular position, strained muscles of mastication and loose ligaments of the joints. Figure 13.20 compares sagittal border movements between a patient with the discs in place, relaxed muscles and stabilized mandibular position (Fig. 13.20E and F) and a prestabilization patient with tight muscles and unstable mandibular position (Fig. 13.20G and H). There is a clear difference between the two patients. Thus, the status of the joints can be assessed by locating THA and by recording border movements of the mandible from THA. It is also possible to evaluate the effect of stabilization of mandibular position by comparing prestabilization and poststabilization mandibular movement records.

Figure 13.21A and B shows a reverse curve in the initial part of mandibular movement from THA. This is an important sign of disc displacement. These recordings are useful in picking up early signs of disc displacement before the clinician can detect clicking with finger palpation.

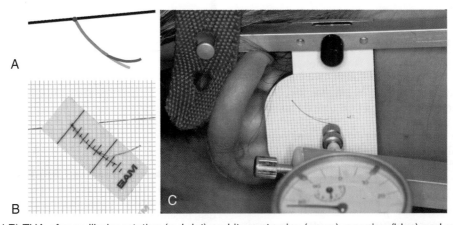

Figure 13.20 (**A** and **B**) THA of mandibular rotation (red dot) and its protrusive (green), opening (blue) and mediotrusive (orange) paths of movement recorded in sagittal plane. The three tracings are superimposed for the first 8 mm before separating when the joint is normal without disc displacement. (**C**) Recording of mandibular border movements in the sagittal plane.

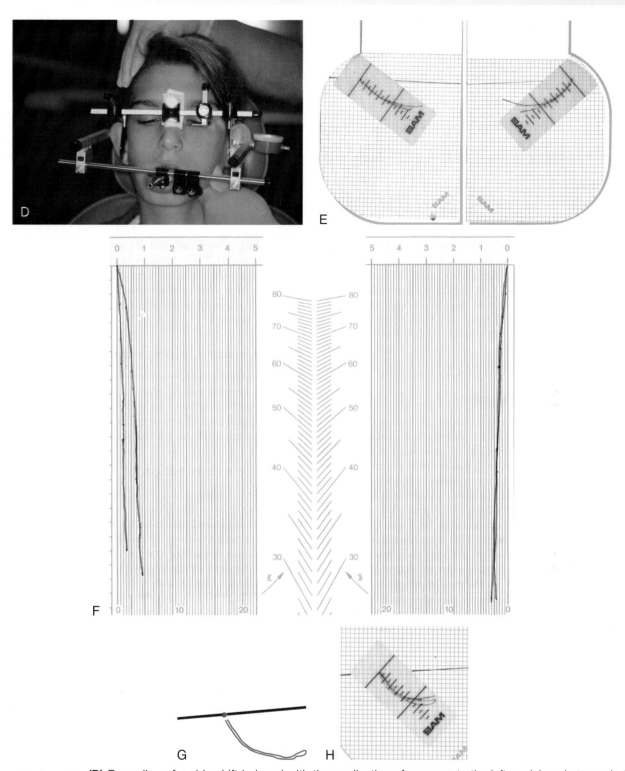

Figure 13.20, cont'd **(D)** Recording of a side shift induced with the application of pressure to the left gonial angle towards the right temporalis. **(E)** Sagittal border movements were recorded for the right and left joints. The line passing through THA (red dot) represents the axis-orbital plane. **(F)** Side shifts in the coronal plane were measured for the right and left joints. Border movement is shown in red and unguided movement is shown in blue. Immediate side shift is less than 0.5 mm, indicating minimal joint laxity. **(G and H)** In a loose joint, three border movements in the sagittal plane are not superimposable.

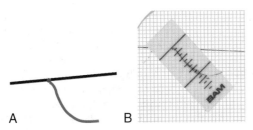

Figure 13.21 (**A** and **B**) A reverse curve is present early during jaw movement. This is typically observed at an early stage of disc displacement.

Immediate side shift

In healthy joints, immediate side shift is small (Fig. 13.20F) and less than 1.0 mm in adults. It increases as the joints get loose. Smaller immediate side shift is more favourable for the health of the gnathic system. Larger immediate side shift, which indicates increased ligament laxity, affects the occlusion at the occlusal surface level, cusp height, groove direction, tooth alignment and arch form. It also increases stress on the periodontium, muscle tension, tooth attrition and cervical tooth loss by abfraction.

Hypermobility of the joint

A study has shown that two-thirds of hypermobile joints have disc displacements and hypermobility accounts for two-thirds of disc displacements.[33] The two conditions are closely interrelated. Joint hypermobility is defined as an excessive range of condylar movement in mouth opening beyond the insertion of the anterior joint capsular attachment, which is the anterior limit of the joint. This anterior limit is located at an average of 4 mm (0–8 mm), anterior to the apex of the eminence. This hypermobility can be felt by careful palpation. The author has witnessed the possibility of reducing the amount of immediate side shift and hypermobility by stabilizing mandibular position, particularly in patients with mild disc displacement.

DISC DISPLACEMENT

In the early 1970s, Farrar's work[34] on internal derangements of the TMJ led to the recognition of disc displacement by clinicians. Disc displacement was perceived as a two-dimensional change in the sagittal plane, predominantly as anterior displacement. One treatment modality derived from this observation was splint therapy for anterior repositioning of the mandible in an attempt to reduce or recapture the disc. Functional appliances were also used for the same purpose. In those days, even Farrar was not aware of the common occurrence of disc displacement. Today, we know that disc displacement occurs three-dimensionally and that simple forward repositioning of the mandible would fail to recapture the disc. In the initial stage of disc displacement, a part of the disc slides off the condyle, commonly in an anterolateral direction at lateral. The rest of the disc still stays on the condyle. The displaced area of the disc increases with time, along with increasing complexity of displacement direction.

MRI is the best imaging modality for diagnosis of disc displacement. A normal disc is depicted as a dark grey biconcave structure interposed between the eminence and condyle on a proton density-weighted image. The posterior disc attachment has a light grey colour on the MRI image in a healthy state. Unstable disc position causes fibrosis of the posterior attachment with the appearance of a dark-grey band. When disc displacement progresses, the posterior band of the disc is no longer at the 12 O'clock position but located further down the slope of the eminence. Along with this change in disc position, the condyle changes its position from the normal superior and anterior position to a slightly posterior and inferior position in the fossa. In this stage of disc displacement, the disc looks black on a T2-weighted MRI image and is surrounded by excessive synovial fluid (joint effusion).[35] This allows better visualization of the disc's shape. The disc has already been deformed by this stage in many cases. In addition to MRI, the following examinations and records help the diagnosis of disc displacement.

Careful history taking regarding

- Trauma to the face, particularly the mandible
- Parafunctional habits, such as clenching and bruxism
- Frequent headache
- Joint sound and character of the sound
- Inability to open the mouth smoothly

Chairside examination of

- Muscles by palpation
- Asymmetry in ramus length
- Fatigue of masticatory muscles during chewing
- Strain of mentalis and obicularis oris
- Mandibular deviation and deflection with opening
- Dental midline deviation
- Tilting of occlusal plane
- Excessive attrition of teeth, particularly canines
- Tooth mobility
- Cervical enamel loss (abfraction)
- Gingival recession around mobile teeth
- Hypersensitivity of teeth
- Torus formation in lower lingual, upper buccal and palatal areas

Cephalometry

Mandibular asymmetry should be checked on a PA cephalogram as disc displacement causes mandibular midline deviation.[36] Antegonial notching should also be noted. It must be kept in mind that disc displacement can exist in all skeletal patterns including mandibular protrusion and low-angle cases. On a lateral cephalogram, attention needs to be paid to double-image appearance of the lower border of the mandible and posterior border of the ramus, which indicates asymmetry.

Tomography and CBCT

Disc displacement affects the position of the condyle in the fossa. Condylar position delineated on corrected tomograms and CT images may, therefore, indicate the presence and direction of disc displacement. In this regard, the CBCT image of optimum condylar position mentioned earlier serves as a very useful standard for the assessment of the patient's disc status. For definitive diagnosis of disc displacement, MRI is required to exclude disc deformation.

- Normal (Fig. 13.22A) and partial disc displacements (Fig. 13.22B).
- Total disc displacement with reduction (Fig. 13.22C).
- Disc displacement without reduction (Fig. 13.22D and E).

Mandibular movement

It is risky to diagnose disc position only based on mandibular movement records (Fig. 13.23). On one hand, a patient with long-standing nonreducing disc displacement may show normal-looking mandibular movement tracings. On the other hand, a reverse curve in the initial part of sagittal mandibular movement tracings, which indicates slight disc displacement, is a helpful tool in confirming the finding of disc displacement when used in conjunction with other diagnostic records. The deviations of mandibular movement tracings, often described

in literature as typical clicking or disc displacement with reduction, have little diagnostic value. Clicking can be detected simply by palpating the joint area.

When three sagittal jaw movement tracings (opening, protrusive and mediotrusive) do not superimpose for the first 8 mm or when mandibular movement does not start from THA, unstable mandibular position or hypermobility can be suspected. These conditions are often associated with disc displacement. It is difficult to feel disc displacement with palpation of the joint from outside when the disc is displaced medially. The separation of mediotrusive movement tracing from opening or protrusive tracing after stabilization may suggest medial or lateral disc displacement.

CONTINUUM OF CHANGE IN DISC DISPLACEMENT

Figure 13.24 shows the continuum of disc displacement progression. The author finds this diagram very useful since it closely represents clinical situations observed in actual patients. Figure 13.25 shows the prevalence rate of temporomandibular disorders (TMD) by age taken from

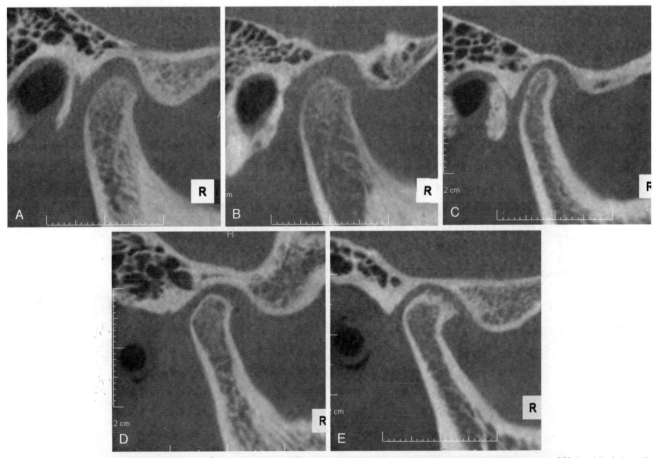

Figure 13.22 **(A)** CBCT image of normal condylar position. **(B)** CBCT image of partial disc displacement. **(C)** In this joint, the entire disc from medial to lateral is displaced but reduced upon opening. The condyle maintains its basic form, though smaller in size. **(D)** An example of disc displacement without reduction. The functional parts of the joint have flattened with altered osseous morphology of the condyle, fossa and eminence. **(E)** A disc displacement without reduction case. Erosion of the functional areas of the joint is noted with a reverse curve in the eminence.

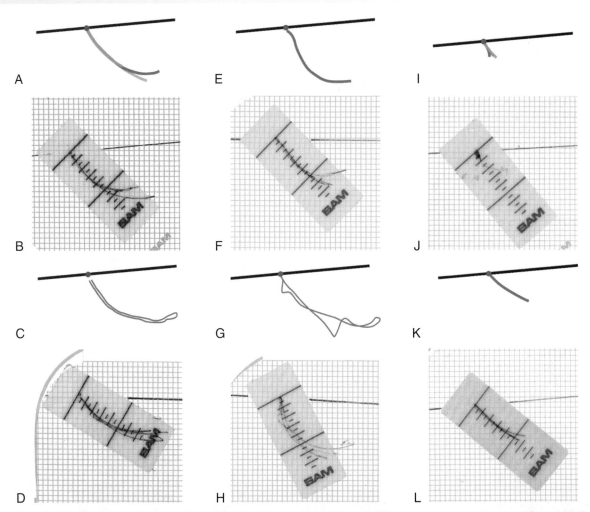

Figure 13.23 (**A** and **B**) Normal function. (**C** and **D**) Hypermobile joint. (**E** and **F**) Partial disc displacement. (**G** and **H**) Partial or total disc displacement with reduction. (**I** and **J**) Locked joint (acute phase). Disc displacement without reduction. (**K** and **L**) Disc displacement without reduction (chronic phase).

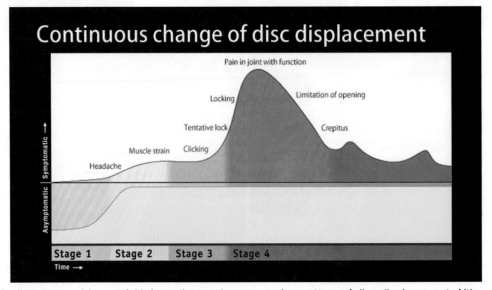

Figure 13.24 This diagram provides useful information on the progression pattern of disc displacement. Although the pace and degree of progression varies from patient to patient, disc displacement typically progresses from partial displacement to total displacement, tentative lock and then lock (Also refer Fig. 13.27).

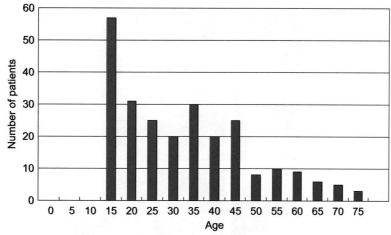

Figure 13.25 This graph shows the number of patients visiting the investigator's clinic with symptomatic disc displacement plotted by age. Prevalence is disproportionately high at age 15, an important finding that should draw orthodontists' attention. (Image courtesy: Isberg A, et al. Oral Surg Oral Med Oral Pathol Oral Radio Endod 1998; 85:252–257).

an article published by Isberg in 1998.[37] It shows a very high TMD prevalence at age 15 years, which is of great interest to orthodontists. The youngest age in this chart is 15. What is the prevalence rate of TMD before this age? Nebbe and Major reported in 2000 that disc displacement was very common among adolescents seeking orthodontic treatment. Approximately 85 and 60%, respectively, of the preorthodontic female and male patients studied had unilateral or bilateral disc displacement (Fig. 13.26).[38] The mean age of the study subjects was 12 years. The author's own clinical experience also supports these findings that disc displacement is prevalent in children.

Disc displacement in children has not drawn much attention because of lack of clinical symptoms in most cases. Now that emerging data suggest a high prevalence of disc displacement in children ready for braces, as well as in younger children, disc displacement is a significant problem that can no longer be disregarded. We need to evaluate the status of the joints before starting treatment, if we are to deliver health services to our patients.

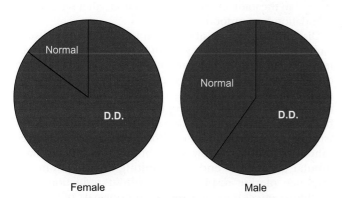

Figure 13.26 Nebbe and Major[38] conducted an MRI study on the prevalence of disc displacement in 138 adolescents who came to a university hospital and a private clinic in Alberta, Canada, seeking orthodontic treatment. Unilateral or bilateral disc displacement was observed in 85% and 60% of the female and male patients, respectively.

Stages of disc displacement

The author classifies disc displacement into the following four stages for diagnostic purposes (Fig. 13.27). Staging helps to specify the type of treatment needed. Stage 1 is the incipient stage where the patient is free of symptoms and extreme care must be taken in palpating the joints. Stage 1 disc displacement is often discovered by chance from follow-up records or during diagnostic assessment of the contralateral joint with more advanced disc displacement. The time may come when MRI imaging becomes more readily available and incorporated as a standard examination, allowing routine detection and even prevention of incipient disc displacement.

Stage 2 is the early stage where the disc is partially displaced. The lateral part of the disc is displaced in a majority of cases, while the medial part is displaced in a few cases. This stage of disc displacement is often seen in children seeking orthodontic treatment. The stage of disc displacement progression in one joint is frequently different from that in the other joint. In this partial disc displacement stage, two-thirds to one-third of the total disc area remains on the condyle and one-third to two-thirds of the total disc area is displaced off the condyle. While the displacement of the lateral part is more common, a few patients have the lateral part 'on' and the medial part 'off'. This stage also includes some lateral or medial shift of the entire disc and slight anterior displacement of the entire disc from the 10 O'clock to the 11 O'clock position.

Stage 3 is a more advanced stage with the entire disc displaced anteriorly, laterally or medially to the 9 O'clock position or below with reduction only during mouth opening. This stage is the trickiest of all four stages. Stage 3 often progresses to locking. Any dental procedure that causes changes in occlusion requires extra attention at this stage. Some cases in transition from Stage 2 to Stage 3 can be reversed to Stage 1 with stabilization splint therapy in the author's experience. Treatment of cases in the beginning of Stage 3 is indeed challenging.

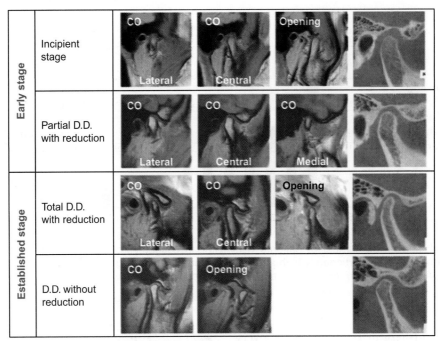

Figure 13.27   The author uses this chart in staging disc displacements based on initial MRI findings.

In the final Stage 4, the disc no longer reduces with mouth opening. This stage is preceded by locking that makes the patient aware of the problem. It is not so difficult to diagnose a patient with locking because of pain induced by mouth opening. The amount of mouth opening increases with time as the condition becomes more chronic. Some patients in this stage have little difficulty or pain with mouth opening. Careful examination is necessary to avoid misdiagnosis. Some early teenage patients are already in this stage of disc displacement without knowing.

DISC DISPLACEMENT AND ORTHODONTIC TREATMENT

How does the presence of disc displacement affect orthodontic treatment? It has been said that orthodontic treatment has no influence on the TMJs. However, the joints respond even to splint therapy, which is a less drastic means of producing occlusal changes than orthodontic treatment. When the patient is monitored for 6 months or more during splint therapy, changes are observed in many areas including the soft and hard tissues of the joints, muscles, mandibular position and tooth mobility. Occlusal changes do have impact on many areas of the gnathic system. This is nothing to be feared. It even implies that orthodontics is an important health service rather than a mere tooth aligning tool. Should orthodontics have no bearing on the TMJs, the orthodontist would not need to pay attention to the patient's disc status. On the contrary, the gnathic system is responsive even to splint therapy that does not involve tooth movement. We orthodontists must keep in mind that unlike other disciplines of dentistry, the procedures we perform produce greater than 99% change in the occlusion. We are thus obliged to develop a deeper

understanding of the TMJ so that we can effect positive changes in the gnathic system.

What is the orthodontic implication of disc displacement? Animal experiments have demonstrated that disc displacement induces changes in the cartilage of the joint. Even slight and short-term displacement of the disc has been shown to affect the cartilage.[39] Clinically, disc displacement is found on the side to which the mandibular midline is deviated in many mandibular asymmetry cases. Orthodontists often encounter unilateral Class II cases with Angle Class II relationship on one side and Class I relationship on the other. Mandibular midline shift is not two-dimensional. The deviation occurs three-dimensionally; vertically and anteroposteriorly. Our job is to eliminate not only the PA discrepancy or Class II problem that can be observed intraorally but also the vertical discrepancy that cannot be seen in the mouth. Most importantly, we must realize that disc displacement causes a three-dimensional change in the joint and the skeletal patterns that serve as the foundation for our tooth alignment.

Disc displacement is also known to cause growth disturbance, if it occurs during growth.[40] An attempt to correct mandibular underdevelopment in the presence of disc displacement in a growing patient may result in the suppression of mandibular growth.[41] In traditional orthodontics, appliances that bring the mandible forward have been widely used in growing patients with mandibular retrusion. Animal studies have shown that these appliances inhibit mandibular growth. Attempts to stimulate mandibular growth will end up inhibiting the growth in the presence of disc displacement without reduction. The inhibitory effect is greater in the anterior part of the condyle, which means that the condyle cannot grow superiorly and anteriorly. The result is clockwise rotation of the chin and further aggravation of mandibular retrusion.

Class II intermaxillary elastics are often used for overjet reduction, but this may cause further progression of disc displacement. The elastics extrude the molars and cause further backward rotation of the mandible, resulting in an increased overjet. The same is true for upper molar distalization with a headgear, especially with cervical type. Its wedge effect may cause clockwise rotation of the mandible. This tendency is increased when the molars are distalized with a cervical headgear that has an extrusive effect on the upper molars.

Patients with unstable mandibular position are predisposed to disc displacement. Occlusal interference or posterior fulcrum created during a dental procedure may promote parafunctional habits, such as bruxism and cause the condyle to deviate posteriorly and inferiorly in the fossa, leading to an even more unstable mandibular position and further progression of disc displacement.

What is the effect of the chin cap that is often used for Class III correction? Against the misconception that TMJ problems are uncommon in Class III patients, the prevalence rate of disc displacement in this patient population is not low. The use of a chin cap in the presence of disc displacement may have a negative effect depending on the stage of disc displacement. The problem lies in the routine use of the appliance without regard to the status of the joint.

Finally, disc displacement is an intra-articular change that is very difficult for us to deal with when we use conventional mechanics. Orthodontic treatment without knowing the stage of the patient's disc displacement is analogous to setting out on a voyage without knowing where we are and where we want to go. We need treatment mechanics based on a new concept of disc displacement. First and foremost, we should realize that the majority of orthodontic patients have disc displacement.

DIAGNOSIS FOR THE PRACTICE OF A FUNCTIONAL ORTHODONTIC TREATMENT

Chairside examination and history

Some patients come to orthodontic offices complaining of TMJ problems. The orthodontist, therefore, needs to obtain a detailed history by asking if the patient has any joint pain, sound or trismus, when the problem started, where it occurred, how long it lasted and what it was like under what circumstances. In particular, history of trauma should be carefully investigated, even those dating back to early childhood. The presence of parafunctional habits, such as bruxism, clenching and nail biting, and headache that occurs once every 2 weeks or more frequently, should be noted. This should be followed by chairside examination that includes the palpation of the masseter and temporalis muscles for tenderness and tightness and external palpation of the joints for tenderness, condylar movement laxity and disc instability. The next step is to have the patient open and close the mouth with the examiner's fingers in the patient's ear canals to determine if the discs are in place. The fingers are then pulled towards the patient's front to check for the presence of tenderness or for any difference in degree of tenderness between the right and the left (Fig. 13.28).

The amount of mouth opening is then examined. Mandibular deviation or deflection upon opening is also assessed, followed by the examination of ramus and mandibular asymmetries, scars and stitches in the chin area and position of the right and left ears (Fig. 13.29).

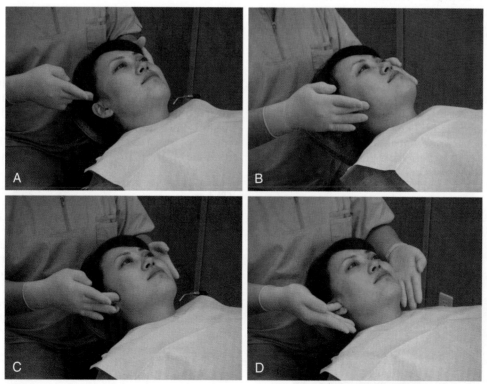

Figure 13.28 **(A)** Palpation of temporalis muscles. **(B)** Palpation of masseter muscles. **(C)** Palpation of TMJ. **(D)** Palpation of the posterior aspect of condyles through ear canals.

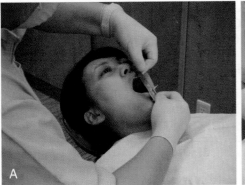
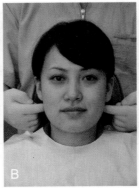
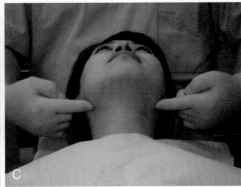

Figure 13.29 **(A)** Measure the maximum mouth opening. **(B)** Check positional difference of the right and left ears. **(C)** Check asymmetry of the mandible.

Instrumentation

Functional orthodontic treatment requires a different set of records from that considered to be the 'traditional orthodontic records', namely hand-held models, lateral cephalograms and intraoral images. Well-trained staff, their skilled assistance and efficient office are also essential to a successful treatment. Once these requirements are met, the amount of information derived from these comprehensive records—which will be described in this section—is much more than that from traditional records. Without a complete set of records, it is very difficult to fully satisfy a patient's request to 'fix the bite'. Each and every one of these records has been taken and used for years in dentistry. Therefore, the information gathered through compilation of these records makes orthodontics compatible with other areas of dentistry, and widens the scope of orthodontic treatment. The fundamentals of such records and methods of record-taking will be described briefly here to facilitate the readers' understanding of the case report contained in this chapter.

Facebow transfer

The photograph shows the recording of a three-dimensional relationship of the maxilla and maxillary teeth to a reference plane. The Panadent system uses the axis-orbital plane as a reference plane, which is defined with the nasion relator and the right and left ear rods placed into the auditory canals (Fig. 13.30).

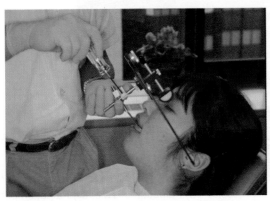

Figure 13.30 Facebow transfer.

CO bite registration

A thin but dimensionally stable piece of wax is used to record the patient's habitual occlusal position or CO. The CO bite is an important record used in quantifying condylar displacement with CPI. Note that this bite is *not* used to mount models on an articulator (Fig. 13.31).

CR bite registration

This wax bite records the patient's *initial* CR, which should not be mistaken for *true* CR. It is extremely difficult to capture one's true CR at chairside during initial visit. This method is used to obtain the best achievable seating of the condyles in the fossae for that day. A true CR can be registered only after the stabilization of condylar position (Fig. 13.32).

Mounting

The upper model is mounted in its appropriate relation to the axis-orbital plane, and the lower model is subsequently mounted using the CR wax bite (Fig. 13.33).

Condylar position indicator

CPI measures the three-dimensional displacement of the condyles using the CO wax bite. This procedure is affected by the accuracy of the CR and CO wax bites, models and their mounting. Thus, each of the preceding steps must be performed, and CPI must be handled carefully as they require a high level of precision (Fig. 13.34).

CPI data

CPI data consists of three graphs: right and left sagittal graphs and a transverse graph. The top two graphs are used to measure condylar displacements in the sagittal plane. The origin of coordinate represents the patient's initial CR position, and the CO position is indicated with red dots. The graph at the bottom quantifies condylar displacement in the frontal plane. A transverse discrepancy of greater than 0.5 mm raises a concern (Fig. 13.35).

CO-CR discrepancy

The intraoral photographs show the patient's habitual occlusal position or CO. Study models of the same patient were mounted in initial CR. Comparing the two

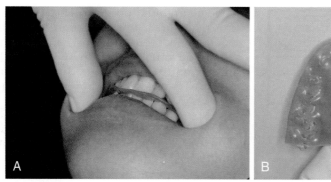
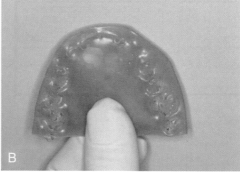

Figure 13.31   (**A** and **B**) CO bite registration.

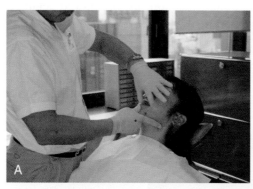
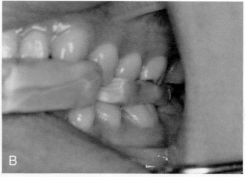

Figure 13.32   (**A** and **B**) CR bite registration.

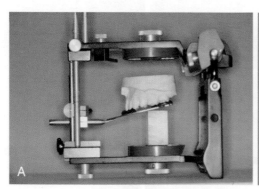
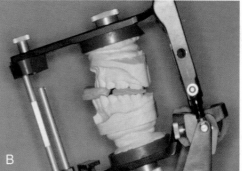

Figure 13.33   (**A** and **B**) Mounting.

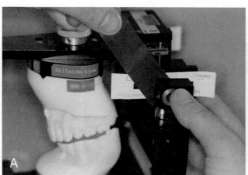
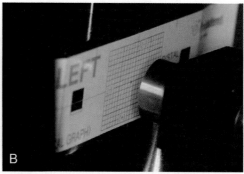

Figure 13.34   (**A** and **B**) Condylar position indicator.

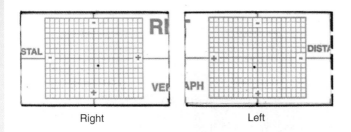

Right   Left

Transverse condylar position

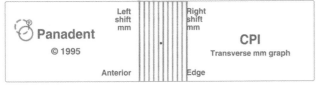

Figure 13.35   CPI data.

records reveals the patient's CO-CR discrepancy. Note how much information can be obtained even from initial CR mounting (Fig. 13.36).

Splint therapy

A stabilization full coverage upper centric splint with a mutually protected occlusion is used to achieve a stable mandibular position. The splint is fabricated on an articulator. Upon closure of the arches, there are simultaneous centric stops with mandibular buccal cusps. The anterior teeth have 0.0005″ clearance. The splint is adjusted to eliminate occlusal interferences in protrusive and lateral movements of the mandible (Fig. 13.37).

Stabilization-type splint

These intraoral photographs show the stabilization-type splint placed in the mouth. Note the smooth surface and rounded shape of the splint for minimal patient discomfort (Fig. 13.38).

Monitoring of condylar position during splint therapy

Once the patient's muscles are relaxed, changes in mandibular position are monitored regularly during splint therapy. The patient is asked to close into wax while the orthodontist supports the chin as shown in the photographs (Fig. 13.39).

The wax bite registrations are placed on the original mounted models of the patient to mark any changes in the position of the condyles in the fossae with CPI (Fig. 13.40).

Changes in condylar position can be monitored with CPI data taken on a regular basis. Data here shows

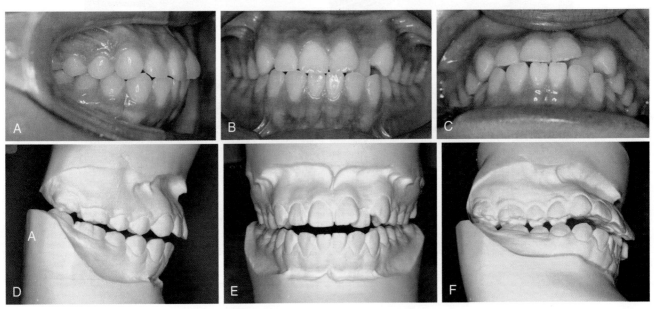

Figure 13.36   (**A–F**) CO-CR discrepancy.

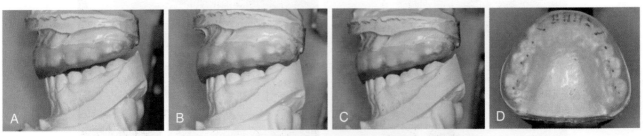

Figure 13.37   (**A**) Left lateral. (**B**) Right lateral. (**C**) Protrusive. (**D**) Occlusal view.

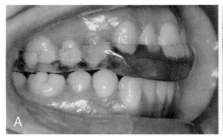
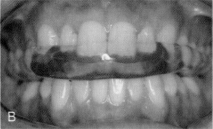
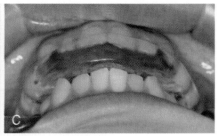

Figure 13.38 (**A–C**) Stabilization-type splint.

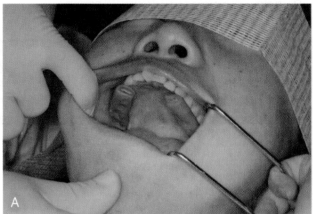
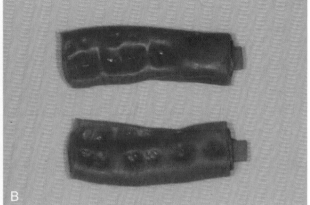

Figure 13.39 (**A** and **B**) Check the patient's bite regularly during splint therapy.

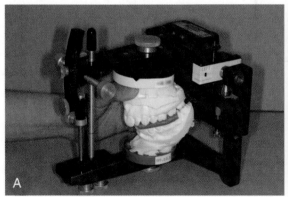
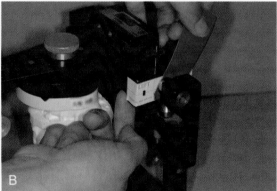

Figure 13.40 (**A** and **B**) Tracking patient's condylar position in the fossae during splint therapy with CPI.

upward and forward seating of the condyles in the fossae from their initial positions (Fig. 13.41).

These are plots of the condylar positional changes recorded with CPI over time in the sagittal and transverse planes and are demonstrating how the condyles are repositioned in the fossae and stabilized (Fig. 13.42).

These photographs show typical intraoral changes seen during splint therapy with initial rapid and dramatic changes followed by slowly occurring minimal changes (Fig. 13.43). For comprehensive analysis, not only intraoral changes and CPI data, but changes in clinical symptoms are also monitored.

Stabilization of mandibular position

When no more change is occurring in condylar position, the same mandibular position can be observed in cephalogram, on mounted models and in patient's mouth (Fig. 13.44). This mandibular position can be recorded with any wax or other bite registration techniques or by any operator.

Recording of mandibular movements

Once condyles are stabilized within the respective fossa, it becomes easy to record the centre of condylar rotation in closing or in CR (provided there is a

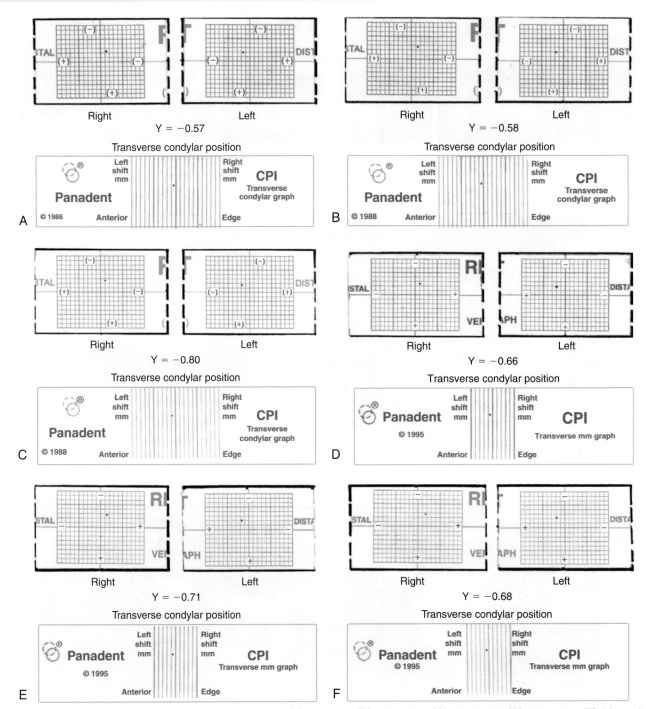

Figure 13.41 Changes in CPI data during splint therapy. **(A)** 7 weeks. **(B)** 13 weeks. **(C)** 16 weeks. **(D)** 18 weeks. **(E)** 20 weeks. **(F)** 24 weeks.

normal disc–condyle relationship). Protrusive and lateral border movements starting from CR and lateral shifts of the condyles in the frontal plane, called *side shifts*, can be recorded with good reproducibility (Fig. 13.45).

Diagnostic record-taking described above is a very efficient clinical method that can accurately identify the three-dimensional condylar position. Once you develop a habit of using this diagnostic method for orthodontic treatment, you would find it virtually

impossible to diagnose a case only with standard orthodontic records. To me, cases diagnosed solely with conventional methods that I see being presented in meetings are like fast food that may be called a meal but is nothing comparable to a sophisticated French cuisine. There is a tremendous difference between this method of diagnosis as described above and the conventional diagnosis in the amount and quality of information gained, as well as in the end result.

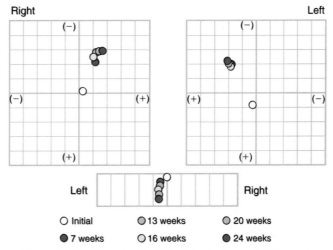

Figure 13.42   Changes in CPI data during splint therapy.

Case summary

A 13-year-old male patient presented with the chief complaint: teeth alignment and seeking information on the need for Phase II treatment (Fig. 13.46). From his family history, his elder sister and father had open bites and unstable jaw positions. The patient reported frequent headaches. The mandible was very difficult to manipulate in bite registration. Intraorally, the molar relationship was Angle Class I on both sides (Figs 13.47–13.51).

Splint therapy, intended to uncover his true mandibular position, revealed Class III tendency on the right side, Class II relationship on the left side and an open bite (Figs 13.52–13.55). As the mandibular position was stabilized and problems were identified (Figs 13.56–13.63), how to treat each specific problem was thought out in advance. This led to efficient occlusal improvement (Figs 13.64–13.73). The occlusion remains very stable post-treatment.

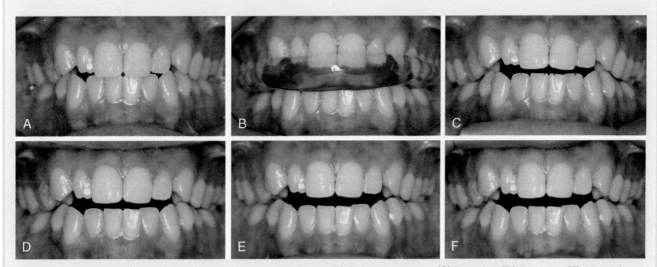

Figure 13.43   Intraoral views during splint therapy. **(A)** Initial. **(B)** Splint placement. **(C)** 3 weeks. **(D)** 7 weeks. **(E)** 20 weeks. **(F)** 24 weeks.

Continued

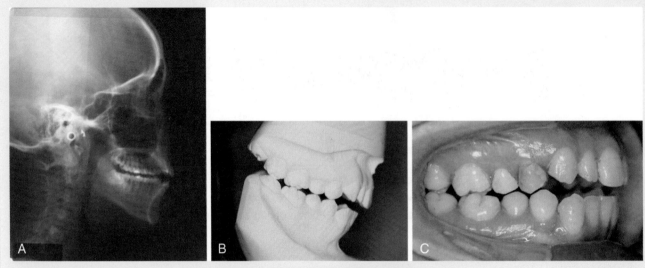

Figure 13.44   (**A–C**) Stabilization of mandibular position.

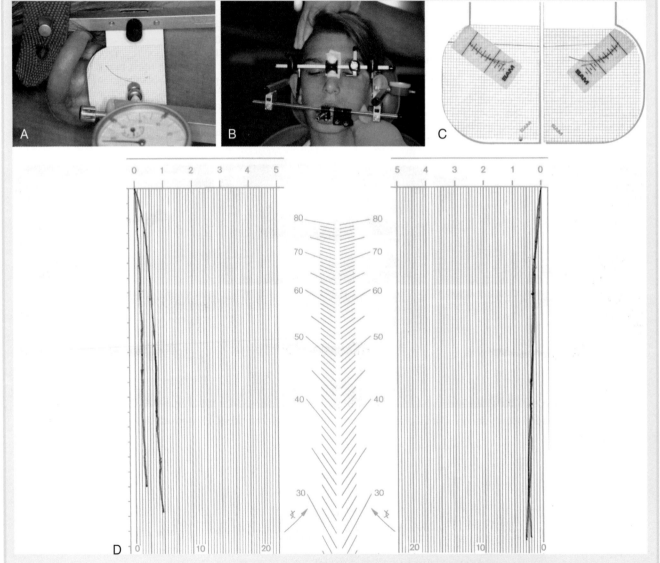

Figure 13.45   (**A–D**) Recording of mandibular border movement.

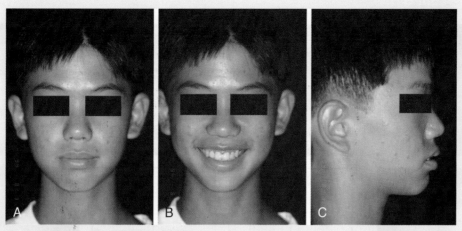

Figure 13.46 (**A–C**) Initial facial photographs (13 years and 4 months).

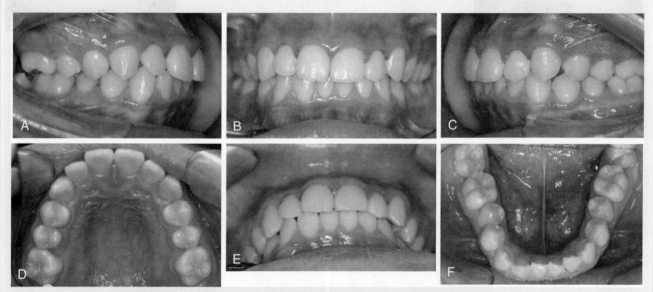

Figure 13.47 (**A–F**) Initial intraoral photographs.

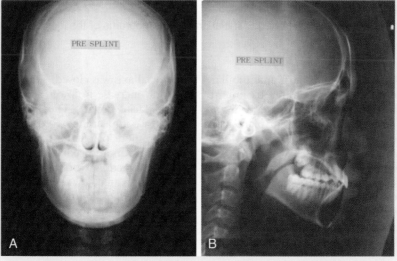

Figure 13.48 (**A** and **B**) Initial PA and lateral cephalograms.

Continued

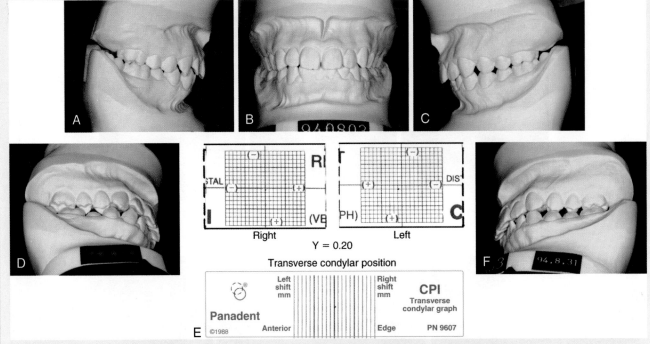

Figure 13.49   (**A–F**) Initial models mounted in CR and CPI data.

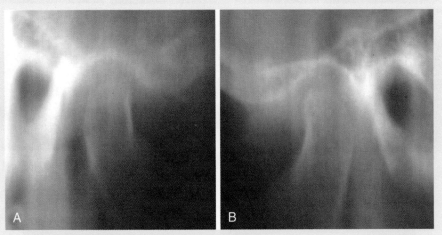

Figure 13.50   (**A** and **B**) Initial oriented tomograms of the joints.

Case discussion

The facial profile, tooth alignment and mandibular position were improved with orthodontic treatment (Figs 13.73–13.76). The patient's problems were identified *first* to strategize with specific treatment plans and sequence, allowing the entire treatment to progress efficiently and smoothly. As a result of adequate vertical control, the PA problem was corrected at the same time (Figs 13.77 and 13.78). The extraction spaces that remained after elimination of crowding were utilized to correct the transverse problem with compliance-dependent diagonal elastics. Very favourable soft tissue changes were produced as the condyles were positioned closer to CR and

the facial axis was closed. The chin was brought forward with no increase in lower facial height, providing a balanced facial profile. The lips became relaxed without protrusive appearance. Recovery of lip competence and improvement of plaque control helped resolve gingival inflammation and redness. It is practically impossible to achieve functional occlusion with the condyles out of place, no matter how well the teeth are aligned. Treating without paying attention to condylar position would adversely affect the tooth alignment, muscles, TMJs, periodontium and teeth in the future, and the occlusion would never be stable (Figs 13.79–13.82).

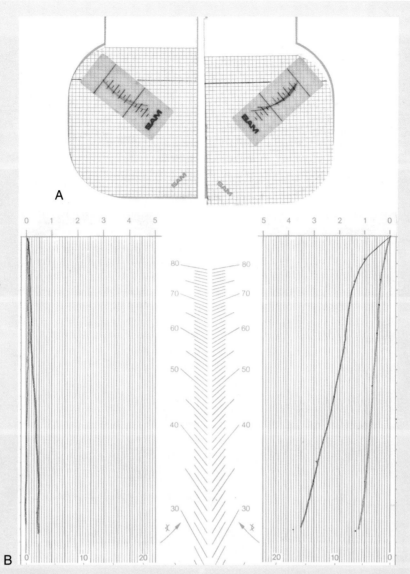

Figure 13.51 (**A** and **B**) Initial mandibular border movement. Note the large immediate side shift on the left.

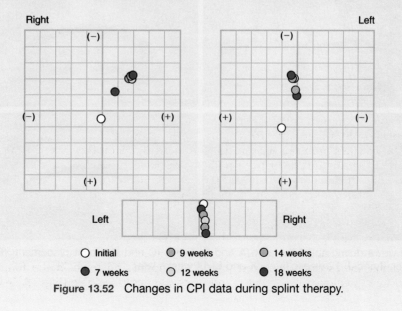

Figure 13.52 Changes in CPI data during splint therapy.

Continued

CASE REPORT—cont'd

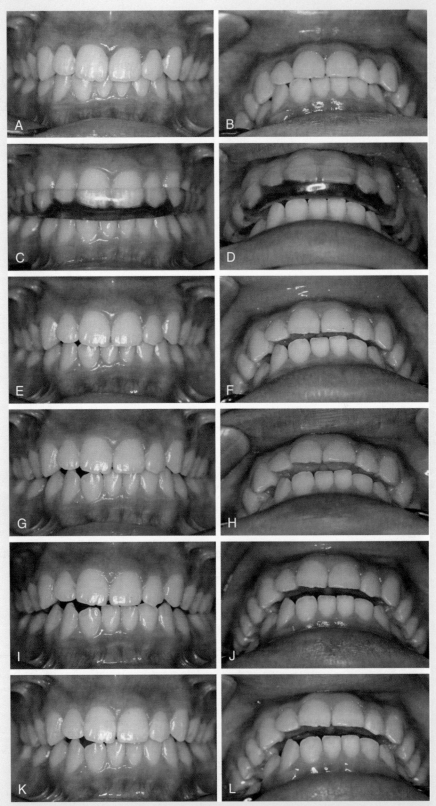

Figure 13.53 Intraoral views during splint therapy. (**A** and **B**) Initial. (**C** and **D**) Splint placement. (**E** and **F**) 5 weeks later. (**G** and **H**) 9 weeks later. (**I** and **J**) 12 weeks later. (**K** and **L**) 14 weeks later.

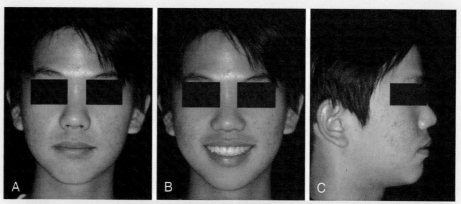

Figure 13.54 (**A–C**) Postsplint facial photographs (14 years and 1 month).

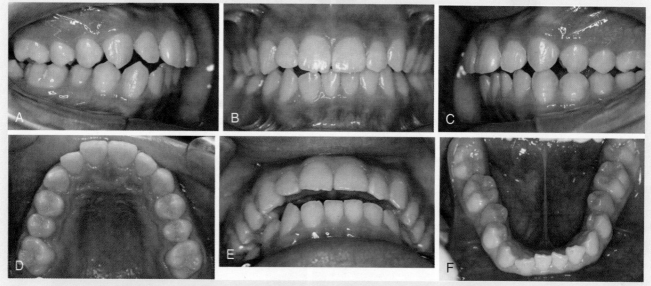

Figure 13.55 (**A–F**) Postsplint intraoral photographs demonstrating Angle Class III relationship on the right, Class II tendency on the left, midline shift and an open bite.

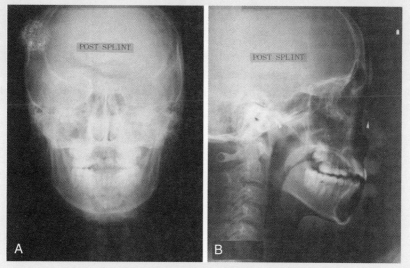

Figure 13.56 (**A** and **B**) Postsplint PA and lateral cephalograms illustrating a slight midline shift to the left and an open bite.

Continued

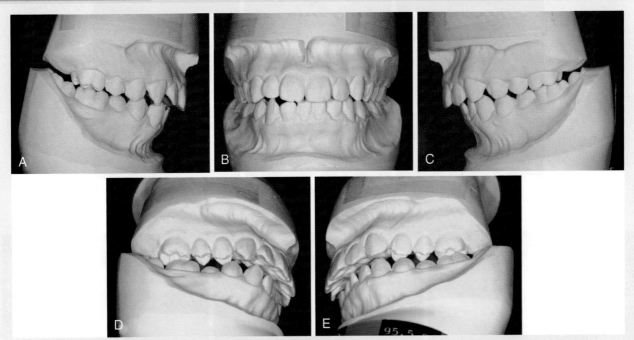

Figure 13.57 **(A–E)** Postsplint hinge-axis mounting. Note the absence of posterior crossbite on the left side.

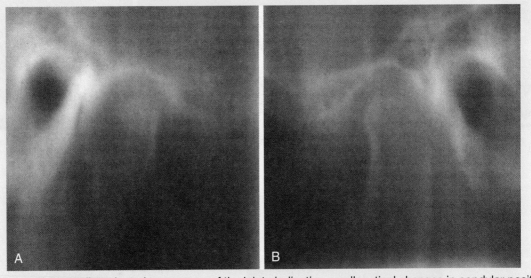

Figure 13.58 **(A and B)** Postsplint oriented tomograms of the joints indicating small vertical changes in condylar position in the fossae and an open bite.

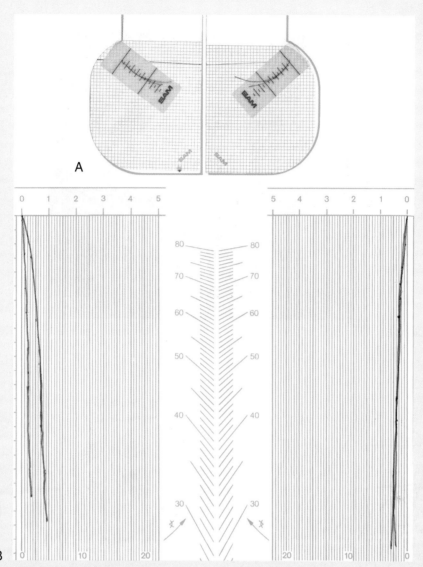

Figure 13.59 (**A** and **B**) Postsplint mandibular border movements. Side shifts were reduced and the lines of protrusive, mediotrusive and opening movements in the sagittal plane are nicely superimposed.

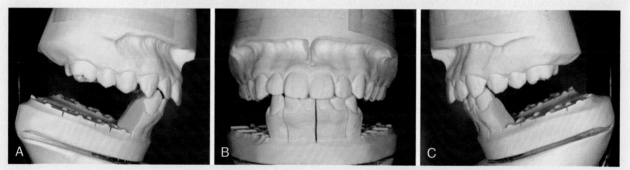

Figure 13.60 (**A–C**) Three-dimensional check on the mounted pin model. Vertical correction eliminates most of the PA problem, leaving the transverse problem to be corrected. Note the canine relationship on the right side.

Continued

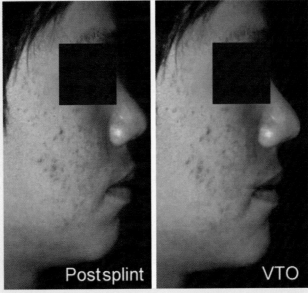

Figure 13.61   Prediction of post-treatment profile based on visual treatment objective (VTO).

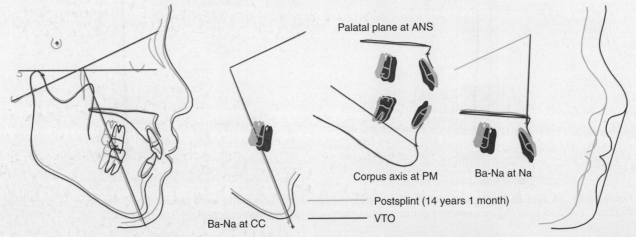

Figure 13.62   Superimposition of VTO and postsplint tracing. The molars need to be controlled in height and moved mesially to close the facial axis, which combined with lingual tipping of the incisors will facilitate lip closure.

Treatment plan	Mechanics
• Vertical control	**Vertical**
• Transverse and midline correction	• Intrusion of upper molars
• Correction of crowding	• Mesializing molars
• Retraction of incisors	• Light force wires to align brackets
• Extraction of four first bicuspids	• Intermaxillary elastics should not be used for this purpose
	Transverse
	• Utilization of extraction spaces
	• Diagonal elastics

A   B

Figure 13.63   **(A)** Treatment plan. **(B)** Mechanics.

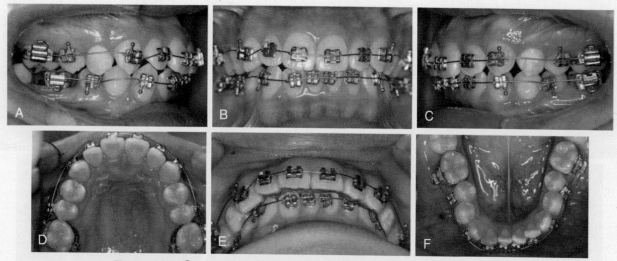

Figure 13.64 Course of treatment. **(A–F)** Appliance placement: ↑↓ 014 Align.

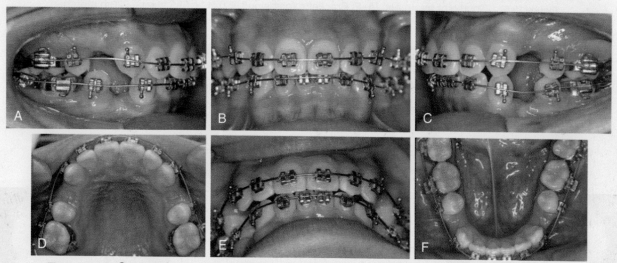

Figure 13.65 Course of treatment. **(A–F)** Bracket alignment: ↑↓ 018 × 025 Neosentalloy: 2nd month.

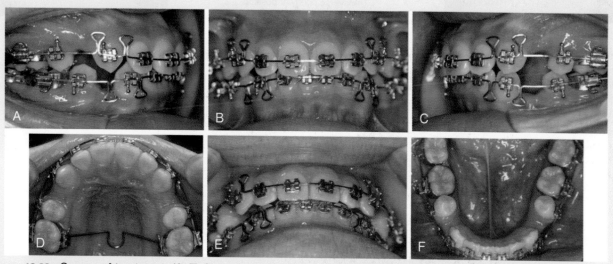

Figure 13.66 Course of treatment. **(A–F)** Closure of extraction spaces: ↑↓ 019 × 025 double key hole loops. Transpalatal arch: 4th month.

Continued

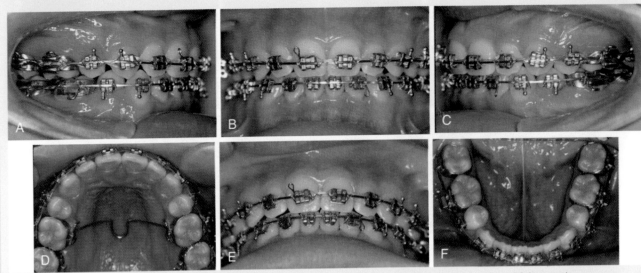

Figure 13.67   Course of treatment. (A–F) Bracket expression: ↓↑ 021 × 025 steel — 20th month.

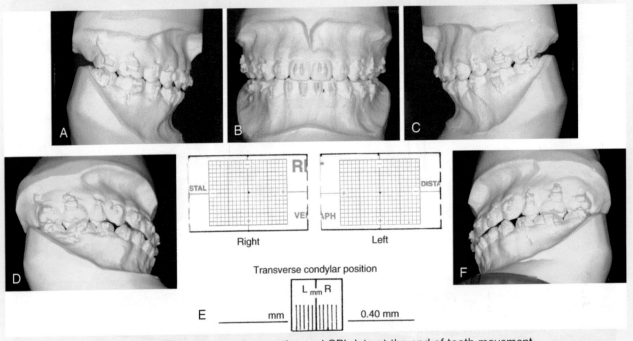

Figure 13.68   (A–F) Hinge-axis mounting and CPI data at the end of tooth movement.

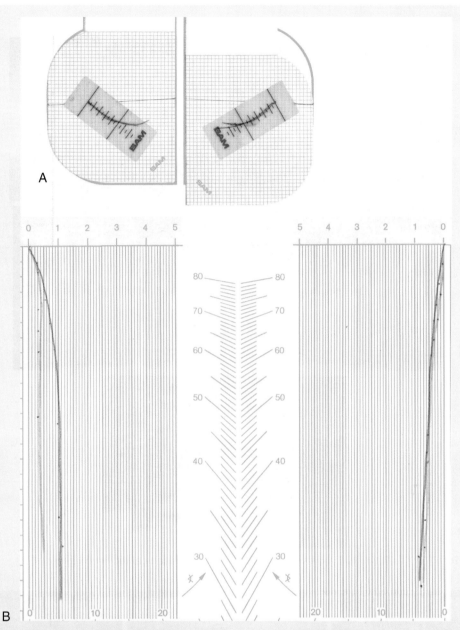

Figure 13.69 (**A** and **B**) Mandibular border movement at the end of tooth movement. These data on mandibular border movements are used to program a semi-adjustable articulator.

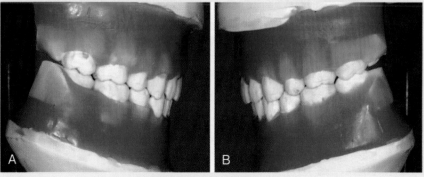

Figure 13.70 (**A–G**)

Continued

CASE REPORT—cont'd

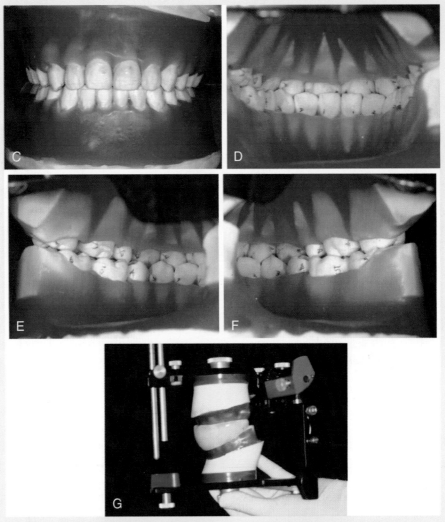

Figure 13.70, cont'd (**A-G**) Setup for gnathological tooth positioner.

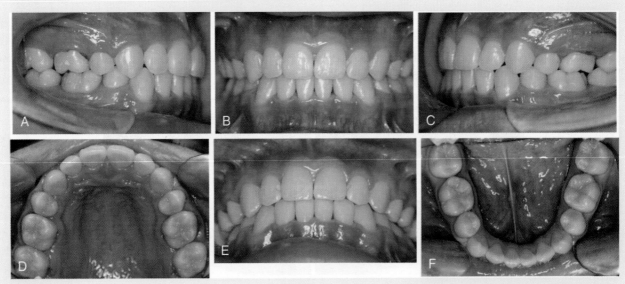

Figure 13.71 (**A–F**) Fixed type appliance removed. Gnathological tooth positioner wear was initiated at this time.

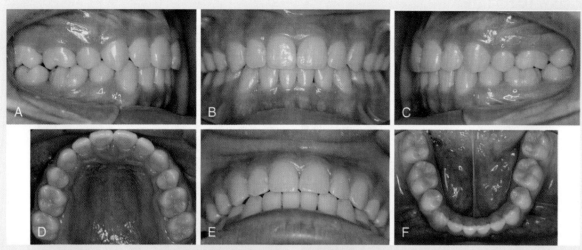

Figure 13.72 **(A–F)** Intraoral photographs after 2 weeks of gnathological tooth positioner wear. The tooth positioner allows proper intercuspation of the upper and lower teeth while removing the overcorrections built into straight wire appliance (SWA) and maintaining condylar position.

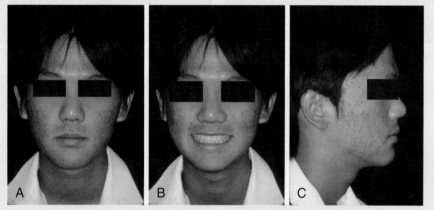

Figure 13.73 **(A–C)** Facial photographs at the end of active treatment (16 years and 5 months).

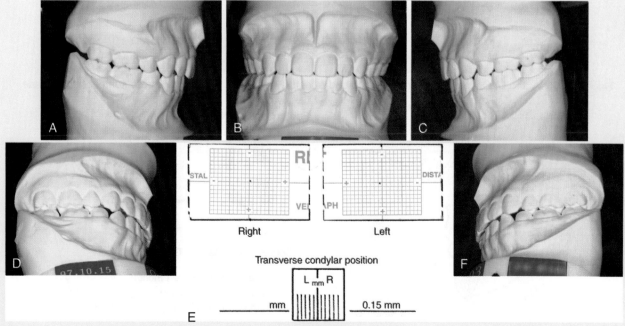

Figure 13.74 **(A–F)** CR mounting and CPI data at the end of active treatment. CO-CR discrepancies are minimal.

Continued

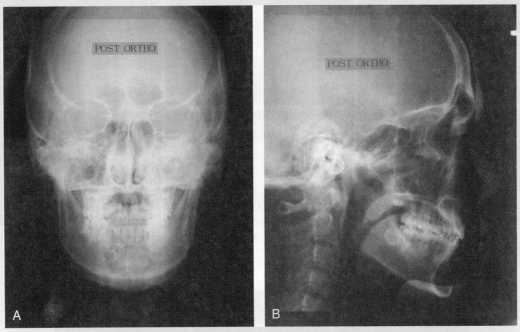

Figure 13.75   (**A** and **B**) PA and lateral cephalograms at the end of active treatment.

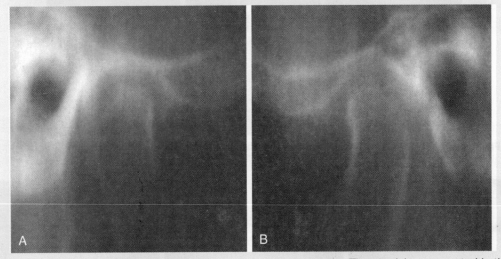

Figure 13.76   (**A** and **B**) Oriented tomograms at the end of active treatment. The condyles are seated in the fossae.

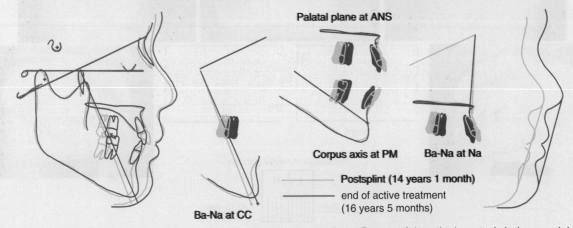

Figure 13.77   Superimposition of pretreatment and post-treatment tracings. Successful vertical control during mesial movement of posterior teeth allowed the facial axis to close and the chin to move forward.

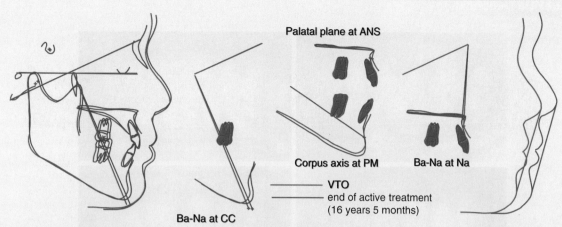

Palatal plane at ANS

Corpus axis at PM   **Ba-Na at Na**

Ba-Na at CC

——— VTO
——— end of active treatment
(16 years 5 months)

Figure 13.78 Superimposition of VTO and post-treatment tracing. The posterior segments were intruded more than that predicted with VTO, resulting in increased closure of the facial axis and favourable facial change as expected.

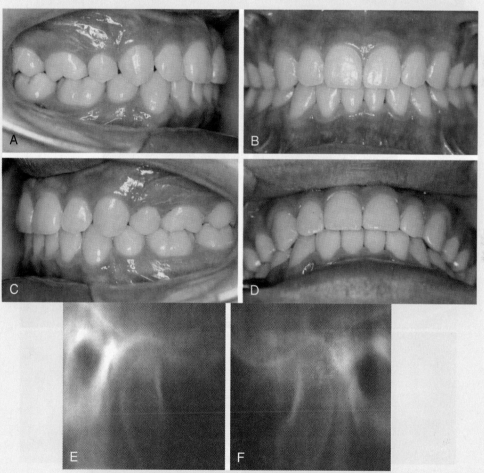

Figure 13.79 Follow-up. **(A–F)** Two years after active treatment (18 years and 9 months).

Continued

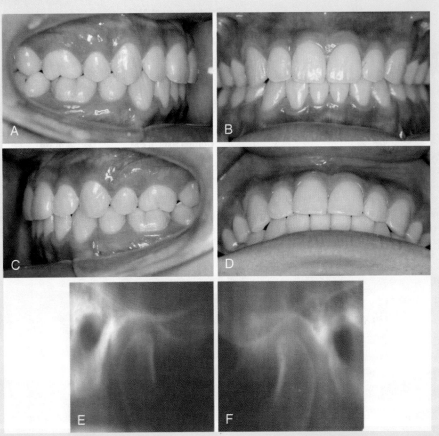

Figure 13.80   Follow-up. (**A–F**) Five years after active treatment (21 years 8 months).

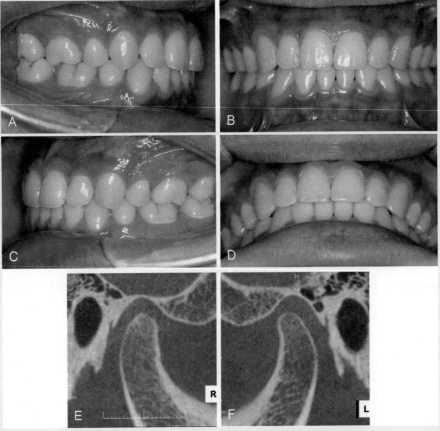

Figure 13.81   Follow-up. (**A–F**) 7 years after active treatment (23 years and 5 months).

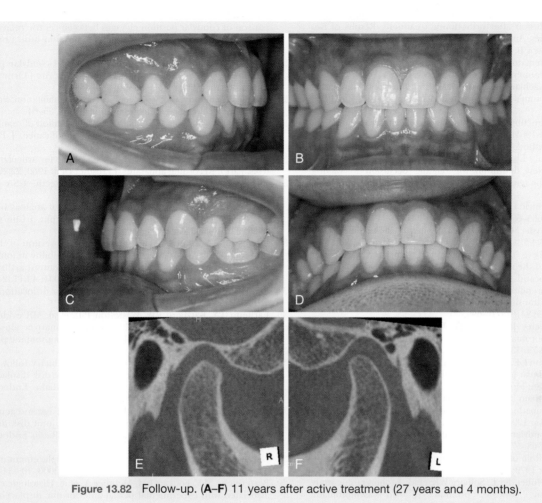

Figure 13.82   Follow-up. (**A–F**) 11 years after active treatment (27 years and 4 months).

CONCLUSION

To transform orthodontics from the study of malocclusions focusing only on tooth irregularity to that promoting the health of the gnathic system, we need to recognize that there is more to the occlusion than just straight teeth and develop the habit of examining the status of the joints, muscles and mandibular movements before checking tooth alignment in the mouth. It is important to realize that occlusal discrepancies observed intraorally at the level of the occlusal surface do not always reflect discrepancies occurring at the joint level. Correct understanding of the relationship between intraoral and intraarticular changes requires careful observation of how the occlusion changes intraorally when condylar position changes three-dimensionally in the fossa, which in turn enables us to appreciate the effect of orthodontic tooth movement on the joints.

Then, it will become increasingly clear that we should shift the emphasis from merely correcting PA jaw relationship to controlling vertical discrepancies. Constant attention to both the occlusion and the TMJs thus marks the first step towards the goal of functional occlusion in orthodontic treatment.

As we develop orthodontic skills to harmonize the occlusion with the joints, we will come to appreciate how relaxed the muscles are when the occlusion and joints are in harmony. The same objective of muscle relaxation can also be accomplished with the use of a stabilization splint. It is these experiences that increase our understanding of the relationship between the occlusion and TMD and the very important role that orthodontics plays in alleviating TMD problems, so that we can ultimately treat patients with TMD in need of orthodontic care.

REFERENCES

1. Angle EH. Treatment of malocclusion of the teeth, 7th edn. Philadelphia: The S.S. white dental manufacturing company; 1907. 1–45.
2. Pullinger AG, Seligman DA, Solberg WK. Temporomandibular disorders. Part: occlusal factors associated with temporomandibular joint tenderness and dysfunction. J Prost Dent 1988; 59:363–367.
3. Egermark-Eriksson I. Mandibular dysfunction in children and in individuals with dual bite. Sweden Dent J 1982; (Suppl. 10):1–45.
4. Reynders RM. Orthodontics and temporomandibular disorders: a review of the literature (1966–1988). Am J Orthod Dentofac Orthop 1990; 97:463–471.
5. Rendell JK, Louis AN, Gay T. Orthodontic treatment and temporomandibular joint disorders. Am J Orthod Dentofac Orthop 1992; 101:84–87.
6. Roth RH. The maintenance system and occlusal dynamics. Dental Clinics of North Am 1976; 20:761–788.

7. Sadowsky C, Polson AM. Temporomandibular disorders and functional occlusion after orthodontic treatment: Results of two long-term studies. Am J Orthod 1984; 86:386–390.

8. Nielsen L, Melsen B, Terp S. TMJ function and the effects on the masticatory system on 14–16-year-old Danish children in relation to orthodontic treatment. Eur J Orthod 1990; 12:254–262.

9. Nickel JC, McLachlan KR, Smith DM. Eminence development of the postnatal human temporomandibular joint. J Dent Res 1988; 67:896–902.

10. D'Amico A. Functional Occlusion of the natural teeth of man. J Prosthet Dent 1961; 11:899–915.

11. Okeson J. Orthodontics current principles and techniques, 4th edn. St Louis: Elsevier Mosby; 2005. 333.

12. Dawson PE. New definition for relating occlusion to varying conditions of the temporomandibular joint. J Prosthet Dent 1995; 74:619–627.

13. Gilboe DB. Centric relation as the treatment position. J Prosthet Dent 1983; 50:685–689.

14. Ramfjord S, Ash M. Occlusion, 2nd edn. Philadelphia: WB Saunders; 1971. 95.

15. Hansson T, Oberg T, Carlsson GE, et al. Thickness of the soft tissue layers and the articular disk in the temporomadibular joint. Acta Odontol Scand 1977; 35:77–83.

16. Shen G, Ali Darendeliler M. The adaptive remodeling of condylar cartilage – a transition from chondrogenesis to osteogenesis. J Dent Res 2005; 84(8):691–699.

17. Durkin JF, Heeley JD, Irving JT. Cartilage of the mandibular condyle. Temporomandibular Joint – Function and Dysfunction. USA: Mosby; 1979. 43–100.

18. Oberg T, Carlsson GE. Macroscopic and microscopic anatomy of the temporomandibular joint. Temporomandibular Joint -Function and Dysfunction. USA: Mosby; 1979. 101–118.

19. Arnett GW, Milam SB, Gottesman L. Progressive mandibular retrusion – idiopathic condylar resorption. Part II. Am J Orthod Dentofac Orthop 1996; 110:117–127.

20. Mongini F. Condylar remodeling after occlusal therapy. J Prost Dent 1980; 43:568–577.

21. Weinberg LA. Role of condylar position in TMJ dysfunction-pain. J Prosthet Dent 1979; 41:636–643.

22. Pullinger AG, Hollender L, Solberg WK, et al. A tomographic study of mandibular condyle position in an asymptomatic population. J Prost Dent 1985; 53:706–713.

23. Ricketts RM. Variations of the temporomandibular joint as revealed by cephalometric laminography. Am J Othod 1950; 36:877–898.

24. Katzberg RW, Westesson P-L, Tallents RH, et al. Anatomic disorders of the temporomandibular joint disc in asymptomatic subjects. J Oral Maxillofac Surg 1996; 54:147–153.

25. Ribeiro RF, Tallents RT, Katzberg RW, et al. The prevalence of disc displacement in symptomatic and asymptomatic volunteers aged 6 to 25 years. J Orofacial Pain 1997; 11:37–47.

26. Utt TW, Meyers CE Jr, Wierzba TF, et al. A three-dimensional comparison of condylar position changes between centric relation and centric occlusion using the mandibular position indicator. Am J Orthod Dentofacial Orthop 1995; 107:298–308.

27. Ikeda K, Kawamura A. Assessment of optimal condylar position with limited cone-beam computed tomography. Am J Orthod Dentofacial Orthop 2009; 135:495–501.

28. Posselt W. The physiology of occlusion and rehabilitation. 2nd edn. London: Blackwell Scientific Publications; 1968. 25–64.

29. Lundeen HC, Shryock EF, Gibbs CH. An evaluation of mandibular border movements: their character and significance. J Prosthet Dent 1978; 40:442–452.

30. Lee R. Jaw movements engraved in solid plastic for articulator controls. Part I. Recording apparatus. J Prosthet Dent 1969; 22:209–224.

31. Lundeen HC, Gibbs CH. The function of teeth. USA: L and G publishers LLC; 2005. 33–35.

32. Slavicek R. Clinical and instrumental functional analysis for diagnosis and treatment planning. Part 5. Axiography. J Clin Orthod 1988; 22:656–667.

33. Johansson A-S, Isberg A. The anterosuperior insertion of the temporomandibular joint capsule and condylar mobility in joints with and without internal derangement: a double-contrast arthrotomographic investigation. J Oral Maxillofac Surg 1991; 49:1142–1148.

34. Farrar WB. Diagnosis and treatment of anterior dislocation of the articular disc. NYJD 1971; 41:348–351.

35. Larheim TA, Katzberg RW, Westesson P-L, et al. MR evidence of temporomandibular joint fluid and condyle marrow alterations: occurrence in asymptomatic volunteers and symptomatic patients. Int J Oral Maxillofac Surg 2001; 30:113–117.

36. Legrell PE, Isberg A. Mandibular height asymmetry following experimentally induced temporomandibular joint disk displacement in rabbits. Oral Surg Oral Med Pathol Oral Radio Endod 1998; 86:280–85.

37. Isberg A, Hagglund M, Paesani D. The effect of age and gender on the onset of symptomatic temporomandibular joint disk displacement. Oral Surg Oral Med Oral Pathol Oral Radio Endod 1998; 85:252–257.

38. Nebbe B, Major PW. Prevalence of TMJ disc displacement in a pre-orthodontic adolescent sample. Angle Orthod 2000; 70:454–463.

39. Berteretche M-V, Foucart J-M, Meunier A, et al. Histologic changes associated with experimental partial anterior disc displacement in the rabbit temporomandibular joint. J Orofacial Pain 2001; 15: 306–319.

40. Legrell PE, Isberg A. Mandibular length and midline asymmetry after experimentally induced temporomandibular joint disk displacement in rabbits. Am J Orthod Dentofacial Orthop 1999; 115:247–253.

41. Bryndahl F, Eriksson L, Legrell PE, et al. Bilateral TMJ disk displacement induces mandibular retrognathia. J Dent Res 2006; 85:1118–1123.

Excellence in Finishing

14

Ashok Karad

Proper finishing is of critical importance in achieving an excellent occlusal result after orthodontic appliance removal, and it has been widely recognized for many years. Stability of the orthodontic treatment result has been a topic of great interest to the profession since the inception of our speciality. The improvements in the position of teeth achieved after great deal of effort may be lost to varying degrees after the removal of orthodontic appliances. Sometimes, changes in tooth positions are noticed even during the period when the patient is using retention appliances.[1] It has been recognized for many years that the stability of orthodontic treatment results at least partially depends on the way cases have been finished.[2] Orthodontic finishing still remains a continual challenge for the orthodontist. Toward the end of the nineteenth century, the great evolutionary process in orthodontics began. A clearer conception of orthodontic problems was gained principally through the careful application of fundamental principles by such interested workers as Farrar, Guildford, Jackson, Case and Angle. Angle's final achievement, the edgewise appliance, was the culmination of many years of effort and many different appliance designs attempting to place the teeth according to his 'line of occlusion'. The basic mechanical component was a metal bracket with a rectangular slot, and the original size of the slot was 0.022″ × 0.028″. Due to the limitations of this appliance system and the existing treatment philosophy, most often the cases were undertreated, exhibiting lack of torque in upper incisors and absence of true Class I molar relationship. This all resulted into occlusion that had the appearance of a 'nice orthodontic result' that looked 'artificial' and compromised long-term stability of the result. Over the years, many changes and modifications have been made by various clinicians in the basic appliance itself. Preadjusted edgewise appliances in their current variations probably represent the biggest step up the orthodontic evolutionary ladder and provide great benefits to orthodontists in all stages of treatment, especially during finishing and detailing. However, in some clinical situations, it requires a great deal of effort and skill to achieve an excellent occlusal result after appliance removal.

This chapter deals with defining finishing goals and achieving them with the appropriate treatment mechanics for optimal aesthetics, function and stability. It highlights certain occlusal (static and dynamic), periodontal and aesthetic parameters that provide useful guidelines for finishing in both the adolescent and adult orthodontic patients. It is author's belief that the orthodontic finishing begins with diagnosis and treatment planning. With advances in treatment mechanics, there is hardly an abrupt stage of complicated wire bending to fine-tune the tooth positions; rather, it is a gradual progression toward finishing. In the management of a routine orthodontic case, it is extremely important for a clinician to define finishing goals at the beginning of treatment and continue to focus on them till the finishing stage in order to achieve them with appropriate treatment mechanics. The commonly accepted orthodontic treatment goals are as follows:[1-3]

1. Normal static occlusal relationships—Class I occlusion with 'six keys',[4] 3 mm of overjet and overbite
2. Normal functional movements—a mutually protected occlusion
3. Condyles in a seated position—in centric relation
4. Relaxed healthy musculature
5. Normal periodontal health
6. Optimal aesthetics
7. Long-term stability of post-treatment tooth positions

The intent of this chapter is to inform the orthodontic clinician of the importance of occlusal, periodontal and aesthetic parameters to finish orthodontic cases to the highest standards. The American Board of Orthodontics (ABO) established guidelines and objective grading system for scoring dental casts and panoramic radiographs containing eight parameters. These include alignment, marginal ridges, buccolingual inclination, occlusal relationships, occlusal contacts, overjet, interproximal contacts and root angulation.[5]

To achieve these goals, precision wire bending and archwire configurations are required during a clearly defined finishing stage of treatment when standard edgewise appliances are used. However, in contemporary orthodontics, with the use of the built-in features of preadjusted appliance and precise bracket placement, moving teeth to their final position begins as soon as the initial archwires are placed. There is a gradual and a progressive movement of teeth toward finishing rather than a well-defined 'finishing stage'.[1,3] The entire discussion of orthodontic finishing with redefined finishing goals and the appropriate treatment mechanics to achieve the same can be outlined as follows:

1. Occlusal parameters—both static and dynamic
2. Optimal aesthetics
3. Periodontal health
4. Long-term stability

OCCLUSAL PARAMETERS

Achieving proper occlusal relationship of maxillary and mandibular teeth at the conclusion of orthodontic treatment has been a fundamental objective of any orthodontic treatment plan. It was generally assumed that when the teeth were aligned properly and orthodontic appliances were taken off, they would settle into good intercuspation and good function would follow. Unfortunately, this was not always the case, as teeth never settled into maximum interdigitation and some instances of excessive wearing of teeth and temporomandibular dysfunction were noted. Therefore, it is extremely important to define finishing goals with respect to occlusal relationships of teeth based on optimal aesthetics, function

and long-term stability and achieve them with the appropriate treatment mechanics before the removal of appliances. The occlusal parameters can be described as follows:

- Static occlusal goals—as observed on dental casts or intraorally
- Functional occlusion goals—as observed during various mandibular movements

Static occlusal parameters

Angle[6] proposed his most famous key to occlusion as a guide to orthodontic diagnosis and treatment planning. It was based on the relationship of the upper first permanent molar to the lower first permanent molar. Andrews[7] proposed his six keys to occlusion, which gave a well-delineated prescription for an ideal intercuspation of the teeth. These all constitute only a static relationship.

Alignment

Proper alignment of teeth has been generally acknowledged to be the fundamental objective of any orthodontic treatment plan. The predebonding evaluation must contain an assessment of tooth alignment in the anterior and posterior segments of maxillary and mandibular dental arches. In assessing the tooth alignment, it is essential to identify the determinants of anterior and posterior tooth alignment.

The ABO[5] further clarified and quantified the static occlusal goals by providing a grading system for study casts and panoramic radiographs. In the maxillary anterior segment, the incisal edges and lingual surfaces of incisors and canines are used to establish anterior alignment. This is based on the fact that these surfaces are the functioning surfaces, and when aligned properly, the anteriors appear to be in their best aesthetic relationship (Fig. 14.1B). In the maxillary posterior segment, mesiodistal central grooves of the premolars and molars are used to attain optimal alignment. Again, these areas are used since they represent the functioning surfaces of the maxillary posterior teeth and are easy to observe intraorally (Fig. 14.1B).

In the mandibular arch, the labioincisal edges of the incisors and canines are the determinants of anterior alignment (Fig. 14.1D). In the mandibular posterior segment, the buccal cusps of premolars and molars represent the functioning surfaces, and they are easy to visualize intraorally. Therefore, these landmarks are used to establish the proper alignment in the posterior teeth within the patient's acceptable archform (Fig. 14.1D).

The alignment of teeth, irrespective of the treatment technique, is carried out during the initial phase of treatment before correction of major elements of malocclusion. It is not considered to be complete until finishing archwires become passive in the brackets. The degree of rotational control of teeth is dependant on the mesiodistal width of the bracket. The greater the width the greater the rotational control. This is achieved, however, at the expense of reducing the interbracket distance

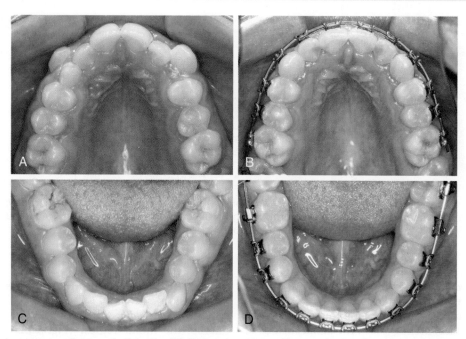

Figure 14.1 Achieving proper alignment of teeth. **(A)** Pretreatment maxillary arch showing crowding and high labially placed canines. **(B)** Proper alignment of anterior and posterior segment teeth with full-size archwire in place. **(C)** Pretreatment mandibular arch showing anterior crowding and rolled-in first molars. **(D)** Well-aligned anterior teeth and uprighted, properly positioned first molars.

that has implications during the subsequent stages of treatment.

Archform coordination

It has been recognized for many years that by the finishing stage of treatment, the maxillary and mandibular archforms should be accurately established with the rectangular archwires. It is a good practice to coordinate the upper and lower arch widths to the patient's original archforms right from the beginning of treatment through the transitional phase to avoid extra efforts and time required to adjust them during the finishing stage. Broomell[8] in 1902 wrote that ' . . . the teeth are arranged in the jaws in the form of two parabolic curves, the superior arch describing the segment of a larger circle than the inferior, as a result of which the upper teeth slightly overhang the lower'. Most clinicians have acknowledged that there are extensive variations in the size and shape of human archform. Chuck[9] noted the variation in human archform and suggested that archforms had been referred to as square, round, oval, tapering, etc. He further stated that while the Bonwill-Hawley[9] archform was not suitable for every patient, it could be used as a template for the construction of individualized archforms. Over the years, the majority of edgewise appliance users used the Bonwill-Hawley[10] archform as a beginning template for the construction of the edgewise archwire. White[11] compared the accuracy of various standardized arch designs with 24 untreated ideal adult occlusions.

He concluded that:

- The catenary curve[6] showed a good fit with 27% of the cases, a moderately good fit with 46% of the cases and a poor fit with 27% of the cases.

- The Bonwill-Hawley[9] archform had a good fit with 8% of the cases, a moderately good fit with 40% of the cases and a poor fit with 52% of the cases.
- The Brader[12] archform had a good fit with 12% of the cases, a moderately good fit with 44% of the cases and a poor fit with 44% of the cases.

From these research studies, it is evident that there are extensive variations in human archforms and there is no single archform that can be used for all orthodontic cases. However, it is universally accepted that there are three basic types of archforms. They are ovoid, tapered and square.

Felton et al[13] evaluated a wide range of manufactured archwires from orthodontic companies. It was observed that the archforms were quite close to ovoid, tapered and square groups. When these archforms are superimposed, they vary mainly in the intercanine width, having a range of approximately 6 mm.

Components of archform

In order to select the specific archform for a patient and modify it to coordinate well to the patient's original archform, it is essential to identify the different components of archform. Understanding various parts of archform would provide a basis for the design of a preformed archwire system and the need for minor adjustments to make it individualized. The components of archform (Fig. 14.2A) are as follows:

1. Anterior curvature
2. Posterior curvature
3. Intercanine width
4. Intermolar width

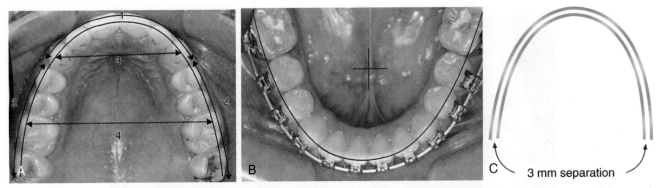

Figure 14.2   Archform coordination. **(A)** Components of archform: (1) anterior curvature, (2) posterior curvature, (3) intercanine width and (4) intermolar width. **(B)** Mandibular archform during finishing stage. **(C)** Maxillary and mandibular archwires should be coordinated by keeping even separation of 3 mm when superimposed.

The anterior curvature. This component of the archform is a smooth curve in the anterior segment extending from canine to canine. Since the labiolingual thickness of the maxillary lateral incisor is less, the labial surface of lateral incisors is more lingually placed when compared with central incisors and canines. The greater labiolingual dimension of the cuspid places its labial surfaces more labially than the central and lateral incisors. However, in a well-finished case, the lingual surfaces of these teeth in the maxillary arch should describe a smooth curve (Fig. 14.2A1). When the intercanine width is narrow, this component of the archform is more tapered; and when the intercanine width is wide, it is more square or flattened.

The posterior curvature. The posterior curvature of the archform extends from the cuspids posteriorly to the second molars. This component exhibits a straight line in the Bonwill-Hawley archform and a significant curvature in the Brader archform. There seems to be a universal acceptance favouring a gradual curvature between canines and second molars. However, it is author's observation that this part of the archform exhibits a gradual curvature from the canine to the mesiobuccal cusp of the first molar and another gradual curvature from this point to the distobuccal cusp of the second molar (Fig. 14.2A2). This is because the mesiobuccal cusp of the maxillary first molar is the most prominent part of the posterior segment, and the buccal surface is also substantially angled, with the distal buccal surface more lingual than the mesiobuccal allowing the distobuccal cusp to occlude properly with the lower first molar.

The intercanine width. This is the distance between the two canines on the maxillary and mandibular archforms (Fig. 14.2A3). This component of the archform is considered to be the most critical, and the strict adherence to the patient's original dimension is highly recommended since significant relapse occurs, if this component is altered. In most of the archform system, the intercanine width varies by 6 mm.

Burke et al[14] used the meta-analysis technique to review 26 previous studies of mandibular intercanine width. They concluded that 'regardless of patient's diagnostic and treatment modalities, mandibular intercanine width tends to expand or increase during treatment in the order of about one to two millimetres, and

to contract postretention to approximately the same dimension'.

Intermolar width. This component of the archform, across the molar region (Fig. 14.2A4), can be altered during treatment depending on the patient's requirement. This is because the treatment changes in this area appear to be more stable than the changes in intercanine width. If the maxillary arch has been expanded, earlier in the treatment, the expansion needs to be maintained during the finishing stage either by expanding the chosen archform in the molar region or by using the square archform.

Archwire coordination

Once the archform has been selected as per the patient's original archform, the maxillary and mandibular archforms should be coordinated throughout the treatment. Whatever changes are done during the initial and transitional stages of treatment, they should be maintained during the finishing stage. Before making any alterations in the chosen archform for desired treatment changes, it is critical to identify the areas for potential relapse. Gardner[15] studied intercanine, interfirst premolar, intersecond premolar and interfirst molar widths, as well as arch length changes in 103 cases. In all, 74 were nonextraction, and 29 were treated with extraction of four first premolars. He concluded that intercanine width increased during treatment but had a strong tendency to return to its original pretreatment width in both nonextraction and extraction cases. Interfirst premolar width showed the greatest treatment increase, with only a minimal amount of post-treatment width decrease. Second premolar width in nonextraction cases showed a significant amount of increase, with a slight tendency for postretention decrease. Second premolar width in extraction cases showed a decrease during treatment and a slight continued decrease postretention. The intermolar width in nonextraction cases showed a significant increase in width during treatment, but the extraction cases showed a significant decrease during treatment. However, there were no changes in intermolar width in either extraction or nonextraction cases postretention. The incisor to intermolar distance decreased with treatment and had a slight tendency to continue to decrease postretention. Archform templates can be used to coordinate maxillary and mandibular finishing arch-wires. When superimposed, the maxillary archwire should be approximately 3 mm wider outside of the mandibular archwire (Fig. 14.2C).

Establishing marginal ridge relationships

The marginal ridges are used as a key to achieve relative vertical positioning of the maxillary and mandibular posterior teeth. During the finishing stage, it is important to make sure that the marginal ridges of adjacent posterior teeth are positioned at the same level (Fig. 14.3A and B). The levelled marginal ridges will position the cusps and fossae of the teeth at the same level, thereby promoting proper occlusal contacts. According to Casko et al,[5] once the marginal ridges of the posterior teeth are positioned at the same relative level, then the cementoenamel junctions are also at the same relative level. This will lead to the bone levels between the adjacent teeth being flat, producing a much healthier periodontal situation for the patient. The precise bracket placement, especially in the vertical plane, has been generally acknowledged to be the critical element in establishing marginal ridge relationships. The vertical bracket height affects the torque and in–out and height of the tooth and, therefore, holds the key to proper vertical crown positioning, marginal ridge relationships and contact points.[16] If there is an error in vertical bracket placement, it will be expressed as abnormal crown position after the initial levelling. At this stage, the bracket should be precisely repositioned to level marginal ridges and to ensure better stability. If this is not performed during the initial phase of treatment, these corrections can be done during the finishing stage of treatment by incorporating some bends in the finishing archwire.

The ABO[5] noted that the most common mistakes in marginal ridge alignment were between the maxillary first and the second molars and between the mandibular first and the second molars. The difficulty in the positioning of posterior attachments due to limited visibility, gingival hypertrophy, variable clinical crown height and delayed eruption of teeth may lead to these errors.[17] The lack of distal root tip in the maxillary second bicuspids, expressed during the finishing stage, leads to discrepancy in the marginal ridge matching between these teeth

and the first molar. This also leads to a lack of occlusal contact in the posteriors.

The levelled marginal ridges are not a good indicator of relative posterior vertical tooth position in a periodontally compromised adult patient. In such clinical situations, it is appropriate to rely on the bone levels between the teeth to determine the proper vertical position of teeth.[18]

Contact points

The importance of proper contact points between the teeth in preventing food impaction and stability of the dental arches after orthodontic treatment has been well understood by all specialists. Interproximal contacts are also used to determine, if all spaces within the dental arch have been closed. During the finishing stage, three-dimensional control of the teeth positions and their relationship with the adjacent teeth are essential to establish the correct location of interproximal contact points. In order to get the proper perspective of their positioning, the contact points should be observed from two aspects: the labial or buccal aspect and the incisal or occlusal aspect. These views will demonstrate the relative positions of the contact points cervico-occlusally, labiolingually or buccolingually.

Contact points or contact surfaces of teeth are generally located in the occlusal one-third of the proximal walls, slightly buccal to the central fossa in the molar and premolar areas with the exception of the maxillary first and second molars [19,20] (Fig. 14.4A–C). The position of contact points in the maxillary anterior segment, when viewed from front, seems to progress from the incisal to the cervical and from the central incisors to the canine (Fig. 14.4A). When viewed from the occlusal aspect, the contact points in the maxillary anterior teeth are centred labiolingually. In the mandibular anterior segment, the contact points are located at the incisal third of the crowns and seem to move toward cervical region from anterior to posterior teeth. Since the molars become progressively shorter from the first to the third, the centres of the contact areas drop cervically when viewed from the buccal aspect (Fig. 14.4C). The contact points in the mandibular anterior and posterior segments are centred labiolingually or buccolingually, when viewed from the occlusal aspect.

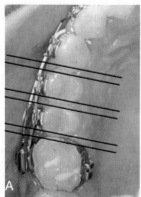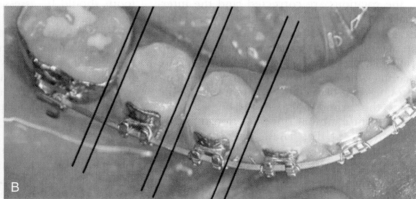

Figure 14.3 Establishing marginal ridge relationships. Proper positioning of marginal ridges in the maxillary right posterior segment **(A)** and in the mandibular right posterior segment **(B)**.

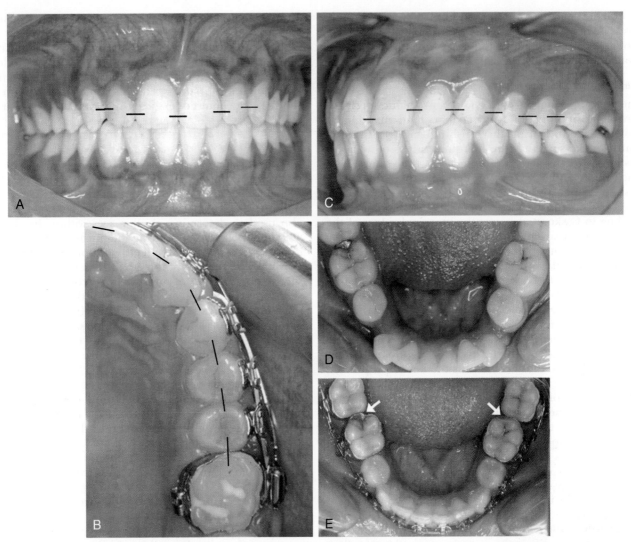

Figure 14.4 Proper location of contact points. **(A)** Contact points in the maxillary anterior teeth progress from incisal to cervical and from central incisor to canine. **(B)** Contact points in the maxillary posterior segment when viewed from the occlusal aspect. **(C)** Contact points when viewed from the buccal aspect. **(D)** Another patient showing normal contact relationship between the mandibular first and second molars pretreatment. **(E)** Abnormal position of contact points between the first and second molars due to built-in offsets in the first molar attachments.

During the finishing stage of treatment, it is important to make sure that the teeth are properly vertically positioned, the rotations are corrected, and the interproximal spaces are closed and maintained to optimally position the contact points. The distal offsets incorporated in the mandibular first molar attachments found in some appliance prescriptions lead to inappropriate or broken contacts between first and second molars.[21] This offset rotates first or second molars to the mesial or can displace the second molars to the lingual creating abnormalities in marginal ridge relationships and contact points (Fig. 14.4E). These discrepancies of treatment must be carefully evaluated and addressed during the finishing stage in order to promote proper proximal contacts, marginal ridges and alignment.

Occlusal relationship

Optimal interarch relationship of maxillary and mandibular teeth at the conclusion of treatment is the prime objective of any orthodontic treatment plan. In order to achieve accuracy in this relationship, each individual tooth should be assessed in anteroposterior, transverse and vertical planes and positioned into its best fit, both anatomically and functionally. Andrews once said that 'We (orthodontists) tend to look at teeth collectively rather than individually'. It is, therefore, essential to define goals for each individual tooth and achieve them with appropriate treatment mechanics before the removal of orthodontic appliances.

Molar position

At the conclusion of orthodontic treatment, the maxillary permanent first molar should be positioned in such a way that its mesiobuccal cusp occludes in a groove between the mesial and the middle cusps of the mandibular permanent first molar.[22] It should have sufficient distal rotation, mesioaxial inclination and buccal root torque, so as to fit the mesiolingual cusp in the central fossa of the mandibular first molar and its distal marginal ridge occluding with the mesial marginal ridge of the mandibular second molar (Fig. 14.5A). Insufficient thickness of maxillary second bicuspid causes first molar to rotate mesially upon initial wire engagement, leading to an increase in Class II tendency and buccal movement of second bicuspid (Fig. 14.5B).

During the finishing stage, it is of paramount importance to evaluate the buccolingual inclination of the posterior teeth to achieve good intercuspation and prevent interferences during mandibular movements. This should be assessed by evaluating the relationship between the buccal and the lingual cusps of the maxillary and mandibular premolars and molars—called the *curve of Wilson*. In normal situation, the lingual cusp should be at the same level or within a millimetre of the same level as the mandibular buccal cusps.[5]

This relationship makes the occlusal tables of posterior teeth relatively flat, therefore, promoting better contact of the maxillary lingual cusps and the fossae of the mandibular posterior teeth (Fig. 14.5D). The extreme amount of mandibular posterior lingual crown torque found in many preadjusted appliance prescriptions results in 'rolled-in' mandibular posterior teeth as a result of

expressed torque (Fig. 14.5C).[23,24] The mandibular molars should be uprighted and progressively torqued with no rotations and spaces.

Bicuspid position

The buccal cusps of the maxillary premolars should be positioned to have a cusp–embrasure relationship with the mandibular premolars (Fig. 14.6A), and the lingual cusps of the maxillary premolars should exhibit a cusp–fossa relationship with the mandibular premolars. Ricketts[25] pointed out that the contact position of the maxillary second premolar is the key to a properly treated malocclusion. The maxillary second bicuspid should have a normal contact relation with the mesial incline of the lower first molar, which produces an interlocking into the corresponding interspaces of the lower premolars (Fig. 14.6D). This relationship causes the tip of the mesiobuccal cusp of the upper first molar to be slightly distal to the mesiobuccal groove of the lower first molar. According to Ricketts, this is the most efficient, self-cleansing and self-preserving relationship in accordance with nature's plan. The maxillary bicuspids should have mesioaxial angulation with the second bicuspid exhibiting distal root tip to promote marginal ridge matching between these teeth and the first molar and for better interocclusal contact (Fig. 14.6F).

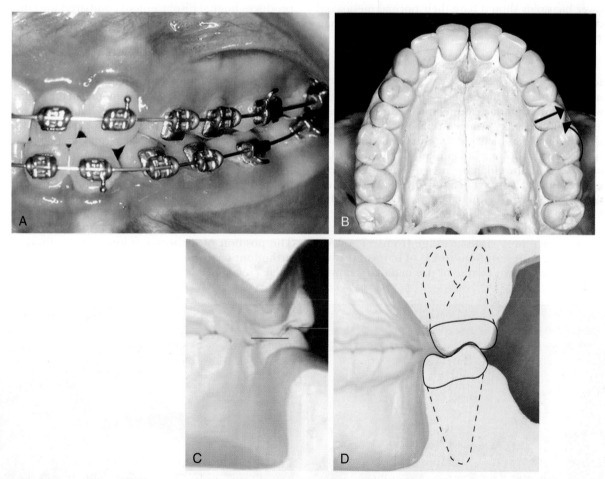

Figure 14.5 Molar position. **(A)** Proper position of maxillary and mandibular first molars with optimal mesioaxial inclination and buccal root torque. **(B)** Insufficient thickness of maxillary second bicuspid causes first molar to rotate mesially and buccal movement of second bicuspid upon initial wire engagement. **(C)** Limited amount of maxillary posterior buccal root torque and the extreme amount of mandibular posterior buccal root torque, leading to improper interdigitation, increased buccal overjet and balancing interferences. **(D)** Improved buccolingual relationship of posterior teeth by reducing the lower posterior torque and by increasing the upper posterior torque.

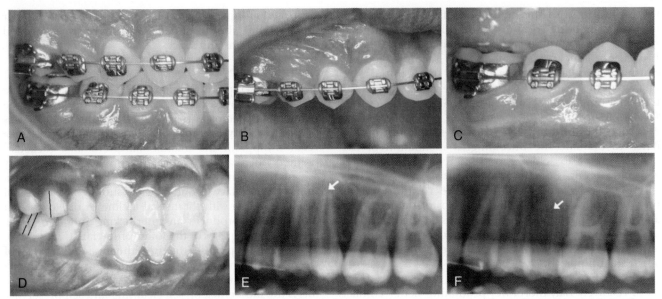

Figure 14.6 Bicuspid position. **(A)** Sagittal, transverse and vertical positioning of maxillary and mandibular bicuspids leading to good intercuspal relationship. **(B)** Maxillary right segment bicuspids. **(C)** Mandibular right segment bicuspids. **(D)** Position of maxillary second bicuspid—a key to a properly treated malocclusion. **(E)** Lack of distal root tip in the maxillary second bicuspid. **(F)** Distal root tip expressed during the finishing stage promotes better marginal ridge relationship and interocclusal contact.

The lower bicuspids should have their normal mesioaxial angulation with proper contact points and levelled marginal ridges.

Canine position

The maxillary canine has a cusp–embrasure relationship with the mandibular canine and first premolar. It should exhibit normal contact relationship with the lateral and the first bicuspid, mesioaxial angulation and optimal length for cuspid guidance. The mandibular cuspid crown should have mesioaxial angulation, proper mesiodistal contact relationship and the cusp tip 1 mm higher than the incisal edges of the mandibular incisors (Fig. 14.7 A and B). It is interesting to note that the torque values for the maxillary canine in various appliance prescriptions range from −7° of Andrews-influenced prescriptions to 17° of bioprogressive. Excessive lingual crown torque of the maxillary canine produces lingual displacement compared with that of the other anterior teeth.[21] A similar situation exists in case of mandibular canines, where the torque values exhibit extreme range from −11° of Andrew's prescriptions to 17° of bioprogressive-based prescriptions.

McLaughlin et al[24] recommended no canine torque for canines that are prominently positioned in the pretreatment archform. This also helps in maintaining the roots within the cancellous bone during retraction mechanics. During the finishing stage, the maxillary and mandibular cuspid positions should be evaluated to make sure that they exhibit mesioaxial angulation, proper proximal contacts and optimal vertical and horizontal overlap for good function.

Incisor position

The position of incisors has long been a focal point of orthodontic diagnosis and treatment planning. It has been recognized by many orthodontists that the

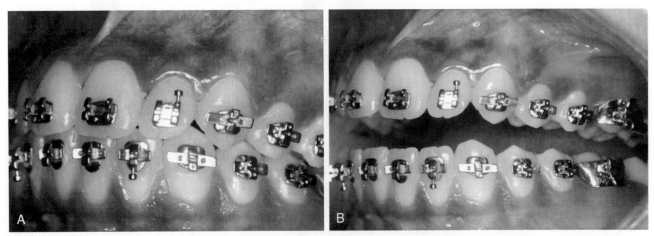

Figure 14.7 Canine position. **(A)** Cusp–embrasure relationship of maxillary and mandibular cuspids. **(B)** Proper position of maxillary and mandibular canines and their relationship with adjacent teeth.

cornerstone of a stable dentition is the proper positioning of maxillary and mandibular incisors. A single ideal position that fits every clinical situation may never be found because of the extreme variations in skeletal and muscular patterns. The search for the ideal position has been almost endless, and even so there is little agreement among orthodontists as to what position is best. Optimal positioning of maxillary and mandibular incisors at the conclusion of treatment is the prime objective of any orthodontic treatment plan. The control of undesirable movement inherent with the routine orthodontic treatment mechanics would reduce the amount of fine tuning of incisor position during the finishing stage. AlQabandi et al[26] reported 6–7° of lower incisor flaring when simply levelling the curve of Spee with fixed appliances. Reports have described the limitations of controlling the labial proclination of lower incisors during levelling, even with rectangular wires, especially when using Class II elastics.[26,27]

The lower incisor flaring, if not controlled during the initial stage of treatment, would require increased labial crown torque of the maxillary incisors to maintain appropriate overjet and overbite. This results into bimaxillary protrusion impairing the facial aesthetics. The overall inclination of the maxillary and mandibular anterior teeth is best evaluated with a lateral cephalometric radiograph. The interincisal angle plays an important role in aesthetics, function and stability and should not be based on averages. Growth direction, aesthetics and overbite should also be considered in determining ideal torque in the maxillary and mandibular arch.[28]

The maxillary central and lateral incisors in their final positions should have no more than 0.5 mm height differential and 5° and 9° mesioaxial inclination, respectively, and they should be adequately torqued (Fig. 14.8A–C). The incisal edges should be 2–2.5 mm below the lip embrasure of the upper and lower lips, when the lips are closed with no lip strain. Raleigh Williams[29] suggested certain guidelines to optimally position mandibular incisors and canines for long-term stability. The mandibular incisors should be aligned contact point-to-contact point with the roots in the same labiolingual plane (Fig. 14.8D). The lower incisor root apices should be spread distally to the crowns, and the apices of the lower lateral incisor must be spread more than those of the central incisors (Fig. 14.8E). They should be positioned at the cephalometric goal of 11 to A-Po. The maxillary and mandibular incisors should have approximately 2.5 mm overjet–overbite relationship; however, it should be proportional to the height of cusps of posterior teeth.

Occlusal contact relationship

After the resolution of malocclusion, the teeth need to be individually settled into their final positions before appliance removal. In the posterior segment, teeth are generally held away from one another in vertical plane due to full-size rectangular steel finishing archwires. The vertical settling of maxillary and mandibular teeth to achieve maximum intercuspation is done by using different configurations of vertical elastics (Fig. 14.9 A and B). The more precise the placement of brackets and tubes, the easier it is to settle the teeth and the less elastics need to be used in this way. The adequacy of posterior teeth interdigitation is evaluated by assessing the contact

relationship between the cusps and the fossae of the molars and premolars. Ricketts[25] suggested that without third molars, 16–24 occlusal stops or centric stops on each side are adequate for a good balanced occlusion (Fig. 14.9C). The lingual cusps of the maxillary premolars and molars should be in contact with the marginal ridges or the fossae of the mandibular premolars and molars.[5] In addition, the buccal cusps of the mandibular premolars and molars should contact the fossae or marginal ridges of the maxillary molars and premolars.[5] Due to lack of an adequate occlusal table, the lingual cusps of the maxillary first premolars may not establish contact with the mandibular first premolar. In the maxillary buccal segments, the palatal cusps of the first and second molars are generally slightly longer and extend slightly more occlusal than the buccal cusp. With the common use of expansion treatment often using overexpanded, commercial arch blanks or limited amount of maxillary posterior expressed buccal root torque, palatal cusps extend occlusally beyond their normal limits. This leads to inappropriate interdigitation between maxillary and mandibular posterior teeth.[17]

Therefore, the buccolingual relationship of posterior teeth should be improved to achieve maximum intercuspation by flattening the curve of Wilson, minimizing or eliminating the discrepancies in the posterior overjet and avoiding the prominence of palatal cusps by reducing the lower posterior torque and by increasing the upper posterior torque.

Vertical dimension

The control of vertical dimension of occlusion is one of the greatest problems faced by orthodontists while treating variety of clinical situations. Quite often, orthodontic treatment mechanics has a tendency to extrude posterior teeth and encourage excess vertical alveolar growth leading to what is termed a *molar fulcrum*.[30] This promotes the development of anterior open bite through the bicuspids and a tongue-thrust swallow. The temporomandibular joint (TMJ) clicking and tightness or stiffness of the mandibular musculature, often associated with pain or discomfort of any combination of mandibular muscles, are some of the common symptoms of this disorder.[30] Also, during various mandibular excursions, the patient may not be able to execute smooth gliding movement without any interference. Any extrusive treatment mechanics, like prolonged use of Class II elastics, overexpansion of the maxillary arch that facilitates overhanging palatal cusps and distal driving of molars in cases with a short ramus or short posterior facial height should be avoided to maintain the vertical dimension.

Dynamic occlusal parameters

In addition to achieving the static occlusal relationships as suggested by Angle[6] and the 'six keys to occlusion' by Andrews,[22] other researchers, like Williamson,[31] Aubrey,[32] Ricketts[33] and Roth,[30] have all expanded the area of knowledge in occlusion to include the neuromuscular and bony structures of the TMJ in establishing orthodontic treatment objectives. In dealing with the various elements of functional occlusion as one of the finishing goals, it is important to achieve stable centric relation of the mandible with maximum intercuspation of the teeth

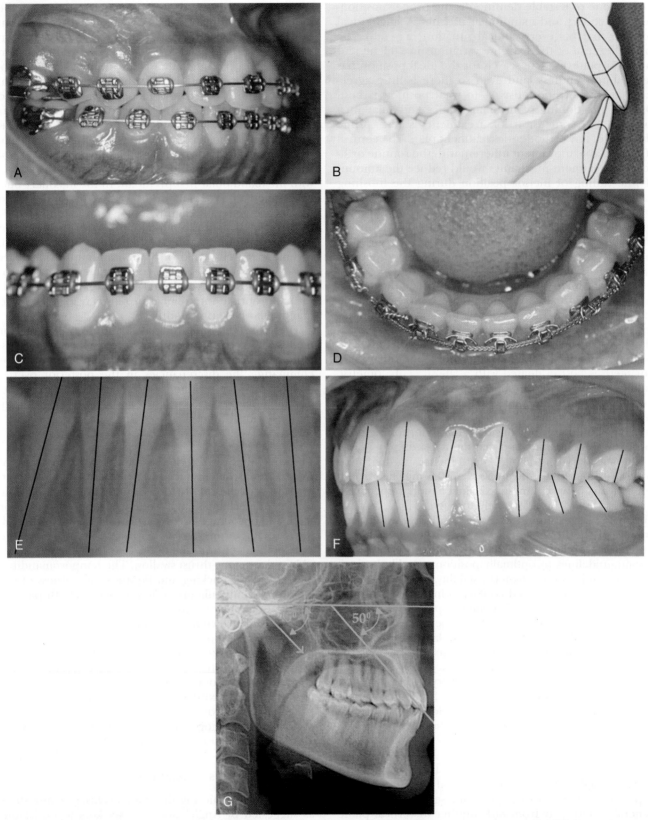

Figure 14.8 Incisor position. **(A)** Normal overjet and overbite relationship. **(B)** Optimal interincisal angle. **(C)** Normal vertical positioning of incisors and their relationship with canines. **(D)** Labiolingual position of mandibular incisors. **(E)** Optimal lower incisor positioning with progressive distal root spread. **(F)** Normal interincisal relationship, overjet and overbite achieved by optimal incisor torque control. **(G)** The ideal angle of disclusion in protrusive is thought to be 5° greater than the condylar disclusive angle.

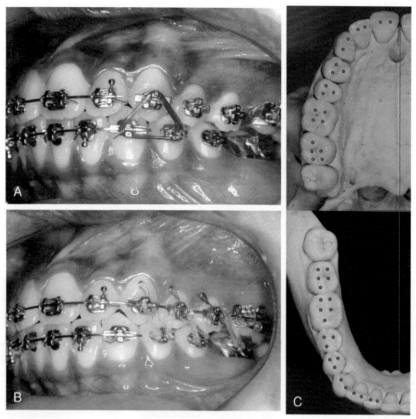

Figure 14.9 Occlusal contact relationship. **(A and B)** Use of different configurations of vertical elastics to settle the posterior teeth into maximum intercuspation. **(C)** Location and the number of occlusal stops or centric stops on each side of arches.

at this position. In the intercuspal position and retruded contact position, the mandible should be situated in the same sagittal plane, the distance between the two positions being less than 1 mm. All the teeth must occlude in maximum intercuspation when the mandible is in the centric relation. The anterior teeth must be positioned to provide separation (disclusion) of the posterior teeth immediately when the mandible leaves its centric relation position to move anteriorly or laterally. When these relationships are achieved, the teeth will not interfere with condylar movement, and no neuromuscular avoidance mechanism will be necessary. Therefore, as the patient nears the end of fixed appliance therapy, the checklist should include careful consideration of three aspects of functional occlusion: centric relation, anterior guidance and stability of posterior tooth arrangement. The occlusal scheme that is most successful in preventing occlusal problems in patients over a long period of time is the mutually protected occlusion.[34]

Anterior guidance

Ideally, in the protrusive excursion of the mandible, there should be harmonious glide path of anterior teeth. These teeth should work against one another to separate or disclude the posterior teeth as soon as the mandible moves out of centric closure. Since the incisors are the teeth farthest from the muscles moving the mandible, they can be expected to receive the least stress. The proper overbite and overjet established after orthodontic treatment should allow for a gentle glide path (Fig. 14.10 J–L). The optimal position of maxillary and mandibular incisors

and their relationship with each other after orthodontic treatment are the key elements of anterior guidance. According to McHorris,[35,36] in the optimal functional occlusion, the anteriors are in very close approximation but do not touch when molars are in occlusion. The lower anteriors engage the lingual incline of the opposing upper anteriors immediately with mandibular movement. The lingual discluding surface of the upper anteriors seems to reflect the anatomical angle or the discluding pathway of the mandibular condyles. The ideal anterior disclusion angle is greater than or equal to 5° than the condylar disclusion angle (Fig. 14.11). The common mistake to achieve anterior guidance is to place insufficient labial crown torque in the maxillary incisors, lack of adequate time for the torque to be sufficiently expressed or treating to an end-to-end incisor position in the conviction that the case is 'overtreated'. All too often, the case stays 'overtreated', and the patient has many posterior interferences. An occlusal interference on the anterior teeth, identified during unforced closure of the mandible, sometimes associated with a distalizing effect in condylar position has been termed *anterior interference*.[37] The axial inclinations of maxillary and mandibular anteriors and the subsequent interincisal angle should be proper in order to avoid anterior interferences after orthodontic treatment.

Lateral excursions

The key tooth in lateral mandibular movements is the mandibular cuspid. It has the best anatomy and is in the best position to provide the main gliding inclines for lateral excursions, with no interferences on the balancing side (Fig. 14.10 G–I and M–O). Ideally, it should be the posterior teeth working against the maxillary cuspid, but under certain situations when maxillary cuspid is missing, it can be made to work satisfactorily with a maxillary bicuspid. If more teeth than the mandibular cuspid on working side are allowed to contact in lateral excursions, uneven wear is likely to occur because each tooth is at different distance from the rotating condyle and therefore, moves on a different arc.[38] Therefore, during the finishing stage of treatment, maxillary and mandibular canine positions should be checked to provide gentle lateral lift during the mandibular lateral excursion. Excessive lateral stress on the cuspids should also be avoided as this may cause lingual movement of the lower cuspids and resultant lower anterior crowding or labial movement of the maxillary cuspids.

To achieve these goals, it is necessary to have three-dimensional tooth control during orthodontic treatment and position each individual tooth as per the static occlusal parameters. It is essential to bond second molars whenever possible so that they may be properly positioned. Occlusal interference involving these teeth can be most damaging because they are located closest to the muscle forces that move the mandible.

PERIODONTAL FACTORS

One of the finishing goals of orthodontic treatment is to achieve optimal periodontal health. As Schweitzer[39] suggested that 'the single goal agreed to by all concepts and theories of occlusion is the preservation, in good health, of the whole masticatory system for the lifespan of the

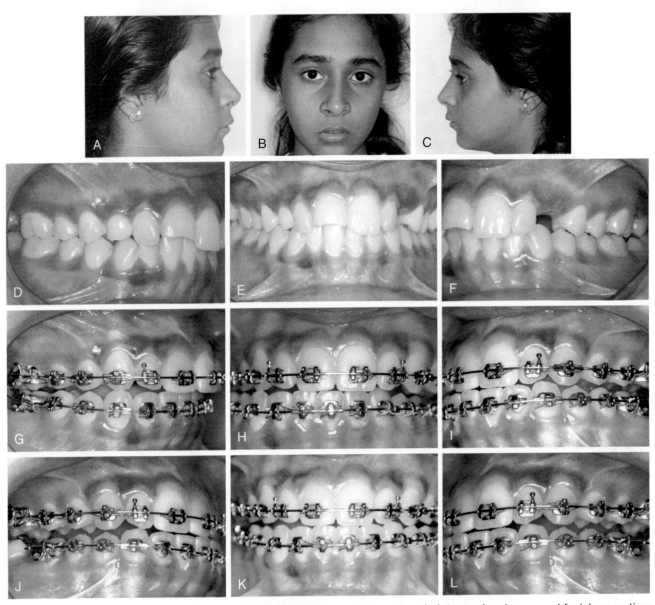

Figure 14.10 Establishing functional occlusal goals. **(A–C)** Pretreatment extraoral pictures showing normal facial proportions and orthognathic profile. **(D–F)** Pretreatment intraoral pictures showing over-retained maxillary right deciduous canine, un-erupted permanent canines and fractured maxillary right central incisor. **(G–I)** Mandibular right lateral excursion. **(J–L)** Protrusive mandibular movement.

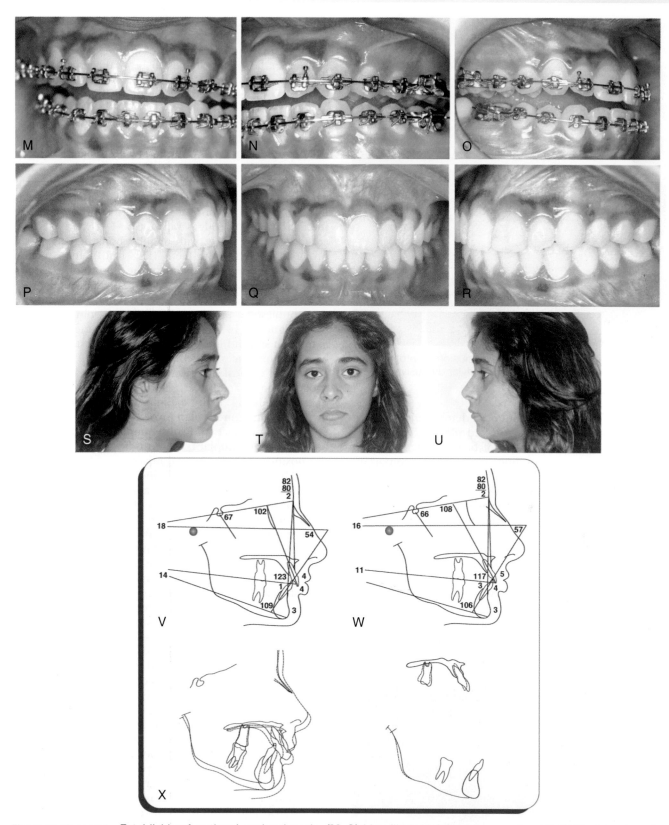

Figure 14.10, cont'd   Establishing functional occlusal goals. **(M–O)** Mandibular left lateral excursion. **(P–R)** Post-treatment intraoral pictures showing static occlusal goals. **(S–U)** Post-treatment extraoral pictures showing orthognathic profile and normal facial proportions. **(V)** Pretreatment lateral cephalometric tracing. **(W)** Post-treatment lateral cephalometric tracing. **(X)** Pretreatment and post-treatment cephalometric superimpositions.

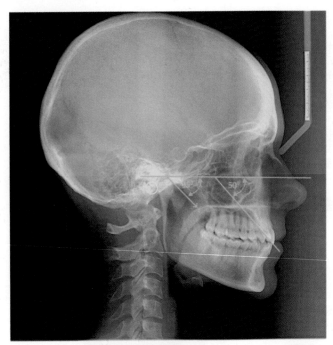

Figure 14.11 The ideal angle of disclusion in protrusive is thought to be 5° greater than the condylar disclusive angle.

individual. This includes minimum deterioration of hard and soft tissues, good function and pleasing aesthetics'. Therefore, during the course of orthodontic treatment and as a part of predebonding evaluation, it is important to check the bone level between adjacent teeth, the parallelism of roots, the morphology of the roots and the health of the supporting soft tissues (Fig. 14.12). In adolescent patients, the bone levels between the adjacent teeth are not a matter of concern, as they generally do not exhibit a periodontal disease that leads to bone destruction. However, in adult patients who have lost bone on individual teeth, the involved tooth should be relieved from occlusion and erupted orthodontically. This controlled, slow-forced eruption improves the bone level and crown-to-root ratio.[40] In adult orthodontic patient with interproximal bone loss, the incisal edges or marginal

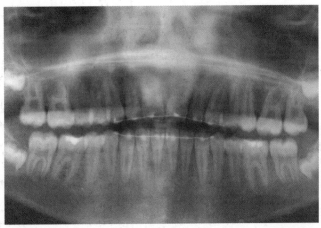

Figure 14.12 Post-treatment radiograph showing even root spacing and optimal bone levels between the adjacent teeth.

ridges should not be used as a guide for vertical positioning of adjacent teeth.[18] In such a situation, it is advisable to align the bone levels rather than the adjacent teeth.

Another factor that needs to be evaluated during the finishing stage is the position of the roots of adjacent teeth that should be parallel to one another. Other factors being normal, if the roots are parallel to one another, there will be sufficient bone between the roots of teeth. It is considered that more interproximal bone will provide greater resistance to periodontal bone loss, if the patient develops periodontal disease in the future. During the finishing stage, if the teeth are not properly uprighted, especially when the second bicuspids or first molars are extracted or missing and the posterior teeth are drifted into that space, then the marginal ridges will not be level and proximal contacts will be faulty, with angular bony defects on the proximal aspect of the teeth (Fig. 14.13). In extraction cases, it is important to maintain the closure of extraction spaces during the finishing stage of treatment with the roots of the adjacent teeth parallel to each other. This eliminates the troublesome problem of spaces reopening postretention. (Figure 14.14 shows tipping of adjacent teeth into the extraction site and uneven root spacing, with the potential of extraction spaces reopening postretention.)

Another clinical situation that demands parallelism of roots of the adjacent teeth is when the maxillary lateral incisor is missing. If the maxillary lateral incisor is missing and the treatment plan involves sufficient opening of lateral incisor space and subsequent restoration with an osseointegrated implant, then it is important to evaluate the position of the roots of adjacent teeth radiographically. The roots of the central incisor and canine should be parallel to each other with adequate space between the roots for implant placement (Fig. 14.15).

All these finishing procedures should be performed with minimum deterioration of supporting hard and soft tissues. The root resorption has been described in the orthodontic literature as an inevitable pathological outcome of orthodontic tooth movement.[41] The aetiology of the external root resorption phenomenon is multifactoral.[42] It can be detected even in the early levelling stages of orthodontic treatment with an increased risk for long, narrow and deviated roots.[43] Intrusion is a critical type of orthodontic tooth movement in relation to external root resorption, and the research has shown that the root resorption is directly proportional to the magnitude of the intrusive force applied[41] (Fig. 14.16 A and B). Even though force magnitude and orthodontic biomechanics are not the sole factors that can lead to external root resorption, heavy forces during intrusion should be used cautiously, especially if this procedure will be carried out over a long period of time. More resorption measured by volumetric analysis is associated with heavy force levels, and it is seen more on the buccal cervical and lingual apical regions of root surfaces than on other regions, suggesting that high-pressure zones are more susceptible to resorption.[44]

AESTHETIC PARAMETERS

Achievement of optimal dentofacial aesthetics is the primary goal of orthodontic treatment. Pretreatment

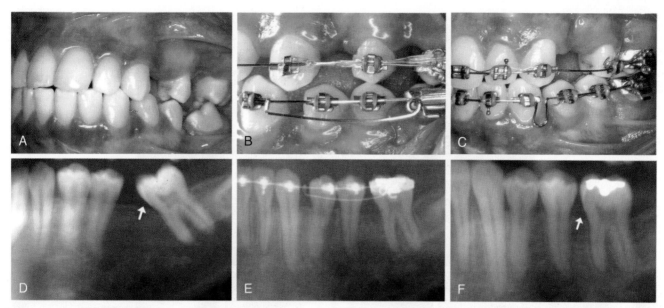

Figure 14.13 Mesially drifted molars. **(A)** Mandibular left first molar is missing, and the second molar is mesially drifted. **(B)** Molar uprighting mechanics. **(C)** Optimal molar position. **(D)** Radiograph showing angular bony defect on the mesial aspect of mesially tipped molar. **(E)** Molar is being uprighted. **(F)** Post-treatment molar position and elimination of bony defect on the mesial aspect of molar.

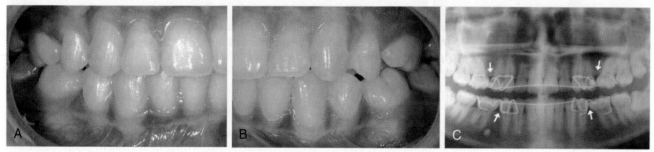

Figure 14.14 Poor orthodontic finish. **(A and B)** Teeth adjacent to the extraction site are not uprighted. **(C)** Radiograph showing tipping of teeth into the extraction site and uneven root spacing.

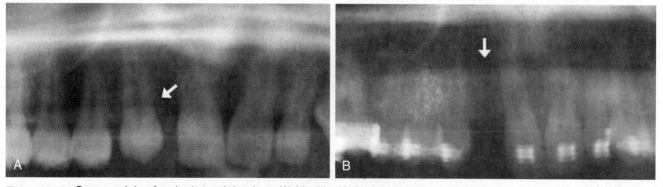

Figure 14.15 Space gaining for single tooth implant. (A) Maxillary right lateral incisor missing and deficient space for restoration. **(B)** Space opened for single tooth implant. Note the parallelism of adjacent roots.

evaluation of facial aesthetics and the projections concerning the desired goal of treatment should be done prior to the beginning of treatment. Its evaluation should be the ongoing process during the stages of orthodontic treatment. Though orthodontists enjoy a high level of patient appreciation, partly because of the impact of aesthetic improvement, quite often, the finished result is short of the finest possible aesthetic result. This

is probably because of disproportions in the crown width, length and abnormal shape of anterior teeth; abnormal gingival architecture, etc.

Crown width discrepancy

Size of the teeth is one of the most important elements of anterior dental aesthetics. Orthodontists are often faced

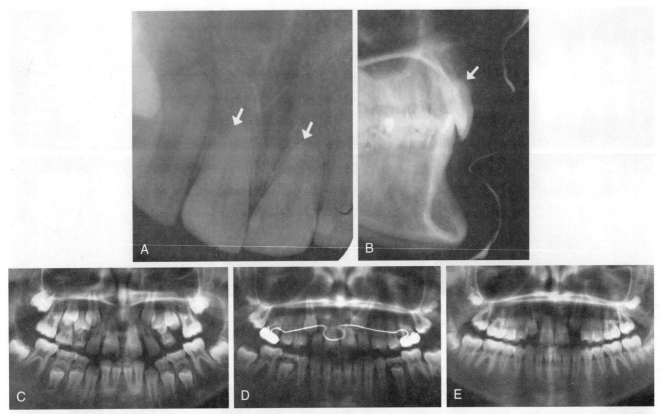

Figure 14.16 Iatrogenic root resorption. **(A** and **B)** External root resorption of maxillary central incisors following their intrusion. **(C)** Another patient during mixed dentition stage showing maxillary canines exerting pressure on the roots of lateral incisors. **(D)** Poor treatment planning and mechanics leading to severe root resorption of lateral incisors. **(E)** Lateral incisors were ultimately extracted.

with disproportionate widths of anterior teeth during treatment. This tooth size discrepancy is commonly found in patients with peg-shaped lateral incisors. Even after getting the teeth perfectly aligned and the archforms properly established with orthodontic treatment, the abnormal shape and smaller size of lateral incisor pose aesthetic problems. Such clinical situations require sufficient space provided by orthodontic treatment to restore the normal width of lateral incisor. If a lateral incisor is of normal shape but only slightly narrower than normal, and the discrepancy is bilateral, it may not be necessary to create space to restore normal widths of lateral incisors. If the discrepancy in the widths of lateral incisors is minimal, the influence on the anterior occlusion and the impact on aesthetics may not be distinguishable.[45] However, if the tooth size discrepancy is unilateral, or if it is quite significant, it affects the anterior occlusion and aesthetics.[46,47] It is, therefore, imperative to restore the size of the malformed lateral incisors after the completion of orthodontic treatment for overall good treatment result. In doing so, it is best advisable to follow the principle of golden proportion, which can be called the building blocks of nature itself. This ratio is an ideal ratio that can be mathematically defined as 1:1.618 (Fig. 14.17 F). It has been observed that when the rule of golden proportion is followed, the result is something that is naturally attractive and pleasing to the eye. Smiles can be made attractive by following these mathematical rules of nature to create harmony, symmetry and proportion.[20,48] The width of

maxillary central incisor is in golden proportion to the lateral incisor width, which in turn is in proportion with the mesial width of the canine.[49] During the finishing stage of orthodontic treatment, if excessive space exists in the anterior segment, it should be redistributed to restore the proper crown width (Fig. 14.17 B and C). If insufficient space exists to restore these teeth, an adequate space should be gained, which will permit the restoration of proper crown width. To determine the space required to restore the crown width, during the treatment planning stage, construction of a diagnostic wax-up is an important step to visualize the final result. After removal of the fixed orthodontic appliances, provisional restorations should be given before final restorations to avoid relapse. When gaining space orthodontically, where should the maxillary lateral incisor be positioned in all three planes of space? Vincent Kokich[50] provided certain guidelines to optimally position malformed lateral incisors for best results. One must remember that the contour of the mesial surfaces of lateral and central incisors is relatively flat. If the lateral incisor is positioned too close to the canine, its mesial surface should be overcontoured to establish normal crown width. Therefore, as far as the mesiodistal position of peg-shaped lateral incisor is concerned, it should be positioned nearer the central incisor for optimal aesthetic result (Fig. 14.17B).

The labiolingual position of the malformed lateral incisor will depend on the type of the subsequent permanent restoration used to restore the appropriate

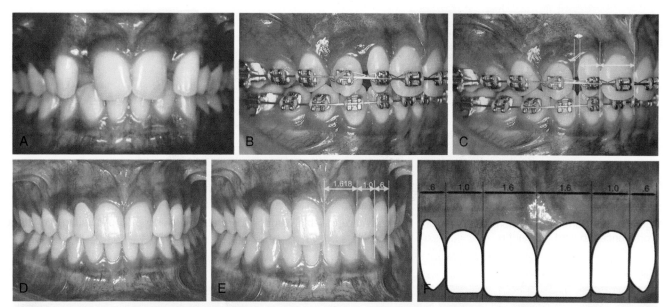

Figure 14.17 Crown width discrepancy. **(A)** Class I malocclusion with disproportionate crown widths of anteriors due to peg-shaped laterals. **(B and C)** Proper distribution of anterior spaces to restore normal widths of lateral incisors. **(D and E)** Peg-shaped laterals are restored with ceramic veneers in a golden proportion with adjacent teeth. **(F)** The golden proportion—an ideal ratio can be mathematically defined as 1:1.618.

crown width. This restoration could be either a porcelain crown or a porcelain veneer. If it is a porcelain crown, the orthodontic treatment should be directed to position the peg-shaped lateral incisor in the centre of the alveolar ridge labiolingually, with approximately 0.50–0.75 mm overjet. This will eliminate the need for additional tooth preparation on the lingual aspect of the lateral. However, if the subsequent restoration is going to be the porcelain veneer, the malformed lateral incisor should be positioned lingually to be in contact with the mandibular incisors. This lingual position should be in proportion with the thickness of the porcelain veneer. During the finishing stage of treatment, it is important to evaluate the gingivoincisal position of the lateral incisor. Ideally, the incisal edges and the gingival margins should be aligned with the contralateral lateral incisor. Orthodontic intrusion or forced eruption will position the peg-shaped lateral incisor at the appropriate level, which in turn will help restore proper length of the tooth.

Role of 'Illusion'

The size and shape of anterior teeth, particularly their length and width, as a result of disproportion, may appear aesthetically compromised. If this disproportion is not very severe, it can be addressed by using optical concepts to create optical illusions of size and shape.[20] As a general rule, visual perception is possible because of the contrast in shape, lines and colour of objects. Therefore, the perception of size and shape is dependant on the reflection or deflection of light from different surface areas of objects. By controlling the phenomenon of light reflection and by altering the surface of a tooth, it is possible to establish proportions because 'our vision is often fooled by optical illusive effects'.[51]

These optical principles can be summarized as follows:[20]

- Increased light reflection increases visibility.
- Increased light deflection diminishes visibility.
- Increased contrast increases visibility.

The key factor here is to control the light reflection or deflection by contouring the tooth surface. Tooth contouring should be limited to mesial and distal inclines, incisal edges, gingival inclines, natural grooves, angles, etc. In case of a wider tooth mesiodistally proportions can be re-established by applying the principles of narrowing illusion. This can be accomplished by adjusting the lateral prominences toward the centre, increasing the curvature of the central prominence mesiodistally, and moderately increasing the length of the central prominence (Figs 14.18 and 14.19).

Aesthetic recontouring

Fine-tuning the position of anterior teeth, both individually and collectively, that leads to proper incisor display upon smile is one of the keys to achieve optimal aesthetics. However, certain abnormalities of teeth like irregular incisal edges, abnormal tooth morphology or attrided anterior teeth interfere with the aesthetic outcome of orthodontic treatment. Dental recontouring or reshaping, also called *odontoplasty* or *enameloplasty*, is a procedure in which small amounts of tooth enamel are removed in order to change the length, shape or surface contours of a tooth. The goal of aesthetic recontouring is to enhance the aesthetic component of orthodontic result by selectively remodelling anterior teeth to correct minor anterior tooth imperfections. However, it should be remembered that it should not be used as a substitute for incomplete orthodontic treatment. Before

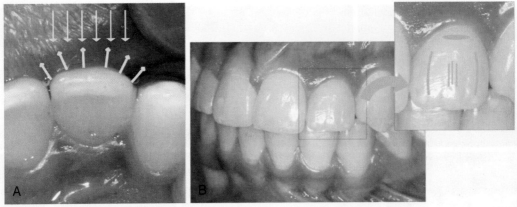

Figure 14.18 Narrowing illusion. **(A)** Increasing the curvature of labial surface (central prominence). **(B)** Adjusting the lateral prominences toward the centre.

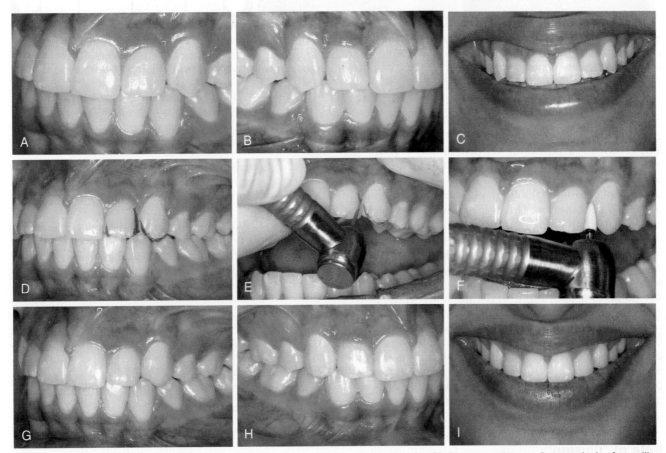

Figure 14.19 Step-by-step procedure for applying the principles of illusion. **(A–C)** Disproportionate (larger size) of maxillary lateral incisors. **(D–F)** Sequential recontouring procedure. **(G–I)** Proportionate width (altered visual perception) of maxillary lateral incisors. Note that the contact points between laterals and centrals and laterals and canines are not disturbed.

performing aesthetic recontouring procedure, the clinician should review the incisor display upon smile to decide on the guidelines that are specific to the feminine and masculine smiles.[52] The characteristic features of youthful, feminine smiles are rounded incisal edges, open incisal and facial embrasures and softened facial line angles. However, the masculine smile is typically characterized by more closed incisal embrasures and prominent incisal angles. Therefore, the morphology

and architecture of the maxillary anterior teeth ennced by aesthetic countouring procedure determined by these principles greatly contribute to the composition of an individual smile. Prior to this procedure, the clinician should review the aesthetic goals of treatment to determine if the finished orthodontic treatment result could be enhanced with recontouring. Once the goals are defined, the procedure should be outlined and sequenced to adequately and conservatively prepare the teeth. The basic tenet of the contouring procedure is to achieve natural, anatomic forms of anterior teeth. The selective remodelling of anterior teeth is done by using high-speed handpiece with intermittent brush strokes, adequate water supply and proper illumination followed by enamel polishing and fluoride application.[52]

It is the author's experience that the proper positioning of anterior teeth with orthodontic treatment combined with intentional changes in tooth morphology by recontouring to correct minor imperfections significantly enhances the final result.

Postdebonding restoration of original enamel surface

Achievement of treatment goals with proper positioning of teeth during the finishing stage of orthodontic treatment is followed by debonding procedure. It involves the proper removal of various orthodontic attachments and the residual composite from the teeth. Incomplete removal of the residual adhesive from the tooth surface after debonding leads to staining and plaque accumulation, demineralization or caries formation and gingival inflammation from contact with rough surface. To enhance the positive impact of orthodontic treatment result, it is essential to establish the pretreatment enamel surface qualities by using proper techniques of debonding and residual composite removal with no introgenic damage to the enamel. It is in fact quite difficult to remove the residual adhesive due to its colour similarity with the enamel. Therefore, choosing the best method of residual composite removal after debonding is a common problem faced by most clinicians. The important step is to identify the residual adhesive sites by drying the tooth to visualize the dull opaque resin remnants on the tooth or by using a probe or an explorer to feel the rough surface as opposed to a smooth enamel finish. The ultrafine diamond bur is the most efficient in the removal of composite remnants, but it produces very rough finished enamel surface.[53] The preferred method is to use dome-tapered tungsten carbide bur in a contra-angle handpiece at approximately 30,000 rpm.[54] Use of water cooling for bulk removal of composite is recommended; however, it should not be used while removing the last traces of adhesive as it reduces the contrast with enamel. The author uses the combination of composite removing pliers and high-speed tungsten carbide bur with water cooling for the bulk removal, low-speed tungsten carbide bur with no water and aluminium oxide polishing points and rubber cups for the removal of last traces, followed by enamel polishing with pumice as the best way to restore the enamel surface to its pretreatment surface quality.

Enamel decalcification

The presence of white spots or areas of enamel demineralization of varying degrees due to noncompliance with oral hygiene instructions has been the problem of great concern to many clinicians. Almost half of the patients undergoing orthodontic treatment with multibonded appliances exhibit the areas of enamel decalcification, with the highest incidence in the maxillary incisors, especially the laterals.[55] These lesions significantly compromise the aesthetic component of orthodontic result, prompting the orthodontist to establish and reinforce the preventive program. In addition to proper tooth-brushing, daily rinsing with dilute (0.05%) sodium fluoride solution along with a regular use of a fluoride dentifrice is recommended as a routine procedure for orthodontic patients.[56] A single application of a fluoride varnish, which is a viscous liquid consisting of 5% sodium fluoride in a base of natural colophony, has been shown to reduce decalcification in vitro by 50%.[57] In comparison with fluoride rinses and dentifrices, fluoride varnish demonstrates a more sustained release of fluoride ions over a longer period of direct contact with the enamel.[58,59] Unlike many other methods of fluoride application, fluoride varnishes do not depend on patient cooperation for their effectiveness in reducing enamel decalcification. After normal prophylaxis, acid-etching and bonding of brackets, cheek retractors are left in place and teeth are air-dried prior to varnish application. A thin layer of varnish is then painted onto enamel surfaces adjacent to the brackets with a sponge applicator or minibrush. The enamel surface between the bracket and the gingival margin on each tooth must be painted with a varnish. The fluoride varnish then sets into yellow–brown waterproof coating after contact with saliva. After the fluoride varnish application, the patient is instructed not to brush for 4–5 h. The discolouration usually abrades away after several weeks of normal brushing and function.

Teeth whitening: the finishing touch to beautiful, straight teeth

Teeth whitening is one of the simplest methods yet can make most dramatic changes to patient's appearance. People feel better about themselves with whiter and brighter teeth, and it has been recognized that people respond to a dazzling, healthy smile in a more positive manner. The majority of the patients are concerned about aesthetics, and they want the best possible smile. Patients who are interested in straight teeth are interested in straight, white teeth.

The orthodontic treatment result, which essentially constitutes straight teeth and good occlusion, can be enhanced by teeth whitening to obtain a brilliantly white smile. Tooth bleaching or whitening that can be performed externally is called *vital tooth bleaching* and that can be done intracoronally in root-filled teeth is called *nonvital tooth bleaching*. It can be performed at-home and in-office. At home, method of tooth whitening is done using custom-fitted trays and diluted concentration of a whitening gel, usually 10% carbamide peroxide. Although this method works well, it is very time consuming and takes a great deal of patience and compliance. However, in-office bleaching technique involves the use of higher concentrations of whitening gel, usually 35% hydrogen peroxide, which in the presence of strong light source, makes a profound difference in discoloured teeth in a shorter time. Tooth sensitivity is a common side effect of external tooth bleaching.[60] Higher incidence of tooth sensitivity from 67 to 78% of the patients was reported after in-office bleaching with hydrogen peroxide in combination with heat.[61] Tooth sensitivity normally persists for up to 4 days after the cessation of bleaching treatment.

It is important to explain to the patient that tooth whitening will last an average of approximately 2 years with periodic at-home touchups. This duration of whitening effect also depends on the patient's personal habits. Smoking, dark foods and drink will diminish the results more quickly.

Replacement of missing laterals with implants

Dental agenesis occurs quite frequently, especially of the maxillary lateral incisors, and it presents a true challenge to an aesthetic solution. For a long time, many clinicians had suggested an alternative treatment approach by moving the entire lateral segment mesially to position the cuspid in the lateral incisor position. However, this approach ends up with compromised results that do not fulfill the aesthetic requirements of good orthodontic treatment. This is because the cuspid has a very different crown and root shape to that of the lateral incisor, and it has a darker shade. When missing lateral incisor space is closed by moving the entire lateral segment mesially, lateral excursions are made using bicuspids, which have shorter, thinner roots; thus, functional requirements are also not fulfilled either.

If restoration is the treatment of choice, it requires reshaping neighbouring teeth, with consequent removal of varying amounts of enamel, and eventual risk of gingival recession, caries, etc. The osseointegrated implant is the most conservative and biological method since the missing tooth can be replaced without damaging the adjacent teeth. If the use of implants is the part of treatment plan for the missing lateral incisors, it is necessary to decide the exact placement of implants and evaluate the smile line and gingival contour. When the lateral incisors are missing, there is usually no adequate space to restore them due to drifting of the adjacent teeth (Fig. 14.20 A and B). In such cases, it is essential to gain adequate space with orthodontics for the placement of implant and for the crown restoration for optimal aesthetic result (Fig. 14.20 I and J). The exact amount of the space created should be according to the proposed size of lateral incisors, which should be proportionate to the width of the central incisors. After opening up of sufficient space, acrylic teeth may be selected closer to the shade of the patient's teeth, bracketed and attached to the archwire for aesthetic purpose. Before the orthodontic appliances are removed, it is important to evaluate the position of the roots of adjacent teeth radiographically. The roots of the central incisors and canines on either side, in case of bilaterally missing laterals, should be parallel to each other with adequate space between the roots for implant placement (Fig. 14.20F). Before removal of orthodontic appliances, quite often, there is adequate space for the prosthesis and inadequate space between the roots of the adjacent teeth for an implant. This usually occurs due to tipping movement of adjacent teeth, which requires proper uprighting of the roots during the finishing stage of orthodontic treatment. The minimum space of 6.5 mm between adjacent roots is required to place a standard implant of 3 mm width.

Gingival architecture

Colour, contour and health of the gingival tissues provide the framework and backdrop for the pleasing smile. Even if the case is well finished with orthodontic treatment, abnormality of the gingiva either in the form of loss of papilla, asymmetrical pattern or excessive display upon smile leads to a poor result.[1] It is, therefore, essential to have proper gingival architecture and display to achieve a maximum aesthetic result. In normal situation, the gingival tissue blends into tooth embrasure that is totally filled from buccal to lingual. The presence of a papilla between the maxillary central incisors is a key element in anterior aesthetics.[45,62] While evaluating the aesthetics related to gingival tissues, it is important to consider two key factors: (1) gingival levels and (2) gingival contour or gingival zenith.

As a general rule, a line drawn at the level of the free gingival margin of the anterior segment will show the free gingival margin of the central incisors and the cuspids to be at the same height and that of the lateral incisors to be slightly coronal (Fig. 14.21C1). The gingival papillary tip should be halfway between the incisal edge and the labial gingival height of contour over the centre of each anterior tooth. The contour of the margins of gingiva should mimic the cementoenamel junctions. The most apical point of the labial gingival contour, called the *gingival zenith*, is located just distal of the long axis of the central incisors and cuspids, whereas the gingival zenith for the lateral incisors coincides with their long axis[20,63] (Fig. 14.21C2). In other words, the height of the gum line across the face of the tooth should be centred on the lateral incisors and positioned in the distal one-third of the face of the tooth for the centrals and canines. This gives the gingiva a semicircular appearance for lateral incisors and an elliptical appearance for central incisors and canines.

During the process of eruption, the whole periodontal apparatus is carried with the erupting tooth. When there is asymmetric eruption of the teeth, it will also result in discrepancies in heights of the underlying crestal bone. This, in turn, results into asymmetries in gingival heights from one side of the arch to the other. This type of a clinical situation can be managed orthodontically by intrusion or extrusion of teeth (Fig. 14.21B).

Anterior aesthetic gingival depigmentation

Exposure of maxillary gingiva of approximately 1–2 mm upon smile is generally considered part of the aesthetic smile. Excessive gingival display 'gummy smile' is one of the major concerns for large number of patients seeking orthodontic treatment. This problem is aggravated in patients with gingival hyperpigmentation, expressed as 'dark gums' leading to compromised gingival aesthetics (Fig. 14.22 A and B). Aesthetic periodontal plastic surgery 'depigmentation' is rewarding in such patients with compromised aesthetics. Therefore, maxillary gingiva of normal colour and maxillary gingiva display of approximately 1–2 mm upon smile should be the goal that should be achieved at the conclusion of orthodontic treatment (Fig. 14.22 C and D).

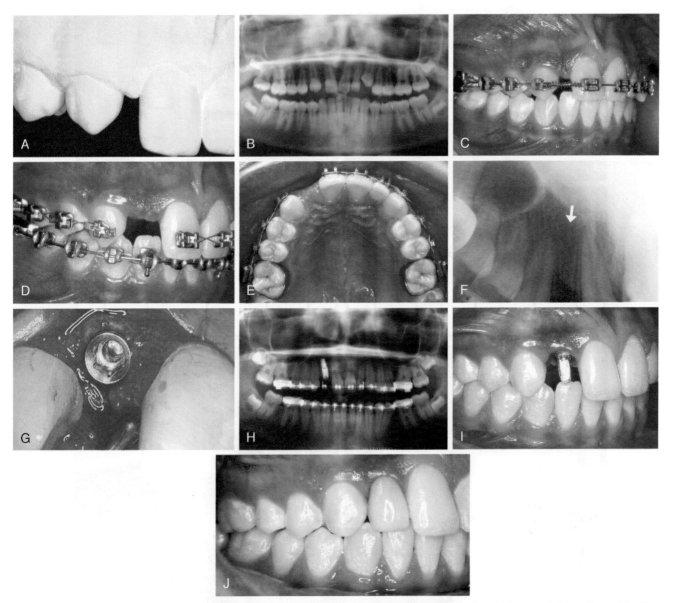

Figure 14.20 Replacement of missing laterals with implants. **(A)** Maxillary lateral incisor is missing, and the adjacent teeth are drifted into the space. **(B)** Inadequate space between the roots of central incisor and canine. **(C)** Orthodontic mechanics to open the space. **(D and E)** Optimal space gained for restoration. **(F)** Intraoral periapical radiograph shows adequate space between the roots of the central incisor and the canine. Note the parallelism of roots of the adjacent teeth. **(G)** Osseointegrated implant placement in the lateral incisor region. **(H and I)** Single tooth implant in place with abutment. **(J)** Final restoration.

Melanin, a brown pigment, is the most common cause of endogenous pigmentation of gingiva.[64,65] Gingival depigmentation is essentially a periodontal plastic surgical procedure carried out to eliminate or reduce the gingival hyperpigmentation. Gingival depigmentation procedure using scalpels involves surgical removal of gingival epithelium along with a layer of the underlying connective tissue to heal by secondary intention. The newly formed epithelium is devoid of melanin pigmentation. Laser depigmentation technique has recently become quite popular and is even preferred over scalpel technique by clinicians. Selection of a specific technique is based on clinical experience and individual preferences. The documented advantages of lasers in periodontal surgery include less bleeding[66] and reduced postoperative pain.

Gingival depigmentation procedure offers a practical solution to dramatically improve patient's smile in case of a display of dark gums due to hyperpigmentation.

Smile

Smile is one of the most effective means by which people convey their emotions.[67] There is no universal 'ideal' smile. One of the most important aesthetic goals of orthodontic treatment is to achieve a 'balanced smile,' which can be described as an appropriate positioning of the teeth and normal gingival architecture within the dynamic display zone.[68]

A balanced smile is an expression of the laws of nature, which can be interpreted in the form of mathematical

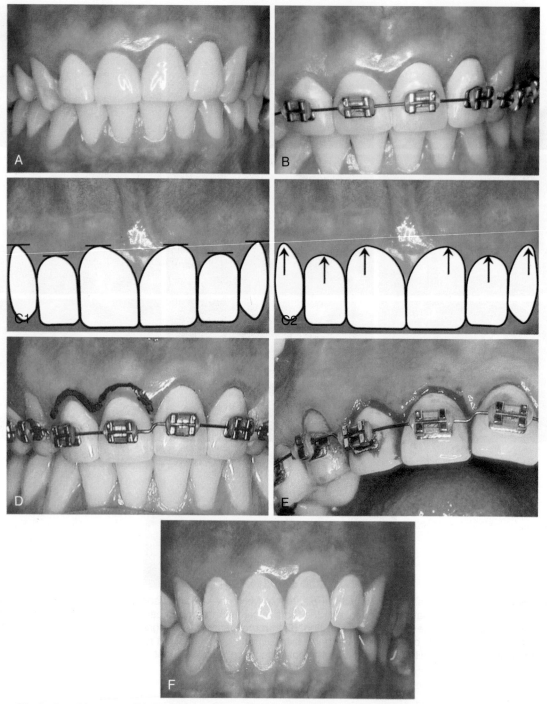

Figure 14.21 Gingival architecture. **(A)** Faulty maxillary anterior restoration violating the biologic width and discrepancy in gingival margins and gingival zenith. **(B)** Forced eruption. **(C1 and C2)** Normal gingival architecture. **(D)** After the differential forced eruption of incisors, the crown extension procedure has been planned on upper right central and lateral incisors to resolve the residual gingival discrepancy. **(E)** Crown extension procedure. **(F)** The combined orthodontic and restorative treatment exhibiting normal gingival architecture with physiologic positioning of finishing margins of anterior restoration.

proportions[20] and visual judgment—falls within the inaccurate purview of evaluator's interpretation.

When viewed from the frontal aspect, the smile begins at the corners of the mouth, extend laterally. The lips may remain at contact except with people having a short upper lip. As smile expands and approaches laughter, the lips separate, the corners of the mouth curve upward and the teeth are exposed to view. Some people show only the maxillary teeth, others show the

mandibular teeth and some show both. As the angles of the mouth extend and the lips separate, the mesial half of the maxillary first molars and the mandibular second premolars may be exposed. The maxillary gingival display of approximately 1–2 mm upon smile is considered part of the aesthetic smile. As the smile approaches a laugh, the jaws separate and a dark space develops between the maxillary and mandibular teeth. This well-formed dark space, called the *negative space*,

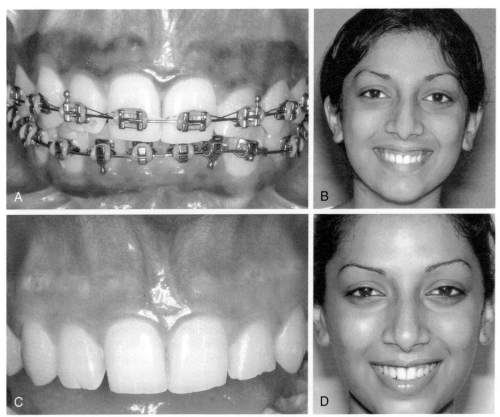

Figure 14.22 Gingival depigmentation. **(A)** Melanin pigmentation expressed as 'dark gums'. **(B)** Gummy smile with gingival hyperpigmentation. **(C)** Restoration of normal pink gingival colour after depigmentation procedure. **(D)** Smile after gingivoplasty and depigmentation procedure.

lends attractiveness to the smile and enhances the appearance of the oral region.[46]

The perfect smile occurs when the maxillary anterior dentition is in line with the curvature of the lower lip, the corners of the lips are elevated to the same height (symmetry), and bilateral negative spaces separate the teeth from the corners of the lips.[69]

Anatomy of the smile

The upper and lower lips frame the display zone of the smile consisting of the teeth and the gingival scaffold as the main components. The soft tissue determinants of the display zone are lip thickness, intercommissure widths, interlabial gap, smile index (width and height) and the gingival architecture. To get adequate information on dentofacial midline, alignment, right–left symmetry of canine and premolar torque, the patient's smile should be observed directly from the frontal view (Fig. 14.23).

What is smile line?

A patient's smile line is determined by the position of the lips during a natural unforced smile. The maxillary teeth follow the contour of the lower lip. This convex curve, known as the incisal curve, produces a radiating symmetry.[70] Lombardi[46] suggested the application of the golden proportion in dentistry. Snow[71] considered a bilateral analysis of apparent individual tooth width as a percentage of the total apparent width of the six anterior teeth. He proposed the golden percentage, wherein

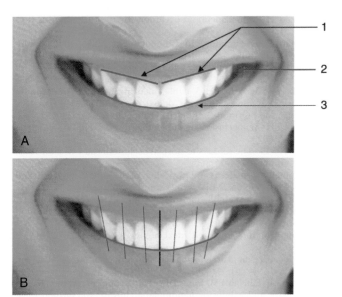

Figure 14.23 Anatomy of the smile. **(A)** (1) Gingival aesthetic line, (2) Buccal corridor and (3) Smile line. **(B)** Axial inclination of teeth in relation to the midline.

the proportional width of each tooth should be: canine 10%, lateral 15%, central 25%, central 25%, lateral 15% and canine 10% of the total distance across the anterior segment in order to achieve an aesthetically pleasing smile.

The anterior and lateral negative spaces act as a border to the dental elements, while the lips represent the frame. The anterior negative space is evident during speech and laughter, while the bilateral space can be observed in a broad smile and provides a cohesiveness to the dentofacial composition.[72] Assessing incisal edge position in both vertical and anteroposterior directions is a fundamental part of the aesthetic diagnosis.[8] Its location can significantly affect aesthetics and function. It is also an important marker to achieve both. Vertical position can be identified with the help of dentolabial phonetics, amount of incisal exposure during speech (ideally 2 mm) and smile line. Anteroposterior position can be evaluated with the help of overjet and overbite and facial profile of the patient. Amount of teeth and gingiva exposed during an active smile would determine the extent of corrections required with a broad smile requiring more aesthetic consideration.

Sarver[73] stresses on the importance of gingival shape and gingival contour in the final aesthetic outcome of orthodontic patients. Gingival shape refers to curvature of the gingival margin of the tooth. For the mandibular incisors and the maxillary laterals, it is a symmetrical curve, while for the maxillary centrals and canines, it is more elliptical. Thus, the gingival zenith (the most apical point of the gingival margin) is located distal to the longitudinal axis of the maxillary centrals and canines. The gingival zenith of the maxillary laterals and mandibular incisors should coincide with their longitudinal axis.[20]

CONCLUSION

Modern orthodontic treatment is aimed at creating the best possible occlusal relationships within the framework of acceptable facial aesthetics and stability of the occlusal result. It is extremely important for a clinician to define finishing goals at the beginning of treatment and continue to focus on them till the finishing stage, in order to achieve them with appropriate treatment mechanics.

This chapter has provided certain occlusal (static and dynamic), periodontal and aesthetic parameters that outline useful guidelines for finishing in both the adolescent and adult orthodontic patients. Also, in patients requiring interdisciplinary treatment, choosing the best possible treatment options from other specialities and combining them as a part of the optimal treatment plan based on scientific rationale should be the aim for the highest standards of orthodontic case finishing.

REFERENCES

1. Ashok Karad. Excellence in finishing: current concepts, goals and mechanics. J Ind Orthod Soc 2006; 39:126–138.
2. Ronald H Roth. Functional occlusion for the orthodontist. JCO 1981; 1:32–50.
3. Richard P McLaughlin, John C Bennett. Finishing with the preadjusted orthodontic appliance. Semin Orthod 2003; 9:165–183.
4. Andrews LF. Straight wire – the concept and the appliance. In: Valleau J, Olfe JT, eds. Straight wire. Los Angeles: Wells; 1989:32–33.
5. Casko J, Vaden J, Kokich V et al. American Board of Orthodontics objective grading system for dental casts and panoramic radiographs. Am J Orthod Dentofacial Orthop 2000; 114:530–532.
6. Angle EH. Malocclusion of the teeth. 7th edn. Philadelphia: S.S. White; 1907.
7. Andrews LF. The six keys to normal occlusion. Am J Orthod 1972; 63:296–309.
8. Broomell IN. Anatomy and physiology of the mouth and teeth. 2nd edn. Philadelphia: P. Blakiston's Son; 1902:99.
9. Chuck GC. Ideal archform. Angle Orthod 1934; 4:312–327.
10. Hawley CA. Determination of the normal arch and its application to orthodontia. Dental Cosmos 1905; 47:541–552.
11. White LW. Individualized ideal arches. J Clin Ortho 1978; 12: 779–787.
12. Brader AC. Dental arch form related to intraoral forces: PR5C. Am J Orthod 1972; 61:541–561.
13. Felton MJ, Sinclair PM, Jones DL, et al. A computerized analysis of the shape and stability of mandibular archform. Am J Orthod 1987; 92:478–483.
14. Burke SP, Silveira AM, Goldsmith LJ, et al. Meta-analysis of mandibular intercanine width in treatment and postretention. Angle Orthod 1998; 68(1):53–60.
15. Gardner SD. Posttreatment and postretention changes following orthodontic therapy. Angle Orthod 1976; 46:151–161.
16. Richard P McLaughlin, John C Bennett. Finishing with the preadjusted orthodontic appliance. Semin Orthod 2003; 9:165–183.
17. Bowman SJ. Addressing concerns for finished cases: the development of the Butterfly bracket system. J Ind Orthod Soc 2003; 36:73–75.
18. Kokich VG. The role of orthodontics as an adjunct to periodontal therapy. In: Newman MG, Carranza FA, Takei H, eds. Carranza's clinical periodontology. 9th edn. chap. 53. Philadelphia: WB Saunders; 2002:704–718.
19. Wheeler RC. Dental anatomy, physiology and occlusion. Philadelphia: WB Saunders; 1984.
20. Claude R Rufenacht. Fundamentals of esthetics. Chicago: Quintessence publishing; 1990:117–120.
21. Sondhi A. An analysis of orthodontic prescriptions: their strengths and weaknesses. 103rd AAO session, Honolulu, HI; 6 May 2003.
22. Andrews LF. The six keys to normal occlusion. Am J Orthod 1972; 63:296–309.
23. Ricketts RM. Bioprogressive therapy. Rocky Mountain Orthodontics: Denver; 1979.
24. Mc Laughlin RP, Bennett JC, Trevisi HJ. Systematized orthodontic treatment mechanics. St. Louis: Mosby; 2001.
25. Robert M Ricketts. Occlusion – the medium of dentistry. J Pros Dent 1969; 1:39–60.
26. AlQabandi A, Sadowsky C, BeGole E. A comparison of the effects of rectangular and round archwires in leveling the curve of spee. Am J Orthod Dentofac Orthop 1999; 116:522–529.
27. Tahir E, Sadowsky C, Schneider BJ. An assessment of treatment outcome in American Board of Orthodontics cases. Am J Orthod Dentofac Orthop 1997; 111:335–342.
28. James J Hilgers. BIOS … A bracket evolution, a systems revolution. Clin Impressions (ORMCO) 1996; 5(4):8–14.
29. Raleigh Williams. Eliminating lower retention. JCO 1985; 5: 342–349.
30. Roth RH. Functional occlusion for the Orthodontist, part III. J Clin Orthod 1981; 15:174–198.
31. Williamson EH. Occlusion – understanding or misunderstanding. Angle Orthod 1976; 46:86–93.
32. Aubrey RB. Occlusal objectives in orthodontic treatment. Am J Orthod 1978; 74:162–175.
33. Ricketts RM. Early treatment (JCO interview). J Clin Orthod 1979; 13:181–199.
34. Stallard H. Organic Occlusion. In Pavone BW, ed. Oral rehabilitation and occlusion. Section II, topic 9. San Francisco: Univ. California; 1972.
35. Mc Horris W. Occlusion, part I. J Clin Orthod 1979; 13:606–620.
36. Mc Horris W. Occlusion, part II. J Clin Orthod 1979; 13:684–702.

37. Anup Sondhi. Anterior interferences: their impact on anterior inclination and orthodontic finishing procedures. Semin Orthod 2003; 9: 204–215.
38. Huffman RW, Regenos TW. Principles of occlusion. London: H and R press; 1973.
39. Schweitzer J. Dental occlusion – a pragmatic approach. DCNA 1969; 13:701–724.
40. Ingber JS. Forced eruption: part I. A method of treating isolated one and two wall infrabony osseous defects – rationale and case report. J Periodontol 1974; 45:199.
41. Harris DA, Jones AS, Darendeliler MA. Physical properties of root cementum: part VIII. Volumetric analysis of root resorption craters after application of controlled intrusive light and heavy orthodontic forces: a microcomputed tomography scan study. Am J Orthod Dentofacial Orthop 2006; 130:639–647.
42. Reitan K. Initial tissue behavior during apical root resorption. Angle Orthod 1974; 44:68–82.
43. Smale I, Artun J, Behbehani F, et al. Apical root resorption 6 months after initiation of fixed orthodontic appliance therapy. Am J Orthod Dentofacial Orthop 2005; 128:57–67.
44. Eugene Chan, Ali Darendeliler. Physical properties of root cementum: part V. Volumetric analysis of root resorption craters after application of light and heavy orthodontic forces. Am J Orthod Dentofacial Orthop 2005; 127:186–195.
45. Kokich VO, Kiyak A, Shapiro PA. Comparing the perception of dentists and lay people to altered dental esthetics. J Esthet Dent 1999; 11:311–324.
46. Lombardi R. The principles of visual perception and their clinical application to denture esthetics. J Prosthet Dent 1973; 29:358.
47. Chiche G, Pinault A. Replacement of deficient crowns. In: Pinault A, Chiche G, eds. Esthetics of fixed prosthodontics. Chicago: Quintessence; 1994:53–73.
48. Gillen RJ, Schwartz RS, Hilton TJ, Evans DB. An analysis of selected normative tooth proportions. Int J Prosthodont 1994; 7(5):410.
49. Bragger U, Lauchenauer D, Lang NP. Surgical lengthening of the clinical crown. J Clin Periodontol 1992; 19(1):58–63.
50. Vincent G Kokich. Excellence in finishing: modifications for the periorestorative patient. Semin Orthod 2003; 9:184–203.
51. Goldstein RE. Esthetics in dentistry. Philadelphia: JB Lippincott; 1976.
52. Epstein MB, Mantzikos T, Shamus IL. Esthetic recontouring. A team approach. NY State Dent J 1997; 63(10):35–40.
53. Hong YH, Lew KKK. Quantitative and qualitative assessment of enamel surface following five composite removal methods after bracket debonding. Eur J Orthod 1995; 17(2):121–128.
54. Zachrisson BU, Artun J. Enamel surface appearance after various debonding techniques. Am J Orthod 1979; 75:121.
55. Gorelick L, Geiger AM, Gwinnett AJ. Incidence of white spot formation after bonding and banding. Am J Orthod 1982; 81:93.
56. Zachrisson BU. Fluoride application procedures in orthodontic practice: current concepts. Angle Orthod 1975; 44:72.
57. Todd MA, Staley RN, Kanellis MJ, et al. Effect of fluoride varnish on demineralization adjacent to orthodontic brackets. Am J Orthod 1999; 116(2):159–167.
58. Arends J, Schuthof J. Fluoride content in human enamel after fluoride application and washing: an in vitro study. Caries Res 1975; 9(5):363–372.
59. Petersson LG. Fluoride gradients in outermost surface enamel after various forms of topical applications of fluorides in vivo. Odont. Revy 1976; 27:25–50.
60. Haywood VB, Leonard RH, Nelson CF, et al. Effectiveness, side effects and long-term status of night guard vital bleaching. J Am Dent Assoc 1994; 125(9):1219–1226.
61. Cohen SC, Chase C. Human pulpal response to bleaching procedures on vital teeth. J Endod 1979; 5:134–138.
62. Kokich V. Anterior dental esthetics: an orthodontic perspective: part I. Crown length. J Esthet Dent 1993; 5:19–23.
63. Sanavi F, Weisgold AS, Rose LF. Biologic width and its relation to periodontal biotypes. J Estheic Dent 1998; 10(3):157.
64. Patsakas A, Demetriou N, Angelopoulos A. Melanin pigmentation and inflammation in human gingiva. J. Periodontol 1981;52(11): 701–704.
65. Cicek Y, Ertas U. The normal and pathological pigmentation of oral mucous membrane: a review. J Contemp Dent Pract 2003; 4(3):76–86.
66. Pick RM, Pecaro BC, Silberman CJ. The laser gingivectomy. The use of the CO_2 laser for the removal of phenytoin hyperplasia. J. Periodontol 1985; 56:492–496.
67. Hulsey CM. An esthetic evaluation of lip-teeth relationships present in the smile. Am J Orthod 1970; 57:132–144.
68. Janzen E. A balanced smile: a most important treatment objective. Am J Orthod 1977; 72:359–372.
69. Irfan A. Geometric considerations in anterior dental esthetics: restorative principles. PPAD 1998; 10(7):813–322.
70. Fradeani M. Evaluation of dentolabial parameters as part of a comprehensive esthetic analysis. EJED 1(1); 2006:62–70.
71. Snow SR. Esthetic smile analysis of anterior tooth width: the golden percentage. J Esthet Dent 1999; 11:177–184.
72. Levin EI. Dental esthetics and the golden proportion. J Prosthet Dent 1978; 40:244–252.
73. Sarver DM. Principles of cosmetic dentistry in orthodontics: part I. Shape and proportionality of anterior teeth. Am J Orthod Dentofacial Orthop 2004; 126:749–753.

15 Retention and Stability: A Perspective

P Emile Rossouw

Longitudinal changes in the untreated person, as well as in the treated orthodontic patient, remain a fascinating area of study. Moreover, the stability following orthodontic treatment has been a topic of interest and great discussion since the inception of the orthodontic speciality. Hence, retention regimens have become an essential part of the contemporary orthodontic treatment plan. Ultimate success depends on a compilation of steps, including appropriate planning, well-controlled treatment mechanics, retention compliance and, in general, an appreciation of the biological limits of tooth movement. This chapter provides an overview of the retention versus stability concept, defines relapse and stability, provides a perspective on the management of stability, shows the difficulty in achieving stability or the lack thereof and ultimately endeavours to elicit discussion and encourage further investigation into this important area of the orthodontic discipline.

The need to obtain developmental and morphologic homeostasis following orthodontic treatment, or in orthodontic terms, the pursuit to understand the fine balance that exists between stability and relapse has resulted in many attempts to identify some significant factor(s) responsible for post-treatment relapse.[1–30] Every time an orthodontist treats a patient with a malocclusion, it is assumed that the outcome will favour success. The possibility of failure is, however, very real and thus the quest for some form of long-term stability has become one of the most significant challenges in orthodontics. Notwithstanding many research efforts, a workable concept that takes into account the complex circumstances dealing with equilibrium and stability versus imbalance and relapse is lacking. At the present time, no mechanical instrument is available to determine or to predict the stability of a dentition. Although attempts in this regard have been reported in the literature, no method presently exists to predict accurately the future status of the post-treatment orthodontic occlusion.[1–5] Taken into account the multifactorial nature of long-term stability, the multivariate regression model (standardized coefficients) is probably at this time the closest to provide an indication of the factors involved in stability.[6]

Fortunately, efforts to improve knowledge and treatment methods in orthodontics have resulted in many excellent investigations into aspects of relapse.[6,14,15,27–29] Despite these important studies, many causes of orthodontic relapse are not fully understood.[20] Many pitfalls that lead to treatment problems exist, and no orthodontist is immune to them.[25,26]

Given the recognized problems associated with orthodontic treatment, certain relapse changes may be anticipated. The patient's original problem, unfavourable cooperation and poor growth are the factors that may forewarn that relapse is a possibility. At other times, relapse will occur unexpectedly and for no obvious

416

reason. Moreover, the fact that a malocclusion is corrected, or for that matter left untreated, is also no guarantee that no further changes will occur as normal untreated occlusions show longitudinal changes. Occlusal stability after orthodontic treatment should be considered a primary goal for every orthodontist.[15] In the search for postorthodontic treatment stability, it may be necessary for an orthodontist to review the diagnosis, consider the potential growth and developmental changes expected, change the treatment regimen or even vary the overall treatment philosophy en route to attain acceptable clinical outcome (Fig. 15.1).

This chapter provides a summary overview of long-term changes and management of these changes to show where the discipline of orthodontics finds itself in respect to contemporary retention and stability; in addition, it shows the difficulty in achieving stability or the lack thereof, elicits discussion and encourages further investigation into this important area of the orthodontic discipline.

REQUIREMENTS FOR RETENTION AND STABILITY

Definition of retention

Retention, according to Joondeph and Riedel,[33] is the holding of teeth in ideal aesthetic and functional positions. Retention is thus the action or fact of holding, retaining or keeping the teeth in a fixed place or position; that is, the condition of being retained.[34] Retention is

accomplished by a variety of mechanical appliances (Fig. 15.2).

It is important to ensure that the retention protocol is in physiological harmony with the function of the masticatory system. The goal of physiological stability seems to be the practical outcome of successful treatment versus a rigid set of treatment parameters that do not ensure long-term stability. Retention requirements thus should be decided at the diagnosis and planning stage of treatment; the following are important to consider at this stage:

1. Correct and detailed diagnosis
2. Logical treatment plan in harmony with craniofacial growth, developmental and clinical parameters (see later)
3. Ideal timing of treatment initiation
4. Objectives directed to ideal aesthetics and function
5. Permanent maintenance; that is, a separate phase of long-term retention and occlusal management
6. Dependent on the original malocclusion, aetiological factors, growth implications and cooperation of the patient with the retention protocol; this long-term retention management could be as simple as no retention advocated by Williams[13] or fixed retention for life by Little et al[19] and Little.[35]

Terms that are commonly used and others less universally known to define or describe relapse or post-treatment changes include relapse, physiologic recovery, developmental changes, growth recovery, rebound, postretention settling, *recidief,* crowding or recrowding, imbrication, stability, retention, metaposition,

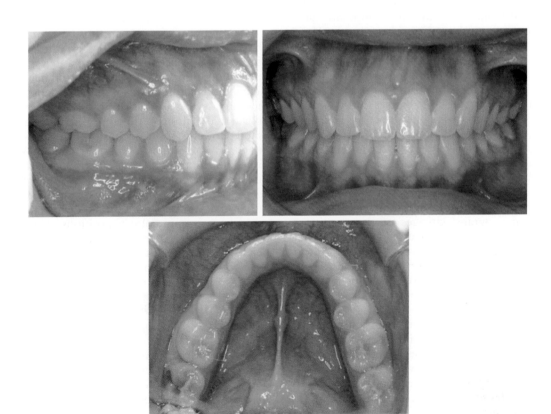

Figure 15.1 Clinical goals for good treatment, according to Tweed,[32] should display an aesthetic, healthy, functional and stable occlusion following treatment. The keys of occlusion described by Andrews[11,12] emphasize these parameters.

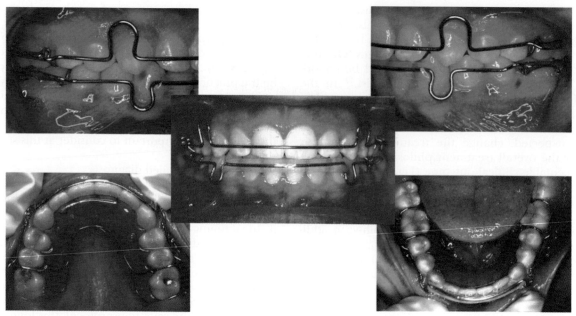

Figure 15.2 The removable retainer is still a popular choice and the favourite retaining appliance used by the author of this chapter.

compensation, adaptation, iatrogenic changes and physiologic stability.[36]

Definition of stability

Stability is the condition of maintaining equilibrium.[34] This refers to the quality or condition of being stable. Some orthodontists may be reluctant to evaluate their patients in the postretention phase of treatment. However, it is only through a retrospective view of treatment that factors, which cause undesirable postretention changes, can be identified. Such discoveries could lead to greater occlusal stability after orthodontic treatment. It is important to recognize that stability is not retention. Therefore, it is necessary to distinguish between relapse, physiologic recovery and developmental changes. The term *relapse* has been used, perhaps erroneously, when referring to all post-treatment changes.[37] This word is usually sensed a failure. However, *physiologic stability* is a term defined by Rossouw[36] and appears to encompass the acceptable changes a clinician can expect; it also includes the normal ageing changes of the dentition, which take place irrespective of treatment outcome. That is; physiologic stability refers to events, such as growth and development, occlusal settling, physiologic influences, rebound effects as a result of the elasticity of the tissues and the more difficult to control neuromuscular influences.

Relapse occurs when the corrected malocclusion slips back or falls back to a former condition, especially after improvement or seeming improvement. Riedel[38] believed that the word was too harsh a description of the changes that follow orthodontic treatment, and he preferred the term *post-treatment adjustment* for these changes. However, poor clinical treatment should not be conducted or condoned under the designation of relapse or under the auspices of one of the other terms noted as

part of the long-term stability problem. It is imperative to be cognizant of the different descriptions of long-term change to enable the clinician to interpret stability of the finished result and also provide adequate communication of possible post-treatment changes to prospective patients. Thus, all orthodontic patients should be well-informed of the expected long-term changes and the need to conform to retention protocol.

The retention process can thus be seen as an another phase of orthodontic care—a phase where the occlusion is observed as it accommodates to a new environment—in addition, minor adjustments can be made in order to facilitate this settling and wean the patient away from the retaining devices as maturity of the adolescent is attained or when the desired outcome goals have been established. However, some occlusions may necessitate permanent retention either to maintain a patient's objective or to negate the influences of aberrant neuromuscular influences. The finalization process should include both active stabilization and passive guidance procedures, rather than rigid fixation of teeth, which after treatment could be in unphysiologic positions. The purist orthodontist or the true occlusionist endeavours to produce a healthy, functional, aesthetic and physiologic stable occlusion that will last for the patient's lifetime (Fig.15.3).

NORMAL CHANGES IN THE UNTREATED DENTITION

One of the most often cited treatment requests is that of the correction of lower incisor crowding, needless to say that it is probably also the most often complaint in respect to changes following orthodontic treatment; that of late lower incisor irregularity. The focus of many studies has been on the mandibular arch, the assumption being that alignment of the lower arch serves as a

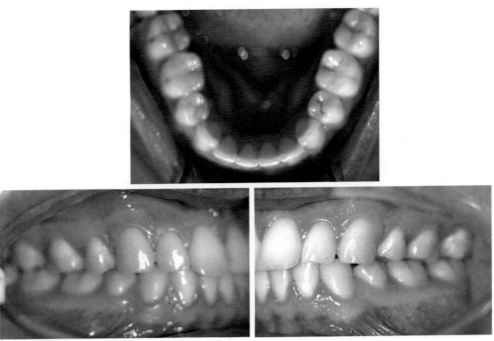

Figure 15.3 An example of a long-term postretention result showing a Class I, well-aligned, healthy, aesthetic, functional and stable occlusion; preferably without full-time retention.

template around which the upper arch develops and functions. The following questions: 'Why is retention necessary?' 'When can retainer use be discontinued, and will significant change follow?' are answered in the most objective manner by observing the long-term changes occurring as a result of normal ageing.

Measurement of lower incisor irregularity

Data from the National Health and Nutrition Examination Survey (NHANES) conducted between 1988 and 1991 in respect to the oral health in the United States shows that 54.5% of children between age 8 and 11 years possess well-aligned lower incisors.[39] A common measurement tool to show the degree of irregularity of the lower incisors is the Little Irregularity Index.[31] This index provides a millimetre number to indicate the discrepancy in contact points between the lower anterior teeth and canine-to-canine (Fig. 15.4).

An adult sample from the NHANES III study (1988–1994) was investigated by Buschang and Shulman[40] in respect to their mandibular incisor irregularity. Buschang and Shulman[40] compiled the clinically relevant information from the evaluation of untreated subjects, 15–50 years of age, from the NHANES III study that is portrayed in Figure 15.5. Note that approximately 39.5% of this sample showed moderate to severe irregularity, thus the group that definitely requires some form of orthodontic treatment. Approximately 50% fall in the clinically acceptable range and may or may not require treatment depending on the compilation of factors.

A study from the Burlington Growth Center at the University of Toronto by Eslambolchi et al[41] provided information as to longitudinal changes that can be

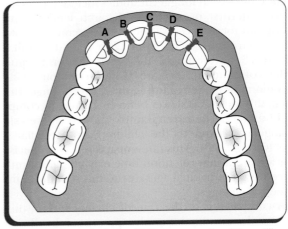

Figure 15.4 Irregularity Index.[31] The aggregate of the millimetre measurements of the discrepancy of the contact points (A + B + C + D + E) provides the score of the Index. Less than 3.5 mm is clinically acceptable, 3.5–5.5 mm indicates moderate irregularity and greater than 5.5 mm indicates severe irregularity.

expected from an untreated sample. Longitudinal or long-term change is mostly recorded as the difference(s) between two intervals, preferably over a long period of time. Time point 1 (T1) represents the beginning of the assessment (in treated evaluations, this will be the beginning of treatment), and time point 2 (T2) normally represents the end of an age interval in untreated measurements or in treatment change evaluation that indicates the end of treatment (post-treatment interval). The third time point (T3) merely indicates another time interval or age interval, and in a treatment change assessment this mostly indicates the postretention interval. In the

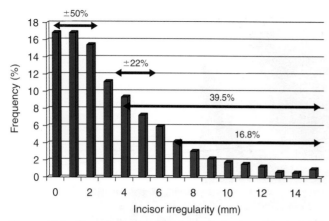

Figure 15.5 Mandibular incisor irregularity in untreated US subjects, 15–50 years of age. The subjects who showed moderate to severe irregularity were 39.5%. Using the irregularity index from Figure 15.4,[31] the various categories of irregularities for the sample is shown. (Modified from Buschang PH, Shulman JD. Angle Orthod 2003; 73:502–508).

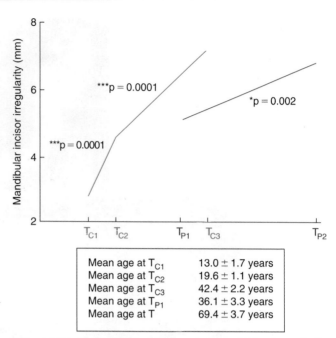

Mean age at T_{C1}	13.0 ± 1.7 years
Mean age at T_{C2}	19.6 ± 1.1 years
Mean age at T_{C3}	42.4 ± 2.2 years
Mean age at T_{P1}	36.1 ± 3.3 years
Mean age at T	69.4 ± 3.7 years

Figure 15.6 Combined changes in the Little Irregularity Index in a sample of untreated children and their parents (Eslambolchi[41]).

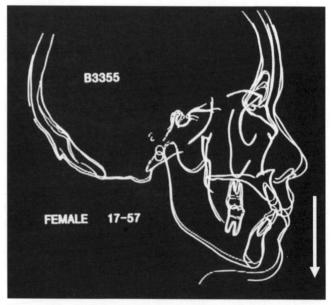

Figure 15.7 Female long-term changes. Note the vertical changes occurring from 17 to 57 years of age. (From Behrents RG. Ann Arbor: University of Michigan; 1985).

above-noted study, longitudinal changes in untreated children (at T1^c= 13y, T2^c= 19,6y and T3^c= 42,4y) and their untreated parents (at T1^p= 36,1 and T2^p= 69,4y) were compared to determine when the tempo of irregularity changes. Parameters that have become measurement standards in long-term studies included intercanine width, interfirst premolar width, arch length, anterior space and total space. All these measurements showed a decrease from T1 to T2, from T2 to T3 and overall from T1 to T3. Interestingly, the lower incisor irregularity index continued to increase. However, an important observation was made regarding the rate of change. In children, this index was slower between T2 and T3 compared to T1 and T2. The parent sample showed an even slower change compared to the children; in particular after age 40 (Fig. 15.6). This rate impacts retention decisions; it is apparent that retention time may be significantly reduced as an individual ages due to this slow down in longitudinal changes.

A comparison of the rate of change in crowding in various longitudinal samples presented by Buschang and Shulman[40] also showed a continual change in irregularity of lower incisors in the long-term. Moreover, the data also confirmed that this continual tempo of increase in the irregularity in the long-term appears to decrease with ageing from approximately the middle of the second decade onwards with some hope of long-term stability.

The latter information thus shows that the untreated dentition appears to show continual changes into adulthood, even into the seventh decade; a fact also confirmed by Behrents[42] in his assessment of longitudinal changes in individuals of the Bolton-Brush growth study. Not only does the dentition change over time but also the entire craniofacial environment including the soft tissues undergo continual changes (Figs 15.7 and 15.8).

Bolton-Brush Growth Sample (Figs 15.7 and 15.8) shows the following general longitudinal changes (Behrents[42]):

1. Considerable craniofacial alteration beyond 17 years in males and females

2. Craniofacial changes continue into the oldest age spans (83 years) in an apparently adaptive but decelerating manner
3. Sexual dimorphism—shown
4. Mandibular plane rotations—occur in a forward direction in males. In backward or vertical direction in females
5. Vertical changes—common in adulthood.
6. Soft tissue changes:
   a. Soft tissue changes—greater than skeletal changes
   b. Changes include—elongation of the nose, flattening of the lips and augmentation of the chin

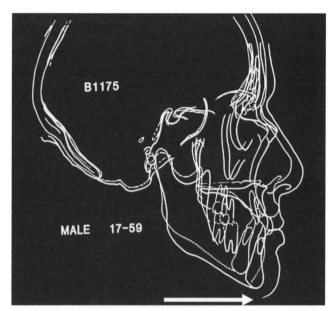

Figure 15.8 Male long-term changes. Note the horizontal changes occurring from 17 to 59 years of age. (From Behrents RG. Ann Arbor: University of Michigan; 1985).

The treated dentition is no more or less susceptible to the above-noted changes. Thus, there is no surprise when authors recommend permanent lifetime retention.[19,44,45] It is important to have an understanding of how the untreated dentition behaves as it can be extrapolated to that of the post-treatment orthodontic occlusion.

Changes in alignment in the untreated lower arch occur at various developmental stages. On average, crowding decreases between 7 and 12 years (mixed dentition development) and increases thereafter (loss of leeway and eventually E-space). According to Richardson,[45] the maximum increase occurs in the teenage years between 13 and 18, little or no change occurs in the third decade and small increases occur later in life. As mentioned previously,[40,41] it appears that the increase in lower incisor irregularity increases rapidly into the third and fourth decades followed by a decrease in the velocity of change after 40 years of age.

Overbite and overjet changes

Other changes may also influence the stability of the occlusion and thus the retention phase of the post-treatment occlusion. Overbite and overjet increase significantly from the mixed to the permanent dentition. During the maturation of the permanent dentition (13–20 years), these changes were reversed, and decreases in overbite and overjet were observed by Barrow and White,[46] Björk,[47] Moorrees,[48] and Sinclair and Little.[49]

Other dental arch changes

Intermolar width remains relatively stable in untreated individuals.[41,48–52] Arch length decreases over time.[41,46,48,49–52] Moreover, longitudinal data show that changes in arch dimensions, as well as lower incisor crowding occur as part of the normal ageing process.[41,42,46,48–52]

One could refer to these changes as the *wrinkling of the teeth*. Late mandibular incisor crowding, thus, may be unrelated to any previous orthodontic treatment. There is no doubt that normal untreated occlusions provide valuable insight into longitudinal changes and thus management of tooth alignment.

Natural space for lower incisor alignment

After eruption of the lower permanent incisors, it appears that there is little or no skeletal growth in the anterior part of the lower jaw at this time.[3,7,32–34] An important means of creating space for incisor alignment is the fact that the lower incisors procline relative to the mandibular plane by an average of 13° between 5 and 11 years.[13] This gain in space is enhanced by an increase in arch width across the canines caused by alveolar growth, just before and during the eruption of the permanent incisors.[2,4,35]

In addition, leeway space or ultimately E-space provides space for the larger permanent incisors; that is the excess space by which the primary molars and canine is larger compared to their permanent successors.[51–60] Any disturbance in establishing the normal occlusion as described could have a detrimental impact on the alignment of the lower incisors.

Anterior component of force resulting in mesial migration of teeth

The cause of increased crowding in the intact lower arch is not fully understood. It is obviously multifactorial, and for this reason, it is difficult to show a cause and effect relationship. Mesial migration of human teeth has been recognized since the late eighteenth century, when it was described by John Hunter,[61] and is shown as the forward movement of the posterior teeth during adolescence. There is evidence to support the view that it is largely responsible for the increase in crowding during the teenage years. Mesial migration may be caused by physiological mesial drift, by the anterior component of the force of occlusion on mesially inclined teeth, by the mesial vectors of muscular contraction or by the contraction of the transseptal fibres of the periodontal ligament.[50,51,53,55,58,62,63]

Role of third molars in the development of mandibular incisor crowding

Third molar agenesis and extraction studies[63–66] suggest that mesial migration is greater in the presence of a developing third molar. This suggestion is strongly reinforced by second molar extraction studies.[67,68] Removal of the second molar effectively isolates the third molar from the rest of the arch. The reduction in crowding and the distal movement of first molars in patients whose second molars have been extracted compared with the increase in crowding and mesial movement of first molars in nonextraction subjects[67,68] provide convincing evidence of the effects of developing third molars on the anterior part of the arch. Other studies on patients treated by extraction of second molars[69–72] reported similar results. It is a mistaken impression that it is only impacted third molars that cause the problem. A third molar that erupts is likely to exert more pressure on the dental arch than the one that remains impacted, and some impacted third molars may exert more pressure than others.[73,74]

Decisions relative to the timing of third molar extraction should be made on the basis of potential development of pathosis, technical considerations of the surgical procedure and long-term periodontal implications rather than potential impact on mandibular incisor crowding.[75] Although erupting mandibular third molars probably exert some force on the dentition,[76–80] most of the scientific studies[81–83] have found no significant correlation between the presence or absence of mandibular third molars and developmental incisor crowding. The effect of mandibular third molars on the dentition, particularly the lower incisors, remains unclear according to Bishara and Andreasen.[84]

Mandibular growth and its effect on late mandibular incisor crowding

Changes in mandibular growth direction and rotation during the post-treatment and postretention periods have also been implicated in the aetiology of late incisor crowding.[85–87] In addition, the vertical development of the mandibular ramus continues until late adolescence (Fig. 15.9A and B, Buschang et al[88]). Crowding of the mandibular incisors was observed in vertical growers as a result of chronic airway obstruction.[89,90]

CHANGES IN THE TREATED DENTITION

Role of extraction or nonextraction treatment on the stability of the treated occlusion

Orthodontists routinely are faced with the dilemma of attaining aesthetic soft tissue profiles versus long-term stability. Moreover, a controversy exists as to which treatment decision, extraction or nonextraction, will eventually lead to orthodontic stability. Extraction of teeth as an aid in the treatment of malocclusion is one of the oldest and most controversial subjects in the history of orthodontics. Dr Edward H Angle's[9] nonextraction influence dominated the discipline of orthodontics for many years; however, a change was eminent when Dr Charles H Tweed,[10,91,103] one of Angle's most ardent supporters, became so discouraged by postretention relapse that he deemed it necessary to include extractions into his treatment regimen to meet his original orthodontic objectives; that being stable, healthy, functional and aesthetic. Tweed[91] subsequently investigated 100 extraction and 100 nonextraction subjects, 25 years postretention and concluded that the extraction cases were more stable than were the nonextraction cases. However, as extraction spaces are closed and the teeth are moved together orthodontically, the adjacent teeth do not move through the gingival tissue but appear to push the gingivae in front of them into a fold of epithelial and connective

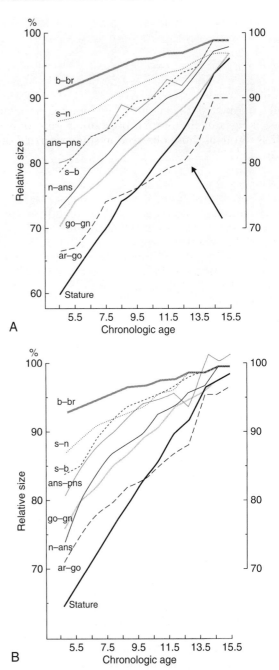

Figure 15.9 **(A)** Craniofacial growth maturity gradient: males 4–16 years (Buschang et al).[88] Note the late vertical maturation of Ar-Go. **(B)** Craniofacial growth maturity gradient: females 4–16 years (Buschang et al).[88] Note the late vertical maturation of Ar-Go.

tissue. This excess tissue can result in the opening of the extraction space that constitutes a common form of relapse of orthodontically treated occlusions. Edwards[92] recommended to remove this tissue surgically so that relapse could be alleviated.

The presence of mandibular incisor crowding indicates that there is a space shortage somewhere in the dental arches. The incisor position[93–96] and facial profile, in combination with a tooth-arch size analysis, provide clues that can help to make a decision whether an extraction or nonextraction treatment protocol must be followed.

Glenn et al[95] studied 28 nonextraction treatment cases, an average of 8 years out of retention. In these patients, who were treated by the same orthodontist, they found that slight incisor irregularity occurred postretention. Sinclair and Little[49] noted that relapse patterns were similar to, but more severe than, those seen in a study conducted in an untreated normal population. The changes in the normal population were only one-half as severe as those observed in studies carried out by Little et al.[19,44]

An evaluation of long-term post-treatment orthodontic changes after at least 10[19] or more years,[44] which included premolar extractions,[97,98] lower incisor extractions,[99] nonextraction cases with generalized spacing and patients treated with arch expansion provided further insight into treated occlusions. Observations from the results of the noted studies were made in comparison to changes occurring in untreated normal control subjects.[5,14] Similar physiologic changes were reported in all the groups, which also conform to other long-term studies published. The changes observed included the following:

1. Arch length decreases after orthodontic treatment.[100–102]
2. Arch width measured across the mandibular canine teeth typically reduces post-treatment, whether or not the case was expanded during treatment.[101]
3. Mandibular anterior crowding during the post-treatment phase is a continuing phenomenon well into the 20-to-40 years age bracket and likely beyond.[97,98]
4. Third molar absence or presence, impacted or fully erupted, seems to have little effect on the occurrence or degree of relapse.[75]
5. The degree of postretention anterior crowding is both unpredictable and variable, and no pretreatment variables either from clinical findings, casts or cephalometric radiographs before or after treatment seem to be useful predictors.

The question thus arises as to what effect the orthodontic technique or appliance management may have on the long-term dental changes. According to Little et al,[19] when lower incisors, measured to the point A-pogonion (APo) line, were proclined an average of 1.4 mm during treatment, they tended to remain stable postretention. Sandusky[15] reported on the postretention stability of 83 extraction cases treated by Tweed and Tweed foundation members. Using Little's Irregularity Index to grade the results, Sandusky[15] found less than 10% relapse of the lower incisors. The general orthodontic treatment philosophy appears to play a role in the long-term occlusal outcome. This was illustrated by Woodside et al[102] in a comparison of serial extraction not followed by active treatment (*driftodontics*) with that of extraction treatment followed by active treatment and concluded that the actual orthodontic treatment appears to influence the long-term changes. The untreated occlusions showed less change.

Tweed[103] suggested that mandibular incisors should, as is found in normal individuals, always be positioned upright over the medullary bone of the jaw. Relapse of orthodontically treated dentitions may be influenced by apical base differences, the subject's age, the time of retention, incisor positions relative to basal bone, post-treatment growth, third molar development, periodontal fibres, habits, occlusal functioning, Bolton discrepancies, continued decrease in arch length and other unknown factors.[19]

A tendency exists in contemporary orthodontics to pursue a completely nonextraction philosophy; that is a dependency on growth and 'arch development'. Friel[104] showed that natural expansion does, however, occur as a result of normal growth and development. It could be incorrect to assume that the appliances used during this growth period were the cause of the expansion. The results of a number of cephalometric studies dealing with the treatment effects of functional appliances on Class II division 1 malocclusions concluded that overjet reduction occurred predominantly as a result of dentoalveolar changes.[105] Dentoalveolar changes also appeared to be largely responsible for overjet relapse, especially when incisors were proclined during treatment.[106–108] Anteroposterior or lateral increase in the mandibular archform usually fails with the dental arch typically returning to the pretreatment size and shape.[109] Haas[110] showed that malocclusions treated by means of rapid maxillary expansion (RPE), however, remained stable, 8 years post-treatment. Haas [110] maintained that his success can be ascribed to a combination of the RPE and to the duration of the retention which he uses.

Moreover, the extraction versus nonextraction debate is still with us as the incidence of nonextraction treatment has shown an increase similar to the 1920s. Based on the available literature, arch expansion as a space-gaining procedure must be approached with caution.[111] Mandibular intercanine width is regarded as a fixed entity, and the early literature recommends that it should not be expanded, if stability is an objective of treatment.[112–115] Expansion of the maxillary arch can be achieved with RPEs[93,110,116–121] and to a lesser extent with archwires.[28,121–124] Postretention, relapse percentages vary after archwire expansion;[28,123,124] average relapse after RPE treatment is approximately 20%.[94,120] Similar to the maxillary arch, expansion of the mandibular arch has been achieved with expansion appliances, such as the lip bumper,[93,124–127] and again, to a lesser extent with archwires.[94,122123] Postretention arch dimensional changes appear to occur regardless of the treatment modality, although more arch width is lost after expansion with archwires alone.[93,95,118,123,124] Blumber et al[128] reported on the short-term postretention stability of the transverse dimension in patients with Class I malocclusion, treated with the Damon System (Ormco, CA). All of the treatment increases in transverse arch dimensions were significant (maxillary arch 2.0–5.6 mm and mandibular arch 2.4–4.6 mm) and greater than expected when compared to untreated controls. Postretention decreases for many of the measurements were significant; however, often less than expected when compared with untreated controls. Moreover, significant net gains remained, especially in the mandibular arch. Occlusal settling occurred following active treatment causing significant improvement in post-treatment outcomes. Retention was for an average of 2.1 ±0.9 years, followed by no retention for an average of 2.3 ±0.9 years.

Simons and Joondeph[129] have reported that irrespective of whether individuals were treated with or without extractions, relapse of overbite, as well as relapse of lower incisor alignment, still occurs after the removal of the appliances. Only about 30% of occlusions treated with first premolar extraction therapy retained good anterior mandibular alignment while two-thirds of the sample relapsed.[19] In comparing the results of a sample showing minimal incisor relapse[130] with a sample showing about two-thirds relapse,[19] Gorman[131] concluded that the orthodontic technique used plays an important role in achieving stability of the post-treatment orthodontic result.

Conlin[132] recalled 1000 subjects and valuated their long-term dental stability and facial aesthetics. He found that there was no real need for extraction cases to appear flat or for nonextraction cases to appear full. Thus, one of the greatest challenges in orthodontics is the need to make a sound diagnosis. No cookbook recipe is available with respect to extraction or nonextraction treatment. Various strategies are used to aid orthodontists in their extraction decisions, including the use of visual treatment objectives.[133,134]

With above 28 years of orthodontic experience, Gorman[131] explained that his perspective on retention has changed from an expectation of universal stability following bicuspid extraction and 2 years of retention to the realization that individual retention plans must be developed for each patient irrespective of the treatment regime (extraction or nonextraction) used. The extraction of teeth, or for that matter nonextraction of teeth, do not necessarily assure long-term stability of the corrected malocclusion, especially lower incisors; however, clinically stable results can be achieved.[102,111,135,136]

Stability of archform has been considered to be one of the most elusive goals of treatment. Diagnosis and treatment of the transverse dimension are important steps on the way to attain a stable treatment outcome. Vanarsdall[137] emphasizes the critical importance of utilizing the Ricketts[138] analysis on the frontal cephalogram (Fig. 15.10) to determine the skeletal differential between the width of the maxilla and the width of the mandible (Table 15.1) irrespective of following an extraction or nonextraction treatment. He refers to this differential as measured on a posteroanterior (PA) cephalogram and emphasizes that undiagnosed transverse discrepancy leads to adverse periodontal response, unstable dental camouflage and less than optimal dentofacial aesthetics. The normal (maxillary and mandibular) values for the Caucasian race (values for all racial and ethnic groups and even genders will vary), but the differential between the width of the maxilla and width of the mandible, is the critical evaluation for the individual patient.

Longitudinal changes in the soft tissue profile and the influence on the dentition

The long-term influence of the oral and facial musculature and other soft tissues on the dentition is not clearly understood.[139–142] Lip pressure on the teeth as a result of the incisor position appears to influence the changes seen in the dentition.

The correctly diagnosed and well-treated occlusion results in a similar soft tissue outcome. Various soft tissue analyses have been proposed to assess the profiles. Amongst the familiar analyses are Steiner,[143] Merrifield,[144] Burstone,[145] Ricketts[138] and Holdaway.[146] Nonextraction

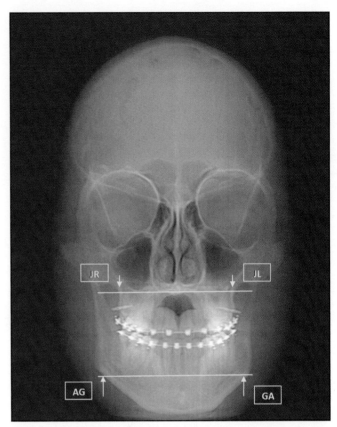

Figure 15.10 The frontal cephalogram showing the effective maxillary width (JR-JL) and effective mandibular width (AG-GA). The expected maxillomandibular difference is defined as the age-appropriate expected AG to GA distance (right and left antegonial notches-mandibular width)—the age-appropriate-expected J point to J point (or Mx) distance (left and right intersections of the maxillary tuberosity and the zygomatic buttress-maxillary width). The actual maxillomandibular difference is defined as the actual AG to GA measurement—the actual J point to J point measurement.[137]

Table 15.1   The mean normal maxillomandibular differentials from Vanarsdall (1999)[137]

	Mean Normal Values		
Age	Mandibular	Maxillary	Difference
9	76.0	62.0	14.0
10	77.4	62.6	14.8
11	78.8	63.2	15.6
12	80.2	63.8	16.4
13	81.6	64.4	17.2
14	83.0	65.0	18.0
15	84.4	65.6	18.8
16 (adult)	85.8	66.2	19.6

Larger values indicate that the mandibular width is much larger compared with the maxillary width, and thus the maxilla requires expansion. Clinical opinion will justify whether surgical, RPE, archwire only or a combination of these will provide adequate expansion for long-term stability.

aesthetics and balance should be equal to that of the extraction occlusion and soft tissue (Fig. 15.11).[21,111,147,148] Many debates as to the influence of extraction versus nonextraction treatment often favours the one or other direction; and often stability of the long-term result comes to question.

The chin, and especially, the nose influence the soft tissue profile outcome.[149] The nose and chin (mandible) appear to maintain growth longer than the other extremities; thus, the lips appear to become retrusive in relation to the nose and chin over the long term according to the soft tissue analyses. Such changes need to be considered in the treatment decision in collaboration with the stability goals. The impacts of these parameters on the long-term postretention soft tissue profile are well illustrated in the comparison of extraction and nonextraction treatments (Figs 15.12–15.14). Bishara et al[149] reported the changes in males and females, between 5 and 45 years of age, to be similar in both magnitude and direction; however, the timing of the greatest changes in the soft tissue profile occurred earlier in females (10–15 years) than in males (15–25 years). In addition, the Holdaway soft

tissue angle (H-angle[146]) progressively decreased over this period of observation. Thus, the upper and lower lips became significantly more retruded in relation to the aesthetic line (E-line[138]) between 15 and 25 years of age; a trend which continued between 25 and 45 years of age.

Soft tissue goals are well described by Holdaway.[132,146] A harmonious soft tissue balance without lip strain and with lip competence should be the clinical goal following treatment. According to Posen,[141] this balance not only determines the extraction or nonextraction treatment choice but also leads to soft tissue balance and occlusal stability. Holdaway[133] proposed his soft tissue visual treatment objective (VTO) to facilitate the planning of the soft tissue profile as noted in relation to the future occlusal goals (Fig. 15.15).

Ideal relationship between the H-angle and the Point A convexity was cited by Holdaway[133] in his description of the use of the soft tissue visual objective. An example of this relationship—H-angle of 10° relates well to Point A convexity of 0 mm. The ideal range of the H-angle is accompanied by a specific Point A convexity; example 11° H-angle with Point A convexity of +1 mm

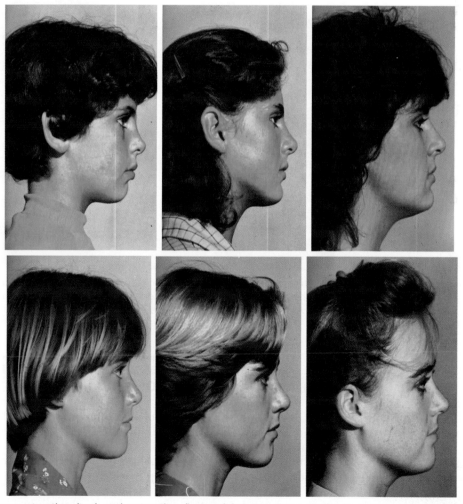

Figure 15.11 The nonextraction (top) and extraction (bottom) images show similar long-term changes (T2–T3; mean 7-year interval).[111] The extraction profile at the T1 appears ahead of the soft tissue profile lines noted in the text. The lips become more retrusive with age in both instances; however, no significant clinical differences are apparent. Thus, in general, extraction equals similar nonextraction soft tissue change outcomes. (Case images courtesy: Dr. R. Melville, Cape Town, SA).

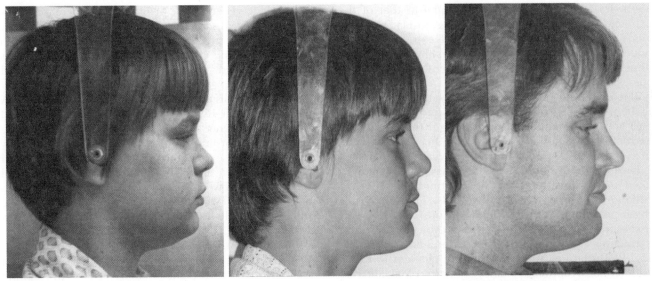

Figure 15.12   A Class II division 1 malocclusion following nonextraction treatment shown 16 years 3 months post-treatment. Note the general lip changes in respect to the nose and chin for this forward rotator and horizontal grower (T1: 11 years 8 months; T2: 14 years 1 month; and T3: 30 years 4 months). An occlusal stable result was attained. (Case images courtesy: Dr Jim Boley, Richardson, Texas, USA).

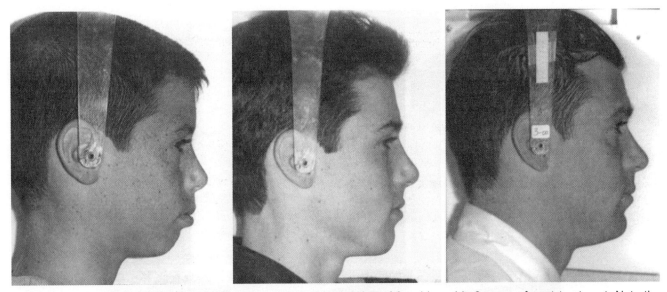

Figure 15.13   A Class II division 1 malocclusion treated with extraction of four bicuspids 9 years of post-treatment. Note the general lip changes in respect to the nose and chin for this forward rotator and horizontal grower (T1: 13 years 2 months; T2: 16 years 8 month; and T3: 25 years 1 months). An occlusal stable result was attained. (Case images courtesy: Dr Jim Boley, Richardson, Texas, USA).

or for an H-angle measurement of 9° for a −1 Point A convexity. The adjustment for this ratio is thus dependent on the H-angle measurement. In a long-term study evaluating extraction and nonextraction treatment stability outcomes between males and females, Rossouw et al[150] observed the changes portrayed in Table 15.2. The group measurement closer to this balance (female group; higher extraction percentage) appeared to have the least long-term lower incisor irregularity. In addition, the female group also showed fuller lips to the profile line with males more retrusive in respect to this measurement.

RETAINERS AND POST-TREATMENT OCCLUSION

The retainers most often prescribed following orthodontic treatment include:

1. Fixed retainers meet the retention requirements well and compliance to wear is not a problem. However, it creates a permanent link to the practice, but if the clinician has a philosophy of long-term post-treatment maintenance, then this also is of no consequence. The fixed retainer should not serve as

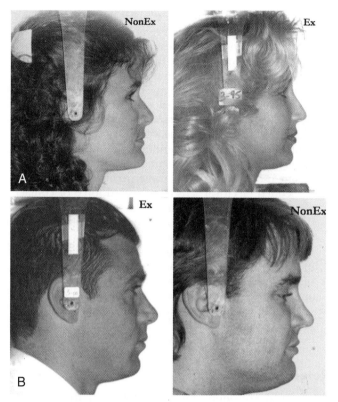

Figure 15.14 A comparison of extraction and nonextraction profiles of stable long-term occlusal results. **(A)** Female nonextraction forward rotator (17 years postretention) versus an extraction backward rotator (13 years postretention). **(B)** Male extraction backward rotator (9 years postretention) versus nonextraction forward rotator (16 years 3 months postretention). **(A)** NonEx (17 years postretention) versus Ex (13 years postretention). **(B)** Ex (9 years postretention) versus NonEx (16 years 3 months postretention). (Case images courtesy: Dr Jim Boley, Richardson, Texas, USA).

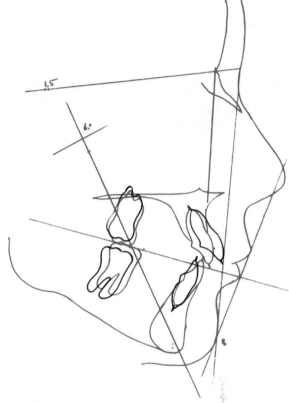

Figure 15.15 An example of a VTO[133] illustrating the soft and hard tissue objectives. The H-angle is in harmony with Point A convexity (Table 15.2).

protection for unlimited expansion. In addition, this form of permanent retention may create a hygiene problem. It is imperative to have an excellent hygiene protocol in place with this type of fixed retainer (Fig. 15.16). Different wire preferences exist for use with the popular fixed intercanine retainer and cover from gold braided to stainless steel braided, to rectangular, to round and to half-round stainless steel wires. Fixed retainer such as noted can

also be used between any number of teeth. When only the canines are bonded, a more rigid wire is normally used and when all the teeth are bonded, a more flexible braided wire is often used. However, this selection varies from clinician to clinician. The important fact is that whatever wire is used, it needs to meet the retention requirements.

2. A fixed mandibular canine-to-canine retainer (0.0215 × 0.027 inch stainless steel rounded rectangular wire) bonded only to the lingual surfaces of the lower canines can be effective in maintaining the long-term alignment of the mandibular anterior teeth in most patients; however, it was shown that a relatively high

Table 15.2 A comparison of Point A convexity and H-angle (Holdaway1983)[146] between extraction and nonextraction groups[151]

	A-convex in mm		H-angle in degrees	
	Extraction group	**Nonextraction group**	**Extraction group**	**Nonextraction group**
T1	3.45 (3.07)	4.08 (2.54)	16.90 (3.79)	16.79 (3.98)
T2	2.33 (2.75)	1.40 (2.47)	13.36 (2.74)	13.76 (3.66)
T3	1.61 (3.04)	0.50 (2.89)	12.37 (3.30)	12.34 (4.08)

Post-treatment interval (T2-T3) 7 years.

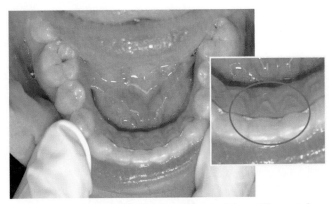

Figure 15.16 Lower fixed intercanine retainer. The retainer used in the illustration was prepared from 0.020″ half-round stainless wire with the flat surface against the tooth surface and bonded to each tooth. Note the presence of calculus on the lingual surfaces. The latter is a common problem with fixed retainers and requires meticulous hygiene control.

percentage can experience a small to moderate increase in the lower incisor irregularity.[152]

3. The flexible spiral wire (0.0195 inch, 3-stranded, heat-treated twisted wire named Wildcat from GAC International, Bohemia, NY) also used from mandibular canine-to-canine and bonded to all lingual surfaces of the six lower anterior teeth often serve as a long-term retainer. It maintains the alignment of the lower anterior segment following orthodontic treatment; however, regular assessment is imperative to ensure that all bonds are intact. Any unnoticed bond failure easily leads to post-treatment lower anterior irregularity.[153]

4. A popular choice in contemporary orthodontic practice is vacuum-formed or suck-down clear retainers, as it can easily be produced in a custom format in-house (Fig. 15.17). Moreover, if a replacement is required, this creates minimal practice time, and in general, is a very cost-effective and efficient appliance. It is removable and thus facilitates hygiene, but if compliance is lacking in respect to wear, then the occlusion is exposed to the changes described in this chapter.

5. The most commonly used retainer is the Hawley retainer or modifications thereof. It is removable and is exposed to the previously noted compliance issues; in addition, it allows freedom to settling of the occlusion as the occlusal surfaces are not covered with the clear overlay retainers.[151] Minor adjustments are thus possible with both (Fig. 15.18).

6. Combinations of the noted retainers are also in use (Fig. 15.19). The post-treatment occlusion was assessed in a study by Lustig[151] using the T-Scan II system (Tekscan of South Boston, MA) to determine what influence the retainers have on post-treatment settling (Fig. 15.20). This system uses a thin (0.004″) interocclusal recorder with embedded electrical sensors to record force of contact, dispersion of contact and timing of contact of the occlusion. It was noted that full coverage worn full time prevents ideal settling. The clear overlay group (Essix, Raintree Essix, New Orleans, LA) showed no change or increase in anterior force and contact area; which indicates a lack of occlusal settling. In contrast, the Hawley group showed an increase in posterior force and area; thus detectable settling. It is recommended that the occlusal parameters as described by Andrews[11,12] and Williams[13] should be established prior to full coverage retainers.

Retention protocol

Taken into consideration that change in the occlusal contacts will occur in the long term, the following example of a retention protocol is recommended.

1. Wear the removable retainers during the first month as much as possible.
2. Drink water to adapt, but remove the retainers when eating.
3. A dental hygiene regimen should be followed without the retainers in place. Moreover, proper hygiene measures must also be in place for the retainers.
4. After the first month, the retainers only have to be worn at home and at night. This is a practical schedule as retainers are then kept at home and misplacement elsewhere will be at a minimum.

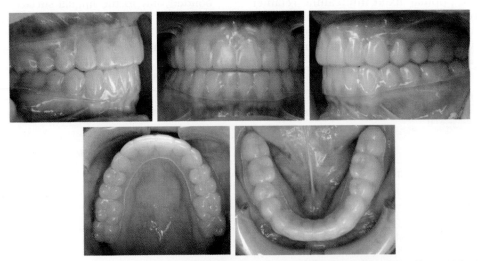

Figure 15.17 Clear overlay retainers (often referred to as Essix® or Invisalign®). Note that all teeth must be included and any teeth not included, such as second molars, may overerupt and create an open bite when the retainers are not in place.

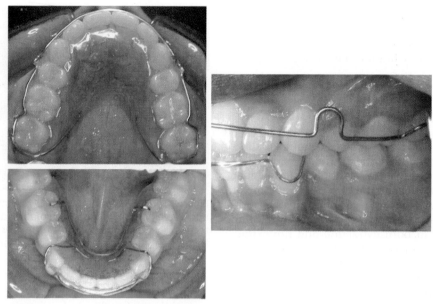

Figure 15.18   Maxillary wraparound modification of the traditional Hawley and an extended spring retainer for the mandibular arch.

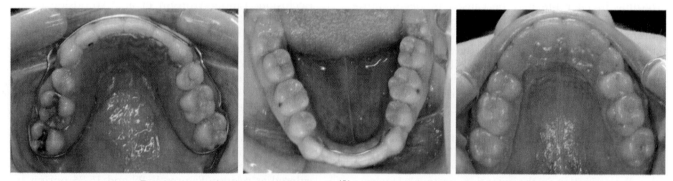

Figure 15.19   Retainer combinations used by Lustig[151] in his study to determine post-treatment settling.

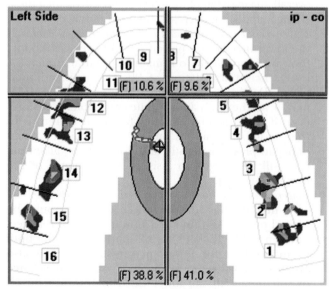

Figure 15.20   An example of the T-Scan II System (Tekscan of South Boston, MA) occlusal contact patterns measured in the post-treatment study.[151]

5. Retention visits are initially scheduled at 6 weeks; 3 months; 6 months; 1 year and then annually.

6. As a rule of thumb, the retainer should be in place at least for the same duration as the treatment time; however, keep in mind that depending on the age at T2, the physiologic changes may be rapid or at a reduced rate (Fig. 15.6).[23,41] Retainer wear should be determined accordingly.

7. A classic regimen also is to wear the retainers full time for half of the treatment time. Then divide the remainder of the treatment time in two periods; the first period is for at home wear and the second period is for night-time wear; thereafter the retainers can be maintained for night-time wear or can be weaned away by alternate night wear until it is worn only to test for a good fit. If there is any difficulty in the fit, then an adjustment or at least night-time wear be maintained.

8. The ultimate goal is no retainers.[13,18] The wean away process as described is thus important. Some

patients prefer to maintain night-time retainer wear, and with no adverse evidence shown for this exercise, it is recommended to maintain night wear until the long-term changes have minimal effect (Fig. 15.6).[23,41]

FACTORS TO CONSIDER IN THE MAINTENANCE OF LONG-TERM STABILITY

It remains unknown why treated patients continue to deteriorate long after retainer removal and untreated malocclusions do not seem to display this same level of instability.

As previously mentioned, an ever-increasing volume of literature reports a variable and unpredictable deterioration in lower arch alignment irrespective of orthodontic treatment regimens, in both extraction and nonextraction, and long-term after retention. It is often claimed that this is caused by the normal physiological process of maturation found in untreated subjects. Nevertheless, it is not unreasonable to expect that teeth that have been moved orthodontically might be more susceptible to the pressures that cause arch length reduction and crowding. The long-term changes in untreated and treated subjects reported in this chapter suggest that increased crowding in later life may be caused by degenerative changes associated with ageing or periodontal disease. Moreover, patients treated early will have completed retention during the late adolescent ages and will be influenced by the same forces responsible for increased crowding in untreated subjects, at their maximum in the teenage years. In subjects completing retention after this age and into adulthood may experience that these forces should be largely decreasing and a degree of stability similar to that found in untreated arches in the third decade[154,155] might be expected. This slowdown in changes impacting the treated dentition may also determine the reduction in the retention protocol. However, it could be argued that retention after the second and third decade may be unnecessary, but it is patently not so, as factors associated with orthodontic tooth movement remain unpredictable and continue to impact the postretention instability although in a lesser extent throughout the ageing process.

Meticulous orthodontic care, including proper diagnosis in order to distinguish between extraction and nonextraction malocclusions, is imperative. Orthodontic technique, including individual retention management, appears to play an important role in achieving physiologically stable results. In order to provide complete orthodontic care, patients must be informed of the benefits and disadvantages of the various treatment regimens, the possible changes in the long term and the importance of adhering to the prescribed protocol, which could be full time, part time or a combination of the two divided between the dental arches.

Long-term observations of untreated and treated dentitions have provided factors, occlusal keys,[11–13] hypotheses and theorems[33] to consider in the pursuit to a physiologic stable occlusion:

1. *Eliminate aetiologic factors:* The impact of aetiological factors on malocclusion has been well documented in the literature.[33,89,90,156–158] An example to illustrate the

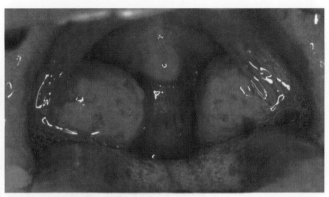

Figure 15.21 The impact of airway obstruction during growth and development of the craniofacial area, such as enlarge tonsils, is well documented in the literature and removal of this cause will prevent or assist in correction of malocclusion.

aetiology of malocclusion is upper airway obstruction (Fig. 15.21), the impact on the vertical dimension and lower incisor irregularity. A normal functioning airway potentially has a lesser impact on the stability of the occlusion. Linder-Aronson et al,[89] Woodside et al[90] and Harvold[156,157] illustrated the phenomenon of an increase in vertical facial height with upper airway obstruction and the consequent influence on the occlusion, which often is shown as an increase in lower incisor irregularity.

2. *Teeth that have been moved tend to return to their former positions.*[33] Studies assessing the changes that occur following the treatment show to a minor or major extent that the teeth have a tendency to undergo rebound or settling changes. Minor changes fall into the category of physiologic stability[1,36] and unacceptable changes can be considered as relapse. Figures 15.22 and 15.23 portray examples of this tendency of treated teeth to return to the original positions. The teeth tend to crowd as a result of these changes, especially the mandibular incisors; the overall image is that of tooth irregularity. Note that these changes appear to decrease in tempo with age.[41]

3. *Lower incisor position should be upright on basal bone:*[32] If the lower incisors are placed upright over basal bone, they are more likely to remain in good alignment. A lower incisor angulation of 90° to the mandibular plane (IMPA), or 65° to the Frankfort plane (FMIA), may be aesthetically appropriate and stable.[32,130] Moreover, if there is any tendency for teeth to return to their original positions and in this instance, a tendency to procline slightly, additional space, albeit minor, will be created to assist in maintenance of the tooth alignment.[130]

4. *Lower incisor position in respect to the point APo line:*[13,138] The incisal edge of the lower incisor should be placed on the APo line or 1 mm in front of it as recommended by Ricketts (1 ±2 mm). This is the optimum position for lower incisor stability.[138] It also creates, according to Williams,[159] optimum balance of soft tissues in the lower third of the face for all the variations in apical base differences within the normal range. The angulation of lower incisors has not proven to be as relevant to their stability as the

millimetre measurement to the APo line.[13] Appliance control is required to achieve optimal positioning of the lower incisor at the end of treatment as shown by Williams and Hosila[160] and Woodside et al.[102] This is especially important in contemporary orthodontics, as we practice clinical orthodontics in an era where prescription appliances are used as the norm. It is thus imperative to treat each patient as a unique individual as all prescriptions may not be appropriate for all, the same as we do not all wear the same size shoes. If the lower incisor is advanced too far beyond the APo line, relapse and crowding will occur. Lower incisors that are overly proclined in treatment (beyond one standard deviation) can only be maintained in such a position with a fixed retainer. The

incisors will move lingually and become crowded when the retainer is removed according to Mills.[161,162] Lower incisor position also dictates when teeth need to be extracted and which ones would be ideal. Moreover, a literature review by Blake and Bibby[163] showed that the most stable positions of the teeth are their pretreatment positions.

5. *Lower incisor mesiodistal inclination or second-order position:* The lower incisor apices should be positioned distally to the crowns more than as generally considered appropriate, and the apices of the lower lateral incisors must be more than those of the central incisors.[11–13] Modern day appliances have this tip (second-order prescription) included in the design of the appliances (Figs 15.24 and 15.25). When the lower incisor roots

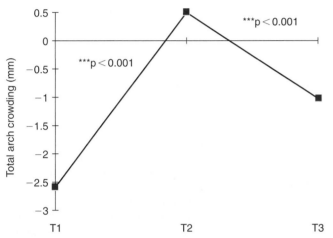

Figure 15.22 Changes in total arch crowding for the entire sample.[6] Note the correction of crowding from T1–T2 with conventional fixed appliance orthodontic treatment; then subsequent return of the problem following treatment (T1: −2.59 ±3.68 mm; T2: 0.49 ±0.67 mm; T3: −1.03 ±1.14 mm; post-treatment T2–T3: 11.97 years).

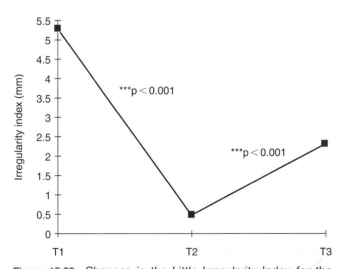

Figure 15.23 Changes in the Little Irregularity Index for the entire sample.[6] Initially there appears to be rapid changes that tapers off as individuals reach maturity towards the third and fourth decades.[41]

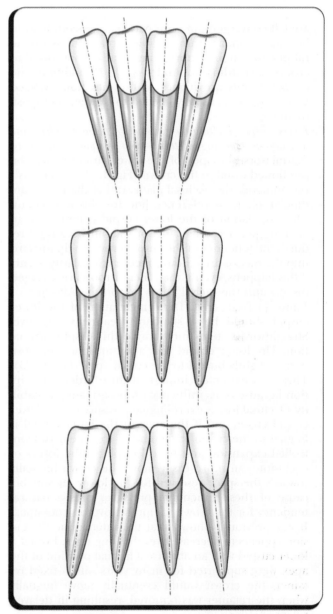

Figure 15.24 Williams[13] emphasizes to have the root apices sufficiently divergent. Most of the contemporary fixed appliances in use provide options in prescription to accommodate this principle. (With permission from Williams R. J Clin Orthod 1985; 19:342–349).

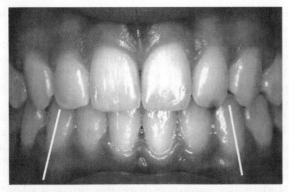

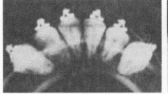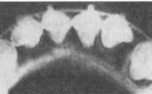

Figure 15.26 Labiolingual plane indicating necessity to align root apices as well as incisal edges. (With permission from Williams R. J ClinOrthod 1985; 19:342–349).

Figure 15.25 Lower canine apices distal to the crown and root buccal to the crown. The panoramic radiograph supports the clinical image.

are left convergent, or even parallel, the teeth tend to become irregular again following treatment as a natural phenomenon of uprighting; that is, roots distal to crowns, according to Andrews.[11,12] In addition, the contact points are higher in this situation. A fixed lower retainer is usually needed to prevent such post-treatment relapse.

6. *Lower cuspid inclination (mesiodistal/second order) and angulation (labiolingual/third order) position:* Similarly to the incisors, the apex of the lower cuspid should be positioned distal to the crown (Fig. 15.25). Williams[13] recommends the occlusal plane, rather than the mandibular plane as reference line for this assessment. This angulation of the lower cuspid is important in creating post-treatment incisor stability because it reduces the tendency of the cuspid crown to tip forward into the incisor area. Lower incisor irregularity occurs if this happens, even if their incisor roots are diverged distally and the incisal edges are on the APo line or 1 mm in front of it. Distal inclination of the lower cuspid should be a standard treatment objective. Straightwire systems incorporate this cuspid inclination. The lower cuspid root apex must also be positioned slightly buccal to the crown apex (Fig. 15.25). This is an extremely important third order prescription because of its influence on post-treatment stability. Occlusal forces exert lingual pressure on the lower cuspid crown and if the apex of the lower cuspid is lingual to the crown at the end of treatment (uncontrolled expansion and buccal tipping), the forces of occlusion can more easily move the crown lingually towards the space reserved for the lower incisors because of these functional pressures plus a natural tendency for the crown to upright over its root apex. It was previously shown that the intercanine dimension appears to decrease over the long term. Even if a lower cuspid with an abnormal lingual position of the apex were supported for many years with a fixed retainer, the crown would eventually move lingually when the retainer was removed, resulting in delayed relapse.[6,13,102,111,135]

7. *Roots, such as for the crowns, must be appropriately aligned:*[13] All four lower incisor apices must be in the same labiolingual plane according to Williams (Fig. 15.26).[13] Alignment of the incisor incisal edges is often

mistaken for adequate incisor alignment. Great care must be given to align also the apices of the incisors mesiodistally and labiolingually. The distal positioning of the apices of the lower incisor roots results in a reciprocal tendency for the crowns to move mesially. Moreover, the contact areas between the incisor crowns move upward towards the anatomical contact points, which are small, rounded and near the incisal edge. This strong mesial pressure on the crowns during the root positioning process (care must be taken with this positioning as the tooth takes up more space in this manner) easily leads to incisor irregularity due to the contact point displacement labiolingually. This results in a reverse movement of the apices linguolabially. Additional space is required for these movements to ensure stability, otherwise the labiolingual apical displacement of the lower incisors and noted subsequent lower incisor post-treatment irregularity will be established. This again emphasizes the meticulous management of the appliance;[102,135,136,160] rectangular archwires control these movements more efficiently than round wires.

8. *Interproximal contact of the lower incisors often requires slenderizing:* The mandibular arch length shows a continued decrease over time.[6,41] This is a biologic occurrence in both treated and untreated dentitions, which ultimately results in an outcome of slipping contacts or an increase in tooth irregularity. This is one factor in the anterior component of force, which with others, such as growth pattern, mandibular plane angle, forward inclination of teeth and forward driving occlusal forces to name some, all collectively facilitate lower incisor crowding or irregularity. The lower incisors should be slenderized as needed after treatment to release tight contacts or any tooth-size discrepancies.[13,18] Lower incisors that have sustained no proximal wear have round, small contact points, which are accentuated if the apices have been diverged for stability. Consequently, the slightest amount of continuous mesial pressure can cause various degrees of contact slippage in either buccal or lingual direction in the lower incisor segment (anterior component of force described by Southard et al[164]). Adverse tooth–jaw relationship is another possible factor in post-treatment changes. This is especially true in extraction treatment; the removal of two, four or more teeth may not provide the perfect solution for tooth-size–jaw-size discrepancy, and it is conceivable that the right combination to provide balance and stability in some instances should be the partial removal of teeth; that is 1¾ teeth when

two are required for extraction or 3¾ teeth when four teeth need to be extracted.[13] Thus, interproximal enamel reduction (Figs 15.27 and 15.28) is essential to facilitate this balance. Sparks evaluated long-term changes following interproximal enamel reduction (IPR). Although some changes occurred, especially in the lower incisors segment, these changes appeared to be less (25% less) than in the occlusions where no IPR was performed. It thus seems to be a valuable method to reduce long-term crowding. Flattening lower incisor contact points by slenderizing or stripping creates flat contact surfaces that help resist labiolingual crown displacement. This treatment also maintains post-treatment alignment, and in some instances, eliminate the need for lower incisor retention.[13,18] The method of enamel reapproximation is well described by Rossouw and Tortorella.[166,167]

9. *Malocclusion should be over corrected as a safety factor:*[33] It is preferable to treat and let the post-treatment changes occur in favour of the norm; thus such parameters as overbite and overjet illustrate this phenomenon well. The over corrected overbite and overjet as indicated in Figures 15.29 and 15.30 allow post-treatment settling to occur towards the normal clinical values described. This goal is also pursued for, especially, the transverse dimension.[110,137]

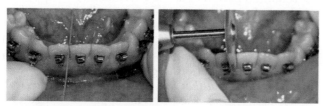

Figure 15.27 Slenderizing using diamond discs (slow handpiece) or metal diamond strips.

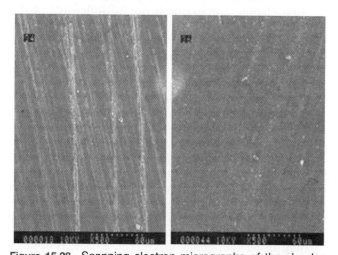

Figure 15.28 Scanning electron micrographs of the slenderizing action followed by 3M polishing discs and strips versus a comparison with the addition of 37% phosphoric acid. Note the scratched enamel surface following the abrasive diamond and polishing slenderizing action versus the smooth enamel surface following the brief acid treatment. The addition of 10% maleic acid attained similar results. (With permission from Rossouw PE, Tortorella A. J Can Dent Assoc 2003; 69(6): 384–388).

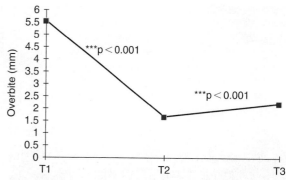

Figure 15.29 Changes in overbite for the Entire Sample.[6] Note the overbite was reduced to a mean of 1.27 mm and then during the post-treatment interval (T2–T3: 11.97 years), it settled at 2.12 mm, which in general is approximately at the norm (T1: 3.28 ± 2.06 mm; T2: 1.27 ± 0.54 mm; T3: 2.12 ± 0.95 mm).

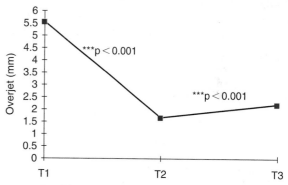

Figure 15.30 Changes in overjet for the Entire Sample.[6] Note the similar change as for overbite in Figure 15.29. The overjet was reduced during treatment to an over corrected position of 1.68 mm and post-treatment settling occurred to a measurement of 2.22 mm, again close to the approximate norm (T1: -5.59 ± 3.07 mm; T2: 1.68 ± 0.41 mm; T3: 2.22 ± 0.71 mm).

10. *Proper interdigitation of the teeth as defined by the Andrews six keys to a normal occlusion:*[11,12] Proper occlusion is a potent factor in holding teeth in their corrected positions and is one of the classic theorems of stability.[33] Pancherz[168] also recommended this factor as a facilitator of long-term stability. He observed Herbst treatment in the correction of Class II malocclusions for many years and concluded that a well-established interdigitated occlusion post-treatment provided long-term stability of the treated result (Fig. 15.31). The correction of the molar and canine to a Class I relationship post-treatment was also illustrated by Rossouw.[21] He observed the changes in the post-treatment measured Class I molar and canine relationships. Table 15.3[21] portrays the correction from T1 to T2 with a subsequent minor change from T2 to T3. Interesting to note that the Class I molar and canine relationships were well maintained in the long term.

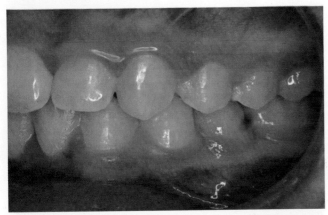

Figure 15.31 Class I occlusion with well-interdigitated teeth with adequate overbite and overjet in the anterior and posterior occlusion.

Table 15.3 Molar and canine changes after a post-treatment interval (T2–T3) of approximately 7 years[21]

Achievement and Maintenance of Class I Molar

	Left Class I	Right Class I
T1	48.9%	42.0%
T2	94.3%	93.2%
T3	90.9%	93.2%

Achievement and Maintenance of Class I canine

	Left Class I	Right Class I
T1	19.3%	20.5%
T2	94.3%	93.2%
T3	90.9%	90.9%

The results indicate that proper occlusion assists in maintenance of a high percentage of the occlusal goals.

11. *Maintain the original archform:*[33] One of the classic theorems of stability[33] tells the clinician to maintain the original archform. It is professed that the mandibular arch, in particular, cannot be permanently altered by appliance therapy. Moreover, according to growth studies, the basal transverse dimension in the anterior part of the mandible increases minimally after the age of 4 years and even less from 10 years to adulthood.[53] Numerous long-term studies of both treated and untreated malocclusions support this claim and have underlined the fact that the original intercanine width should be maintained as a continued decrease appears to occur in the long term. Two groups from a clinically stable sample were identified after a long-term evaluation of the outcome of treatment.[6] It was noted that the group that had more intercanine expansion, albeit nonsignificant, showed more post-treatment intercanine width decrease (Fig. 15.32).[6] A recent long-term evaluation of the post-treatment stability of combined RPE and lip bumper therapy, as part of an early phase of treatment (Phase 1) followed by fixed appliance treatment (Phase 2), showed that mild and moderate arch width increases during the mixed dentition maintained a net increase in the long term.[169] The arch width increase and long-term stability was mostly in the posterior segments.

12. *Time must be allowed for reorganization of hard and soft tissues:* Orthodontics is a 'game of patience'. Not all tissues react similarly at the same time; moreover, teeth move into new positions and then have to be maintained in order to allow time for the other tissues to 'catch-up' with their reorganization. Thus, not strange to have a classic theorem of stability stating that bone and adjacent tissues must be allowed time to reorganize around newly positioned teeth.[33] Reitan[170] showed that the rearrangement of the bone and principal fibres in the middle and apical regions of the root may occur even after removal of the retainers. He illustrated that the supra-alveolar structures in dogs still undergo displacement after a retention period of 232 days. Thilander[171] supported these changes in a publication on the biology of relapse. It is thus recommended that the teeth be aligned in their ultimate positions as a primary goal and then maintained as a secondary goal through the treatment period (Fig. 15.33).

13. *The further teeth that have been moved appear to create less likelihood of relapse:*[33] The apparent image created by a large movement followed by a small change versus a small movement followed by a small change shows the first as more stable. The first change apparently is not as noticeable as the second where the small change represents a larger percentage of the overall small initial tooth movement. The outcome here is the impact of the net effect of the treatment following the post-treatment recovery changes.

14. *Corrections carried out during periods of growth are less likely to relapse:*[33] This classic theorem is well supported by the controversial Phase1 versus Phase 2 treatments. A net gain in arch width was shown in the long term following expansion during the mixed dentition followed by a second fixed appliance phase of treatment.[169] Gianelly[172] reported in a publication on one-phase versus two-phase treatment that crowding can be resolved in 73% of patients in the mixed dentition stage of development, simply by preserving and using the leeway space (Fig. 15.34). It appears that preventative interventions early prove to provide more favourable long-term outcomes; both for hard and soft tissues (Fig. 15.35: Class II div 2 correction example). It is also apparent that intervention was necessary during a period where critical growth changes were occurring, making it essential to

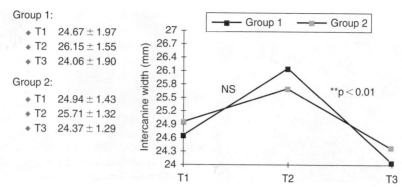

Group 1:
- ♦ T1   24.67 ± 1.97
- ♦ T2   26.15 ± 1.55
- ♦ T3   24.06 ± 1.90

Group 2:
- ♦ T1   24.94 ± 1.43
- ♦ T2   25.71 ± 1.32
- ♦ T3   24.37 ± 1.29

Figure 15.32   Changes in mandibular intercanine width[6]: Group 1 (mean Little Irregularity Index[31] decreased, T1–T2: 5.6 to 0.5 mm, and increased after approximately 12 years; T2–T3: 0.5 to 4.4 mm) versus Group 2 (mean Little Irregularity Index[31] decreased, T1–T2: 5.0 to 0.4 mm, and increased after approximately 12 years T2–T3: 0.4 to 1.7 mm). Both groups had intercanine expansion during treatment, albeit a nonsignificant ($p > 0.05$) difference; Group 1 had more expansion. The clinically significant observation occurred in the long-term where both groups showed the traditional decrease in width, but here the differences were statistically significant ($p < 0.01$) with Group 1 decreasing more in comparison to Group 2.

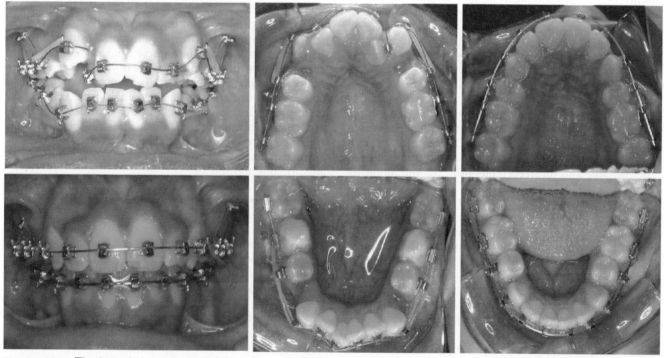

Figure 15.33   The irregularly aligned teeth are aligned as soon as possible during the early phase of the treatment and then basically retained during the arch coordination and consolidation phase towards finishing. The 1-year treatment progress images portrayed in this treatment of a malocclusion show the complete alignment of the teeth. Thus, for the remainder of the treatment, the aligned teeth are 'in retention'. Note the glass ionomer bite pad to disclude and facilitate alignment.

make use of such natural phenomena as the primate spaces, leeway space, arch width increases and incisor movement into ideal relationships. This shows early treatment at its best in an effort to help with physiologic stability.

15. *Mandibular backward rotation appears to influence long-term change:* Long-term studies on stability mostly show that no single predictor for lower incisor stability exists; moreover, no significantly strong correlations could be established.[136] However, two studies found that the vertical dimension could influence stability.[6,173,174]

THE PHASE OF MAINTENANCE: PHASE 3

An overview of the retention and stability literature as portrayed in this chapter shows that there are continual changes taking place over time. It is thus natural to expect patients to return to a practice with the request to perform some revision due to changes that may have occurred as a result of no retention, a retention regimen being stopped to soon or no compliance to the retention protocol following treatment. However, to

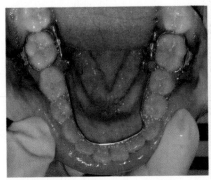 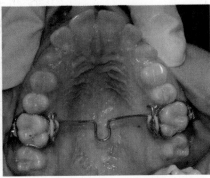

Figures 15.34 Maintenance of natural spaces, such as the leeway space or E-space, utilizing lingual arches and transpalatal arches appear to provide clinicians with options to treat borderline extraction cases with a nonextraction regimen and ultimately achieve a more ideal soft tissue balance. Note that the author prefers to use removable arches as shown in the images, as these can be removed easily for adjustments and replaced for further applications.

some patients, a very minor change impacts on their quality of life. An example of this long-term maintenance can be seen in the following revision case (Fig. 15.36).

CLINICAL TREATMENT RECOMMENDATIONS

The mandibular dental arch dimensions decrease longitudinally in both treated and untreated malocclusions; a normal physiologic phenomenon. The degree of arch length reduction, constriction and resultant crowding is quite variable and unpredictable; however, the following clinical guidelines are suggested:

1. Treat to ideal standards; utilize the contemporary clinical and radiological parameters to obtain the best possible occlusion, oral health and function.
2. Maintain lower arch dimensions whenever possible; consider enlargement only if a narrow arch width with lingually tipped teeth are due to a treatable aetiologic factor, if mandated by facial profile concerns or to harmonize the occlusion with maxillary palatal expansion for crossbite correction.
3. Use the patient's pretreatment archform as a guide for the future treated arch shape.
4. Retain the archform long term and continue to monitor patient response into and throughout adult life.
5. Obtain the highest quality pretreatment records to ensure proper diagnosis and treatment planning; moreover, also pursue quality post-treatment records and continue to use them to assess patient progress and more importantly, evaluate personal clinician growth in the establishment of better treatment and physiologic stability.
6. Consider a Phase 3 of long-term care to ensure physiologic stability.

THE FUTURE

The future holds additional promise: Retention and stability may be enhanced by the accelerated tooth movement created by alveolar corticotomies, and in some instances combined with osteotomies, in an effort to produce the so-called regional acceleratory phenomenon (RAP),[180,181] which individuals have mentioned as possibly more stable over the short term. However, more studies in this respect must be completed to provide substantial evidence that is a future possibility in our quest for less retention and more stability. Bisphosphonates[182] have been experimentally used to provide anchorage in laboratory animals. It is still difficult to maintain this in specific areas, but similar to the RAP this also may be a future consideration in respect to retention and stability. Clinical excellence may only be limited by our imagination; thus, the future may bring exciting adjunct treatment to complement our existing armamentarium.

FINAL COMMENTS

An orthodontic philosophy that is conducive to stability is required to obtain a physiologic stability. Thus, a complete 'Orthodontic Technique' should *not* include only brackets and wires! Moreover, it should include the following:

1. A complete orthodontic system that is focused on,
   a. Diagnosis, and
   b. A detailed treatment plan.
2. It must obey the laws of nature, which provide a limit or border for our treatment.
3. Long-term care with or without retention, which allows for maturational changes; thus a management phase to evaluate these changes and incorporate the needed refinements in the retainers where applicable.
4. Relapse should be reserved for poor treatment or lack of adequate cooperation during treatment and also following treatment in the retention phase.
5. Revision thus may be needed due to physiologic stability.

Long-term change is a biological occurrence, and orthodontists thus accept that this change will occur during and following treatment, as a normal event of maturation. Some consider this as relapse and other condone it as poor or inadequate treatment as such. The term *relapse* should mean a return toward an original condition, but it has taken on a broader meaning to

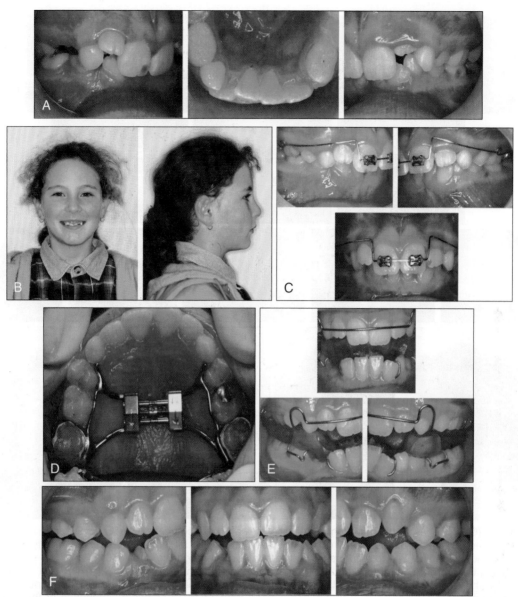

Figure 15.35 The early intervention of this Class II div 2 malocclusion proved to be advantageous. Initially, it is apparent that there is a deep bite and a minor overjet, very typical for this type of malocclusion, and also a beginning of crowding through early space loss following the premature exfoliation of a primary lower canine. Should this be left in the present state and natural development occurs, this malocclusion easily turns into an extraction treatment with detrimental effects on the nonextraction type soft tissue profile. **(A)** The Class II division 2 malocclusion with crowding due to premature exfoliation of primary lower canine. **(B)** The 'ugly duckling' stage as portrayed in the smile image. A retrognathic mandibular position is shown in the sagittal image with the lower lip behind the Ricketts E-line.[134,138] Ideally, the lower lip should be close or ahead of the E-line in the young individual. It was noted earlier that the lips become more retrusive with age in relation to the profile line. **(C)** The Phase 1 treatment plan included a decompensating phase of treatment, which included the proclination of the upper incisors; thus creating a Class II div 1 malocclusion. Overjet was established to allow space for regaining the lost space in the lower arch following the early loss of the primary canine. Note the narrow buccal segments that require some expansion to allow correction for the Class II posterior segment into Class I. **(D)** A number of classic growth hypotheses were presented early in the evolution of the orthodontic speciality. These hypotheses were an endeavour to show the impact of certain factors on the developing craniofacial morphology. These hypotheses were each based on certain premises, and the one being utilized in this treatment is that of Moss,[173,174] cited as the functional matrix hypothesis. Carter and McNamara[175] provided an interfirst maxillary molar width of approximately 33–35 mm in adults; less for females than for males. It was thus imperative to follow the prescriptions of the latter and improve the functional oral environment meeting Moss' requirements, as well as enlarge the arch according to McNamara. RPE was implemented but with a slow adjustment (0.25 mm/quarter turn per day). **(E)** Following adequate arch gaining as previously described, the Phase 1 was completed using the Clark Twin Block Class II correcting functional appliance.[176] **(F)** End of the Phase 1 treatment; interim phase of retention with an anterior inclined bite plate to maintain the over correction until Phase 2 treatment is able to commence. Note a super Class I was established showing overcorrection of the molar segments into a Class III relationship and anterior edge - edge relation (see previous factor 9). Adequate space for the erupting permanent canines was established during Phase 1.

Continued

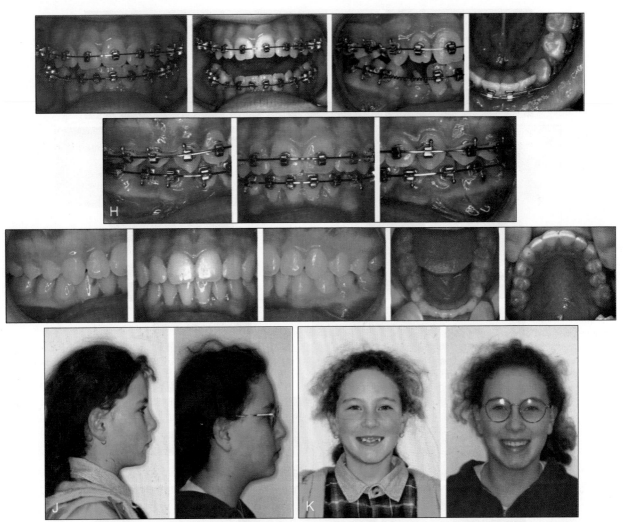

Figure 15.35, cont'd **(G)** The Phase 2 treatment entailed a short fixed appliance phase (018″ SPEED appliance, Strite Industries, Cambridge, ON Canada). Note the modified retainer with the anterior inclined biteplate which served initially as transition during Phase 1 and 2. The lower canine was rotated firstly using a cantilever through the 016″ × 016″ auxiliary slot of the appliance and then engaged in the archwire on route to arch coordination and establishment of Class I. **(H)** The end of Phase 2 fixed appliance treatment with the Class I goal attained. **(I)** Retention commenced utilizing a conventional Hawley maxillary retainer and a fixed intercanine retainer. **(J)** The soft tissue profile comparison from T1 to T3 shows maintenance of the soft tissue profile balance. The early intervention prevented possible extractions to gain space for the correction that would almost be a certainty if this preventive intervention was not pursued. Moreover, the nonextraction regimen followed as a consequence of the early intervention assisted in the normalization of the profile measurements according to Ricketts.[138] **(K)** The smile aesthetic change, over the treatment period underlines the soft tissue balance.

include almost any post-treatment irregularity. However, patients may appear to accept these changes, but they mostly do not as they want to have well-aligned teeth. In addition, to attain this ideal alignment necessitates a great deal of time, effort and money. Moreover, patients have the reasonable expectation that their well-aligned teeth following treatment will be maintained. Since change, to a minor or a major degree, will occur in both treated and untreated cases, orthodontists need to ensure that patients are well informed of these changes; patients can choose the removable or fixed retainers to provide artificial stability or enhance this by a management phase where corrections are maintained with or without retention as another phase of treatment or dental care. Patients thus can elect to continue to see the orthodontist indefinitely, if they so wish. Consider this in the same manner as patients consulting their general practitioner for a prophylaxis.

Clinicians who fully grasp the underlying principles of retention, who appreciate its difficulties and who are able and willing to devote to it that high order of mechanical skills which adequate retaining devices demand, will find few things in dentistry which bring quite the satisfaction and permanent pleasure as the branch they have chosen to practice (orthodontia).

—CALVIN CASE (1908)

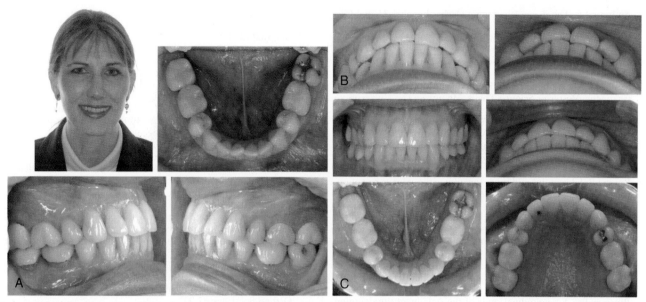

Figure 15.36   An example of long-term maintenance; revision or a Phase 3 where no retention was in place following treatment. **(A)** An adult patient consults the author with a request to align the irregular lower incisors that seem to have changed and is now causing an irritation to her tongue. The occlusion presents in a stable Class I relationship with accompanying soft tissue harmony; in general, the average adult patient with good occlusion and acceptable long-term physiologic stability. The research data[177,178] showed that this is an acceptable long-term change; however, our commitment to excellence is long-term care. Hence, evaluation of the occlusion and determination of a concomitant treatment plan is recommended. **(B)** An evaluation of the morphology of the teeth showed: (1) Minor irregularity of the lower central incisors. (2) Maxillary incisors show enlarged lingual mesial and distal ridges. (3) Upper palatal irregularity and especially the mesial and distal ridges match lower incisor irregularly, in particular the buccal irregularity. (4) A Bolton tooth size discrepancy[179] exists with the mandibular anterior segment (canine–canine) fractionally larger compared to the maxillary anterior segment. (5) The Little Irregularity Index by Little[31] measures a clinically very acceptable long-term result. (6) The treatment plan for this revision or phase 3 was set to: (a) focus on revision of the alignment and adjustment of the maxillary incisor palatal anatomy, (b) lower interproximal enamel reduction to correct the Bolton discrepancy and (c) clear aligner treatment (Invisalign, CA) to provide alignment of the teeth. **(C)** The end of successful treatment following uncomplicated clear aligner treatment (Invisalign). Note the corrected incisor palatal anatomy attained through enameloplasty that allows the establishment of an ideal upper palatal to lower incisor relationship. This is a showcase of successful long-term orthodontic care within the realm of physiologic stability. Note the difference in interincisor occlusion between Figure 15.36 B and C. Clear retainer options as previously discussed instigated.

CONCLUSION

This chapter provided insight into the dilemma of long-term change and the subsequent retention phase. Material was presented for consideration in attaining physiologic stability; it could be as simple as a fiberotomy for prevention of rotations or more involved and lead to over correction during treatment. This part of orthodontic care entails such a wide field that it was impossible to address every aspect; however, it is envisaged that the information provided in this chapter will serve to engender discussion, enhance the clinical outcome of treatment in the long term and serve as a basis for further investigations by all students of orthodontics.

REFERENCES

1. Rossouw PE. Introduction to retention and stability.Semin Orthod 5(3); 1999. 135–137.
2. Lombardi AR. Mandibular incisor crowding in completed cases. Am J Orthod 1972; 61:374–383.
3. Peck H, Peck S. An index for assessing tooth shape deviations as applied to the mandibular incisors. Am J Orthod 1972; 61:384–401.
4. Keene A, Engel G. The mandibular dental arch. Part IV. Prediction and prevention of lower anterior relapse. Angle Orthod 1979; 49:173–180.
5. Little RM. Stability and relapse of dental arch alignment. In: Hosl E, Baldauf A, eds. Retention and long-term stability, 8th International conference for Orthodontists. Heidelburg: HutigbuchVerslag; 1993. 83–94.
6. Franklin S. A longitudinal study of dental and skeletal parameters associated with stability of orthodontic treatment. Diploma Thesis. Toronto: University of Toronto; 1995.
7. Mentz DD. Alongitudinal study of soft tissue in subjects during and after orthodontic treatment. Diploma Thesis. Toronto: University of Toronto; 1996.
8. Angle EH. Classification of malocclusion. Dent Cosmos 1899; 41:248–264, 350–357.
9. Angle EH. Treatment of malocclusion of the teeth. 7th edn. Philadelphia: S.S. White Dental Manufacturing Co.; 1907.
10. Tweed CH. Indications for the extraction of teeth in orthodontic procedure. Am J Orthod Oral Surg 1944; 30:405–428.
11. Andrews LE. The six keys to normal occlusion. Am J Orthod 1972; 62:296–309.

12. Andrews LE. The diagnostic system: Occlusal analysis.Dental Clin North Am 1976; 20:671–690.

13. Williams R. Eliminating lower retention. J Clin Orthod 1985; 19:342–349.

14. Little RM. Stability and relapse of dental arch alignment. Br J Orthod 1990; 17:235–241.

15. Sandusky WC. Along-term postretention study of Tweed extraction treatment. Master of Science Thesis. Memphis: The University of Tennessee; 1983.

16. Sanin C, Savara BS. Factors that affect the alignment of the mandibular incisors: a longitudinal study. Am J Orthod 1973; 64:248–257.

17. Siatkowski RE. Incisor uprighting: mechanism for late secondary crowding in the anterior segments of the dental arches. Am J Orthod 1974; 66:398–410.

18. Boese LR. Fiberotomy and reproximation without lower retention, nine years in retrospect: part I and II. Angle Orthod 1980; 50:88–97, 169–78.

19. Little RM, Wallen TR, Riedel RA. Stability and relapse of mandibular anterior alignment: First premolar extraction cases treated by traditional edgewise orthodontics. Am J Orthod 1981; 80: 349–365.

20. Owman G, Bjerklin K, Kurol J. Mandibular incisor stability after orthodontic treatment in the upper arch. Eur J Orthod 1989; 11:341–350.

21. Rossouw PE. A longitudinal study of the stability of the dentition following orthodontic treatment. PhD Thesis. University of Stellenbosch, Republic of South Africa; 1992.

22. Shearer D. Evaluation of post retention mandibular incisor stability in premolar extraction cases treated by serial extraction without subsequent fixed orthodontic mechanotherapy. Diploma Thesis. Toronto: University of Toronto; 1994.

23. Eslambolchi S. A serial study of mandibular incisor alignment from age 20 to 70 years. Diploma Thesis. Toronto: University of Toronto; 1994.

24. McKnight MM, Daniels CP, Johnston LE Jr. A retrospective study of two-stage treatment outcomes assessed with two modified PAR indices. Angle Orthod 1998; 68:521–526.

25. Strang RHW. Treatment problems:their origin and elimination. Am J Orthod 1954; 40:765–774.

26. Rubin RM. New developments in orthodontics.Va Dent J 1988; 65:17–20.

27. Sadowsky C, Sakols EI. Long-term assessment of orthodontic relapse. Am J Orthod 1982; 82:456–463.

28. Bishara SE, Cummins DM, Zaher AR. Treatment and posttreatment changes in patients with Class II Division Imalocclusion after extraction and nonextraction treatment. Am J Orthod Dentofac Orthop 1997; 111:18–27.

29. King EK. Relapse of orthodontic treatment. Angle Orthod 1974; 44:300–315.

30. Bresonis WL, Grewe JM. Treatment and posttreatment changes in orthodontic cases: overbite and oveijet. Angle Orthod. 1974; 44:295–299.

31. Little RM. The irregularity index: a quantitative score of mandibular anterior alignment. Am J Orthod 1975; 68:554–563.

32. Tweed CH. Clinical orthodontics. Vol.1 and 2. St.Louis: Mosby; 1966.

33. Joondeph DR, Riedel RA. Retention. In: Graber TM, Swain BF, eds. Orthodontics. Principles and techniques. St. Louis: Mosby; 1985. 857–898.

34. The shorter Oxford English dictionary, vol.II. 3rd edn. (1944) revised with corrections in 1975. Ely House, London, Great Britain: Oxford University Press; 1975.

35. Little RM. Stability and relapse of dental arch alignment. Br J Orthod 1990; 17:235–241.

36. Rossouw PE. Terminology: semantics of postorthodontic treatment changes in the dentition. Semin Orthod 5; 1999. 138–141.

37. Ricketts RM. The stabilization and guidance of metapositioning. Part I and II. In: Hosl E, Baldauf A, eds. Retention and long-term stability. 8th International conference for orthodontists. Heidelberg: Huthig; 1993. 111–59.

38. Riedel RA, Richard A. Riedel on retention and relapse. Interview by Brandt S. J Clin Orthod 1976; 10:454–472.

39. Brunelle JA, Bhat M, Lipton JA. Prevalence and distribution of selected occlusal characteristics in the US Population, 1988—1991. J Dent Res 1996; 75(special issue):706–713.

40. Buschang PH, Shulman JD. Incisor crowding in untreated persons 15–50 years of age: United States, 1988—1994. Angle Orthod 2003; 73:502–508.

41. Eslambolchi S, Woodside DG, Roossouw PE. A descriptive study of mandibular incisor alignment in untreated subjects. Am J Orthod Dentofac Orthop 2008; 133:343–353.

42. Behrents RG. Growth in the aging craniofacial skeleton. Monograph 17 Craniofacial Growth Series. Centre for Human Growth and Development. Ann Arbor: University of Michigan; 1985.

43. Kaplan RG. Mandibular third molars and postretention crowding. Am J Orthod 1974; 66:411–430.

44. Little RM, Reidel RA, Artun J. An evaluation of changes in mandibular anterior alignment from 10 to 20 years postretention. Am J Orthod Dentofac Orthop 1988; 93:423–428.

45. Richardson ME. A review of changes in lower arch alignment from seven to Fifty years. Semin Orthod 1999; 5:151–159.

46. Barrow GV, White JR. Developmental changes of the maxillary and mandibular dental arches. Angle Orthod 1952; 22(1):41–46.

47. Björk A. Variability and age changes in overjet and overbite. Am J Orthod. 1953; 39:774–801.

48. Moorrees CFA. The dentition of the growing child. Cambridge: Harvard University Press; 1959.

49. Sinclair PM, Little RM. Maturation of untreated normal occlusions. Am J Orthod. 1983; 83(2): 114–123.

50. Lundstrom A. Changes in crowding and spacing of the teeth with age. Dent Practit 1969; 19(6):218–224.

51. Cryer BS. Lower arch changes during the early teens. Trans Eur Orthod Soc 1966; 87:99.

52. Moorrees CFA. The dentition of the growing child. Cambridge, MA: Harvard University Press; 1959.

53. Van der Linden FPGM. Transition of the human dentition. Monograph 13, Craniofacial Growth Series. Center for Human Growth and Development, University of Michigan. Ann Arbor, MI, 1984.

54. Clinch LM. Variations in the mutual relationships of the upper and lower gum pads and the teeth. Trans Br Soc Study Orthod 1932; 91–107.

55. Baume LJ. Physiological tooth migration and its significance for the development of occlusion. III The biogenesis of the successional dentition. J Dent Res 1950; 29:338–348.

56. Silhnan JH. Dimensional changes of the dental arches: longitudinal study from birth to 25 years. Am J Orthod 1964; 50:824–842.

57. Adams CP, Richardson A. An assessment of the relationship of pre and posteruptive lower incisor position to the facial pattern by serial cephalometric radiography. Trans Eur Orthod Soc 1967; 213–223.

58. Baume LJ. Physiological tooth migration and its significance for the development of occlusion. I The biogenetic course of the deciduous dentition. J Dent Res 1950. ; 29:123–132.

59. Moorrees CFA, Chadha BDS. Available space for the incisors during development-a growth study based on physiological age. Angle Orthod 1965; 35:12–22.

60. Clinch LM. Analysis of serial models between three and eight years of age. Dent Rec 1951; 71:61–72.

61. Hunter J. The natural history of the human teeth. 2nd ed. London: England Johnson; 1778. 81.

62. Richardson ME. Late lower arch crowding: facial growth or forward drift? Eur OrthodJ 1979; 1:219–225.

63. Bergstrom K, Jensen R. The significance of third molars in the aetiology of crowding. Trans Eur Orthod Soc 1960; 84–96.

64. Vego L. A longitudinal study of mandibular arch perimeter. Angle Orthod 1962; 32:187–192.

65. Schwarze CW. The influence of third molar germectomy-A comparative long term study. London: Transactions of the Third International Orthodontic Congress; 1975. 551–562.

66. Lindqvist B, Thilander B. Extraction of third molars in cases of anticipated crowding in the lower jaw. Am J Orthod 1982; 81: 130–139.

67. Richardson ME. The effect of lower second molar extraction on late lower arch crowding. Angle Orthod 1983; 53:25–28.

68. Richardson ME, Mills K. Late lower arch crowding: the effect of second molar extraction. Am J Orthod Dentofac Orthop 1990; 98:242–246.

69. Brenchley ML, Ardouin DGF. Investigations into changes in some mandibular arches in the postdeciduous dentition. Trans Br Soc Study Orthod 1968; 50–58.

70. Schwarze CW. Nachunterst,chungsbefunde bei Patientenmit Extraktion zweiter Molaren. Fortschr Kieferorthop 1980; 41:105–128.

71. Hart AJ, Springate SD. Mandibular permanent second molar extraction: effect on lower incisors. Br Soc Dent Res Abs 1989; 98.

72. Orton HS, Battagel JM, Ferguson R, et al. Distal movement of buccal segments with the "en masse" removable appliance: its value in treating patients with mild Class II, Division 1 malocclusion. Part II: The model measuring system and results. Am J Orthod Dentofac Orthop 1996; 109:379–385.

73. Richardson ME. The development of third molar impaction and its prevention. IntJ Oral Surg 1981; 10(suppl 1):122–30.

74. Richardson ME. The aetiology of late lower arch crowding alternative to mesially directed forces: a review. Am J Orthod Dentofac Orthop 1994; 105:592–597.

75. Ades AG, Joondeph DR, Little RM, et al. Along-term study of the relationship of third molars to changes in the mandibular dental arch. Am J Orthod Dentofac Orthop 1990; 97(4):323–335.

76. Dewey M. Some principles of retention. Am Dent J 1917;8:254.

77. Bergstrom K, Jensen R. Responsibility of the third molar for secondary crowding. Dent Abstr 1961; 6:544.

78. Vego L. A longitudinal study of mandibular arch perimeter. Angle Orthod 1962; 32:187–192.

79. Lindqvist B, Thilander B. Extraction of third molars in cases of anticipated crowding in the lower jaw. Am J Orthod 1982; 81(2):130–139.

80. Richardson ME, Mills K. Late lower arch crowding: the effect of second molar extraction. Am J Orthod Dentofac Orthop 1990; 98(3):242–246.

81. Fastlicht J. Crowding of mandibular incisors. Am J Orthod 1970; 58(2):156–163.

82. Solomon AG. The role of mandibular third molars in the aetiology of mandibular incisor crowding and changing growth patterns in the dentofacial complex. Diploma Thesis, University of Toronto; 1973.

83. Kaplan RG. Mandibular third molars and postretention crowding. Am J Orthod 1974; 66(4):411–430.

84. Bishara SE, Andreasen G. Third molars: a review. Am J Orthod 1983; 83(2):131–137.

85. Björk A. The significance of growth changes in facial pattern and their relationship to changes in occlusion. The Dental Record 1951; 71:197–208.

86. Björk A. Prediction of mandibular growth rotation. Am J Orthod 1969; 55(6):585–599.

87. Björk A, Skieller V. Facial development and tooth eruption: An implant study at the age of puberty. Am J Orthod 1972; 62:339–383.

88. Buschang PH, Baume RM, Nass GG. A craniofacial growth maturity gradient for males and females between 4 and 16 years of age. Am J Phys Anthrop 1983; 61:373–381.

89. Linder-Aronson S, Woodside DG, Hellsing E, et al. Normalization of incisor position after adenoidectomy. Am J Orthod Dentof Orthop 1993; 103(5):412–427.

90. Woodside DG, Linder-Aronson S, Stubbs DO. Relationship between mandibular incisor crowding and nasal mucosal swelling. Proc Finn Dent Soc 1991; 87(1):127–138.

91. Tweed CH. Interview with Dr. D.S. Brandt. J Pract Orthod 1968; 2:11–19.

92. Edwards JG. The prevention of relapse in extraction cases. Am J Orthod 1971; 60:128–141.

93. Ferris T, Alexander RG, Boley J, et al. Long-term stability of combined rapid palatal expansion lip bumper therapy followed by full Fixed appliances. Am J Orthod Dentofacial Orthop 2005; 128:310–325.

94. Gardner D, Chaconas S. Posttreatment and postretention changes following orthodontic therapy. Angle Orthod 1976; 46:151–161.

95. Glenn G, Sinclair P, Alexander RG. Non-extraction orthodontic therapy: posttreatment dental and skeletal stability. Am J Orthod Dentofacial Orthop 1987; 92:321–328.

96. Haas AJ. Long-term posttreatment evaluation of rapid palatal expansion. Angle Orthod 1980; 50:189–218.

97. McReynolds D, Little R. Mandibular second premolar extraction-Postretention evaluation of stability and relapse. Angle Orthop 1991; 61:133–144.

98. Little R, Riedel R, Engst E. Serial extraction of first premolars-Postretention evaluation of stability and relapse. Angle Orthod 1990; 60:255–262.

99. Haruki T, Little R. Early versus late treatment of crowded first premolar extraction cases: postretention evaluation of stability and relapse. Angle Orthod 1998; 68:61–68.

100. Riedel R, Little R, Bui T. Mandibular incisor extraction-postretention evaluation of stability and relapse. Angle Orthod 1992; 62:103–116.

101. Little R, Riedel R, Stein A. Mandibular arch length increase during the mixed dentition: postretention evaluation of stability and relapse. Am J Orthod Dentofac Orthop 1990; 97:393–404.

102. Woodside DG, Rossouw PE, ShearerD. Postretention mandibular incisor stability after premolar serial extractions. Semin Orthod 1999; 5:181–190.

103. Tweed CH. The Frankfort-mandibular plane angle in orthodontic diagnosis, classification, treatment planning, and prognosis. Am J Orthod Oral Surg 1946; 32:175–221.

104. Friel S. Occlusion. Observation on its development from infancy to old age. Int J Orthod 1927; 13:322–341.

105. Mills JRE. Clinical control of craniofacial growth: a skeptic's view point. In: McNamara JA, Ribbens KA, Howe RP, eds. Clinical alteration on the growing face, Monogram 14, Craniofacial Growth Series. Ann Arbor: University of Michigan; 1983.

106. Weislander L, Lagerstrom L.The effect of activator treatment on Class II malocclusions. Am J Orthod 1979; 75:20–26.

107. Clavert FJ. An assessment of Andresen therapy in Class II division 1 malocclusions. Brit J Orthod 1982; 9:149–153.

108. Hunt NP, Ellisdon PS. The Belle Mandsley memorial lecture1984. The Bionator: Its use and 'abuse', part I and II. Dent 1985; 12: 51–61, 129–132.

109. Little RM. Stability and relapse of dental arch alignment. Br J Orthod 1990; 17:235–241.

110. Haas AJ. Long-term posttreatment evaluation of rapid palatal expansion. Angle Orthod 1980; 50:189–217.

111. Rossouw PE, Preston CB, Lombard C. A longitudinal evaluation of extraction versus nonextraction treatment with special reference to the posttreatment irregularity of the lower incisors.Semin Orthod 1999; 5:160–170.

112. McCauley DR. The cuspid and its function in retention. Am J Orthod 1944; 30:196–205.

113. Howes AE. Case analysis and treatment planning based upon the relationship of the tooth material to its supporting bone. Am J Orthod Oral Surg 1947; 33:499–533.

114. Steadman SR. Changes of intermolar and intercuspid distances following orthodontic treatment. Angle Orthod 1961; 31:207–215.

115. Strang R. The fallacy of denture expansion as a treatment procedure. Angle Orthod 1949; 19:12–22.

116. Herold J. Maxillary expansion: a retrospective study of three methods of expansion and their long-term sequelae. Brit J Orthod 1989; 16:195–200.

117. Adkins MD, Nanda RS, Currier GF. Arch perimeter changes on rapid palatal expansion. Am J Orthod Dentofacial Orthop 1990; 97:194–199.

118. Sadowsky C, Schneider BJ, BeGole EA, et al. Long-term stability after orthodontic treatment: Non-extraction with prolonged retention. Am J Orthod Dentofacial Orthop 1994; 106:243–249.

119. Moussa R,O'Reilly MT, Close JM. Long-term stability of rapid palatal expander treatment and edgewise mechanotherapy. Am J Orthod Dentofacial Orthop 1995; 108:478–488.

120. McNamara JA Jr, Baccetti T, Franchi L, et al. Rapid maxillary expansion followed by fixed appliances: a long-term evaluation of changes in arch dimensions. Angle Orthod 2003; 73:344–353.

121. Isik F, Sayinsu K, Nalbantgil D, et al. A comparative study of dental arch widths: extraction and non-extraction treatment. Eur J Orthod 2005; 27:585–589.

122. Kim E, Gianelly A. Extraction vs nonextraction: arch widths and smile esthetics. Angle Orthod 2003; 73:354–358.

123. Taner T, Ciger S, EIH, et al. Evaluation of dental arch width and form changes after orthodontic treatment and retention with a new computerized method. Am J Orthod Dentofacial Orthop 2004; 126:464–476.

124. Solomon MJ, English JD, Magness WB, et al. Long-term stability of lip bumper therapy followed by Fixed appliances. Angle Orthod 2006; 76:36–42.

125. Osborn WS, Nanda RS, Currier GF. Mandibular arch perimeter changes with lip bumper treatment. Am J Orthod Dentofacial Orthop 1991; 99:527–532.

126. Werner SP, Shivapuja PK, Harris EF. Skeletodental changes in the adolescent accruing from use of the lip bumper. Angle Orthod 1994; 64:13–22.

127. Vargo JA. Treatment effects and short-term relapse of maxillo mandibular expansion during the early-mid mixed dentition. M.S. 1998. The Texas A&M University System-Baylor College of Dentistry.

128. Blumber K, Rossouw PE, Buschang PH. Stability of the transverse dimension after damon orthodontic treatment. J Dent Res 2007; 86 (spec issue A):107.

129. Simons ME, Joondeph DR.Change in overbite: a ten-year postretention study. Am J Orthod 1973; 64:349–367.

130. Sandusky WC. A long-term postretention study of Tweed extraction treatment. Master of Science Thesis. Memphis: The University of Tennessee; 1983.

131. Gorman JC. The effects of premolar extractions on the long-term stability of the mandibular incisors. In: Nanda B, ed. Retention and stability in orthodontics. Philadelphia: W.B. Saunders Co; 1993. 81–95.

132. Conlin RT. Finished cases and their faces. J Clin Orthod 1989; 23:751–754.

133. Holdaway RA. A soft-tissue cephalometric analysis and its use in orthodontic treatment planning. Part II. Am J Orthod 1984; 85:279–293.

134. Ricketts RM, Bench RW, Gugino CF, et al. Bioprogressive therapy. Book 1. Denver: Rocky Mountain Orthodontics; 1979. 52–262.

135. Rossouw PE, Preston CB, Lombard C, et al. A longitudinal evaluation of the anterior border of the dentition and its relationship to stability. Am J Orthod Dentofac Orthop 1993; 104(2):146–152.

136. Little RM. Stability and relapse of mandibular anterior alignment: university of Washington studies. Semin Orthod 1999; 5:191–204.

137. Vanarsdall RL. Transverse dimension and long-term stability. Semin Orthod 1999; 5:171–180.

138. Ricketts RM. Perspectives in the clinical application of cephalometrics, the First Fifty years. Angle Orthod 1981; 51:115–150.

139. Tomes CS. The bearing of the development of the jaws on irregularities. Dental Cosmos 1873; 15:292–296.

140. Strang R. The fallacy of denture expansion as a treatment procedure. Angle Orthod 1949; 19:12–22.

141. Posen AL. The in fluence of maximum perioral and tongue force on the incisor teeth. Angle Orthod 1972; 42(4):285–309.

142. Thuer U, Ingervall B. Pressure from the lips on the teeth and malocclusion. Am J Orthod Dentof Orthop 1986; 90(3):234–242.

143. Steiner CC. Cephalometrics for you and me. Am J Orthod 1953; 39:729–755.

144. Merrifield LL. The profile line as an aid in critically evaluating facial esthetics. Am J Orthod 1966; 52:804–822.

145. Burstone CJ. Lip posture and its significance in treatment planning. Am J Orthod 1967; 53:262–284.

146. Holdaway RA. A soft-tissue cephalometric analysis and its use in orthodontic treatment planning. Part I. Am J Orthod 1983; 84:1–28.

147. Paquette DE, Beattie JR, Johnston LE. A long-term comparison of non-extraction and premolar extraction edgewise therapy in 'borderline' Class II patients. Am J Orthod Dentofac Orthop 1992; 102(1):1–14.

148. Bishara SE, Cummins DM, Jakobsen JR, et al. Dentofacial and soft tissue changes in Class II, Division 1 cases treated with and without extractions. Am J Orthod Dentofac Orthop 1995; 107:28–37.

149. Bishara SE, Jakobsen JR, Hession TJ, et al. Soft tissue profile changes from 5 to 45 years of age. Am J Orthod Dentofac Orthop 1998; 114:698–706.

150. Rossouw PE, Preston CB, Lombard CJ. Longitudinal change in male and female orthodontic subjects and its value in assessing postorthodontic stability. In: James A. McNamara Jr, Carroll-Ann Trotman, eds. Orthodontic treatment: the management of unfavourable sequilae. Craniofacial Growth Series, No. 31. Ann Arbor: University of Michigan; 1996. 389–437.

151. Lustig JR. Short-term evaluation of postorthodontic occlusion with a wrap-around and clear overlay retainer. Master's Thesis, Texas A&M University Health Science Center Baylor College of Dentistry; 2003.

152. Renkema AM, Al-Assad, Bronkhorst E, Weindel S, Katsaros C, Lisson J. Effectiveness of lingual retainers bonded to the canines in preventing mandibular relapse. Am J Orthod Dentofacial Orthop 2008; 134:179.e1–179.e8.

153. Renkema AM, Renkema A, Bronkhorst E, Katsaros C. long-term effectiveness of canine-to-canine bonded flexible spiral wire lingual retainers. Am J Orthod Dentofacial Orthop 2011; 139:614–621.

154. Richardson ME. Lower arch crowding in the young adult. Am J Orthod Dentofac Orthop 1992; 101:132–137.

155. Richardson ME, Gormley JS. Lower arch crowding in the third decade. Eur J Orthod 1998; 20:597–607.

156. Harvold EP, Chierici G, Karin Vargervik K. Experiments on the development of dental malocclusions. Am J Orthod 1972; 61: 38–44.

157. Harvold EP, Chierici G, Karin Vargervik K. Primate experiments on oral sensation and dental malocclusions. Am J Orthod 1973; 63:494–508.

158. Linder-Aronson S, Woodside DG, Hellsing E, Emerson W. Normalization of incisor position after adenoidectomy. Am J Orthod Dentofac Orthop 1993; 103(5):412–427.

159. Williams R. The diagnostic line. Am J Orthod 1969;55:458–467.

160. Williams R, Hosila FJ. The effect of different extraction sites upon incisor retraction. Am J Orthod 1976; 69:388–410.

161. Mills RJE. The long term results of proclination of lower incisors. Br Dent J 1966; 120:355–363.

162. Mills JRE. A long-term assessment of the mechanical retroclination of the lower incisors. Angle Orthod 1967; 37:165–174.

163. Blake M, Bibby K. Retention and stability: a review of the literature. Am J Orthod Dentofac Orthop 1998; 114:299–306.

164. Southard TE, Behrents RG, Tolley EA. The anterior component of occlusal force: part II. Relationship with dental malalignment. Am J Orthod Dentofac Orthop 1990; 97:41–44.

165. Sparkes AL. Interproximal enamel reduction and its effect on the long-term stability of the mandibular incisor position. Master's Thesis, University of Alabama at Birmingham; 2001.

166. Rossouw PE, Tortorella A. Enamel Reduction Procedures in Orthodontic Treatment. J Can Dent Assoc 2003; 69(6):378–383.

167. Rossouw PE, Tortorella A. A Pilot Investigation of Enamel Reduction Procedures. J Can Dent Assoc 2003; 69(6):384–388.

168. Pancherz H. The Herbst appliance—its biologic effects and clinical use. Am J Orthod 1985; 87:1–20.

169. Ferris T, Alexander RG, Boley J, et al. Long-term stability of combined rapid palatal expansion–lip bumper therapy followed by full fixed appliances. Am J Orthod Dentofac Orthop 2005; 128:310–325.

170. Reitan K. Clinical and histologic observations on tooth movement during and after orthodontic treatment. Am J Orthod 1967; 53:721–745.

171. Thilander B. Biological basis for orthodontic relapse. Sem Orthod 2000; 6:195–205.

172. Gianelly AA. One-phase versus two-phase treatment. Am J Orthod Dentofac Orthop 1995; 108:556–559.

173. Moss ML. The functional matrix. In: Kraus B, Riedel R, editors, Vistas in orthodontics. Philadelphia: Lea and Febiger; 1962. 85–98.

174. Moss ML, Salentijn L. The primary role of functional matrices in facial growth. Am J Orthod 1969; 55:566–577.

175. Carter GA, McNamara JA. Longitudinal dental arch changes in adults. Am J Orthod Dentofac Orthop 1998; 114:88–99.

176. Clark WJ. The twin block technique: a function alappliance system. Am J Orthod Dentofac Orthop 1988; 93:1–18.

177. Franklin GS, Rossouw PE, Woodside DG. A longitudinal study of dental and skeletal parameters associated with stability of orthodontic treatment. Am J Orthod Dentofac Orthop 1996; 109:1, 109.

178. Driscoll-GillilandJ,Buschang PH, Behrents RG. An evaluation of growth and stability in untreated and treated subjects. Am J Orthod Dentofac Orthop 2001; 120:588–597.

179. Bolton WA. Disharmony in tooth size and its relation to the analysis and treatment of malocclusion. Angle Orthod 1958; 28:113–130.

180. Frost HM. The regional accelerating phenomenon. Orthop Clin North Am 1981; 12:725–726.

181. Wilco WM, WilckoT, Bouquot JE,et al.Rapid Orthodontics with alveolar reshaping: two case reports of decrowding. Int J Periodontics Restorative Dent 2001; 21:9–19.

182. Igarashi K, Mitani H, Adachi H, et al. Anchorage and retentive effects of a bisphosphonate (AHBuBP) on tooth movements in-rats. Am J Orthod Dentofac Orthop 1994; 106:279–289.

Optimizing Orthodontic Treatment

Ashok Karad

The science and art of orthodontics continues to receive significant contributions, both from research and clinical innovations. With the focus on high-quality treatment results, there is growing need for awareness that treatment of complex dentofacial problems requires carefully assessed diagnosis, well-designed and properly implemented treatment plan, and sophisticated appliances in skilled hands. In contemporary clinical practice, efficiency is an absolute requirement for optimal patient care, which leads to practice growth through increased productivity. However, it should be recognized that in dealing with the human body, which is a biological mechanism, the overall goals should be efficient and effective treatment with minimum deterioration of hard and soft tissues, good function and pleasing aesthetics.

It should be recognized that facial orthopaedic and orthodontic treatment modalities influence four main elements of the dentofacial complex—skeleton, dentition, facial soft-tissues, and function (Fig. 16.1). In an average growing individual; skeleton, dentition, and function mature in different ways and at varying speeds. However, they will be in balance, with each part being situated within the range of normal variation.[1]

The function, which also includes soft-tissues, exhibits more limited range of variation than other two parts. Also, function plays a more dominant role in the entire dentofacial complex than the other two elements (skeleton and dentition).

The present scenario is marked by technological advances in appliance designs, absolute anchorage, imaging, etc. Considering the present appliance systems and available prescriptions, no single prescription is ideal for all, since there are a lot of variations in the morphological characteristics of the patient population. Therefore, all individuals vary in amount of tooth movement required. In the author's opinion, what will drive orthodontics in the future will be individualized diagnosis, customized treatment and care. With respect to the available bracket systems, how do we overcome discrepancies as a result of individual patient variations, inherent deficiencies associated with the appliance system itself, or the problems associated with clinician's treatment mechanics? The built-in features of the preadjusted edgewise appliances (PEA) in their present variations allow the clinicians to achieve fairly good results. However, in the author's opinion, few adjustments are still required during the finishing stage of treatment to treat patients to highest standards possible. In other words, individualized diagnosis, treatment planning, treatment mechanics, and results.

SPECIFIC FEATURES OF ORTHODONTIC TREATMENT

A major goal of contemporary orthodontics is to make treatment easier and more convenient for the patient. While refined orthodontic appliance systems and mechanics are

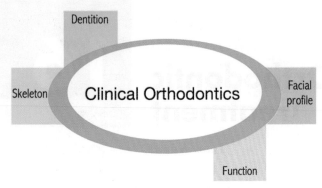

Figure 16.1 Clinical orthodontics influences four main elements of dentofacial complex: skeleton, dentition, facial profile and function.

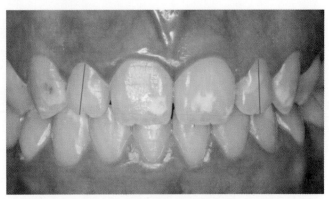

Figure 16.2 Unnecessary prolonged treatment duration leading to patient 'burn-out' and poor compliance that resulted in 'forced debonding', leaving out correction of maxillary lateral incisor tip.

being used to bring about efficient tooth movement, it is essential to understand the specific features of orthodontic treatment to get the delivery of orthodontic care to the next level.

Treatment duration

Efficient tooth movement is the prime goal of orthodontic treatment. It is the result of optimal biologic response to the orthodontic force system. This essentially involves the physiologic activity of alveolar bone resorption and deposition to produce tooth movement induced by the mechanical stimulus through the delivery of orthodontic force systems. A well-defined treatment goal, proper execution of treatment plan and appropriate mechanics are critical to prevent unnecessary prolonged treatment time. The prolonged treatment may ultimately 'burn out' the patient and subsequently results in poor compliance.[2]

Patient compliance

Patient compliance remains to be an integral part of orthodontic treatment. Lack of compliance in all age groups, especially in the adolescent population, has been a matter of concern for the practising orthodontists, having a significant impact on the treatment outcome (Fig. 16.2). Over the past few years, the percentage of patients exhibiting poor compliance has been increased tremendously, with only about 10% demonstrating excellent compliance.[3] It should also be recognized that the patient compliance usually decreases when longer duration treatment is required. Certain measures, like patient motivation, reduction of treatment duration, involvement of patient and parent in treatment decision and the use of noncompliance treatment mechanics, are important to improve patient cooperation.

Pain and discomfort

Mild pain and discomfort during orthodontic treatment are common, and are often reported during the first day(s) of treatment. When an orthodontic force is applied to a tooth, quite often, patients experience some discomfort or mild pain for the initial one or two days. In general, the intensity of pain increases with time at 4 hours and 24 hours, however, it settles down to normal level at 7 days.[4,5]

In an ideal scenario, orthodontic treatment should be without any pain or discomfort. Though this is not always possible, the clinician should strive to minimize any risk or cause of pain. In the author's opinion, certain degree of pain can be avoided by careful application and adjustment of orthodontic appliances, and by performing every treatment procedure with the risk of pain in mind.

Treatment-induced enamel colour alterations

The stability of original tooth colour shades is of profound importance because any alterations produced after orthodontic treatment may impact the overall treatment outcome. Enamel colour alterations may occur as a result of irreversible penetration of resin tags into the enamel structure at depths reaching 50 μm.[6] Since debonding and cleaning procedures cannot remove the impregnated resin in the enamel structure, it is common to observe enamel discolouration due to direct absorption of food colourants and corrosion of fixed appliances.[7] Also, post-debonding residual composite removal, if not done properly, alters enamel surface properties, which may adversely affect the final enamel colour (Fig. 16.3). This is because the final enamel surface is mainly composed of abraded enamel infiltrated by resin tags at the sites of enamel rods dissolved from acid etching. This contributes to the altered refractive index of the region, modifying the diffusely reflected light, thus affecting the enamel colour parameters.

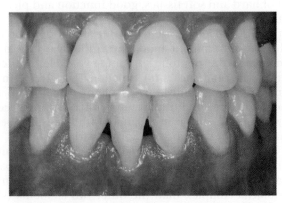

Figure 16.3 Treatment-induced enamel colour alterations.

Enamel decalcification

Fixed orthodontic appliances can create iatrogenic effects on the tooth; of particular importance is the enamel decalcification and caries (Fig. 16.4).[8,9] Various components of the fixed appliances cause obvious visual obstruction, leading to the development and progression of carious lesion. The existing irregularities of teeth coupled with the presence of fixed appliances results into development of more plaque retention sites making it difficult for the patient to maintain oral hygiene. It has been shown that fixed orthodontic appliances induce a rapid increase in the volume of dental plaque, also the lower resting pH than that in non-orthodontic subjects.[10,11] These plaque retentive sites predispose orthodontic patients to high levels of cariogenic activity even on the labial surfaces, where carious lesion usually does not develop.

Root resorption

Orthodontically-induced root resorption, with variable frequency, has been a matter of concern for the clinician (Fig. 16.5). It has been found that apical root resorption involved one-fourth of the original root length in 1.5% of maxillary central incisors and 2.2% of lateral incisors.[12] There are individual variations between patients and between different teeth in the same patient. Tooth mobility and loss of supporting bone may result as a consequence of extensive apical root resorption.[13] Considering these sequelae, the clinician must develop a strategy to minimize treatment-induced root resorption, and establish a plan for follow-up before the commencement of orthodontic treatment.

Adverse effects on periodontal tissues

Bacterial plaque at the gingival margin area is the most significant factor in the development of gingival inflammation (Fig. 16.6). During orthodontic treatment, fixed appliances tend to increase retention sites for microbes responsible for gingivitis. Patients undergoing fixed appliance therapy have significantly higher total number of *Streptococcus mutans* and lactobacilli than nonorthodontic population.[14,15]

Also, higher periodontal pocket depths and gingival bleeding have been associated with molars with

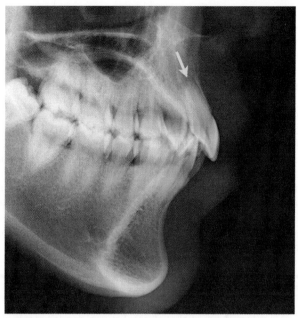

Figure 16.5   Orthodontic treatment-induced maxillary incisor root resorption as evident in lateral cephalogram.

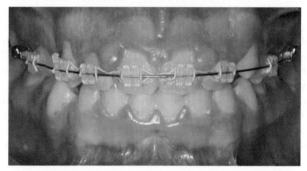

Figure 16.6   Gingival inflammation due to retention of bacterial plaque around the brackets.

orthodontic bands than with bonded attachments.[16] Loss of attachment is also more commonly found in molars with orthodontic bands. Orthodontic appliances, under specific conditions, have the potential to damage supporting structures of the teeth. The incidence and the magnitude of reduction in marginal bone support is significantly higher in treated than untreated teeth.[17] Patients having difficulties with the oral hygiene regimen during the treatment demonstrate more damage to the marginal bone support. In the presence of bacterial plaque, tipping and intrusion of teeth may shift a supragingival bacterial plaque into a subgingival position; thereby converting a gingival inflammation into a lesion associated with attachment loss and infrabony pockets.

Temporomandibular disorders (TMDs)

Temporomandibular disorders are complex in nature encompassing a variety of signs and symptoms. These conditions have countless pathologic and functional

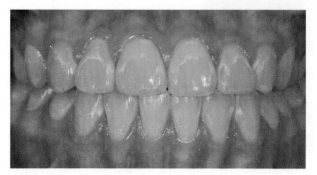

Figure 16.4   Post-treatment enamel white spot lesions.

manifestations on the stomatognathic system. Considering this, orthodontists should possess adequate relevant knowledge and experience to establish accurate diagnosis and also to identify the patients at risk. In a broader perspective, orthodontic treatment produces gradual changes in an environment which are generally adaptive. If orthodontic therapy interferes with the ability of the stomatognathic system to adapt to the changes produced, it may predispose the patient to TMD or it may aggravate an existing dysfunction (Figs 16.7–16.9). Certain clinical situations, like inappropriate post-treatment occlusal relationships, severe mandibular displacement and muscle hyperactivity, should be avoided to prevent iatrogenic effects. Significant orthodontic relapse leading to a functional imbalance between the occlusion, muscles and TMJ may contribute to the development of signs and symptoms of TMD in some cases.

PRACTICE ENVIRONMENT

The management of the clinical practice ultimately determines the degree of efficiency and effectiveness with which the clinician resolves individual patient problems. It is generally considered that a thorough knowledge of theoretical aspects and technical skills provide the basis for orthodontic practice. However, overall outcome of the treatment (treatment success) quite often also depends on the administrative efficiency of the practice, procedural control, and quality assurance. It should be recognized that the practice management skills should not be limited to those who maintain a high volume of practice, rather they are applicable even to practices of any size for better efficiency and quality control. Orthodontists are trained to high level of technical abilities and they generally tend to ignore the essential management skills that create better environment for the expression of their technical aptitudes.

Only technical skills and systems cannot function efficiently and sustain for a longer time unless they operate in a well-organized and managed set-up.

For effective and efficient orthodontic treatment, it is important that the tasks involved must be simplified. They must be converted into an integrated set of related procedures (quality systems), designed and coordinated to accomplish well-defined treatment goals (standard of care). There are four essential ingredients for maintaining a high-quality orthodontic practice:

1. Accurate diagnosis
2. Proper treatment
3. Prevention of complications
4. Satisfactory treatment outcome.

Orthodontic services should be committed to the pursuit of excellence and high quality of care. Determination of quality requires the development, implementation, and maintenance of an effective quality assessment and performance improvement program. This requires regular and systematic assessment and evaluation of the processes involved in providing orthodontic care, and measurement of outcomes using validated instruments for data collection and analysis.

Quality systems

Excellence in orthodontic practice requires expertise in the clinical management of problems in multiple domains, supported by efficient management systems that furthers the goal of care and supports practitioners. The clinical set-up should establish, document, implement and maintain a quality management system and continually improve its effectiveness.[18]

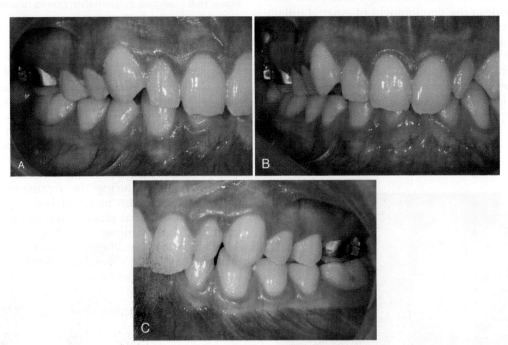

Figure 16.7 This patient was referred to the author's clinic as he developed the symptoms of TMD after maxillary molar distalization.

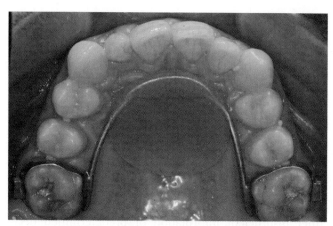

Figure 16.8 Maxillary left first molar was displaced palatally causing prematurity in the posterior region, leading to unstable occlusion.

It is important to make sure that quality improvement activities are routinely followed and regularly assessed to determine their influence on clinical practice. When required, these systems should be collaborative and interdisciplinary. No matter how practice systems are used, the goal should be the same: to improve patient care; and better patient care means better outcomes. This is what clinical quality is all about. Practice systems/operating procedures should be dynamic and evolving; they must change to keep pace with new scientific knowledge and advances in technology.

Evidence-based orthodontic practice procedures promote rational, informed clinical decision-making that reflects the best available scientific information and insights. Effective treatment strategies should be based on researched and rigorously crafted clinical guidelines as valuable tools for improving quality and efficiency. Quality, as reflected in patient outcomes, should be the basis for professional accountability.

In an effort to maintain a high-quality orthodontic practice, the clinician should establish well-designed clinical practice systems; the following principles then become critical to their use.

- *Redefined practice goals:* The guidelines should represent goals that orthodontic services should strive to attain, as opposed to minimal or lowest acceptable practice.
- *Quality standards:* The clinical practice guidelines should follow established practice standards and requirements for quality, such as high-quality patient records, prevention of adverse effects of the treatment, efficient patient scheduling, etc.
- *Code of ethics:* There should be strict adherence to establish professional and organizational codes of ethics.
- *Ongoing revision:* The practice guidelines should be revised over time, reflecting current body of scientific information and updating.
- *Speciality care:* This refers to the provision of services by professionals within an interdisciplinary team, whose

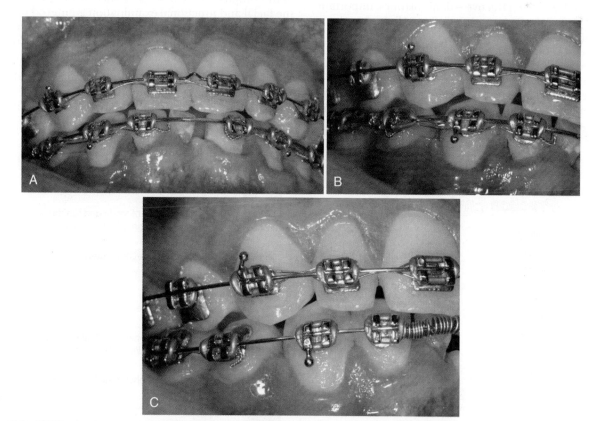

Figure 16.9 TMD symptoms were improved at this stage of treatment, however, patient did complain of occasional pain in the pre-auricular region on mandibular movement. **(A and B)** Increased overjet in the right canine region. **(C)** Improved maxillary and mandibular canine relationship.

work reflects substantial involvement in the care of patients with complex dentofacial problems.

This approach emphasizes understanding and operating the orthodontic practice as a whole rather than focusing on limited parts or isolated areas of practice environment. It underlines the importance of one element, however small it may be, can have dramatic effects on other elements of the system, thereby influencing the overall outcome (Fig. 16.10).

Standard of care

High-quality orthodontic care should have the following ingredients:

- Highly predictable relationship between the goal and the result.
- A well documented, properly analyzed diagnostic criteria system that establishes a definitive treatment plan, with treatment sequencing and monitoring the treatment progress.
- Proper timing—delivered to the right patient at the right time
- Non-compliance therapy
- Reduction of chair time to a minimum
- Achievement of optimal facial aesthetics
- Achievement of goals for patients of any age
- Patient-centred—based on the goals and preferences of the patient.
- Appliance system and mechanics engineered to meet the requirements of an individual patient.
- Beneficial and/or effective—demonstrates important patient outcomes or processes of care linked to desirable outcomes.
- Elimination of abnormal habits
- Improvement in doctor–patient inter-relationship (and level of confidence)
- Services based on evidence-based guidelines representing a systematic rational approach to clinical orthodontics because they are more rigorously grounded in science.

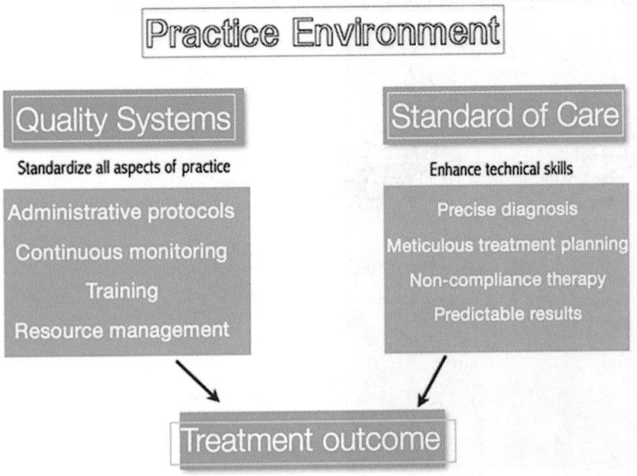

VARIABLES AFFECTING TREATMENT OUTCOME

For efficient orthodontic practice, it is important to simplify both technical and management procedures involved.

Organized approach to diagnostic decision making

The process of setting up the jaw framework, positioning the teeth in appropriate positions on the normally related jaws, and defining treatment goals requires that the diagnosis is accurate. Improper diagnosis is often the result of either insufficient information or predetermined decisions made in order to adapt the case to a specific type of treatment modality. A common mistake is to think in terms of mechanotherapy and related factors at this stage. An accurate diagnosis is established by carefully studying the diagnostic information, without any preconceived ideas. An astute clinician must consider other factors besides mechanical aspects and cephalometric criteria.

It is recommended to define sequential steps involved in making each patient diagnosis to identify the relevant information and leave out the extraneous.

The author follows the same sequence in establishing each diagnosis as outlined below. The diagnostic procedures are typically performed in two steps (Fig. 16.11).

Step 1 involves initial consultation and the patient interview. This is aimed at understanding patient's main concern, enthusiasm for orthodontic treatment, and the patient compliance. A brief summary of the findings from the facial and functional examination is entered in patient data file for quick reference. Care should be taken not to miss out on TMDs or CO-CR discrepancy. The step 2 of the diagnostic procedure involves the following sequence:

1. The relevant findings from step 1 are reviewed.
2. Patient's orthopantomogram and intraoral periapical radiographs are examined to assess overall tooth position, bone condition, and dental health.

Figure 16.10 Good practice environment consisting of quality systems and standard of patient care to produce optimal results.

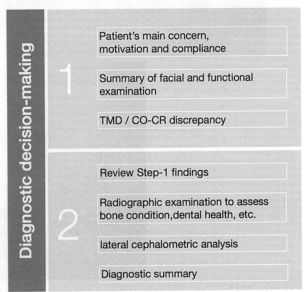

Figure 16.11 Diagnostic decision-making process involves two main steps.

3. The arch length discrepancy is measured next. The study models are carefully analyzed. Considering archform, rotations, tooth size discrepancies, proclination, etc.

4. The next step is to 'eyeball' the lateral cephalogram to understand the overall position and inter-relationship of various components of craniofacial complex. The procedure for visually assessing lateral cephalogram should involve sequential study of: a) soft-tissue profile, b) maxillary skeletal base, c) maxillary dentition, d) mandibular dentition, e) mandibular skeletal base, f) temporomandibular joint area, and g) cranial base.

5. The final step is to write down the diagnostic summery.

A well-designed, properly implemented treatment plan

An accurate diagnosis is critical. It allows for the development of a treatment plan that addresses the patient's chief complaint, medical and dental history; and dental, skeletal, facial, functional, and/or psychosocial problems. Such a plan will facilitate coordination of the treatment objectives and the various methods available to achieve them. The treatment plan should also include a detailed sequence of mechanics, time estimates, and other factors, such as missing teeth or unfavourable growth patterns that might complicate the mechanics.

A well-planned treatment strategy should consist of treatment goals, appliance selection, sequencing and timing of treatment, coordination with other health care providers, and retention (Figs 16.12–16.17). This plan should be periodically reassessed throughout treatment. The reassessment should take into consideration various limiting factors and establish short- and/or long-term objectives. A 'nutshell' description of the problem should be written on the patient treatment chart for quick reference. Reducing the huge amount of patient data to this concise description focuses attention of the clinician on the essence of treatment. This also allows the clinician to refresh the memory of the case quickly, thereby preventing needless paperwork.

Selection of appliance system

Most orthodontists consider both the treatment planning and delivery of orthodontic care as limited to the simple process of bonding brackets to the teeth and following a predetermined sequence of archwires. It is interesting to note that orthodontic procedures involving incisor intrusion for bite opening, correction of rotations, management of sagittal, vertical and transverse discrepancies, space closure in extraction approach and anchorage requirement represent almost 80% of treatment procedures in the authors practice. The best of the pre-adjusted edgewise brackets available today offer no advantage over the conventional bracket systems in these procedures. It should be recognized that the design of the orthodontic bracket should not dictate the final outcome of treatment, rather it should facilitate its achievement. The treatment should be dictated by the individual patient's problem and diagnosis.[19]

Lack of compliance in the present orthodontic patient population has been a major concern for the orthodontists. Considering this diminished compliance trend, it would be appropriate to design treatments and use appliances that minimize the need for compliance.

The clinician needs to design his treatment mechanics to achieve end-of-treatment goals which should be dynamic, not based on statistical norms. The diagnosis and treatment goals defined at the beginning of treatment should guide the clinician in selection and use of appropriate mechanotherapy. It is best to instill the concept of goal-oriented orthodontic therapy, and not to settle for or be limited in the final result by whatever brackets, tubes, wires and other auxiliaries can produce. While designing a mechanotherapy, it is critical to consider 'physiologic rebound' after the removal of appliances. It is not the orthodontist's goal to maintain the final occlusion for the rest of the patient's life. A realistic goal is to accept small post-treatment changes that still result in a healthy overall stomatognathic function.

Precision bracket positioning

Precise bracket placement is critical determinant of efficient, predictable tooth movement and high-quality case

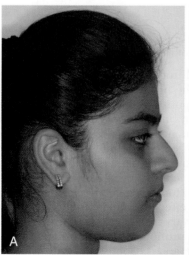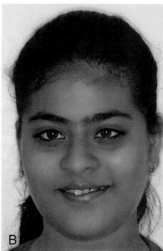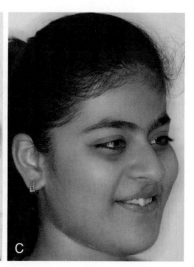

Figure 16.12 Pretreatment facial features.

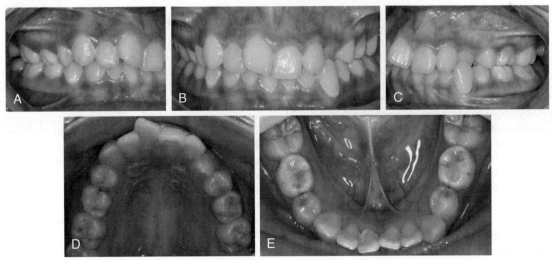

Figure 16.13 Pretreatment occlusion. (Image courtesy: Karad A, Chhajed S. Evaluation of treatment changes associated with maxillary molar distalization with the distal jet appliance. APOS Trends Orthod 2014;4:9–15).

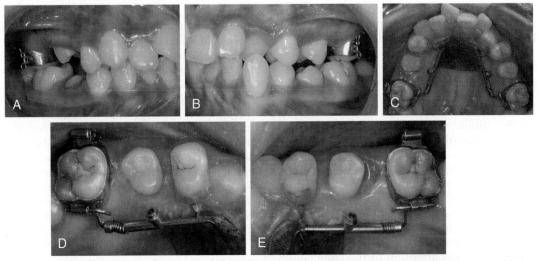

Figure 16.14 Maxillary molar distalization with the distal jet appliance. The maxillary molars have been driven distally in a pre-determined direction with good three-dimensional control over molar position. (Image courtesy: Karad A, Chhajed S. Evaluation of treatment changes associated with maxillary molar distalization with the distal jet appliance. APOS Trends Orthod 2014;4:9–15).

finish. When brackets are not placed at the correct location, the prescription values built into the bracket will not be properly expressed and the final tooth positions will be compromised. The accuracy of bracket placement, the compensations for occlusal interferences, and the adaptability of the bracket bases all affect final tooth positions.

Principles of bracket positioning

1. Placing a bracket in the correct position during the first bonding appointment will help save time during the subsequent phases of treatment. When brackets are placed accurately, fewer wire bends and repositions are required.
2. Properly positioned bracket means well-adapted bracket base to the tooth surface, and therefore, fewer bond failures.

3. Accurate bracket placement promotes efficient, predictable tooth movement and high-quality case finish.

Individual tooth morphology will clearly have an impact on the first-order movement. Our ability to vary mesiodistal position of molar tubes is quite limited. This will have an impact on the first order movements, thereby influencing the position of contact points with the adjacent teeth. It should be recognized that it is the effective torque that matters to the clinician. The degree of convexity on the facial surface of the tooth, tooth morphology/tooth type will influence the effective torque. The effect of changes in the vertical position of a bracket will vary from tooth to tooth. The effects appear to be more pronounced on the maxillary canines and mandibular molars. Some detailing of archwire is still required for most patients but precise bracket placement

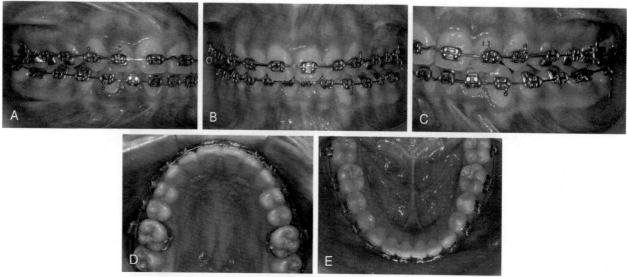

Figure 16.15   Post-distalization fixed appliance therapy to effectively utilize the 'space gained' after molar distalization and to resolve pretreatment dental discrepancy.

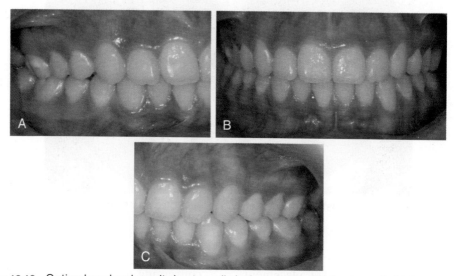

Figure 16.16   Optimal occlusal result due to well-designed, properly implemented treatment plan.

will minimize this. The treatment should be planned and the mechanics should be designed to incorporate maximum number of variables, and the necessary adjustments should be made to compensate for certain factors, like abnormal tooth morphology, occlusal wear, etc. While proper placement of various orthodontic attachments does not guarantee the establishment of normal interarch relationships, improper positioning of brackets can certainly compound their achievement. The correction of tooth positions with faulty bracket placement tends to be extrusive in nature. This is because, orthodontic extrusion of teeth seems to occur significantly more easily than any other direction, therefore, lowest bracketed tooth will tend to move up to the level of highest adjacent bracketed tooth.

• In the presence of abnormal tooth/crown morphology, either congenital or as a result of wear or trauma,

the functional parts of the crown should be used as primary references. Marginal ridges and/or interproximal contact points are primary references while the incisal edges or maxillary buccal cusps as secondary references.

• It is a good practice not to position brackets to compensate for dental deep or open bites, as it requires compensating wire bends to avoid teeth irregularities.

• When direct bonding brackets, it is important to firmly press the bracket on to the tooth to minimize bracket drift, maximize bond strength, minimize resin excess, maintain bracket in-out relations and minimize rotation errors. Since visualizing the bracket angulation is difficult, it is useful to view from the incisal/occlusal aspects using a mouth mirror. It is also useful to have the patient's diagnostic study models at hand to further assist in visualizing all three

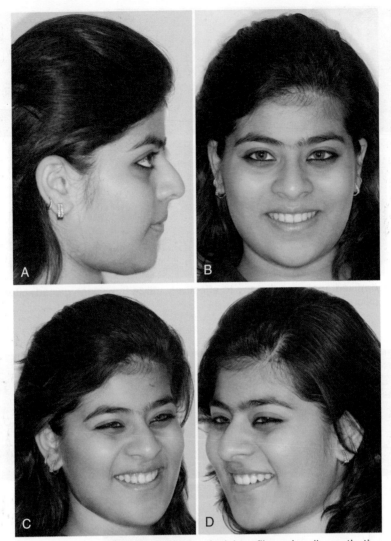

Figure 16.17   Post-treatment pleasing facial profile and smile aesthetics.

dimensions to facilitate precise bracket placement. Irrespective of the prescription used, the bracket positioning criteria are fairly generic and should be applicable to all appliance prescriptions.

Common errors in bracket placement

1. *Maxillary central incisors:* When placing brackets on maxillary central incisors, the most common errors are observed in bracket angulation. Increased mesioincisal angulation of the brackets can create root proximity, flared crowns, and an open incisal embrasure with mesial contact point being positioned too far to the gingival. However, excessive distoincisal angulation of the brackets can create too far incisally placed mesial contact point, the central incisors occupy more space in the arch (false tooth-size discrepancy), and increased overjet.

2. *Maxillary lateral incisors:* Improper bracket angulation and vertical position are the most prevalent errors in maxillary lateral incisor bracket positioning. Due to the difficulty in visualizing the long axis of lateral incisors and their variable morphology, it is common to see cases with lateral incisor root converging with the central incisors during the finishing stage. The maxillary lateral incisor brackets are often placed too far incisal resulting in lateral incisors that are positioned high above the occlusal plane. This leads to gingivally positioned contact points and compromised aesthetics.

3. *Maxillary cuspids:* When positioning brackets on maxillary canines, the most common errors appear to be related to mesiodistal positioning and bracket angulation. With the labial surface of the canine exhibiting the mid-developmental ridge significantly to the mesial, the brackets are commonly placed too far distally. This leads to rotational errors and abnormal interproximal contacts.

4. *Maxillary first and second bicuspids:* It is commonly observed that second bicuspid brackets are positioned too far occlusal. This is because second bicuspids are often the last teeth to erupt in adolescent patients, and attempting to bond brackets on partially erupted second bicuspids leads to this positioning error. This results in a marginal ridge height discrepancy between the bicuspid and first molars.

5. *Maxillary first molars:* When these teeth are banded and not bonded, molar tube positioning problems are usually reflected in height, angulation and rotation, and are often the result of faulty band placement. Band size and its adaptation to the tooth greatly influence the height of the buccal tube. Molar bands that are too small in size will prevent proper seating and subsequently place the buccal tube too far occlusal. On the other hand, when molar bands are too large, it will position the tubes too far gingival. Another commonly observed error in tube positioning results from the tendency for the first molar bands to seat towards the distal. This will either create a mesial rotation or prevent the correction of mesially rotated first molars, due to reduction in the distal offset.

6. *Maxillary second molars:* The main problem in proper positioning of maxillary second molar tubes is due to the difficulty in gaining access to bond these distal teeth. This contributes to vertical placement errors often leading to the extrusion of second molars.

7. *Mandibular incisors:* In deep bite cases, incisor brackets are often bonded gingivally to avoid interference with the opposing teeth. This creates minor vertical placement errors, especially height discrepancy between the cuspids and incisors, which become apparent after initial alignment and levelling. Inability of the clinician to position incisor brackets properly mesiodistally in a crowded dentition leads to minor imperfection in incisor positions. A similar situation is created when bracket base is not completely seated on the labial surface or when brackets are not firmly pressed on to the tooth while bonding.

8. *Mandibular cuspids:* Like maxillary cuspids, with the mid-developmental ridge of the mandibular cuspids often slightly mesial, brackets are placed too far distally. This creates a rotational error and improper proximal contacts.

9. *Mandibular first and second bicuspids:* Bonding brackets early to the partially erupted mandibular second bicuspids leads to a gross vertical placement error. The resultant occlusally positioned brackets create a marginal ridge height discrepancy between the bicuspids and first molars and a compromised occlusion.

10. *Mandibular first molars:* When mandibular first molars are banded, the size of the bands and their adaptation will greatly influence the vertical buccal tube placement. Too large molar bands are usually placed more gingivally, causing gingival placement of the buccal tubes. This leads to extrusion, increased torque and lingual crown tipping. Sometimes molar bands are also placed more gingivally on the mesial than the distal aspects. This leads to distal crown tipping of the first molar with resultant marginal ridge discrepancy with the bicuspid and occlusal dysfunction.

11. *Mandibular second molars:* One of the problems in bonding mandibular second molar tubes is to position them more gingivally in an attempt to avoid occlusal interferences and bond failure. This causes extrusion of the second molar, height discrepancy with the first molar, bite opening, and occlusal prematurity.

Efficient tooth movement

Understand the boundaries

Efficient and effective mechanics is essential to achieve/produce good treatment results, however, it is equally important to recognize the boundaries to the maxillary and mandibular dentition (Fig. 16.18). The resolution of existing dental abnormalities must take place within the framework of critical anatomic limits.

The maxilla and the mandible differ from each other in terms of their bone structure. The thin cortices and trabecular bone of the maxilla offers less resistance to resorption as against the thick cortices and more coarse trabecular pattern of the mandible. The point 'A' is the anterior border for the maxillary incisor roots, and the maxillary tuberosity is the posterior boundary of the maxilla. The tuberosity region increases in length on an average 1.5 mm per year on each side up to age 16 years for girls and 18 years for boys. The maxilla is a laminated structure with cortical bone supporting four cavities: the oral, nasal, sinus and orbital cavities. For the purpose of support, all of these cavities are lined with cortical bone. It should be recognized by the clinician that during orthodontic treatment, this cortical bone support, along with the cortical bone on the facial aspect and the palatal aspect of the alveolar process influences the maxillary teeth movement. Therefore, to plan a tooth movement in the maxillary arch, it is critical to determine the location of the roots in relation to the cortical bone supporting the cavities and the alveolar process.

The point 'B' forms the anterior boundary for the mandibular incisor roots, and the anterior borders of the ascending ramus is the posterior boundary of the lower arch. The growth in the retromolar region increases the arch length by 1.5 mm per year on each side up to age 16 years in girls and 18 years in boys. It is important to note that the point 'B' follows the lingual movement of incisor roots, however, once it is moved posteriorly, it cannot be moved anteriorly again. Wherever possible, the clinician should avoid cortical bone support and direct the roots through the less dense and more vascular trabecular bone. The force levels should be kept ultra-light to encourage a good blood supply necessary for the physiological response and efficient tooth movement. However, in a situation where supporting cortical bone cannot be avoided, it must be remodelled by using even lighter forces. In an adult orthodontic patient, even the cribriform plate of the socket wall is more dense like the cortical bone, therefore, it demands a lighter force initially to allow an adequate blood supply for efficient tooth movement.

A vertical limit does exist. Extrusion of posterior teeth is disastrous to facial balance and harmony in sagittal plane, except in low-angle deep bite cases.

Therefore, orthodontists must recognize these anatomic limitations and design treatment to conform to the dimensions of the maxilla and mandible in sagittal, vertical and transverse planes.

Orthodontic tooth movement

When a moderate, continuous load ranging from 20 to 50 g is applied through orthodontic appliances, a typical

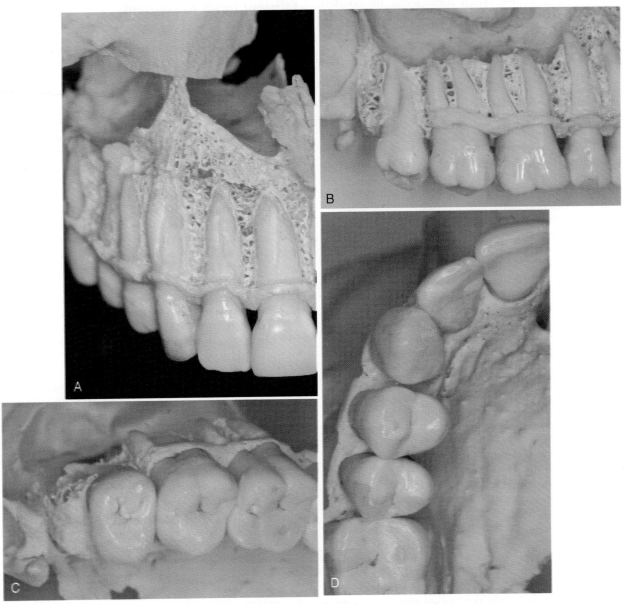

Figure 16.18   Anatomic limits [boundaries] of dentition.

tooth movement response will consist of essentially three elements: initial strain, lag phase, and progressive tooth movement. The first phase of tooth movement, initial strain, due to periodontal ligament displacement (strain), bone strain and tooth extrusion, will range from 0.4 to 0.9 mm and occurs in about one week.[20,21] The initial deformation response occurs within seconds.[22,23] However, actual compression of the periodontal ligament takes place after 1 to 3 hours.[24]

Due to areas of periodontal ligament necrosis (hyalinization), the initial phase of tooth displacement stops in about one week. This lag phase usually lasts 2 to 3 weeks; however, it may be as long as 10 weeks.[20] This is followed by the restoration of vitality of the necrotic areas by undermining resorption, leading to progressive tooth movement phase. The patient's age, the extent of PDL necrotic areas and the density of alveolar bone determine the duration of lag phase.

With coordinated series of events of bone resorption and bone formation, the alveolus drifts in the direction of tooth movement. Efficient mechanics and regular reactivations of orthodontic appliances at about 4-week intervals are essential for optimal rates of tooth movement.[25]

Tooth movement seems to be directly related to light, continuous forces in order to sustain a coordinated bone resorptive response. It should also be recognized that maximal cell proliferation in the periodontal ligament occurs during the resting hours—day time for rats, night time for human beings.[26] In osteoblast differentiation, differentiation to preosteoblasts occurs during the late resting and early arousal periods.[27]

Orthodontic appliance system

In order to bring about a desired tooth movement, light, continuous forces need to be applied in a predetermined direction to teeth. These forces are produced by the orthodontic appliance consisting of brackets, archwires, springs, etc. which are clinically managed and periodically activated by the clinician. Many different appliances and techniques are being used in orthodontics to resolve dentofacial problems. However, there has been no universal agreement regarding the ideal appliance and the specific technique to produce optimal results. This is because the teeth and their supporting structures do not recognize the bracket design, type of archwire alloy, wire shape, etc. and their response with a complex biologic reaction that ultimately results in tooth movement is mainly based on the stresses and strain in the periodontium.

Anchorage

Anchorage is an integral part of appliance system. Resolution of each orthodontic problem requires that the amount of available anchorage is first carefully assessed to treat the case successfully. Fundamentally, anchorage is considered in terms of controlling and stabilizing the anchor units against various movements of teeth occurring during the various stages of orthodontic treatment to effectively resolve underlying discrepancy. Though anchorage is a commonly used parameter in every case, it is arbitrarily defined.

The anchorage value of a specific tooth is determined by the volume of surrounding bone that must undergo resorption for a tooth to move a given distance.

In assessing the anchorage of a tooth, the clinician should consider the density of surrounding alveolar bone, surface area of the roots being exposed to movement and the type of tooth movement. However, mandibular molars offer more resistance to movement than maxillary molars due to thick cortices and more coarse trabeculae. Also, the leading root of mandibular molars being translated mesially forms bone that is far more dense than the bone formed by the translating maxillary molars mesially.[28]

In clinical practice, control of the molar position is an obvious necessity, and an inadvertent anchorage loss prevents the complete correction of the existing discrepancy and also prolongs the treatment duration. Since there are variations in the morphological characteristics of an individual and severity of a problem, anchorage requirements of an individual treatment plan varies from absolutely no mesial movement of the posterior teeth to a desired amount of protraction of the posterior teeth in extraction cases.

Extrusion and tipping are easy movements, however, intrusion and bodily movements are relatively difficult. The difficulty of orthodontic case is directly related to how much change the clinician intends to achieve. In other words, it is the difference between the pretreatment problem and the treatment goal.

The degree of severity of the pretreatment problem is quantified as a function of several contributing variables in sagittal, vertical and transverse planes. Based on the severity of malocclusion and the type of tooth movements required, the clinician should critically assess the anchorage requirements as against the anchorage available to reach a desired goal.

Role of friction

Sliding tooth movement is an integral part of orthodontic practice and requires complete understanding of the complexities involved. When a tooth slides along the archwire, the clinician must recognize the magnitude of friction occurring at the bracket slot–archwire interface. Therefore, when the force is applied to a tooth, a part of it is dissipated as friction and the residual is then transferred to supporting structures of the tooth to mediate tooth movement. Friction occurs due to the relative roughness of two surfaces in contact. In a clinical situation, there are so many variables that can directly or indirectly contribute to the frictional force levels generated at the bracket slot–archwire interface.

1. **Orthodontic archwires:**
   Wire alloy: Stainless steel archwires have the smoothest surface, followed by Co-Cr, Beta-Ti, and NiTi wires in order of increasing surface roughness.[29] However, there is no correlation between surface roughness and coefficient of friction.[30] Despite the smoothest surface demonstrated by stainless wires, it has higher friction than cobalt chromium wires.

2. **Wire size:** An increase in archwire size is associated with increased friction at the bracket slot–archwire interface.[31,32] Therefore, the clinician can control the amount of friction by selecting various archwire shapes and sizes. An adequate play between the bracket slot and the archwire should be provided to prevent binding to reduce the friction. Generally, the rectangular wires produce significantly higher friction than round wires.

3. **Brackets:** New bracket designs, materials and manufacturing techniques have been introduced in the quest for minimal archwire–bracket slot friction and ultimate strength. For most archwire sizes, the sintered stainless steel brackets produce significantly lower friction than cast stainless steel brackets due to smoother surface texture of the sintered stainless steel material. For most archwire sizes and alloy combinations used in both 0.018″ and 0.022″ bracket slot sizes, ceramic brackets demonstrate higher frictional forces than with stainless steel brackets.[33]

Bracket width. Orthodontic literature on the effect of bracket width on friction has been controversial, with some demonstrating no effect on frictional resistance due to altered bracket width,[34] while others demonstrating increased levels of friction with increased bracket width.[31] Also, bracket width is closely associated with interbracket distance which determines the archwire stiffness having an indirect effect on friction at bracket slot–archwire interface.

4. **Second-order archwire deflection:** Achieving complete levelling of bracket slots is a critical factor in reducing friction as the bracket slides along the archwire. Second-order archwire deflections even of a smaller magnitude between brackets can significantly contribute to increased frictional resistance. It has been found that increased angulation between bracket and archwire leads to greater friction.[34,31]

5. **Ligation method:** The ideal clinical situation is created when no friction exists between bracket and archwire. Practically, this does not exist since the ligatures used to hold archwire in the bracket slots exert some force which significantly influences the determination of frictional resistance developed in the appliance. The forces exerted by ligatures have been estimated to be between 50 and 300 gm.[31,35,36]

Self-ligating brackets

To bring about efficient tooth movement and to have good three-dimensional tooth control during the course of treatment, it is essential to establish desired archwire–bracket slot interface. This is possible when archwire is properly engaged and maintained in the bracket slot with either elastomeric ties, steel wire ligatures or a clip that opens and closes in self-ligating brackets. Predictable and secure ligation is the key. However, each method of ligation will have advantages and disadvantages, and it is critical to use the one that is efficient, as 'efficiency'

has become a very important and integral part of any orthodontic practice. Efficiency is influenced essentially by three factors: decreased chairside time, fewer patient appointments and efficient mechanics.

In an ideal scenario, the method of ligation should provide full archwire engagement, have less friction between the brackets and the archwire, promote good oral hygiene and faster archwire change as seen in self-ligating brackets (Figs 16.19–16.23).

It should be recognized that, biologic principles do not change when the specific orthodontic appliance and mechanics are used. The clinician's knowledge, experience and experties are the main elements to effective and efficient treatment with any self-ligation system. A thorough knowledge of specific features of a self-ligating appliance, archwire properties and resultant tissue response is essential to optimize tooth movement. Considering accelerated tooth movement and shorter overall treatment times with the self-ligating appliance, the long-term stability needs to be critically assessed.

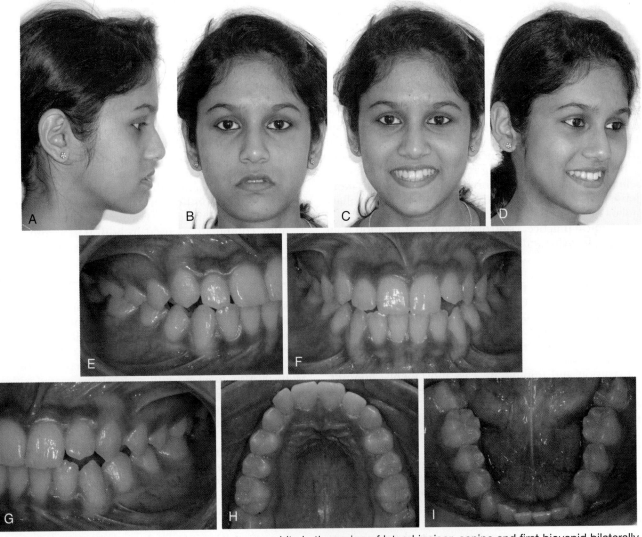

Figure 16.19 Pretreatment records demonstrate open-bite in the region of lateral incisor, canine and first bicuspid bilaterally.
Continued

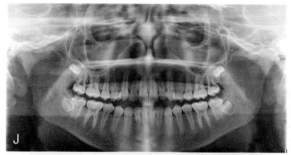

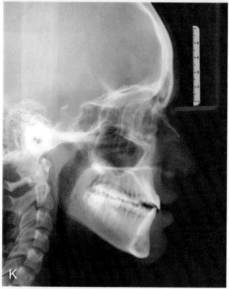

Figure 16.19, cont'd Pretreatment records demonstrate open-bite in the region of lateral incisor, canine and first bicuspid bilaterally.

Quality of ligation

Once the archwire is placed in the bracket slot, the system should possess a secure and robust ligation method. When elastomeric ties are stretched around the bracket wings, subsequent degradation of elastic properties does lead to a significant loss of full archwire engagement. The force decay in elastomerics has been well documented in orthodontic literature.[37] Steel ligatures are good in this respect, but the resultant secure ligation is usually at the cost of an increase in friction. However, they produce substantially lower friction than elastomeric ties.[38] The self-ligating bracket systems eliminate the problems and risks associated with stainless steel or elastomeric ties.

Full archwire engagement

With the experience and clinical observations, it is evident that a full and definitive archwire engagement in the bracket slot does impact the speed of the alignment and levelling. It is, therefore, important to ensure and maintain full archwire engagement in the bracket slot. The archwire ligation with steel ligatures is rigid, and once ligated securely, does not cause its loss subsequently unless the ligature wire breaks. Quite often, the elastomerics do not exert sufficient force to fully engage even a resilient archwire; and due to force decay, there is subsequently loss of full engagement.

Friction

It has been recognized that the rate of tooth movement increases with increase in force levels up to a certain point, after which increased force levels do not result in an appreciable increase in tooth movement.[39] The routine

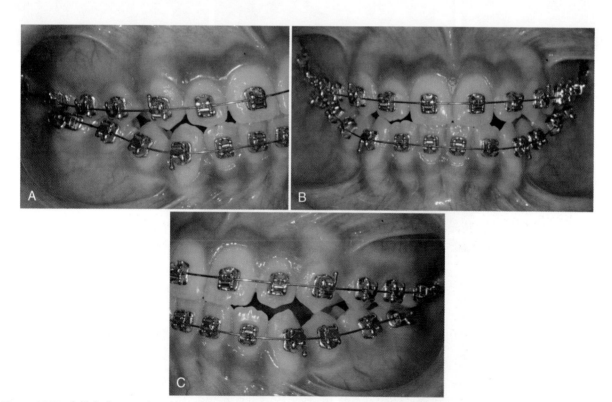

Figure 16.20 Initial alignment and levelling in progress using self-ligating appliance (0.018″ slot—American Orthodontics Empower® self-ligating brackets).

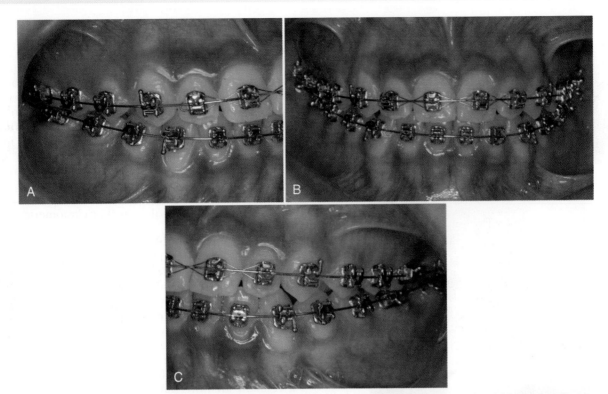

Figure 16.21   Transitional phase of treatment. An improvement in the settling of open bite, and better levelling.

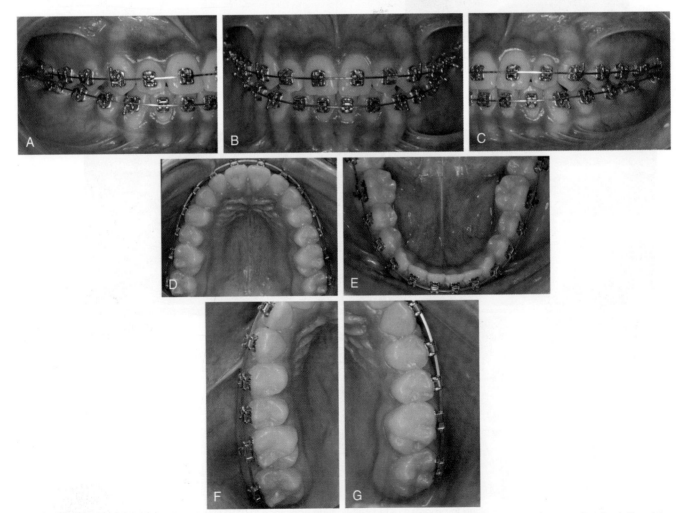

Figure 16.22   Finishing stage of treatment demonstrating optimal individual tooth positioning, proper interocclusal relationships and contact points.

Continued

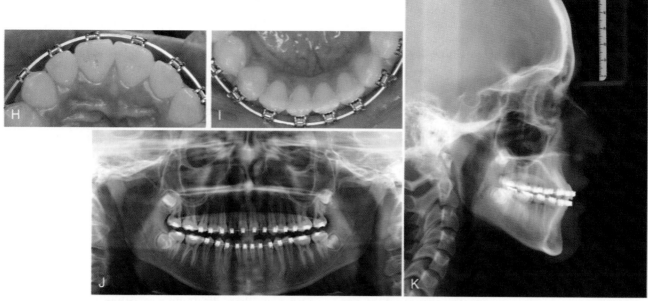

Figure 16.22, cont'd   Finishing stage of treatment demonstrating optimal individual tooth positioning, proper interocclusal relationships and contact points.

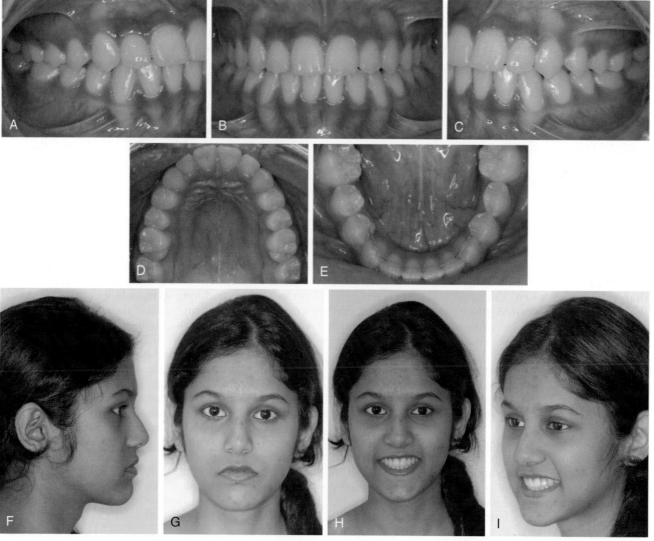

Figure 16.23   Post-treatment records exhibiting achievement of individualized treatment goals.

orthodontic treatment mechanics involves relative movement between the archwire and bracket, and friction occurs at the bracket slot–wire interface. Therefore, to achieve optimal biological tissue response, it is critical that orthodontic appliances generate force levels that adequately overcome friction and also lie within the optimal force range required for efficient tooth movement. Friction depends on what extent the archwire–bracket–ligature are pressed together. It is interesting to note that both 'low friction' and 'close contact' are requirements for controlling tooth position. Initial tooth alignment and sliding of teeth along an archwire require as little contact between archwire and bracket slot as possible. However, close contact is required to prevent the wire from disengaging from the slot, to control tipping, rotation and torquing of the tooth. Stainless steel ligature wires produce lower levels of friction than elastomeric ligatures. The use of an elastomeric module for archwire ligation generates a force of approximately 50 gm of friction per bracket.[40]

A combination of low friction and full archwire engagement associated with self-ligating brackets is the most advantageous feature in the alignment of very irregular teeth and the resolution of severe rotations.[41]

Speed of ligation

Archwire ligation with steel wire ligatures is secure and robust, however, it is a time-consuming procedure which is the main reason for the decline in their use. It takes less time to ligate and release an archwire using self-ligating brackets than with conventional brackets and elastomeric ligatures.[42]

Oral hygiene

Elastomeric ties accumulate more plaque than steel wire ligatures.[43] The use of steel ligatures is associated with less bleeding on probing of the gingival crevice when compared with elastomeric ties.[44]

Identify areas of concern for stability

Stability of tooth positions following orthodontic treatment is an essential component of the contemporary orthodontic treatment plan (Figs 16.24–16.34; Tables 16.1–16.3). The goal of retention plan should not be to hold the tooth positions still maintained by rigid rectangular finishing wires producing orthodontic occlusion that is released when the appliances are removed. Rather, once the desired tooth positions have been achieved, teeth should be held with more resilient wires allowing the process that sustains and guides the settling under the influence of occlusal and muscular forces from orthodontic occlusion into final functioning occlusion. The retention plan must consider the long-term influences involving growth changes, continuous tooth eruption, and function, specific to individual facial type.

An accurate diagnosis and proper treatment plan is the first step towards long-term stability. With regards to specific malocclusions, in children treated early with the orthodontic or functional appliances, the author uses modified activator to maintain the correction. However, no comparative studies have proved the advantages of this type of retention. It has been recognized that the supracrestal gingival fibres take the longest amount of time to reorganize, prolonged retention of rotated teeth may be useful in minimizing relapse. As most rotational relapse occurs within 4–6 years of appliance removal, an adjunctive circumferential supracrestal fiberotomy may be effective in reducing the relapse during this period.[45] Increase in mandibular incisor irregularity occurs throughout life in a large proportion of both treated and untreated subjects. Most changes usually take place by the middle of the third decade.[46] Therefore, prolonged retention of the mandibular anterior segment until the end of the facial growth may reduce the post-treatment relapse. Maintaining the correction of a very deep overbite is challenging for the clinician. The author establishes proper interincisal angle during the finishing stage and uses the maxillary anterior bite plate until the completion of facial growth, especially in patients with anterior mandibular growth rotation.

Pretreatment generalized interproximal spacing and a median diastema are other challenging situations that are difficult to maintain after their correction, and will require long-term retention. Following the correction of anterior and posterior crossbites, retention is usually not required, provided that the clinician establishes adequate incisor overbite and maximum intercuspation.

In patients with root resorption or crestal bone loss, there is an increased risk of deterioration of mandibular incisor alignment post-retention.[47]

The stability of anterior open bite correction is highly unpredictable. The author uses retainers with posterior bite blocks to control vertical position of posterior teeth for treated anterior open bite cases, however, there are no controlled studies for their usefulness.

It is important to maintain the lower arch dimensions whenever possible. It is best to use the patient's pretreatment archform as a guide for the post-treatment arch shape. Patients should be treated to their individualized treatment goal as they vary in morphological pattern.[48]

High-quality finishing

Every clinician should aim for the highest levels of dentofacial aesthetics, stomatognathic function, healthy periodontium and long-term stability of orthodontically treated case. Idealizing a case tests all the skills of the orthodontist. Most of the errors due to improper bracket positioning, inaccurate diagnosis established at the beginning of treatment and improper adjustments made during the transitional phase of treatment get magnified during the finishing stage. In the author's opinion, "finishing is much more than merely positioning an ideal bracket in the perfect position and filling the slot. If it were just to bond orthodontic attachments and follow a predetermined sequence of archwires, orthodontics would not be a speciality".

Orthodontic finishing should begin with diagnosis and treatment planning. A carefully assessed diagnosis, and a well designed, properly implemented treatment plan are the best orthodontist's tools for proper finishing.

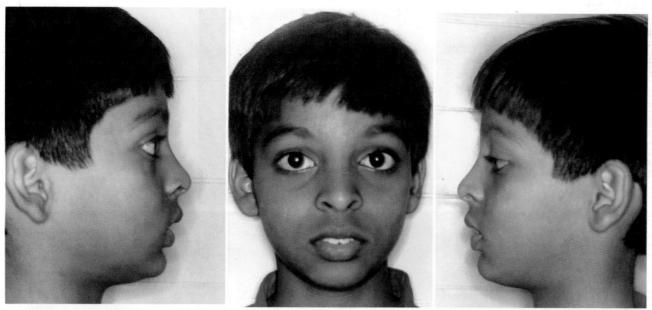

Figure 16.24 Pretreatment extraoral photographs of 11 years 8 months old patient showing convex profile, incompetent lips and deep mentolabial sulcus.

The key here is to avoid cutting short the diagnosis and spontaneous treatment planning. Orthodontic diagnosis is a three-dimensional exercise as dentofacial problems exist in sagittal, vertical and transverse planes. It is of paramount importance for the clinician to be able to clearly define treatment goals before any tooth movement begins. Since orthodontic treatment influences facial soft tissues, treatment plan based solely on the analysis of hard tissues may not produce desired facial aesthetic changes.

The application of specific and individualized orthodontic treatment goals, coupled with the use of a precision appliance system, makes orthodontic finishing faster, easier and more predictable for both the patient and the orthodontist.

With a well-organized and planned approach, most cases finish a little easier, while others require a great deal of efforts and time. It is easier to seat and detail the occlusion when patient's individual muscular pattern is utilized. Patients with strong muscular patterns allow more flexibility in the finishing process and the post-treatment occlusion seems to improve thereafter. However, in vertical growth patterns, it is difficult to hold the occlusion over a period of time and may just deviate from the final result over a period of time.

Orthodontists are often faced with unstable occlusion (Figs 16.35–16.38), with deviations and discrepancies that cause functional and aesthetic problems. The patient's potential problems and limitations must be considered in formulating realistic treatment goals. In such patients, it is important to focus on optimal temporomandibular joint form and function, which is the seated condylar position, defined as superior, anterior and mid-sagittal (centred transversely) position. Diagnostic study models mounted in the seated condylar position provide more accurate and adequate information than hand-held models trimmed in the habitual occlusal position, and allow measurement of the mandibular functional shift from the seated to the unseated (teeth directed) condylar position in all three planes of space. With the use of a simple semiadjustable articulator and facebow, a reasonably accurate mounting of the patient's diagnostic models in the centric relation position can be obtained. The facebow orients the maxillary model to the articulator's condylar hinge axis almost in the same three-dimensional relationship as the patient's maxillary teeth are to his condylar hinge axis (Fig. 16.39). The occlusal plane is also properly related to the upper member of the instrument which is approximately parallel to the patient's Frankfort horizontal plane. Such an orientation of the maxillary and mandibular models enables the clinician to view them in the same perspective as when looking into the patient's mouth. Once the patient's models are precisely mounted in the centric relation, the clinician should evaluate the true nature of the discrepancy between centric relation and maximum intercuspation.

To achieve these goals, it is essential to have the ability to control tooth movement in all three planes of space. Whenever possible, the second molars should be bonded to position them properly. Occlusal interferences in the second molar region can be most damaging since they are located closest to the muscle forces which move the mandible. A well-organized predebonding check-list should facilitate achievement of patient's individualized treatment goals (Fig. 16.40).

Retention is the critical aspect of orthodontic treatment and its importance as the final step in treatment should not be underestimated. Removing orthodontic attachments after the successful completion of active treatment and placing retainers does not necessarily

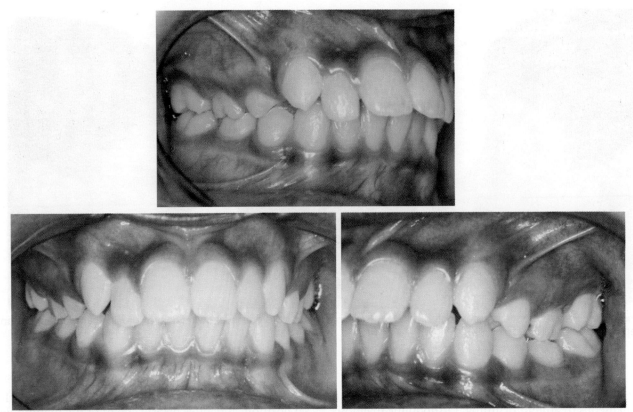

Figure 16.25 Pretreatment intraoral photographs showing increased overjet and overbite, labially placed maxillary canines, class II canine and molar relationships.

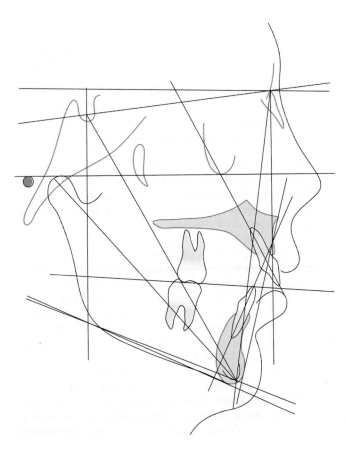

Figure 16.26 Pretreatment lateral cephalometric tracing. (Image courtesy: APOS Trends in Orthodontics[48]).

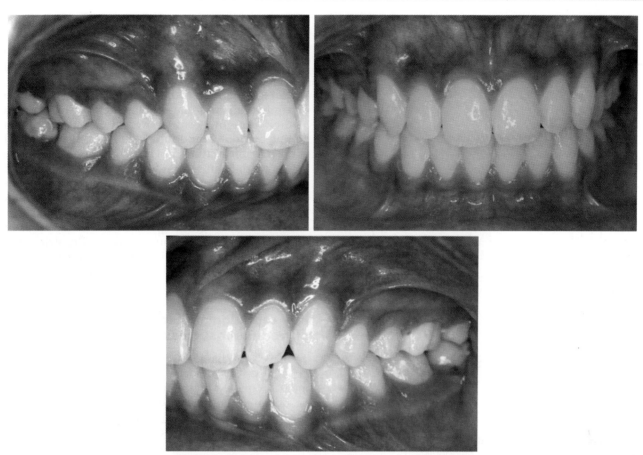

Figure 16.27   Post-treatment intraoral photographs showing normal occlusal relationships.

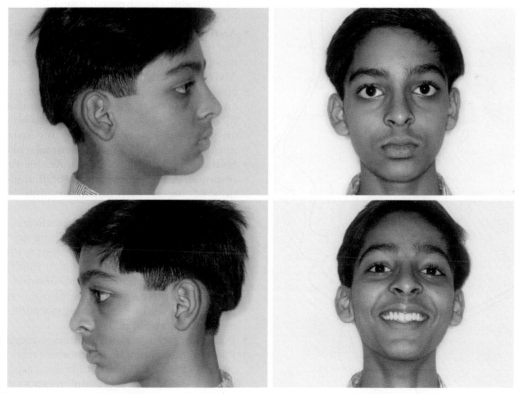

Figure 16.28   Post-treatment extraoral photographs demonstrating improvement in facial profile, lip competence and pleasing aesthetics.

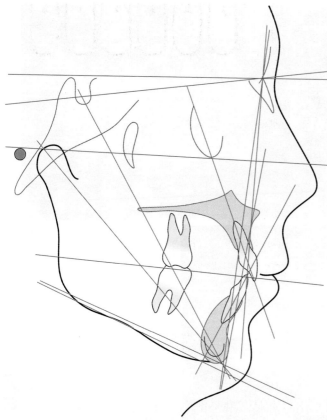

Figure 16.29 Post-treatment lateral cephalometric tracing. (Image courtesy: APOS Trends in Orthodontics[48]).

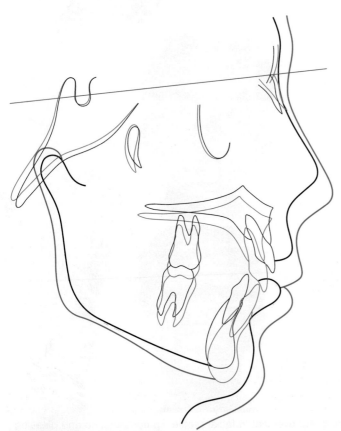

Figure 16.30 Pre-and post-treatment lateral cephalometric superimpositions. (Image courtesy: APOS Trends in Orthodontics[48]).

mean that the teeth are well settled and maintained during the retention phase. The meticulous care as implemented while establishing a diagnosis and during the course of entire treatment should continue through the retention phase.

Quite often, even if the dental arches have not been expanded and the mandibular incisors are corrected to their upright position over the basal bone, maintaining a good orthodontic result can be the most difficult part of treatment. This is because of forces acting on teeth from several sources may disrupt the final tooth positions leading to relapse. Unfavourable muscle forces as a result of tongue thrust habit or abnormal tongue posture can eventually overcome the stability of even highest quality occlusal relationships despite careful retention protocol. Resolving these problems either prior to or concurrently with the orthodontic treatment will greatly contribute to the stability of the result.

Key cephalometric Indicators of treatment success

To make sure that the treatment proceeds smoothly and efficiently, it is important to closely monitor the treatment progress. Mid-treatment lateral cephalogram may be obtained and analyzed to see the key indicators of treatment success (Fig. 16.41).

- **Mandibular plane angle:** In high-angle patients, successful treatment is associated with a favourable counter-clockwise rotation of the mandible by a reduction of mandibular plane angle. However, in low-angle patients, good treatment is determined by a favourable clockwise rotation of the mandible by an increase in mandibular plane angle.
- **ANB angle:** The ANB angle is an indicator of a skeletal discrepancy correction. A successful orthodontic treatment is associated with an improvement in existing ANB discrepancy.
- **Nasolabial angle:** In most situations, the nasolabial angle indicates the dentoalveolar and soft-tissue profile response. A successful treatment is associated with an improvement in the soft-tissue balance and harmony and reduction in the dentoalveolar protrusion.
- **SNB angle:** The SNB angle indicates the mandibular response. An improvement in SNB angle is an indication of better mandibular response, suggesting a successful treatment.
- **Occlusal plane:** Occlusal plane indicates the control of treatment. As extrusion and tipping are relatively easy movements, orthodontic treatment is often associated with the extrusion of molars and flaring of the mandibular incisors, causing the occlusal plane to tip forward. This is an indication of poor control of treatment. Successful treatment is associated with a flattening of the occlusal plane.
- **Posterior facial height to anterior facial height ratio:** Posterior facial height to anterior facial height ratio is an indicator of the mandibular response. In most clinical situations, successful treatment is associated with an increase in posterior facial height than the anterior facial height, leading to an increase in this ratio.

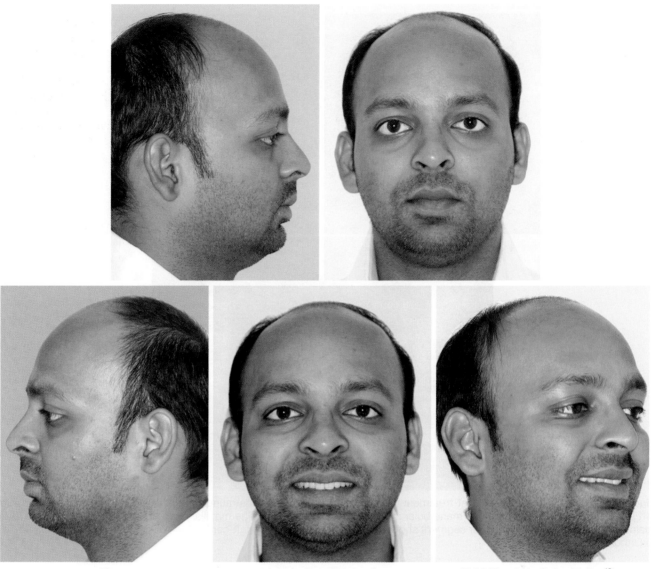

Figure 16.31 Twenty-year post-treatment extraoral photographs. (Image courtesy: APOS Trends in Orthodontics[48]).

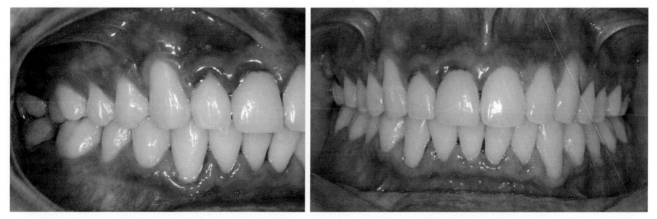

Figure 16.32 Twenty-year post-treatment intraoral photographs demonstrating right side class I interarch relationship, left side end-on relationship, and the mandibular midline shift to the left side. The maxillary and mandibular archforms are well-maintained. The mandibular anterior segment shows distolabial rotation of the left central incisor. (Image courtesy: APOS Trends in Orthodontics[48]).

Continued

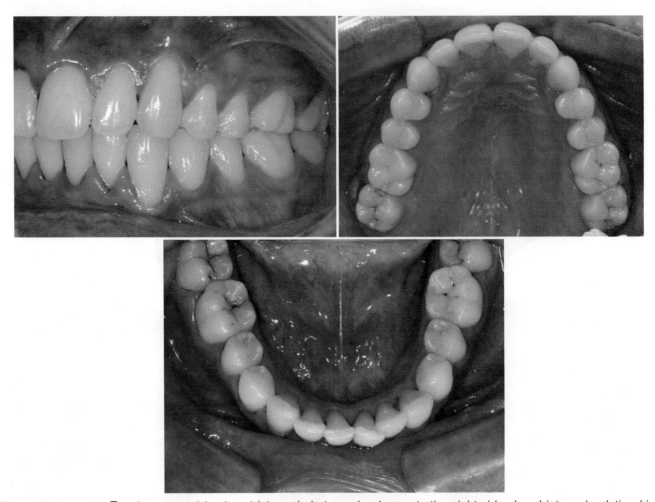

Figure 16.32, cont'd   Twenty-year post-treatment intraoral photographs demonstrating right side class I interarch relationship, left side end-on relationship, and the mandibular midline shift to the left side. The maxillary and mandibular archforms are well-maintained. The mandibular anterior segment shows distolabial rotation of the left central incisor. (Image courtesy: APOS Trends in Orthodontics[48]).

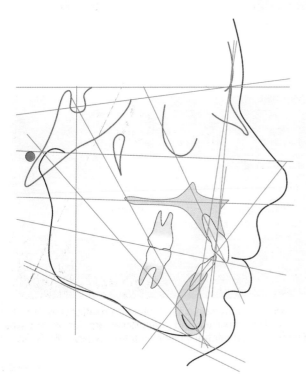

Figure 16.33   Twenty-year post-treatment lateral cephalometric tracing. (Image courtesy: APOS Trends in Orthodontics[48]).

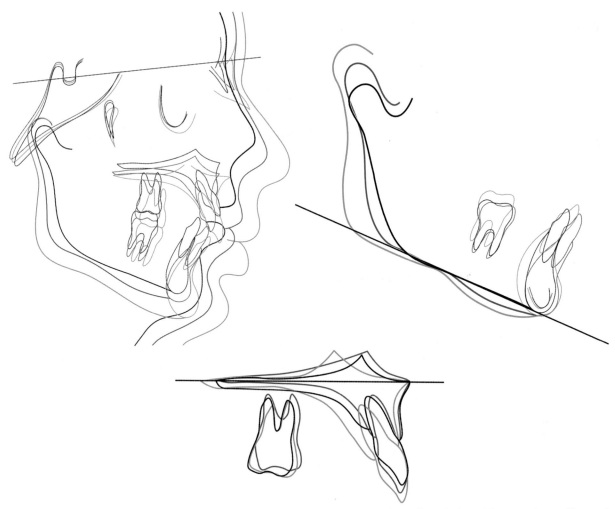

Figure 16.34 Pretreatment, post-treatment and twenty-year post-treatment lateral cephalometric superimpositions. (Image courtesy: APOS Trends in Orthodontics[48]).

Table 16.1   Cephalometric data

	Pretreatment	Post-treatment	20 years post-treatment		Pretreatment	Post-treatment	20 years post-treatment
Maxillary				**Vertical**			
SNA	84°	80°	81°	SN-GoGn	27°	30°	28°
Co-A	91 mm	94 mm	98 mm	FMA	23°	23°	25°
ANS-PNS	52 mm	54 mm	56 mm	SN-PP	6°	7°	6°
Mandibular				Occl-FMA	4°	4°	9°
SNB	76°	77°	78°	LAFH	68 mm	66 mm	71mm
Co-Gn	110 mm	117 mm	123 mm	S-Go	121 mm	125 mm	?
Go-Gn	67 mm	74 mm	82 mm	Y-axis	60°	58°	58°
Maxillo-mandibular				**Maxillary–dentoalveolar**			
ANB	8°	3°	4°	U1-SN	111°	104°	104°
Wits	10 mm	4 mm	2.5 mm (AO ahead of BO)	U1-PP	27 mm	28 mm	32 mm
Co-A / Co-Gn	0.82	0.80	0.79	U6-PP	24 mm	23 mm	26 mm

Continued

Table 16.1   Cephalometric data—cont'd

	Pretreatment	Post-treatment	20 years post-treatment		Pretreatment	Post-treatment	20 years post-treatment
Mandibular–dentoalveolar				L6-MP	30 mm	32 mm	34 mm
IMPA	92°	94°	102°	Dental			
L1-MP	39 mm	39 mm	41.5 mm	Overjet	10 mm	3 mm	4.5 mm
L1-APog	7 mm	5 mm	?	Overbite	5 mm	3 mm	3 mm

(**Source:** APOS Trends in Orthodontics[48])

Table 16.2   Model analysis data

Parameters		Pretreatment	post-treatment	20 years post-treatment
1. Molars				
Right side		class II 4.4mm	class I	class I
Left side		class II 3.83 mm	class I	End on 1.78mm
Intermolar width	Mx	46.5 mm	46.5 mm	48 mm
	Md	40 mm	39.5 mm	40.5 mm
2. Incisors				
Overjet		10.5mm	2.5mm	4mm
Overbite		7.1mm	1.31mm	3.35mm
3. Canines				
Right side		class II 5.19mm	class I	class I
Left side		class II 5.80mm	class I	End on 2.4mm
Intercanine width	Mx	32.5 mm	34 mm	35 mm
	Md	28 mm	27 mm	26 mm
4. Proclination				
Mx. anterior		7.1 mm	4.37 mm	5.12 mm
5. Crowding		-	-	1.39mm
6. Rotations		35, ml	-	31 dl
7. Midlines		2.6mm to lft	-	u- 0.79mm onpt's rt.
8. Arch symmetry		u/l asymm.	symm.	u/l asymm
9. Archform		u/l tapered /oval	u/l oval	u/l oval
10. Curve of Spee		1.03mm	omm	2.18mm
11. Arch length	Mx	33 mm	28 mm	27 mm
	Md	24 mm	24 mm	22 mm

(**Source:** APOS Trends in Orthodontics[48])

Table 16.3 Archform analysis

Parameter (in mm)	Pretreatment	Post-treatment	20 years post-treatment
Maxillary			
Intermolar width	46.5	46.5	48
Intercanine width	32.5	34	35
Arch length	33	28	27
Mandibular			
Intermolar width	40	39.5	40.5
Intercanine width	28	27	26
Arch length	24	24	22

(**Source:** APOS Trends in Orthodontics[48])

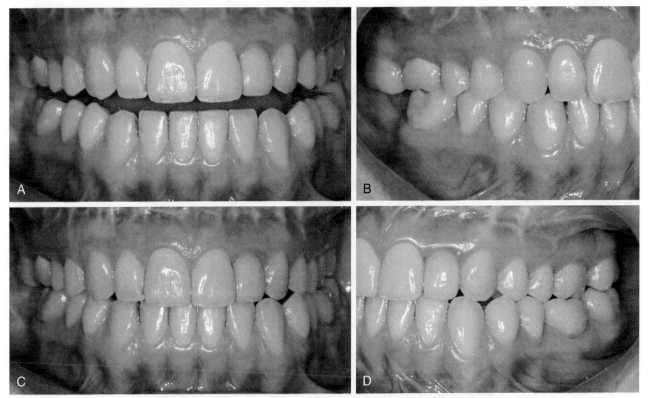

Figure 16.35 (A–D) Pretreatment photographs of unstable occlusion. **(A)** Coincidence of dental midlines in the rest position of mandible; **(C)** Dental midline shift in habitual occlusion due to mandibular shift.

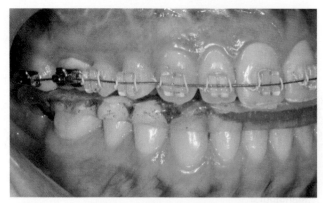

Figure 16.36 Continuation of use of interocclusal splint during the initial stage of orthodontic treatment.

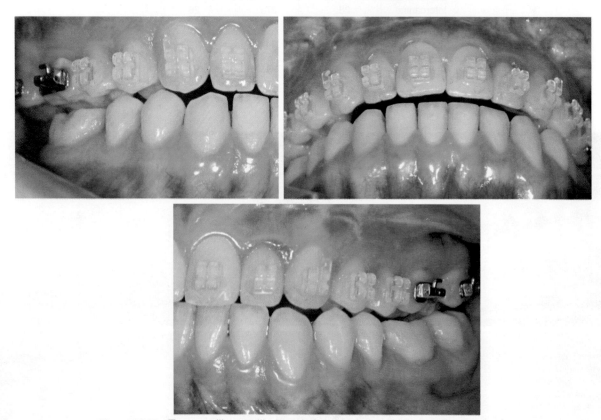

Figure 16.37 True maxillomandibular relationship (unmasking the discrepancy).

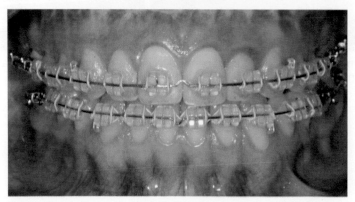

Figure 16.38 Settling of occlusion in stable mandibular position.

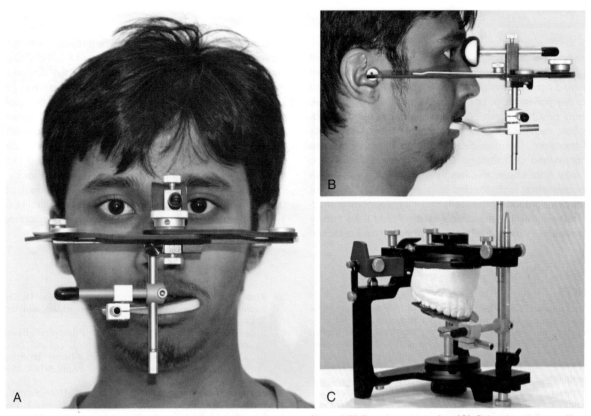

Figure 16.39 Transferring the patient's occlusion to the articulator. **(A** and **B)** Facebow transfer; **(C)** Orienting the maxillary model to the articulator's condylar hinge axis. (Panadent Corporation, USA [www.panadent.com]).

PRE-DEBONDING CHECK-LIST

Occlusion

Class I Molar position
Proper Overjet
Proper overbite
No spacing
Leveled marginal ridges
Proper proximal contacts
Co-ordinated archforms

Skeletal bases

Proper maxillary position
Proper Mandibular position
Maxillo-mandibular relation

Facial profile

Orthognathic profile
Normal naso-labial angle
Competent lips
Normal mento-labial sulcus
Proper chin position

Function

Good TMJ health
Teeth-together swallowing
Relaxed facial muscles
No abnormal habits

Periodontal health

Proper biologic width
Normal gingival health
Proper tooth position
(cancellous bone)

Long-term stability

Original Md intercanine width
Optimal interincisal relation
Elimination of etiological factor
Normal TMJ function

Figure 16.40 Pre-debonding checklist.

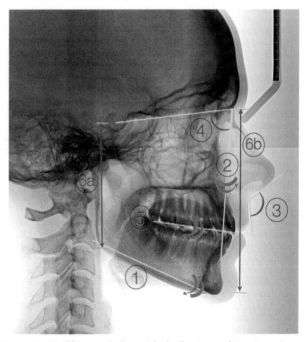

Figure 16.41 Key cephalometric indicators of treatment success. 1. Mandibular plane, 2. ANB angle, 3. Nasolabial angle, 4. SNB angle, 5. Occlusal plane, 6a. Posterior facial height, and 6b. Anterior facial height.

CONCLUSION

One of the greatest values of contemporary orthodontic treatment should be to visualize and establish specific treatment results from the very beginning. The individualized treatment plan should consider morphological and functional variations among the patient population which dictate incisor torque, archforms and final tooth positions. Good treatment results, quite often, require patient's commitment and motivation towards treatment. This should be constantly reinforced by the orthodontist and staff through effective communication. The single most goal of any treatment plan should be to achieve optimal aesthetics, function, and long-term stability with no or minimal deterioration of the teeth and their supporting structures. This requires that the clinical set-up should have quality control systems in place for better performance and outcome.

To bring about efficient and effective three-dimensional tooth movement, the clinician should recognize critical anatomic limits, and design treatment to conform to the dimensions of the maxilla and mandible. It should be recognized that the accuracy of the placement of all components of the appliance system, compensations for occlusal interferences, adaptability of the bracket and molar tube bases and proper clinical management all affect final tooth positions. A carefully assessed diagnosis, well-designed and properly implemented treatment plan, sophisticated appliance system and mechanics engineered to meet the requirements of an individual patient, coupled with good practice environment and quality control systems remain the key elements for optimizing orthodontic treatment.

REFERENCES

1. Vander Linden FPGM. The development of long and short faces, and their limitations in treatment. In: McNamara JA, ed. The enigma of the vertical dimension. Vol.36. Craniofacial growth series. Ann Arbor: Center for human growth and development. University of Michigan. 1999; 61–73.
2. Karad A. Craniofacial growth, diagnosis and treatment planning. In: Ashok Karad, ed. Clinical Orthodontics: current concepts, goals and mechanics, first Edition. New Delhi: Elsevier; 2010. 1–48.
3. Michaud PA, Frappier JU, Pless IB. Compliance in adolescents with chronic disease. Arch FrPediatr 1991; 48:329–336.
4. Fernandes LM, Ogaard B, Skoglund L. Pain and discomfort experienced after placement of a conventional or a superelastic NiTi aligning archwire. A randomized clinical trial. J Orofacial Orthop 1998; 59:331–339.
5. Ngan P, Kess B, Wilson S. Perception of discomfort by patients undergoing orthodontic treatment. Am J Orthod Dentofacial Orthop 1989; 96:47–53.
6. Silverstone LM, Saxton CA, Dogon IL, Fejerskov O. Variation in the pattern of acid etching of human dental enamel examined by scanning electron microscopy. Caries Res 1975; 9:373.
7. Maijer R, Smith DC. Corrosion of orthodontic bracket bases. Am J Orthod Dentofacial Orthop 1982; 81:43–48.
8. Zachrisson BU, Zachrisson S. Caries incidence and orthodontic treatment with fixed appliances. Scand J Dent Res 1971; 79:183–192.
9. Ogaard B. Prevalence of white spot lesions in 19-year-old: A study on untreated and orthodontically treated persons 5 years after treatment. Am J orthod Dentofacial Orthop 1989. 96:423–427.
10. Chatterjee R, Kleinberg I. Effect of orthodontic band placement on the chemical composition of human incisor plaque. Arch Oral Biol 1979; 24:97–100.
11. Gwinnett JA, Ceen F. Plaque distribution on bonded brackets. Am J Orthod Dentofacial Orthop 1979; 75:667–677.
12. Philips JR. Apical root resorption under orthodontic theraphy. Angle Orthod 1955;25:1–22.
13. Levander E, Malmgren O. Long-term follow-up of maxillary incisors with severe apical root resorption. Eur J Orthod 2000; 22:85–92.
14. Lundstrom F, Krasse B. *Streptococcus mutans* and lactobacilli frequency in orthodontic patients: The effect of chlorhexidine treatment. Eur J Orthod 1987; 9:109–116.
15. Rosenblom RG, Tinanoff N. Salivary *Streptococcus mutans* levels in patients before, during and after orthodontic treatment. Am J Orthod Dentofacial Orthop 1991; 100:35–37.
16. Boyd R, Baumrind S. Periodontal considerations in the use of bonds or bands on molars in adolescents and adults. Angle Orthod 1992; 62:117–126.
17. Hollender L, Ronnerman A, Thilander B. Root resorption, marginal bone support, and clinical crown length in orthodontically treated patients. Eur J Orthod 1980; 3:197–205.
18. Quality management systems – requirements. International Standards ISO 9001. 2008. E.
19. Chaconas SJ. Orthodontic diagnosis and treatment planning. J Oral Rehabil 1991; 18:531–545.
20. Reitan K. Biomechanical principles and reactions. In Graber TM, Swain BF, eds. Orthodontics: current principles and techniques, St Louis, 1985, Mosby.
21. Roberts WE, Garetto LP, Katona TR. Principles of orthodontic biomechanics: metabolic and mechanical control mechanisms. In Carlson DS, Goldstein SA, eds. Bone biodynamics in orthodontic and orthopedic treatment. Ann Arbor, Mich, 1992, University of Michigan Pres.
22. Burstone CJ, Pryputniewicz RJ, Bowley WW. Hotographic measurement of tooth mobility in three dimensions. J Periodontal Res 1978; 13:283.
23. Rygh P, Moxham BJ, Berkovitz BKB. The effects of external forces on the periodontal ligament: the response to horizontal loads. In Berkovitz BKB, Moxham BJ, Newman HN, eds. The periodontal ligament in health and disease, Oxford, 1982, Pergamon Press.
24. Roberts WE, Ferguson DJ. Cell kinetics of the periodontal Ligament. In Norton LA, Burstone CJ, eds. The biology of tooth movement, Boca Raton, Fla, 1989, CRC press.
25. Roberts WE, Goodwin WC, Heiner SR. Cellular response to orthodontic force. Dent Clin North Am 1981; 25:3.
26. Robert WE et al. Circadian periodicity of the cell kinetics of rat molar periodontal ligament. Am J Orthod Dentofacial Orthop 1979; 76:316.
27. Roberts WE, Morey ER. Proliferation and differentiation sequence of osteoblast histogenesis under physiological conditions in rat periodontal ligament. Am J Anat 1985; 174:105.
28. Roberts WE, Arbuckle GR, Analoui M. Rate of mesial translation of mandibular molars utilizing implant-anchored mechanics. Angle Orthod 1996; 66:331.
29. Kusy RP, Whitley JQ, Mathew MJ, Buckthal JE. Surface roughness of orthodontic archwires via laser spectroscopy. Angle Orthod 1988; 58:33–45.
30. Prososki RP, Bagby MD, Erickson LC. Static frictional force and surface roughness of nickel-titanium archwires. Am J Orthod Dentofac Orthop 1991; 100:341–348.
31. Frank CA, Nikolai RJ. A comparative study of frictional resistances between orthodontic bracket and archwire. Am J Orthod Dentofac Orthop 1980; 78:593–609.
32. Bednar JR, Gruendeman GW, Sandrik JL. A comparative study of frictional forces between orthodontic brackets and archwires. Am J Orthod Dentofac Orthop 1991; 100:513–522.
33. Angolkar PV, Kapila S, Duncanson MG Jr, Nanda RS. Evaluation of friction between ceramic brackets and orthodontic wires of four alloys. Am J Orthod Dentofac Orthop 1990; 98:499–506.
34. Peterson L, Spencer R, Anderson GF. Comparison of frictional resistance of Nitinol and stainless steel wires in Edgewise brackets. Quint Inter Digest 1982; 13:563–571.
35. Drescher D, Bourquel C, Schumacher H. Frictional forces between bracket and archwire. Am J Orthod Dentofac Orthop 1989; 96:249–254.
36. Popli K, Pratten D, Germane N, Gunsolley J. Frictional resistance of ceramic and stainless steel orthodontic brackets. J Dent Res 1989; 68:275 (A747).

37. Taloumis LJ, Smith TM, Hondrom SO et al. Force decay and deformation of orthodontic elastomeric ligatures. Am J Orthod Dentofac Orthop 1997; 111:1–11.

38. Shivapuja PK, Berger J. A comparative study of conventional ligation and self-ligation bracket systems. Am J Orthod Dentofac Orthop 1994; 106:472–480.

39. Quinn RB, Yoshikawa DK. A reassessment of force magnitude in orthodontics. Am J Orthod Dentofac Orthop 1985; 88:252–260.

40. Meling TR, Odegaard J, Holthe K, et al. The effect of friction on the bending stiffness of orthodontic beams: a theoretical and in vitro study. Am J Orthod Dentofac Orthop 1997; 112:41–49.

41. Haradine NWT. The history and development of self-ligating brackets. Semin Orthod 2008; 14:5–8.

42. Turnbull NR, Birnie DJ. Treatment efficiency of conventional versus self-ligating brackets: effect of archwire size and material. Am J Orthod Dentofac Orthop 2007; 131:395–399.

43. Forsberg C, Brattstrom V, Malmberg E, Nord CE. Ligature wires and elastomeric rings: two methods of ligation, and their association with microbial colonization of *Streptococcus mutans* and lactobacilli. Eur J Orthod 1991; 13:416–420.

44. Turkkahraman H, Ozgur SM, Yesin BF, et al. Archwire ligation techniques, microbial colonization, and periodontal status in orthodontically treated patients. Angle Orthod 2005; 75: 231–236.

45. Edwards JG. A long-term prospective evaluation of the circumferential supracrestal fiberotomy in alleviating orthodontic relapse. Am J Orthod Dentofac Orthop 1988; 93:380–387.

46. Richardson ME, Gormley JS. Lower arch crowding in the third decade. Eur J Orthod 1998; 20:597–607.

47. Sharp W, Reed B, Subtelny JD. Orthodontic relapse, apical root resorption, and crestal alveolar bone levels. Am J Orthod Dentofac Orthop 1987; 91:252–258.

48. Karad A, Dhanjani V, Bagul V. Twenty-year post-treatment assessment of class II division 1 malocclusion treated with non-extraction approach. APOS Trends Orthod 2013; 3:31–41.

Management of an Orthodontic Practice

Karen Moawad

Every orthodontist spends years of learning how to be an excellent clinician. We can move teeth in all directions and correct complex malocclusions, but how we take care of our patients ultimately affects the success of our practice. Enhancing efficiency and profitability should be an ongoing process of incremental improvements to existing office systems. Every attempt should be made to modify or discard the systems that are not efficient and effective. It should be recognized that patients expect exceptional service in everything nowadays and spend substantial amount where they receive extraordinary attention.

This chapter discusses some of the elements in managing an ideal orthodontic practice. The emphasis will be on principles of efficient patient scheduling, analysis of 'the numbers' of your practice, practice building, patient compliance and cost containment. The data and ideas were drawn from orthodontic practice in North America, and some information may not be applicable to an orthodontic practice in other countries.

SCHEDULING

Before developing an ideal schedule, it is important to know what kind of a practice you wish to create. We are not talking about mission statements or philosophical goals, but ask yourself 'How many days do I want to work each month?' Or 'How much money do I want to net each month?' If an orthodontist determines how many days a month he or she is willing to see patients and what net income is desired, it is simple mathematics to calculate everything else.

GOAL SETTING

For example, let us say that our doctor wants to net $75,000 a month from his or her primarily full treatment practice (a Phase I or a Phase II practice is calculated a little differently). We'll assume that the full treatment fee is $4850, and the overhead is running approximately 55% a month. Of course, one can always play with the fee and work on lowering the overhead, but for simplicity sake, we'll take those as given.

Generally, we create a situation where the practice (unless it is new or growing quickly) produces (charges out) 15% more than anticipated collections. This formula doesn't work immediately but should kick in after approximately 6 months following a major change in production.

If overhead is 55%, the gross collections must be approximately $167,000 a month to net $75,000. If production should be 10–15% higher than collections, to generate this collection figure, a schedule must be built to produce $192,000 a month. If the treatment fee is $4850, one must start 40 full cases a month.

Let us also assume that our doctor wants to see patients 14 days a month. This means starting the treatment of three new patients a day. Allowing for no shows but anticipating a 75% conversion rate on exams, the practice should schedule four exams a day (plus two recall patients who fit into exam slots), totalling an average of 84 exam slots a month.

If the rotation is 8 weeks and the patients are seen for approximately 14 visits throughout active treatment, the practitioner will see approximately 100 patients a day. From this information, one can determine that this practice, when correctly scheduled 14 days a month, will benefit from two scheduling coordinators, one treatment coordinator, six clinicians, one financial coordinator and possibly a records technician who helps with sterilization. The choice of having in-house laboratory staff is up to the doctor. The number of clinicians is best determined by how the orthodontist practices—utilization of technology, rotation between visits, extent of expanded duties, percentage of patients beyond their estimated completion date, number of emergencies per day, etc.

A well-crafted schedule that ensures that the doctor is only needed in one place at a time is the secret to success in an orthodontic practice. You can have highly skilled staff with wonderful attitudes, but without a schedule to support them and the practice goals, even the best staff are inefficient.

Prior to implementing a doctor-time schedule, the following problems are observed in most orthodontic practices:

- Nonscheduled procedures are frequently added during an appointment.
- Nonscheduled emergencies are taken care of anytime they come.
- Doctor is often on the telephone when needed clinically.
- The clinic chairs become expensive waiting room chairs, as the patients sit waiting for the doctor to come and check.
- Treatment on patients and communication with the patients are often disjointed, as one staff member starts the patient and another finishes the patient.
- Staff are not at the chair when the doctors arrive at the chair.
- The ratio of patients beyond their estimated completion date is higher than in a practice that runs on a doctor-time schedule.
- Patients are not as aware of cooperation contests as they are when the same chairside starts the patient and finishes the patient.
- Staff are not always certain which procedure they should do, so they wait to be told.
- Procedures to be accomplished at the next visit are not defined at the current visit.

A doctor-time schedule is based on templates that are fully mastered with all the appointments needed during the day. Each schedule has the same number of columns as there are clinical auxiliaries treating patients plus a column for each treatment coordinator and a column for the records technician. Chairsides stay in their own column and see the patients listed in that column. The doctor is available at his/her chair whenever needed.

Step 1 in designing a schedule is to list the outcome you want. Let's say you always want to run on time, you want the doctor to be available when needed to minimize the time that chairside auxiliaries spend waiting for the doctor, you want someone to be available to take records following each exam, you want adequate time to complete each procedure, you want patients finished with treatment by their estimated completion date, you want emergencies minimized, you want the correct number of exams and starts to feed the production level you desire and you want an exemplary level of communication among patients, parents and staff.

Then, you must make some basic decisions about treatment in your practice:

- In a multiple doctor office, will doctors share patients?
- Will patients be assigned to the same clinical team throughout their treatment?

Step 2 is to set the foundation so the practice cannot fail. Here is a checklist:

- Make sure that each person has the materials and equipment needed.
- Help each chairside to understand the 'why' of what is being done.
- Determine your policy for emergencies, late patients and changes in treatment on the day of the appointment and share the information so that everyone knows.
- Allow adequate time in each procedure for staff to relate with each patient, check for loose brackets, explain contests, evaluate hygiene, complete the procedure, record treatment, talk with mom and clean up.

Step 3 involves taking a critical look at how you deliver orthodontics. How many visits does each treatment plan take? How efficient are you at performing all the procedures necessary at each visit? Are emergencies taking too much of your clinical time during the day? Is your rotation in sync with the capability of the brackets and wires you are using?

Step 4 is to list all the procedures that you perform. Then, time these procedures and agree on common timings among the chairsides. These timings (also referred to as configurations or types) will become the basis of your schedule. You don't want to choose the fastest timings unless all chairsides can accomplish the procedure in that time. And you don't want to choose the longest, for your faster auxiliaries will become impatient with the schedule.

Configurations (or types) will reflect how long the chairsides take to complete a procedure in 5-min increments and how long the doctor takes in 1.33 min increments. (Each doctor-time increment is 1.33 min.) When you are timing your procedures, I suggest you add 5 min at the end of each procedure to allow time to chat with mom and clean up. Thus, if a procedure takes 15 min of chairside time with 3 min of doctor time after the first 5 min, the actual configuration will be 20 min with 3 min of doctor time after the first 5 min.

Of course, each practice must develop its own timings. Step 5 is to combine these timings so there are as few configurations as possible. In other words, minimize the number of different configurations by combining as many procedures as possible into the same configuration. Even if you have to increase the doctor time by 1.33 min to accommodate an increased number of procedures, it may be worth it to minimize the number of configurations. The more procedures that fit into one configuration, the more times that configuration is offered during the day, and thus, the more choices a patient has.

The configuration list shows different configurations and their corresponding appointments (Exhibit 17.1).

Step 6 is to tally procedures so that you know how many times each procedure is performed in a month. If 12 different procedures are grouped into one configuration, add up the counts for all 12 procedures, and that is the total number of times that configuration must occur in a month. Once you know the number of times a configuration should be available in a month, it is a simple task to determine how many times that configuration must be available each day. If you use the computer to count procedures, remember that this information is based on patients who are checked out as having had that procedure. You may need a higher count of each configuration because patients often make an appointment and cancel or do not show and still need another appointment of the same configuration later.

Also remember that sometimes you do two or more procedures at one visit. The combination of the most frequently done multiprocedures should be given a name and be linked to a configuration that reflects the time needed to perform all the procedures.

APPOINTING RULES

Before developing the doctor-time schedules or grids for each day, determine the appointing rules you wish to follow. Your appointing rules may look like this:

- No appointments longer than 30 min after 3:30 p.m.
- Only appointments 20 min or less at the last hour of the day
- Fifteen minutes of clean up time each day in each column
- Equalize the start and deband appointments among the first four columns and make the fifth column an easier column for training purposes
- Set aside time for records after every exam in order to facilitate the one-step exam process

Any rules that the physical plant requires should also be listed in preparation for building your scheduling standards or grids. If you must take records in the exam room, for example, the schedule cannot place two exams back to back. But your rules may also indicate that the treatment coordinator should take the records rather than records technicians since their room is unavailable for any other appointment anyway.

BUILDING THE STANDARDS OR GRIDS

Once you have the configurations, the counts and the appointing rules, encourage the chairsides to help build

the schedule. They are a wise group who can bring much to the discussion as to which procedures should go into which columns, etc. The scheduling coordinators should offer their talents as well, for they know what time of day certain appointments are needed. For example, you might want to offer 45 min of short appointments at the start of each day before starting the longer appointments.

Configurations are fit together so that the doctor stays busy throughout the day but is never needed in more than one place at a time. If an appointment calls for just 1.5 min of the doctor's time, then it is possible to be at another column (or even two other columns) during that same 5-min period since only 1.5 min is needed in the first appointment.

If you want to keep the doctors busy and use their time efficiently, you must have five or even six chairsides (depending on the configurations in the practice). Note that when studying this sample schedule (Exhibit 17.2), the x indicates the doctor time. As you can tell from the three xs across almost every 5 min, the doctor time is almost maximized.

It is best to create three grids every time you revise the schedule. If you are scheduling for 14 days a month, one grid can be used five times a month (A), the other grid five times a month (B) and the last grid four times (C). The configurations should be placed at different times on each grid, so there is flexibility in choices of times available. The two starts might be at 9:00 A.M. and 10:30 A.M. on Grid A but at 9:30 A.M. and 10:10 A.M. on Grid B. Maybe you would want to offer an afternoon start on Grid C.

Enter the grids into the computer to reflect hours, number of chairsides and doctors, etc. for each day alternating among Grids A, B and C. The corresponding list with the procedures and their matching configurations should also be entered into the computer so that the procedures and configurations (searches) are linked.

The list of procedure codes is called a *buck slip*. This list also indicates the start codes that are posted when a contract is posted to indicate the start of treatment (Exhibit 17.3).

When procedures are correctly posted in the computer, you can easily retrieve valuable information indicating the number of times each procedure occurred in a day, month and year. You can also verify that all production has been 'charged out'. Posting procedures changes statuses automatically when appropriate. Also, charges and letters are generated from these same postings.

Determine when to start using the new grids at some point in the future when the schedule is not too heavy. Print the days that will be revised so that you have a record of which patients are already scheduled when and for which procedure. Delete those schedules, load the new grids and then reenter the already scheduled patients into the new schedule using searches. Some appointments will 'fall in' at the same time; others must be given a new time.

NOTIFY PATIENTS OF CHANGE IN NEXT APPOINTMENT

If you have more than 50 appointments to change, it is a good idea to order and send postcards with the office

Exhibit 17.1   Configuration list

E1
Code	Description
001	Exam Child
002	Exam Adult
202	Recall Ready

(\75)

EY
Code	Description
OO5	Young Person Exam (6 and under)

(\30)

L1
Code	Description
200	Recall Observation
201	Phase II Pending Recall
004	Second Opinion (Patient in Treatment)

(\15)

C1
Code	Description
300	Phone/Coop Consultation

C2
Code	Description
301	In Office Consultation

D1
Code	Description
704	Debond 2 arches, fixed lingual, imp
705	Debond 2 arches, imps

(\90)

AA
Code	Description
607	Aligner Tray Delivery, IPR (not start)

(\15)

A1
Code	Description
602	Check Appliance (Quad/LA/HG/RPE/Habit)
611	Retainer Check #1, 10 weeks later
612	Retainer Check #2, 4 months later
613	Retainer Check #3, 6 months later, Dismiss Pt.
614	Retainer Check Extra
615	Check Retainer after Inactivation (with fee)
620	Retie
700	Remove Cemented Appliance(s)

(\15)

B2
Code	Description
103	Progress Records, Adjustment
400	Bond/Rebond/Reposition 1-4 Bo, 1 Arch
410	Cement 1-2 Bands, 1 Arch
411	Cement 2-4 Bands, 2 Arches
412	Fit Bands, Imp for Lingual Arch
413	Fit Bands, Imp for Quad Helix
414	Fit Bands, Imp for RPE/Pendulum (1 arch)
416	Remove RPE/Quad/Nance/LA and Reband 6's
420	Bond Lingual Retainer, 1-2 Arches
501	Deliver Upper and Lower RPE

(\35)

B3
Code	Description
401	Bond/Rebond/Reposition 5-12 Bo, 1 Arch
402	Bond/Rebond/Reposition 2-12 Bo, 2 Arch
403	Bond/Rebond/Reposition 13-24 Bo, 2 Arch
404	Full Bonding, 1 Arch (2nd arch)
421	Fit Bands, Imp for RPE (2 arches)
512	Deliver Invisalign, Reprox and Attachments (Start Only)
624	Wire change with Mid Treatment Review
625	Place Surgical Hooks
626	Place Pontic, Change Wires
422	IDB One Arch

(\40)

B5
Code	Description
406	Full Band, Bond 1 Arch (first arch)
407	Full Band, Bond 1 Arch with appliance
415	Rem Herbst: Band, Bond Remaining (follow by B6 same day)
417	621, 1 or 2 Arches
418	621, 1 or 2 Arches with appliance
508	Deliver/Adjust Splint
706	Phase I Debond (Records)

Continued

Exhibit 17.1, cont'd

Code	Description		Marks
		R1	
102	Pan/Ceph/Photos	＼15	
		R2	
104	Impression 1-2 Arches		X
105	Impression to Deliver Hawley/Bite Plate		
106	Impression to Deliver Functional Appliance		
107	Imp to Repair Appliance	＼20	
		RR/R3	
100	Impressions, Ceph	＼25	
		R4	
101	Invisalign Records		
108	Indirect Impressions	＼40	
	(unlabeled)	＼30	X X X / X X X

Code	Description		Marks
		A2	
513	Deliver Replacement Hawley		
514	Deliver Replacement Clear Retainer		X
515	Deliver Rem Appliance (Schwartz/MG/Pos)		
701	Remove Cemented Appliance(s), Imp	＼20	
		A3	
509	Deliver Headgear		
622	1 or 2 AW changes		
623	Detail 1-2 Wire		X
707	End of Invisalign Treatment (Records)	＼30	X
		A4	
500	Deliver Upper RPE		X
502	Deliver Quad		X X
503	Deliver Pendulum		
504	Deliver Nance		
505	Deliver Lingual Arch		
507	Deliver Habit Appliance		
517	Deliver Retainer and Final Photos		
603	Check to Deband, Final Adjustment	＼30	
		B1	
506	Deliver Functional Appliance		
511	Deliver Invisalign, Reprox (Start Only)		X X
608	Occlusal Equilibrate/Reproximation		X
702	Partial Debond		X X
703	Debond 1 arch	＼30	X

Code	Description		Marks
405	Full Bonding, 2 Arches		
408	Full Band, Bond 2 Arches		
409	Full Band, Bond 2 Arches with appliance		
419	621, 1 or 2 Arches with headgear		
423	IDB, 2 arches		
424	IDB, 2 arches with appliance		X
425	Remainder of Remove Herbst, BB Remaining		X X
516	Deliver Herbst	B6	X X
513	Deliver Replacement Hawley		
514	Deliver Replacement Clear Retainer	＼60	
		S1	
350	Seps		
600	Check OH	＼10	
		S2	
601	Check Cooperation (Elastics/Headgear)		
800	Repair Short (clip wire)		X
801	Repair Long (Bracket, Appl)	＼20	

Exhibit 17.2 Sample schedule

Time	#1	#2	#3	#4	#5	#6	TC	TC
8:00								
8:05	A3	A3	A3	S1	A2	R2	E1	EY
8:10				\10				
8:15				S1				
8:20				\10	\20	\20		
8:25	\30	\30	\30					
8:30								\30
8:35	S1	S2			B3			E1
8:40	\10		A4					
8:45				B1				
8:50		\20						
8:55			\30					
9:00	B6	B2						
9:05			B3					
9:10				\30				
9:15				B5		RR		
9:20					\40		E1	
9:25								
9:30			\40			\20		
9:35		S1			D1			
9:40		\10						
9:45						RR		
9:50								
9:55						\20		\75
10:00		B6						
10:05			A1	\60				E1
10:10			\15	S1				
10:15				\10				
10:20							\75	
10:25	\90		B6					
10:30	A4			B2	\90	RR	E1	E1
10:35					B5			
10:40				\35				
10:45						\20		
10:50								
10:55	\30							
11:00		\90				R4		
11:05	D1	B2						
11:10				B3				
11:15								
11:20								
11:25		\90						
11:30		B2		\40				
11:35								
11:40								

Continued

Exhibit 17.2, cont'd

	45	\				\				\ 90								\	X	X	X	\				\				\					45
	50	\				\				A1				S2				\	X	X	X	\ 40				\				\ 75					50
	55	\				\ 35				\	X	X		\			X	\				RR				\									55
12	00	\	X	X	X					\ 15				\				\				\				\								12	00
	05	\	X	X	X	A1								\ 20				\ 60				\				\									05
	10	\				\	X	X		A3				A3				A3				\ 20				\				L1					10
	15	\				\ 15				\				\				\								\ 75				\	X	X	X		15
	20	\								\			X	\			X	\			X	RR								\15					20
	25	\ 90				AA				\	X			\	X			\	X			\													25
12	30					\	X	X	X	\				\				\				\												12	30
	35					\15				\ 30				\ 30				\ 30				\ 20													35
	40																																		40
	45																																		45
	50																																		50
	55																																		55
1	00																																	1	00
	05																																		05
	10																																		10
	15																																		15
	20																																		20
	25																																		25
1	30																																	1	30
	35																																		35
	40																																		40
	45																																		45
	50																																		50
	55																																		55
2	00									S1				A3				S1				R2		X		E1				L1				2	00
	05	B2				A1				\ 10				\				\ 10				\				\				\	X	X	X		05
	10	\				\	X	X		A1				\			X	S1				\				\				\15					10
	15	\				\ 15				\	X	X		\	X			\ 10				\ 20				\									15
	20	\	X	X	X					\ 15				\				S1				R4				\									20
	25	\				A3								\ 30				\ 10				\				\	X	X	X						25
2	30	\				\				A3				A3				A1				\				\	X	X	X	E1				2	30
	35	\ 35				\			X	\				\				\	X	X		\				\				\					35
	40					\	X			\			X	\			X	\ 15				\				\				\					40
	45	A1				\				\	X			\	X							\				\				\					45
	50	\	X	X		\ 30				\				\				S1				\				\				\					50
	55	\ 15				S1				\ 30				\ 30				\ 10				\ 40				\				\	X	X	X		55
3	00	A3				\ 10				AA				A3				A3				R1				\				\	X	X	X	3	00
	05	\				S1				\	X	X	X	\				\				\				\				\					05
	10	\			X	\ 10				\15				\			X	\			X	\ 15				\ 75				\					10
	15	\	X			A4				S1				\	X			\	X			RR								\					15
	20	\				\	X	X	X	\ 10				\				\				\								\					20
	25	\ 30				\				A4				\ 30				\ 30				\								\					25
3	30	AA				\				\	X	X	X	A3				A3				\ 20				E1				\				3	30
	35	\	X	X	X	\				\				\				\								\				\					35

Time		Col 1	Col 2	Col 3	Col 4	Col 5	Col 6	Col 7	Col 8
40		\75	–	RR	X / –	X / –		\30	\15
45			–	–	X / –	X / –	–	S2	A1
50			–	–	\30	\30	\30	–	–
55			–	\20	A3	S2	A2	–	\15
00	4		–		–	–	–	\20	A3
05			–		–	X / –	\20	X / –	X / –
10		L1 X	–	R3	X / –	\20	A3	S2	–
15		– X	–	–	\30	S1	–	–	–
20		\15 X	–	–	A3	\10	X / \20	\20	–
25			–	\25	–	A3	A3	A4	\30
30	4		\75	S1	–	X / –	–	X / –	A3
35				\10	–	X / –	–	X / –	–
40		C2 X X		RR	\30	A3	\30	–	–
45		– X X		–	X / –	–	A1 X X	–	X / –
50		– X X		–	–	–	X / X	–	–
55		–		\20	–	\30	\15	\30	\30
00	5	–							
05		–							
10		–							
15		–							
20		\30							

name and address. ('Due to a schedule change in our office, your appointment, originally scheduled for_____, has been changed to_____. If this is inconvenient for you, please call our office to reschedule. Thank you'.)

APPOINTING POLICY

It is a good idea to develop an appointing policy to give to patients and parents prior to the date the new schedule 'kicks in' so that the patients understand the need to be on time for their visits. You can place this sample on the next page on your stationery or adapt your own.

SAMPLE APPOINTING POLICY FOR NEW PATIENTS

Appointments

In an effort to honour our patients' time and minimize the time spent waiting in our office, we ask patients to brush their teeth and check in prior to their scheduled

Exhibit 17.3 List of procedure codes

New		Description	Srch	Status	Ltrs	Fee
		EXAMS				
001		**Exam Child (7–17)**	E1			
005		**Exam Young Child (6 and under)**	EY			
	900	Initial Exam Child, Records Taken, Start Sched		Start Sched		
	901	Initial Exam Child, Records Taken, Cons Sched		Start Needed		
	902	Initial Exam Child, Records Taken, Start Needed (Susp)		Start Needed		
	903	Initial Exam Child to Recall		Observation		
	904	Initial Exam Child, No Recs, Pending (no ceph, imp)		Pending		
	905	Initial Exam Child, No Tx Needed/Declined		Inactive		
	906	Initial Exam Child, Refer to Specialist/GP		Specialist		
002		**Exam Adult**	E1			
	910	Initial Exam Adult, Records Taken, Start Sched		Start Sched		
	911	Initial Exam Adult, Records Taken, Cons Sched		Rx Taken		
	912	Initial Exam Adult, Records Taken, Start Needed (Susp)		Start Needed		
	913	Initial Exam Adult, No Recs, Pending (no ceph, imp)		Start Needed		
	914	Initial Exam Adult, No Tx Needed/Declined		Inactive		
	915	Initial Exam Adult, Refer to Specialist/GP		Referred		
004		**Second Opinion (Patient in Treatment)**	L1			$50
		RECORDS AND IMPRESSIONS				
100		Impressions, Ceph	R3			
101		Invisalign Records	R4			
102		Pan / Ceph / Photos	R1			
103		Progress Records, Adjustment	B2			
104		Impression 1-2 Arches	R2			
105		Impression to Deliver Hawley / Bite Plate	R2			$
106		Impression to Deliver Functional Appliance	R2			$
107		Imp to Repair Appliance	R2			
108		Indirect Impressions	R4			
		RECALL				
200		Recall Observation	L1	Observation		
201		Phase II Pending Recall	L1	Ph II Pending		
202		**Recall Ready**	E1			
	930	Recall Ready, Records Taken, Start Scheduled		Start Sched		
	931	Recall Ready Records Taken, Cons Scheduled		Rx Taken		
	932	Recall Ready to Recall		Observation		
	933	Recall Ready, Start Needed (Suspense)		Start Needed		
	934	Recall Ready, Tx Declined		Inactive		
	935	Recall Ready, Refer to Specialist/GP		Specialist		
		CONSULTS				
300		Phone / Cooperation Consultation	C1			
301		**In Office Consultaton**	C2			
	940	Consultation, Start Scheduled		Start Sched		
	941	Consultation, Start Appointment Needed (Suspense)		Start Needed		
	942	Consultation to Recall		Observation		
	943	Consultation, Refer to Specialist		Specialist		
	944	Consultation, Tx Refused		Inactive		
		SEPS				
350		Seps	S1			
FA		Financial Arrangements to be confirmed				

New	Description	Srch	Status	Ltrs	Fee
	STARTS				
S1	**Phase 1 Start**		**Phase I**		
S2	**Phase II Start**		**Phase II**		
S3	**Early / Limited Treatment Start**		**Limited**		
S4	**Full Treatment Start**		**Full**		
S5	**TMD Start**		**TMD**		
S6	**Surgery Patient**		**Surgery**		
S7	**Retreatment**		**Retreat**		
S8	**Invisalign Start**		**Invisalign**		
	BAND / BOND				
400	Bond / Rebond / Reposition 1-4 Bonds 1 arch	B2			
401	Bond / Rebond / Reposition 5-12 Bonds 1 arch	B3			
402	Bond / Rebond / Reposition 2-12 Bonds 2 arches	B3			
403	Bond / Rebond / Reposition 13-24 Bonds 2 arches	B3			
404	Full Bonding, 1 Arch (2nd arch)	B3			
405	Full Bonding, 2 Arches	B6			
406	Full Band, Bond, 1 Arch (1st arch)	B5			
407	Full Band, Bond 1 Arch with appliance	B5			
408	Full Band, Bond, 2 Arches	B6			
409	Full Band, Bond 2 Arches with appliance	B6			
410	Cement 1-2 Bands, 1 Arch	B2			
422	IDB 1 Arch	B3			
423	IDB 2 arches	B6			
424	IDB 2 arches, with appliance	B6			
425	Remainder of Remove Herbst, BB Remaining	B6			
411	Cement 2-4 Bands, 2 Arches	B2			
412	Fit Bands, Imp for Lingual Arch	B2			
413	Fit Bands, Imp for Quad Helix	B2			
414	Fit Bands, Imp for RPE / Pendulum (1 arch)	B2			
415	Remove Herbst and Band, Bond Remaining (follow by B6 same day)	B5			
416	Remove RPE / Quad / Nance / LA and Reband 6's	B2			
417	621, 1 or 2 Arches	B5			
418	621, 1 or 2 Arches with appliance	B5			
419	621, 1 or 2 Arches with headgear	B6			
420	Bond Lingual Retainer, 1-2 arches	B2			
421	Fit Bands, Imp for RPE (2 arches)	B3			
	DELIVERIES				
500	Deliver Upper RPE (AM Only)	A4			
501	Deliver Upper and Lower RPE	B2			
502	Deliver Quad	A4			
503	Deliver Pendulum	A4			
504	Deliver Nance	A4			
505	Deliver Lingual Arch	A4			
506	Deliver Functional Appliance	B1			
507	Deliver Habit Appliance	A4			
508	Deliver / Adjust Splint	B5			
509	Deliver Headgear	A3			
511	Deliver Invisalign, Reprox (Start Only)	B1			
512	Deliver Invisalign, Reprox and Attachments (Start Only)	B3			
513	Deliver Replacement Hawley	A2			
514	Deliver Replacement Clear Retainer	A2			
515	Deliver Removable Appliance (Schwartz / Mouthgard / Positioner)	A2			
516	Deliver Herbst	B6			
517	Deliver Retainer and Final Photos	A4			
	CHECK / ADJUST				
600	Check OH	S1			
601	Check Cooperation (Elastics / Headgear)	S1			
602	Check Appliance (Quad / LA / HG / RPE / Habit)	A1			
603	Check to Deband, Final Adjustment	A4			
611	Retainer Check #1, 10 weeks later	A1	R		
612	Retainer Check #2, 4 months later	A1	R		

Continued

Exhibit 17.3, cont'd

New	Description	Srch	Status	Ltrs	Fee
	CHECK / ADJUST Continued				
613	Retainer Check #3, 6 months later, Dismiss Pt.	A1	I		
614	Retainer Check Extra	A1	R	ltr	
615	Check Retainer after Inactivation (with fee)	A1	I		$48
607	Aligner Tray Delivery, IPR (not start)	AA			
608	Occlusal Equilibrate / Reproximation	B1			
	ARCH WIRES				
620	Retie	A1			
622	1 or 2 AW changes	A3			
623	Detail 1-2 Wires	A3			
624	Wire change with Mid Treatment Review	B3			
625	Place Surgical Hooks	B3	Surgery		
626	Place Pontic, Change Wires	B3			
	REMOVE / DEBOND				
700	Remove Cemented Appliance(s)	A1			
701	Remove Cemented Appliance(s), Imp	A2			
702	Partial Debond	B1			
703	Debond 1 arch	B1	?	?	
704	Debond 2 arches, fixed lingual, imp	D1	Retention	ltr	
705	Debond 2 arches, imps	D1	Retention	ltr	
950	End of Phase I		Phase II Pending	ltr	
706	Phase I Debond (Records)	B5	Phase II Pending	ltr	
707	End of Invisalign Treatment (Records)	A3	Retention	ltr	
	EMERGENCIES				
800	Repair Short (clip wire)	S1			
801	Repair Long (Bracket, Appl)	S2			
960	Unscheduled Emergencies				
961	Scheduled Emergencies				
	MISCELLANEOUS CHARGES OR STATUS CHANGES				
970	Miscellaneous Charge				Range
971	Poor Oral Hygiene			ltr	
972	Poor Cooperation			ltr	
973	Update Parent				
974	Patient Dismissed		Inactive		
975	Transfer Out		Inactive		
976	Mouthguard				
977	Maintenance Only		Maintenance		

appointment time. We will make every effort possible to schedule appointments at your convenience. For this reason, we see patients on teacher workdays and some holidays (Martin Luther King Day, Veteran's Day, etc.).

Appointment confirmation

Our computerized confirmation system will telephone you 1–2 days prior to your appointment to confirm the date and time.

Late arrivals

If a patient arrives after the scheduled start time, we may need to reschedule your appointment in order to perform all the necessary orthodontic procedures you need and still stay on schedule for the rest of our patients. Our intention is to value your time, as well as ours. Our staff work very hard, and we want them to be able to have lunch and to go home promptly at the end of the day. Please arrive *on time* for your scheduled appointment.

Orthobucks

Our Orthobucks program is designed to reward patients for good hygiene, good cooperation, being on time for appointments and wearing their office t-shirts. Orthobucks are only given at regular adjustment appointments and are not given for comfort visits.

Comfort visits

Comfort visits are scheduled, if the need arises between regular appointments to alleviate discomfort or to repair a broken appliance. These appointments need to be scheduled in advance. Walk-ins will be seen on a space available basis only or may have to wait or be rescheduled another day.

Arrival time

Each appointment will be scheduled with a technician who specializes in the procedure you are having. You may see a patient arrive after you who is called into the

---

Sample appointing policy explaining new scheduling system to current patients

Dear Patients and Parents,

We are very excited about some changes in our office that we would like to share with our patients and families. As a part of our continuing effort to provide the best quality service in our office, we have developed a new scheduling system. Please take a few minutes and carefully read over the brief details highlighting the new changes you will see starting December 1, 20——. Good communication is vital to successful and timely treatment. Whenever possible, we ask one parent to accompany school-aged patients to their appointment. This allows us to inform the responsible party on the procedure performed and the next appointment needed.

In an effort to accommodate as many patients as possible and minimize excessive time away from school and work, we schedule only relatively short appointments during the afternoons between 2:30 p.m. and 4:00 p.m. Longer appointments are, therefore, scheduled in the morning or early afternoon. A suggestion for school-aged patients is to arrange longer appointments during study hall, easier classes or during the lunch period.

The success of the new schedule is reliant on patients arriving on time. In order to see every patient on time, we cannot squeeze in late patients. We will offer a late arrival the choice of either waiting for an opening or rescheduling for another day and time.

To assist our patients in reaching their completion date in a timely fashion, we strongly encourage that original appointments be kept. To wait several weeks for another after school appointment may result in unfavourable movement and longer treatment.

Lastly, we are committed to excellence, both in our orthodontic treatment results and in the creation of an environment that is warm, friendly, and fun. The service we provide our patients and parents is extremely important to all of us. We welcome comments, concerns, and questions. Together through mutual respect and teamwork, we will work through any adjustment period. As always, we thank you for your confidence, trust, and support!

---

clinic before you. This is because the technician working with you is not yet ready. We want to run on time and give you the very best care possible. Please understand.

Pager

Our technicians carry a pager so we can help patients who have emergency situations that may arise on weekends or after hours. Please call the pager, if you have experienced trauma to the mouth, have a loose expander or have other discomfort that cannot wait until normal office hours_____.

A doctor-time schedule should be reevaluated every 6 months to incorporate growth, new procedures, new techniques, etc. Which configurations should be shortened, lengthened or the doctor-time changed? Make new timings for those configurations you are unsure of. Should some configurations be offered at other times of day? Which configurations were you short of? Which configurations did you have too many of?

START SLOTS

When actually scheduling patients into a doctor-time schedule, be sure all start slots are filled *only* with starts. Make filling the start slots a priority. Determine with the treatment coordinator or a scheduling coordinator who will take responsibility for this important function. If a start slot has not been scheduled 2 days prior to the actual appointment, only then can that slot be used for another configuration, but one must be cognizant of doctor time when filling a start slot with something else.

Remember, a start slot that goes unfilled or filled with an appointment other than a start can never be recaptured. The opportunity to reach your goal is compromised.

ELECTRONIC SIGN-IN

Electronic sign-in, where the patient signs in at the front desk upon arrival, allows the operatory staff to know who has arrived and tracks whether the patient was late or early and by how many minutes. This tool greatly facilitates decision making about whether or not a loose bracket can be replaced. The chairsides need to only look at the screen in the operatory to know how many patients are waiting.

ELECTRONIC TREATMENT CARD

Electronic treatment card is also a helpful tool in scheduling. The chairsides enter what procedures were performed today and what is needed at the next visit, as well as the rotation, and that information is electronically sent to the front desk in preparation for scheduling.

In some offices, on electronic treatment card, the chairsides, since they have a computer at their chairs, schedule adult patients but send minors to the front since they need their mothers involved when scheduling the next appointment.

A light system, whether part of the software package or a separate entity, facilitates the doctor moving through the operatory area. When the chairsides need the doctor at their chair, they hit their light, and the first light lit flashes. The doctor follows the flashing lights.

STAYING ON TIME

It is the chairsides' responsibilities to keep their column running on time and to see that the doctor comes to their chair precisely when they need the doctor's help. If something is loose or broken, it is that chairside's responsibility (in conjunction with a clinic coordinator, if there is one) to decide if the bracket can be repaired right then and there, if the patient should wait for an opening within the next hour or if the patient should be reappointed.

With regard to regular treatment visits, it should be a rule that at a minimum, ties should be changed at every appointment, even if the patient comes late.

Before the end of each visit, the doctor should have determined which procedure is to be done at the next visit, and the chairside will request that procedure code. Before the doctor comes to the chair, the chairside should write down on the bracket table cover what we are doing today, how much time the doctor has, what time the patient should be leaving, the cooperation grade and whether the patient is ahead or behind in treatment time.

CHANGES AT THE FRONT DESK

When scheduling, there is no need to enter appointment dates on the patient chart, if your practice is not on electronic treatment card. It is too time consuming to pull charts every time an appointment is made on the telephone. Anyone needing to check next appointments can look in the computer.

It is always a good idea to print the schedule every Friday for the next 8 weeks, just in case the computer goes down. Additionally, because scheduling coordinators working with a doctor-time schedule normally schedule by search and do not often go into the actual schedule, scanning the printout also gives a good perspective of any unevenness in the schedule.

MORNING MEETING REPORT

The morning meeting is a way of communicating how well the starts are filling and whether they are booked too far into the future. Other significant appointments, such as exams and debands, are also analyzed at this time. This meeting should be run by the scheduling coordinator. It takes 10 min. Everyone must be present.

If the morning meeting report indicates that starts are more than 2 weeks into the future or that there are no exam slots for the next 10 days, it is time to make an adjustment. Do you want to work an extra day doing just exams and starts? Or do you want to change one of the grids to include an additional exam or start? If you decide to work an additional day just to see exams and starts, you must create a start schedule with just start and exam configurations. This handy grid is inserted in a day, whenever necessary.

Remember that though carefully monitored, you will reach your goals without working an additional day. The basic grids should be designed and redesigned to ensure that you reach your goal. Any adjustment you make is not about reaching your goal (for your schedule has already been set up to do that) but may be in response to taking the very best care of referral sources by seeing their patients in a timely manner.

At the morning meeting, chairsides are told which column is theirs for the day. They can stay in their normal chair or move around, but regardless, they do not have to have the same column each day—they may be column 1 on Monday and column 3 on Tuesday just to prevent monotony.

The only exception to this flexibility is the 'Patient Manager' concept when patients are assigned to a chairside team and must always be scheduled with the same chairsides. In this case, the chairsides must stay in their same columns.

RED-DOT, GREEN-DOT CALENDAR

Another helpful tool is the 'red-dot, green-dot' calendar. This computerized year at a glance calendar (easily to download from Microsoft) invites you to place green dots on all patient days, red dots on holidays and yellow dots on nonpatient work days (Exhibits 17.4A 2007 and 17.4B 2008). With careful planning, this process allows the group to manipulate the patient days so as to create as many week-long vacations as they wish. For example, if the practitioner is going to see patients only 14 days a month, normally doctor and staff agree on which 14 patient days throughout the month. Make those green. Paid holidays are red, and the rest of the week days are yellow.

However, a clever team could see patients two 5-day weeks and one 4-day week and take the next 12 days off as yellow-dot days! If they are really astute, they can schedule their patient days late in the following month, and add the yellow-dot days of the second month to the yellow-dot days of the first month for an extended vacation!

Obviously, not everyone is eligible for vacation, but this flexibility is appealing to the doctor and the long-term staff who are eligible for four or more weeks of vacation.

There should be a minimum of one yellow day a month (preferably two or three) so that the staff can have a staff meeting or catch up on side jobs in support of green patient days. In many offices, the group decides during a staff meeting what is to be accomplished during the yellow-dot days the following month, and the staff are given a written assignment at the beginning of each yellow-dot day as to what they must accomplish.

Although some staff only work on (green) patient days, normally staff are supposed to work on yellow-dot days as well. However, if a staff member wishes to take a yellow-dot day off, it is considered either a vacation day or an unpaid day. In order to take an unpaid day, his/her work must be up to date, and he/she must have cleared his/her request with the doctor or the manager.

The 'red-dot, green-dot' calendar is normally created in September or October for the following year. Staff members appreciate knowing the patient days a year in advance so that they can plan their vacations without missing patient days.

VERTICAL CALENDAR

The vertical calendar, originated by Dr Harry Hatasaka, California, shows the rotation of patient visits. It is also a

Exhibit 17.4A Red-dot, green-dot calendar

2007

JANUARY

S	M	T	W	T	F	S
	1	2	3	4	5	6
7	8	9	10	11	12	13
14	15	16	17	18	19	20
21	22	23	24	25	26	27
28	29	30	31			

FEBRUARY

S	M	T	W	T	F	S
				1	2	3
4	5	6	7	8	9	10
11	12	13	14	15	16	17
18	19	20	21	22	23	24
25	26	27	28			

MARCH

S	M	T	W	T	F	S
				1	2	3
4	5	6	7	8	9	10
11	12	13	14	15	16	17
18	19	20	21	22	23	24
25	26	27	28	29	30	31

APRIL

S	M	T	W	T	F	S
1	2	3	4	5	6	7
8	9	10	11	12	13	14
15	16	17	18	19	20	21
22	23	24	25	26	27	28
29	30					

MAY

S	M	T	W	T	F	S
		1	2	3	4	5
6	7	8	9	10	11	12
13	14	15	16	17	18	19
20	21	22	23	24	25	26
27	28	29	30	31		

JUNE

S	M	T	W	T	F	S
					1	2
3	4	5	6	7	8	9
10	11	12	13	14	15	16
17	18	19	20	21	22	23
24	25	26	27	28	29	30

JULY

S	M	T	W	T	F	S
1		3	4 2	5	6	7
8	9	10	11	12	13	14
15	16	17	18	19	20	21
22	23	24	25	26	27	28
29	30	31				

AUGUST

S	M	T	W	T	F	S
			1	2	3	4
5	6	7	8	9	10	11
12	13	14	15	16	17	18
19	20	21	22	23	24	25
26	27	28	29	30	31	

SEPTEMBER

S	M	T	W	T	F	S
						1
2	3	4	5	6	7	8
9	10	11	12	13	14	15
16	17	18	19	20	21	22
23	24	25	26	27	28	29
30						

OCTOBER

S	M	T	W	T	F	S
	1	2	3	4	5	6
7	8	9	10	11	12	13
14	15	16	17	18	19	20
21	22	23	24	25	26	27
28	29	30	31			

NOVEMBER

S	M	T	W	T	F	S
				1	2	3
4	5	6	7	8	9	10
11	12	13	14	15	16	17
18	19	20	21	22	23	24
25	26	27	28	29	30	

DECEMBER

S	M	T	W	T	F	S
						1
2	3	4	5	6	7	8
9	10	11	12	13	14	15
16	17	18	19	20	21	22
23	24	25	26	27	28	29
30	31					

Exhibit 17.4B   Red-dot green-dot calendar

2008

JANUARY						
S	M	T	W	T	F	S
		1	2	3	4	5
6	7	8	9	10	11	12
13	14	15	16	17	18	19
20	21	22	23	24	25	26
27	28	29	30	31		

FEBRUARY						
S	M	T	W	T	F	S
					1	2
3	4	5	6	7	8	9
10	11	12	13	14	15	16
17	18	19	20	21	22	23
24	25	26	27	28	29	

MARCH						
S	M	T	W	T	F	S
						1
2	3	4	5	6	7	8
9	10	11	12	13	14	15
16	17	18	19	20	21	22
23	24	25	26	27	28	29
30	31					

APRIL						
S	M	T	W	T	F	S
				3	4 2	5
6	7	8	9	10	11	12
13	14	15	16	17	18	19
20	21	22	23	24	25	26
27	28	29	30			

MAY						
S	M	T	W	T	F	S
				1	2	3
4	5	6	7	8	9	10
11	12	13	14	15	16	17
18	19	20	21	22	23	24
25	26	27	28	29	30	31

JUNE						
S	M	T	W	T	F	S
1	2	3	4	5	6	7
8	9	10	11	12	13	14
15	16	17	18	19	20	21
22	23	24	25	26	27	28
29	30					

JULY						
S	M	T	W	T	F	S
		1	2	3	4	5
6	7	8	9	10	11	12
13	14	15	16	17	18	19
20	21	22	23	24	25	26
27	28	29	30	31		

AUGUST						
S	M	T	W	T	F	S
					1	2
3	4	5	6	7	8	9
10	11	12	13	14	15	16
17	18	19	20	21	22	23
24	25	26	27	28	29	30
31						

SEPTEMBER						
S	M	T	W	T	F	S
	1	2	3	4	5	6
7	8	9	10	11	12	13
14	15	16	17	18	19	20
21	22	23	24	25	26	27
28	29	30				

OCTOBER						
S	M	T	W	T	F	S
			2	3 1	4	
5	6	7	8	9	10	11
12	13	14	15	16	17	18
19	20	21	22	23	24	25
26	27	28	29	30	31	

NOVEMBER						
S	M	T	W	T	F	S
						1
2	3	4	5	6	7	8
9	10	11	12	13	14	15
16	17	18	19	20	21	22
23	24	25	26	27	28	29
30						

DECEMBER						
S	M	T	W	T	F	S
	1	2	3	4	5	6
7	8	9	10	11	12	13
14	15	16	17	18	19	20
21	22	23	24	25	26	27
28	29	30	31			

Exhibit 17.5 Vertical calendar

2008 Vertical Calendar — Eight-Week

Oct 29, 2007	Nov 5	Nov 12	Nov 19	Nov 26	Dec 3	Dec 10	Dec 17
30	6	13	20	27	4	11	18
31	7	14	21	28	5	12	19
1	8	15	22	29	6	13	20
2	9	16	23	30	7	14	21

Dec. 24	Dec. 31, 2007	Jan. 07	Jan 14	Jan 21	Jan 28	Feb 4	Feb 11
25	1	8	15	22	29	5	12
26	2	9	16	23	30	6	13
27	3	10	17	24	31	7	14
28	4	11	18	25	1	8	15

Feb 18	Feb 25	Mar 3	Mar 10	Mar 17	Mar 24	Mar 31	Apr 7
19	26	4	11	18	25	1	8
20	27	5	12	19	26	2	9
21	28	6	13	20	27	3	10
22	29	7	14	21	28	04	11

Apr 14	Apr 21	Apr 28	May 5	May 12	May 19	May 26	Jun 2
15	22	29	06	13	20	27	3
16	23	30	07	14	21	28	04
17	24	1	8	15	22	29	05
18	Apr 25	2	9	16	23	30	06

Jun 9	Jun 16	Jun 23	Jun 30	Jul 7	Jul 14	Jul 21	Jul 28
10	17	24	1	8	15	22	29
11	18	25	2	9	16	23	30
12	19	26	3	10	17	24	31
13	20	27	04	11	18	25	1

Aug 4	Aug 11	Aug 18	Aug 25	Sep 1	Sep 8	Sep 15	Sep 22
5	12	19	26	2	9	16	23
6	13	20	27	3	10	17	24
7	14	21	28	4	11	18	25
8	15	22	29	5	12	19	26

Sep 29	Oct 6	Oct 13	Oct 20	Oct 27	Nov 3	Nov 10	Nov 17
30	7	14	21	28	4	11	18
1	8	15	22	29	5	12	19
2	9	16	23	30	6	13	20
3	10	17	24	31	7	14	21

Nov 24	Dec 1	Dec 8	Dec 15	Dec 22	Dec. 29, 2008	Jan. 5, 2009	Jan 12
25	2	9	16	23	30	6	13
26	3	10	17	24	31	7	14
27	4	11	18	25	1	8	15
28	5	12	19	26	2	9	16

helpful tool from several points of view. Have you noticed that the pleasure you gain from time out of your office is often diminished by the too-busy days that immediately precede and follow those vacation days or that your schedule is lightly appointed exactly 8 weeks following your vacfation week?

The vertical calendar is a method of organizing the interval in which you see patients and balance their treatment needs with your continuing education and vacation schedule. If you see patients 52 weeks a year, you do not need to use the vertical calendar. In this case, we suggest a good therapist! However, if you are a typical orthodontist, you take a significant amount of time away from the office. The vertical calendar will decrease the frustration of going away and reduce your stress when you return. If you choose, you can organize your vacation time so that you have a week off every 6, 8 or 10 weeks throughout the year without missing a beat.

Each calendar is formatted so that it divides the year into a series of work weeks that cycle on the normal appointment. Calendars are available for 4-, 5-, 6-, 7-, 8-, 9-, 10- and 12-week rotations reflecting your choice for your normal rotation (Exhibit 17.5). The weeks are arranged in vertical columns. Patients seen in any particular week are seen in the week just below in the same column (if their rotation is not interrupted by an office vacation). Arrows indicate that the week patients are next appointed (Exhibit 17.6).

Just keep in mind that no matter which vertical calendar you use, you will have some rotations that are 1 week longer and some 1 week shorter. And if you take 2 weeks off at the same time (normally recommended the last week of one month and the first of another month), you may have a 2-week variance from the ideal rotation.

Once you have chosen the vertical calendar(s) you wish to use, keep the original and make several copies to work with. Determine how many days will be patient days in the upcoming year. Or, conversely, determine how many nonpatient days you wish to have. If you have completed a red-dot, green-dot calendar, simply copy the information into the vertical calendar.

First, yellow-out (or shade) the complete weeks you will not be seeing patients. Then, yellow-out (or shade) individual days or parts of weeks you will not be seeing patients. The shaded areas are for all normal workdays that are taken off, such as holidays, management days, vacations and continuing education courses.

Exhibit 17.6 Vertical calender

2008 Vertical Calendar — Eight-Week

Oct 29, 2007	Nov 5	Nov 12	Nov 19	Nov 26	Dec 3	Dec 10	Dec 17
30 / 31 / 1 / 2	6 / 7 / 8 / 9	13 / 14 / 15 / 16	20 / 21 / 22 / 23	27 / 28 / 29 / 30	4 / 5 / 6 / 7	11 / 12 / 13 / 14	18 / 19 / 20 / 21
Dec. 24	**Dec. 31, 2007**	**Jan. 07**	**Jan 14**	**Jan 21**	**Jan 28**	**Feb 4**	**Feb 11**
25 / 26 / 27 / 28	1 / 2 / 3 / 4	8 / 9 / 10 / 11	15 / 16 / 17 / 18	22 / 23 / 24 / 25	29 / 30 / 31 / 1	5 / 6 / 7 / 8	12 / 13 / 14 / 15
Feb 18	**Feb 25**	**Mar 3**	**Mar 10**	**Mar 17**	**Mar 24**	**Mar 31**	**Apr 7**
19 / 20 / 21 / 22	26 / 27 / 28 / 29	4 / 5 / 6 / 7	11 / 12 / 13 / 14	18 / 19 / 20 / 21	25 / 26 / 27 / 28	1 / 2 / 3 / 04	8 / 9 / 10 / 11
Apr 14	**Apr 21**	**Apr 28**	**May 5**	**May 12**	**May 19**	**May 26**	**Jun 2**
15 / 16 / 17 / 18	22 / 23 / 24 / Apr 25	29 / 30 / 1 / 2	06 / 07 / 8 / 9	13 / 14 / 15 / 16	20 / 21 / 22 / 23	27 / 28 / 29 / 30	3 / 04 / 05 / 06
Jun 9	**Jun 16**	**Jun 23**	**Jun 30**	**Jul 7**	**Jul 14**	**Jul 21**	**Jul 28**
10 / 11 / 12 / 13	17 / 18 / 19 / 20	24 / 25 / 26 / 27	1 / 2 / 3 / 04	8 / 9 / 10 / 11	15 / 16 / 17 / 18	22 / 23 / 24 / 25	29 / 30 / 31 / 1
Aug 4	**Aug 11**	**Aug 18**	**Aug 25**	**Sep 1**	**Sep 8**	**Sep 15**	**Sep 22**
5 / 6 / 7 / 8	12 / 13 / 14 / 15	19 / 20 / 21 / 22	26 / 27 / 28 / 29	2 / 3 / 4 / 5	9 / 10 / 11 / 12	16 / 17 / 18 / 19	23 / 24 / 25 / 26
Sep 29	**Oct 6**	**Oct 13**	**Oct 20**	**Oct 27**	**Nov 3**	**Nov 10**	**Nov 17**
30 / 1 / 2 / 3	7 / 8 / 9 / 10	14 / 15 / 16 / 17	21 / 22 / 23 / 24	28 / 29 / 30 / 31	4 / 5 / 6 / 7	11 / 12 / 13 / 14	18 / 19 / 20 / 21
Nov 24	**Dec 1**	**Dec 8**	**Dec 15**	**Dec 22**	**Dec. 29, 2008**	**Jan. 5, 2009**	**Jan 12**
25 / 26 / 27 / 28	2 / 3 / 4 / 5	9 / 10 / 11 / 12	16 / 17 / 18 / 19	23 / 24 / 25 / 26	30 / 31 / 1 / 2	6 / 7 / 8 / 9	13 / 14 / 15 / 16

Chapel Hill | Pittsboro | Holiday | Non Patient

To place the arrows correctly, start at the top of the vertical calendar. Arrows normally go straight down until shaded out days or weeks interfere.

The goal is to keep the number of patient days balanced from week to week. Three patient days can go into a week with two patient days, three patient days or four patient days. But we do not recommend putting three patient days from the previous rotation into a week with only one patient day or with five patient days. The former would not fit, and the latter would not be productive enough.

Note that 1 day during a week out of the office (such as Labour Day) does not affect the vertical calendar.

It is easier to read the vertical calendar, if the rotation arrows are colour-coded. We recommend highlighting 7-week arrows with one colour (blue), 8-week arrows with another colour (black) and 9-week arrows with a third colour (red). In our example, 6-week rotations are pink.

The vertical calendar only works, if you plan your time off at least 6 months in advance.

Coordinate your appointment book with the vertical calendar. Block out appointment dates as the vertical calendar indicates.

At each morning meeting, the receptionist will announce whether to use a 5-, 6-, 7- or 8-week rotation (for example) for patients being seen that day, based on the arrows on the vertical calendar.

KEY PERFORMANCE INDICATORS

Over the past 10 years, Hummingbird Associates has been tracking financial and clinical numbers of participating offices, as well as Key Performance Indicators (KPIs), and providing participants with a quarterly report so that they can see how they are doing over time and can compare their numbers with those of other participating offices. Note that ratios provide a vehicle so that small practices and large practices can be compared. The KPI is a useful tool for comparing your practice to industry standards.

It is important to point out that the numbers analysis includes solo practitioners, multiple doctor offices, satellites, main offices, etc. Therefore, rather than production or collection figures, the *ratios* offer the best method of comparison, so small practices and large practices can be evaluated in relation to each other. For example, it is not of any value to compare the number of full starts in a satellite with the number of full starts in a three-doctor practice. But if you compare the conversion rate (exams to starts) in both these practices, the information is worthy of evaluation and study.

As an example, the current median for the derived value of collections divided by patients seen is $167.37. If you were to take your average net collections for a year and divide that figure by all the patient visits throughout the year, your ratio should be at least $150. However, many offices have a number lower than $140, and others have a much higher number. Feedback, such as this, gives a practice a roadmap to use to make corrections.

One of the most insightful ratios is collections per orthodontist hour. What does the practice collect for every hour in a month the orthodontist is treating patients? $1441.13 is the current average, with some practices collecting above $3000 per hour.

Offices are encouraged to be diligent about good data, to study their numbers when the report is received, to take action on the feedback from the numbers analysis report and to celebrate their progress.

PRACTICE BUILDING

How many of our patients, parents or referral practices are disappointed with some aspect of their experience but never say anything? How many feel no one at the orthodontic office even knows their name? How many policies are adopted for the convenience of the practice without checking with the patients as to how the change might impact them? How many opportunities to exceed someone's expectations do we miss? How accessible are we to listen to a patient or parent's unhappiness? What do we do to return the satisfaction level to the high level it should be?

Think of the last time you had a poor customer service experience. Perhaps, it was in the grocery store, at an airport, in a shop or in a telephone conversation. Recall your frustration in trying to have your concerns heard and then acted upon to your satisfaction. What would have taken to turn around the situation? There usually is something that someone could have said or done to make it alright.

As customers, we don't want to be unhappy. We want to find suppliers and vendors we can use with confidence, over and over again. We are looking to be loyal.

Think about an exceptional customer service experience—one where they got it just right! These tend to stand out in our memories. With your staff make a list of what made the experiences so positive. The same kinds of things will be written on each list: they listened to me, they were honest with me, they acted like they truly cared, they took decisive and timely action, they made me feel appreciated and they made me feel special.

Donna Panucci, Charleston, WV, insists that her chairsides prompt her when she walks to the chair as to a topic to discuss with that patient. 'Johnny just got back from Orlando, Doctor'. Or the chairside may say, 'Susie won her soccer game yesterday, and she scored a goal'.

The bottom line in outstanding customer service is that we are made to feel special. Never mind that there are over 6 billion of us on the planet. We don't want to feel that we are just a name on a schedule; we want to feel that the person working with us is completely committed to our personal satisfaction—whatever that may look like. We have got to let our patients and referral sources know from the very first contact that they are special to us—not just a number or a name.

Hummingbird consultant, Jodi Peacock, teaches several courses on improving customer service. When the entire team gathers at Jodi's horse ranch for a weekend to focus on customer service, they come away committed to making every interaction customer based. They realize that it's the little things that count. From how the telephone is answered to how a staff member discusses the lack of patient cooperation with the parent, we have opportunities to improve client relations or harm them.

At a Hummingbird client meeting, Dr Steve Sherman, who practices in Baton Rouge, LA, shared an activity from one of his staff retreats. One by one he held up photos of patients and gave a prize to the staff member who could correctly write down the highest number of names.

When staff are asked how customer service can be improved, they discuss that they have the freedom to give gifts when a mistake has been made, accessibility after hours and an attitude of 'Of course we can do what you are requesting—let me do that for you'. This 'can do' attitude goes far in providing white glove customer service.

Sometimes, customer service is invoked with how things are said. It is not always easy to fit patients into a doctor-time schedule. And yet talented scheduling coordinators use phrases such as 'Let's see how we can make that work for you'. Or, 'We want to schedule this appointment at a time that doesn't conflict with an important class—what time is Susie's lunch or free period?' Or 'I have a calendar of the school holidays right here—let's see if we can't take advantage of one of those'. Customer service in action!

PATIENT COMPLIANCE

Hygiene grading should be consistent from chairside to chairside. We often use these definitions to improve consistency: Excellent indicates no food on the teeth as a result of regular and thorough plaque removal and no swelling of the gums. Nightly flossing is usually necessary to receive an excellent grade.

Good indicates no food or visible plaque on the teeth, but minor inflammation of the gums is present. This usually indicates insufficient brushing or flossing to properly remove the plaque.

Poor indicates food or plaque present on the teeth at the time of the adjustment appointment. Damage to the teeth and gums becomes a possibility when a poor level hygiene is not improved.

Then, a series of letters are used to communicate with the parent when noncompliance is an issue.

FINISHING PATIENTS ON TIME

One of the practice goals should be to complete patients during their estimated treatment time. An estimated completion date creates a goal by which the patient should move into the retention phase. When patients languish in active treatment past the estimated completion date, the schedule fills with nonpaying patients, patients become impatient that they are still in treatment and goals are compromised.

A treatment efficiency monitor, with entries made after every deband, will, in time, offer important data indicating whether or not there is a problem with more visits than anticipated, more months of treatment than anticipated and a lower than anticipated collections per visit ratio. A Phase I, Phase II patient with combined fees of $5600 may have 3 visits before Phase I, 12 Phase I visits, 6 visits in observation before Phase II and 14 Phase II visits. These 35 visits divided into the $5600 fee means $160 per visit.

In the following Excel form, the highlighted columns are calculated automatically in the computer (Exhibit 17.7)

If patients are not finishing on time, we strongly recommend a midtreatment review. Suggested questions to consider include the following.

Oral hygiene letter 1 (first poor grade): Intraoral photo is included with the letter

Dear_____

_____ seems to be having difficulty with her oral hygiene. As you will recall from the initial consultation, decalcification, cavities and gum disease are particular concerns when a patient is in braces; thus meticulous daily oral hygiene practices are essential during active treatment. The photo on this letter was taken today during _____'s appointment. As you can see, her hygiene is a problem.

Braces do not cause decay or marks on the teeth. Poor oral hygiene will cause decalcification (soft white marks) around the braces, primarily on the gum side of the braces and between the teeth. Poor oral hygiene also can inflame gum tissue. _____can eliminate this problem by cleaning her teeth properly and avoiding excessive refined sugars. It can take five minutes to brush teeth in order to completely clean them while wearing braces, and_____ should do so after every meal. Drs_____ and_____ recommend a soft-bristled toothbrush, and they ask that you replace it every three months or as the bristles begin to fray. _____also may use a fluoride rinse daily.

We would appreciate your help in monitoring _____'s oral hygiene. Please watch for plaque—a white, milky film of bacteria and food debris that, if left on the teeth, causes tooth decay (initially, white spots on the teeth known as *decalcification*)—and for gum disease (initially puffy, bleeding gums). Please remember that _____should brush thoroughly around the teeth and braces. Proper tooth-brushing, flossing and use of the proxabrush will result in a healthy mouth.

We will, as usual, check _____'s oral hygiene at her next appointment. We hope to see improvement so that she can continue treatment without the risk of decalcification and decay. If you have any questions, please don't hesitate to call.

Sincerely,
Patient Manager

Oral hygiene letter 2 (second poor grade): Intraoral photo is included with the letter

Dear_____

_____ still seems to be having difficulty with her oral hygiene. We are very concerned about the potential of decalcification, cavities and gum disease; scrupulous oral hygiene is essential during active treatment.

We have discussed concerns regarding decalcification, cavities and gum disease with her in the past. However, despite the fact that techniques for good oral hygiene have been reviewed extensively with _____,we find little evidence of improvement in the care she gives her teeth and gums. The photo on this letter was taken today during _____'s appointment. As you can see, her hygiene is still a problem. We would appreciate your help in monitoring _____'s oral hygiene. Please watch for plaque—a white, milky film of bacteria and food debris that, if left on the teeth, causes tooth decay (initially, white spots on the teeth known as *decalcification*)—and for gum disease (initially puffy, bleeding gums). Thorough brushing and flossing is essential. We request you schedule an appointment with Dr _____ for a hygiene visit. We are sending a copy of this letter to Dr _____.

We will, as usual, check _____'s oral hygiene at her next appointment. We hope to see improvement so that she can continue treatment without the risk of decalcification and decay. If you have any questions, please don't hesitate to call.

Sincerely,
Patient Manager

Oral hygiene letter 3 (third poor grade)

Dear_____

_____ is still having difficulty with her oral hygiene. As you know, we have discussed concerns regarding decalcification, cavities and gum disease with her in the past. However, despite the fact that techniques for good oral hygiene have been reviewed extensively and repeatedly with _____, we find little evidence of improvement in the care she gives her teeth and gums. The photo on this letter was taken today during _____'s appointment. You can see the lack of improvement.

We have removed _____wires to make it easier for her to clean her teeth. Unfortunately, removal of the wire will delay her treatment progress. We will replace the wire at her next visit.

We now must also insist that she see Dr _____ for regular cleanings every three months in order to continue orthodontic treatment.

We continue to ask for your help in monitoring _____'s oral hygiene. Please watch for plaque—a white, milky film of bacteria and food debris that, if left on the teeth, causes tooth decay (initially, white spots on the teeth known as *decalcification*)—and for gum disease (initially puffy, bleeding gums). Thorough brushing and flossing is essential.

We will, as usual, check _____'s oral hygiene at her next appointment. We hope to see improvement so that she can continue treatment. **Unless there is improvement, we will recommend removal of the braces before decay destroys the teeth and infection of the gums produces periodontal disease.**

If you have any questions, please don't hesitate to call.

Sincerely,
Patient Manager

Oral hygiene letter 4 (fourth poor grade)

Dear_____

It is with deep regret that we send this letter. As you know, _____has been having considerable difficulty with her oral hygiene. At today's visit, we found her oral hygiene still unimproved. She is at a great risk for decalcification (white spots on the teeth that are the initial stages of tooth decay) and gum disease (bleeding, puffy, painful gums that eventually require gum surgery).

We take this matter so seriously that we do not feel comfortable proceeding with _____'s orthodontic treatment. **We have scheduled a deband appointment to remove _____'s braces on_____.**

In the future, if _____demonstrates a commitment to a clean, healthy mouth and fastidious care of her teeth and gums, may be we can consider resuming treatment.

We will ask that you sign a *Consent Form for Early Removal of Braces* which indicates a less than optimal or ideal result.

If you have any questions, please don't hesitate to call.

Sincerely,
Patient Manager

Exhibit 17.7   Treatment efficiency monitor

	NAME OF PATIENT (Enter on Deband Day)	Sex	Age at Deband	Diag Class	Comprehensive Tx Fee	Estimated Months in Tx	Actual Months in Tx	Months over / under Est Tx	Number of Tx Visits	Number of Emergency Visits	Appts Prior to Tx	Total Appts (except retention)	$ Per Tx Visit	$ Per Total Visits	Notes
1								0.00				0			
2								0.00				0			
3								0.00				0			
4								0.00				0			
5								0.00				0			
6								0.00				0			
7								0.00				0			
8								0.00				0			
9								0.00				0			
10								0.00				0			
11								0.00				0			
12								0.00				0			
13								0.00				0			
14								0.00				0			
15								0.00				0			
16								0.00				0			
17								0.00				0			
18								0.00				0			
19								0.00				0			
20								0.00				0			

12-MONTH REVIEW, STAFF TO ASK

1. Extractions complete? (Yes, no, reevaluate in future in _____months, N/A)
2. Permanent teeth erupted? (Yes, no)
3. Impacted teeth? (Yes, _____, no)
4. Need panoramic radiographs? (Yes, no)
5. Reposition needed? (Yes, no)
6. Level and alignment complete? (Yes, no)
7. Rotations corrected? (Yes, no)
8. Spaces? (Closed, being closed, keeping space for prosthetic)
9. Method of closing spaces? (Chain, closing coils)
10. Growth in normal range (Yes, no)
11. Need for any additional appliance? (Yes, no)
12. Is there a change in treatment plan? (Yes, no) (If so, change the treatment plan)
13. Treatment progress—are we ahead, behind or on track? (Ahead, behind, on schedule)
14. Oral hygiene? (Good, fair, poor)
15. Elastics cooperation? (Yes, no)
16. Keeping appointments? (Yes, no)
17. Cooperation letters needed (Not needed, elastics, OH, appliance breakage, missed appointments, other)
18. Anticipated visits to completion? (_____)
19. Treatment intervals in future (8, 6, 4 weeks)
20. Doctor notes (also in the treatment card)
21. Have patients had their teeth cleaned at their family dentist? (Yes, no)

A letter is created from these answers to give or mail to the parent.

OVERHEAD ANALYSIS/COST CONTAINMENT

One practice in Toronto, Canada, did a detailed cost analysis. All practitioners can learn a great deal about cost containment from studying the following report. It is impossible to evaluate what to change, if you don't know what you are currently spending (Exhibit 17.8).

Exhibit 17.8A A detailed overhead analysis (A-F)

Supplier	Product	Description	Units per Box	Qty. per Patient	Unit Cost	Full 18–24	%
	FULL TREATMENT + PHASE II						
	Total Fee	Full				6,130.00	100.0%
	Materials						
	Consultation						
Ink Fleet	Pans and Ceph	Machine depreciation (20%) / 2,101 exams			10.47	10.47	0.2%
Ink Fleet	Printed Pan	1 box of 50 sheets $16.93	50	2	0.38	0.76	0.0%
	Camera depreciation	$1,300 every 2 years / 2,101 exams times 2			0.33	0.00	0.0%
Ink Fleet	Ink	8 cartridges per month / (2101/12)		1	2.24	2.24	0.0%
Print	Exit Package	Folder + Information		1	3.44	3.44	0.1%
Budget	Sani Cloth Large	1 bottle $10.25	160	2	0.07	0.14	0.0%
Budget	Mask Blue	1 box of 50 masks $9.00		1	0.19	0.19	0.0%
Wayne	Gloves	1 box Vinyl $3.35	100	2	0.03	0.07	0.0%
Patterson	Sterilization Bag	1 box of 1,000 bags $34.95	1,000	1	0.04	0.04	0.0%
EC Print	Informed Consent	1,000 forms $160.00	1,000	1	0.18	0.18	0.0%
Central Printing	Business card	$0.41 cents per card	500	2	0.41	0.82	0.0%
EC Print	Davis Dollar sheet	2,000 sheets for $180.00	2,000	1	0.10	0.10	0.0%
Central Printing	Letterhead	7000 pieces $2,585	7,000	2	0.41	0.83	0.0%
Postal	Stamp	$0.51 per stamp		2	0.51	1.02	0.0%
Central Printing	Envelope	5,000 envelopes $1,985	5,000	2	0.44	0.89	0.0%
	Pen	*Rainbow Optical Fiber Pen $3 per pen*	1	1	3.35	3.35	0.1%
Central Printing	Magnet	*750 magnets $635*	750	1	1.02	1.02	0.0%
Budget	Tray Cover	1 box $19.95	1,000	2	0.02	0.04	0.0%
	Subtotal Consultation					25.59	0.4%
	Braces on +Treatment						
3m Unitek	Brackets 3M Unitek	Full set = $141.70 us	One set	26	162.96	162.96	2.7%
Clinical Research Dental	Etch	*$99.95 20 syringes, 1 syringe for 2.5 patients*		0.4	5.02	2.01	0.0%
3m Unitek	Transbond Primer	1 bottle us $45.5 us for 15 patients	1	0.07	52.33	3.49	0.1%
Patterson	Disposable Prophy Angle	1 box $343.35	1,000	1	0.34	0.34	0.0%
OSC	Pumise	1 bottle $31.45	200	1	0.17	0.17	0.0%
Budget	Micro-brush	1 box $6.5	100	1	0.07	0.07	0.0%
Budget	Tray Cover	1 box $19.95	1,000	1	0.02	0.02	0.0%
Budget	Saliva Ejector	1 box $29.95	1,000	1	0.03	0.03	0.0%
Budget	Bib	1 box $20.95	500	1	0.05	0.05	0.0%
Wayne	Gloves	1 box Latex $4.70	100	6	0.05	0.28	0.0%
Budget	Sani Cloth Large	1 bottle $10.25	160	4	0.07	0.28	0.0%
Ortho Arch	Bite Turbos	1 box US 53.5	10	2	6.15	12.31	0.2%
Patterson	Durafill	1 Syringe $111.25 for 10 turbos	1	0.2	11.13	2.23	0.0%
EC Print	Consent Forms	*2,250 forms $190.00*	2,250	1	0.09	0.09	0.0%
EC Print	Financial Agreement	500 forms $125.00	500	1	0.28	0.28	0.0%
Central Printing	Business card	$0.41 cents per card	500	1	0.41	0.41	0.0%

Continued

Exhibit 17.8A, cont'd

Supplier	Product	Description	Units per Box	Qty. per Patient	Unit Cost	Full 18–24	%
Central Printing	Progress Report	5,000 cards $225	5,000	1	0.05	0.05	0.0%
Central Printing	Davis Dollars (bills)	7,500 bills $ $360	7,500	3	0.05	0.64	0.0%
	Goody bag:						
OSC	Relief Wax	100 units $92.00	100	1	0.99	0.99	0.0%
Sunstar Butler	Floss	144 units $65.50	144	1	0.49	0.49	0.0%
Sunstar Butler	Floss Threaders	100 envelopes $34.40	100	1	0.37	0.37	0.0%
Patterson	Compact Interdental brush	24 units $35.70	24	1	1.61	1.61	0.0%
Lips	Lip balm	500 units $500	500	1	1.08	1.08	0.0%
Patterson	Toothbrush	24 tootbrushes $10.95	24	1	0.49	0.49	0.0%
	Subtotal Braces On + Treatment					190.73	3.1%
	Braces off (Deband)						
Budget	Bib	1 box $20.95	500	1	0.05	0.05	0.0%
Patterson	Disposable Prophy Angle	1 box $343.35	1,000	1	0.34	0.34	0.0%
Budget	Saliva Ejector	1 box $29.95	1,000	1	0.03	0.03	0.0%
Patterson	Prophy Paste (Fluorhide)	$74.10 200 units	200	1	0.40	0.40	0.0%
Patterson	Gold Flame	100 burs $379.50	100	1	4.10	4.10	0.1%
Brasseler	Deband Burr	$13.49 each	5	0.25	13.49	3.37	0.1%
Patterson	2 Impressions	10 bags of 1lb. $84.81 1lb = 9 patients	10	0.11	8.48	1.88	0.0%
Ferraro	MD 3-3 with tray	1 unit	1	1	22	22.00	0.4%
Ferraro	Max Hawley Retainer	1 unit	1	1	61	61.00	1.0%
Ferraro	2-2	1 unit	1	1	20	20.00	0.3%
Clinical Research Dental	Etch	$99.95 20 syringes, 1 syringe for 15 patients		0.07	5.02	0.33	0.0%
3m Unitek	Transbond Light Cure	1 bottle us $45.50 for 40 patients	1	0.025	52.78	1.32	0.0%
Budget	Micro-brush	1 box $6.5	100	1	0.07	0.07	0.0%
Sunstar Butler	Floss Threaders	100 envelopes $34.40	100	1	0.37	0.37	0.0%
Patterson	Disposable Prophy Angle	1 box $343.35	1,000	1	0.34	0.34	0.0%
3m Unitek	Transbond LR Paste	$69 us 25 capsules, 3 patients per capsule	25	0.33	3.17	1.05	0.0%
Budget	Cotton Roll Medicom	$19.95 per 1000 units	1,000	1	0.02	0.02	0.0%
Maxill	Imprinted Retainer Box	$1.15 each	1	1	1.28	1.28	0.0%
Budget	Mask Blue	1 box of 50 masks $9.00		1	0.19	0.19	0.0%
Central Printing	Letterhead	7000 pieces $2,585	7,000	2	0.41	0.83	0.0%
Postal	Stamp	$0.51 per stamp		2	0.51	1.02	0.0%
Central Printing	Envelope	5,000 envelopes $1,985	5,000	2	0.44	0.89	0.0%
	Davis Dollars (prize)	40 davis dollars = $10.00 average		10	1.00	10.00	0.2%
Ink Fleet	Smile Certificate	1 box of 50 sheets $16.93	50	1	0.38	0.38	36.1%
	Goody bag (candy or champagne)	Champagne or candy $3.55		1	3.55	3.55	0.1%
	Subtotal Braces Off (Deband)					134.81	2.2%
	Total Materials					351.13	5.7%
	Labour						

					Amount	%
Doctors					750	12.2%
Hygiene					382.39	6.2%
Front Desk					128.01	2.1%
Repairs & Maintenance					47.90	0.8%
Financial Coordinators					79.91	1.3%
Instruments Coordinators					28.41	0.5%
Management					81.52	1.3%
Dental Assistants					67.57	1.1%
Treatment Coordinators					107.70	1.8%
Marketing					35.68	0.6%
Total Labour					1,709.09	27.9%
Total Direct Cost					2,060.23	33.6%
Gross Margin	Full Treatment				4,069.77	66.4%
Generic Overhead						
Marketing Doctors					22.78	0.4%
Marketing Patients					58.03	0.9%
Auto Expenses					1.48	0.0%
Bank Charges & Interest					72.49	1.2%
Doctor's Professional Development					16.96	0.3%
Equipment Expense					265.96	4.3%
Facility Expense					334.71	5.5%
Fees & Dues					110.24	1.8%
Professional Fees					118.72	1.9%
Staff Expenses					149.65	2.4%
Bad Debts					8.37	0.1%
Total Overhead					1,159.40	18.9%
Net Profit before Tax	Full				2,910.38	47.5%

Exhibit 17.8B

Supplier	Product	Description	Units per Box	Qty per Patient	Unit Cost	LOWER LINGUAL ARCH	%	TWIN BLOCK	%	RAPID PALADEL EXPANDER	%	HAWLEY WITH SPRINGS	%	TONGUE CRIB	%
	PHASE I														
	Total Fee					1,800.00	100.0%	1,800.00	100.0%	1,200.00	100.0%	1,800.00	100.0%	1,200.00	100.0%
	Materials														
	Consultation														
	Pans and Ceph	Machine depreciation (20%) / 2,101 exams			10.47	10.47	0.6%	10.47	0.6%	10.47	0.9%	10.47	0.6%	10.47	0.9%
Ink Fleet	Printed Pan	1 box of 50 sheets $16.93	50	2	0.38	0.76	0.0%	0.76	0.0%	0.76	0.1%	0.76	0.0%	0.76	0.1%
	Camera depreciation	$1,300 every 2 years / 2,101 exams times 2			0.33	0.00	0.0%	0.00	0.0%	0.00	0.0%	0.00	0.0%	0.00	0.0%
Ink Fleet	Ink	8 cartridges per month / (2101/12)		1	2.24	2.24	0.1%	2.24	0.1%	2.24	0.2%	2.24	0.1%	2.24	0.2%
Print	Exit Package	Folder + Information		1	3.44	3.44	0.2%	3.44	0.2%	3.44	0.3%	3.44	0.2%	3.44	0.3%
Budget	Sani Cloth Large	1 bottle $10.25	160	2	0.07	0.14	0.0%	0.14	0.0%	0.14	0.0%	0.14	0.0%	0.14	0.0%
Budget	Mask Blue	1 box of 50 masks $9.00		1	0.19	0.19	0.0%	0.19	0.0%	0.19	0.0%	0.19	0.0%	0.19	0.0%
Wayne	Gloves	1 box Vinyl $3.35	100	2	0.03	0.07	0.0%	0.07	0.0%	0.07	0.0%	0.07	0.0%	0.07	0.0%
Patterson	Sterilization Bag	1 box of 1,000 bags $34.95	1,000	1	0.04	0.04	0.0%	0.04	0.0%	0.04	0.0%	0.04	0.0%	0.04	0.0%
EC Print	Informed Consent	1,000 forms $160.00	1,000	1	0.18	0.18	0.0%	0.18	0.0%	0.18	0.0%	0.18	0.0%	0.18	0.0%
Central Printing	Business card	$0.41 cents per card	500	2	0.41	0.82	0.0%	0.82	0.0%	0.82	0.1%	0.82	0.0%	0.82	0.1%
EC Print	Davis Dollar sheet	2,000 sheets for $180.00	2,000	1	0.10	0.10	0.0%	0.10	0.0%	0.10	0.0%	0.10	0.0%	0.10	0.0%
Central Printing	Letterhead	7000 pieces $2,585	7,000	2	0.41	0.83	0.0%	0.83	0.0%	0.83	0.1%	0.83	0.0%	0.83	0.1%
Postal	Stamp	$0.51 per stamp		2	0.51	1.02	0.1%	1.02	0.1%	1.02	0.1%	1.02	0.1%	1.02	0.1%
Central Printing	Envelope	5,000 envelopes $1,985	5,000	2	0.44	0.89	0.0%	0.89	0.0%	0.89	0.1%	0.89	0.0%	0.89	0.1%
Central Printing	Pen	*Rainbow Optical Fiber Pen $3 per pen*	1	1	3.35	3.35	0.2%	3.35	0.2%	3.35	0.3%	3.35	0.2%	3.35	0.3%
Central Printing	Magnet	*750 magnets $635*	750	1	1.02	1.02	0.1%	1.02	0.1%	1.02	0.1%	1.02	0.1%	1.02	0.1%
Budget	Tray Cover	1 box $19.95	1,000	2	0.02	0.04	0.0%	0.04	0.0%	0.04	0.0%	0.04	0.0%	0.04	0.0%
	Subtotal Consultation					25.59	1.4%	25.59	1.4%	25.59	2.1%	25.59	1.4%	25.59	2.1%
	Treatment														
Ferraro	Lab Fee			1		64.00	3.6%	170.00	9.4%	84.00	7.0%	86.00	4.8%	80.00	6.7%
3M Unitek	2 Molar Bands	$158.19 us for 28 molar bands	28	2	6.50	12.99	0.7%	12.99	0.7%	12.99	1.1%	12.99	1.1%	12.99	1.1%
	1 Impression	10 bags of 1lb. $84.81 1lb = 9 patients	10	0.11	8.48	0.94	0.1%	0.94	0.1%	0.94	0.1%	0.94	0.1%	0.94	0.1%
	2 Impressions	10 bags of 1lb. $84.81 1lb = 9 patients	10	0.11	8.48			1.88	0.1%						
Patterson	Wax	1 box $32	100	0.01	32.00			0.32							
3M Unitek	Cement	US 99.44 1 unit = 30 patients	1	0.03	114.36	3.81	0.2%			3.81	0.3%	3.81	0.3%	3.81	0.3%
Maxill	Imprinted Retainer Box	$1.15 each	1	1	1.28			1.28	0.1%			1.28	0.1%	1.28	0.1%
EC Print	Consent Forms	2,250 forms $190.00	2,250	1	0.09	0.09	0.0%	0.09	0.0%	0.09	0.0%	0.09	0.0%	0.09	0.0%

EC Print	Contract	500 forms $125.00	500	1	0.28	0.28	0.0%	0.28	0.0%	0.28	0.0%	0.28	0.0%	0.28	0.0%
Central Printing	Business card	$0.41 cents per card	500	1	0.41	0.41	0.0%	0.41	0.0%	0.41	0.0%	0.41	0.0%	0.41	0.0%
Central Printing	Progress Report	5,000 cards $225	5,000	1	0.05	0.05	0.0%	0.05	0.0%	0.05	0.0%	0.05	0.0%	0.05	0.0%
Central Printing	Davis Dollars (bills)	7,500 bills $ $360	7,500	3	0.05	0.16	0.0%	0.16	0.0%	0.16	0.0%	0.16	0.0%	0.16	0.0%
	Subtotal Treatment					82.74	4.6%	174.48	9.7%	102.74	8.6%	89.22	5.0%	98.74	8.2%
	Remove Retainer														
Budget	Bib	1 box $20.95	500	1	0.05	0.05	0.0%	0.00	0.0%	0.05	0.0%	0.00	0.0%	0.00	0.0%
Patterson	Disposable Prophy Angle	1 box $343.35	1,000	1	0.34	0.34	0.0%	0.00	0.0%	0.34	0.0%	0.00	0.0%	0.00	0.0%
Budget	Saliva Ejector	1 box $29.95	1,000	1	0.03	0.03	0.0%	0.00	0.0%	0.03	0.0%	0.00	0.0%	0.00	0.0%
Patterson	Prophy Paste (Fluorhide)	$74.10 200 units	200	1	0.40	0.40	0.0%	0.00	0.0%	0.40	0.0%	0.00	0.0%	0.00	0.0%
Budget	Cotton Roll Medicom	$19.95 per 1000 units	1,000	1	0.02	0.02	0.0%	0.00	0.0%	0.02	0.0%	0.00	0.0%	0.00	0.0%
Budget	Mask Blue	1 box of 50 masks $9.00	1,000	1	0.19	0.19	0.0%	0.00	0.0%	0.00	0.0%	0.00	0.0%	0.00	0.0%
Central Printing	Letterhead	7000 pieces $2,585	7,000	1	0.41	0.41	0.0%	0.41	0.0%	0.41	0.0%	0.41	0.0%	0.41	0.0%
Postal	Stamp	$0.51 per stamp		1	0.51	0.51	0.0%	0.51	0.0%	0.51	0.0%	0.51	0.0%	0.51	0.0%
Central Printing	Envelope	5,000 envelopes $1,985	5,000	1	0.44	0.44	0.0%	0.44	0.0%	0.44	0.0%	0.44	0.0%	0.44	0.0%
	Davis Dollars (prize)	40 davis dollars = $10.00 average		10	1.00	10.00	0.6%	10.00	0.6%	10.00	0.8%	10.00	0.6%	10.00	0.8%
	Subtotal Remove Retainer					12.40	0.7%	11.37	0.6%	12.21	1.0%	11.37	0.6%	11.37	0.9%
	Total Materials					120.73	6.7%	211.44	11.7%	140.54	11.7%	126.17	7.0%	135.70	11.3%
	Labour														
	Doctors					500.00	27.8%	375	20.8%	375	31.3%	375	20.8%	375	31.3%
	Hygiene					277.17	15.4%	138.58	7.7%	138.58	11.5%	138.58	7.7%	138.58	11.5%
	Front Desk					128.01	7.1%	128.01	7.1%	128.01	10.7%	128.01	7.1%	128.01	10.7%
	Repairs & Maintenance					47.90	2.7%	47.90	2.7%	47.90	4.0%	47.90	2.7%	47.90	4.0%
	Financial Coordinators					28.46	1.6%	28.46	1.6%	28.46	2.4%	28.46	1.6%	28.46	2.4%
	Instruments Coordinators					16.04	0.9%	16.04	0.9%	16.04	1.3%	16.04	0.9%	16.04	1.3%
	Management					32.84	1.8%	32.84	1.8%	32.84	2.7%	32.84	1.8%	32.84	2.7%
	Dental Assistants					23.45	1.3%	23.45	1.3%	23.45	2.0%	23.45	1.3%	23.45	2.0%
	Treatment Coordinators					32.78	1.8%	32.78	1.8%	32.78	2.7%	32.78	1.8%	32.78	2.7%
	Marketing					31.59	1.8%	31.59	1.8%	31.59	2.6%	31.59	1.8%	31.59	2.6%
	Total Labour					1,118.24	62.1%	854.66	47.5%	854.66	71.2%	854.66	47.5%	854.66	71.2%
	Total Direct Cost					1,238.98	68.8%	1,066.10	59.2%	995.20	82.9%	980.83	54.5%	990.36	82.5%

Continued

Exhibit 17.8B, cont'd

Supplier	Product	Description	Units per Box	Qty. per Patient	Unit Cost	LOWER LINGUAL ARCH	%	TWIN BLOCK	%	RAPID PALADEL EXPANDER	%	HAWLEY WITH SPRINGS	%	TONGUE CRIB	%
	Gross Margin					561.02	31.2%	733.90	40.8%	204.80	17.1%	819.17	45.5%	209.64	17.5%
	Overhead														
	Marketing Doctors					22.78	1.3%	22.78	1.3%	22.78	1.9%	22.78	1.3%	22.78	1.9%
	Marketing Patients					58.03	3.2%	58.03	3.2%	58.03	4.8%	58.03	3.2%	58.03	4.8%
	Auto Expenses					1.48	0.1%	1.48	0.1%	1.48	0.1%	1.48	0.1%	1.48	0.1%
	Bank Charges & Interest					72.49	4.0%	72.49	4.0%	72.49	6.0%	72.49	4.0%	72.49	6.0%
	Doctor's Professional Development					16.96	0.9%	16.96	0.9%	16.96	1.4%	16.96	0.9%	16.96	1.4%
	Equipment Expense					265.96	14.8%	265.96	14.8%	265.96	22.2%	265.96	14.8%	265.96	22.2%
	Facility Expense					334.71	18.6%	334.71	18.6%	334.71	27.9%	334.71	18.6%	334.71	27.9%
	Fees & Dues					110.24	6.1%	110.24	6.1%	110.24	9.2%	110.24	6.1%	110.24	9.2%
	Professional Fees					118.72	6.6%	118.72	6.6%	118.72	9.9%	118.72	6.6%	118.72	9.9%
	Staff Expenses					149.65	8.3%	149.65	8.3%	149.65	12.5%	149.65	8.3%	149.65	12.5%
	Bad Debts					8.37	0.5%	8.37	0.5%	8.37	0.7%	8.37	0.5%	8.37	0.7%
	Total Overhead					1,159.40	64.4%	1,159.40	64.4%	1,159.40	96.6%	1,159.40	64.4%	1,159.40	96.6%
	Net Profit before Tax	Phase I				-598.37	-33.2%	-425.49	-23.6%	-954.60	-79.5%	-340.23	-18.9%	-949.76	-79.1%
		Phase II > 12 months				1,843.51	39.4%	1,843.51	39.4%	2,443.51	46.3%	1,843.51	39.4%	2,443.51	46.3%
		Phase II 12 - 18 months				1,777.27	38.0%	1,777.27	38.0%	2,377.27	45.0%	1,777.27	38.0%	2,377.27	45.0%
		Phase II 18 - 24 months				1,460.38	31.2%	1,460.38	31.2%	2,060.38	39.0%	1,460.38	31.2%	2,060.38	39.0%
		Phase II 24 - 30 months				1,393.44	29.8%	1,393.44	29.8%	1,993.44	37.8%	1,393.44	29.8%	1,993.44	37.8%
		Phase I + II > 12 months				1,245.13	19.2%	1,418.01	21.9%	1,488.91	23.0%	1,503.28	23.2%	1,493.75	23.1%
		Phase I + II 12 - 18 months				1,178.89	18.2%	1,418.01	21.9%	1,422.67	22.0%	1,437.03	22.2%	1,427.51	22.0%
		Phase I + II 18 - 24 months				862.01	13.3%	1,034.89	16.0%	1,105.78	17.1%	1,120.15	17.3%	1,110.62	17.1%
		Phase I + II 24 - 30 months				795.06	12.3%	967.95	14.9%	1,038.84	16.0%	1,053.21	16.3%	1,043.68	16.1%

Exhibit 17.8C

Supplier	Product	Description	Units per Box	Qty. per Patient	Unit Cost	Full <12 <10 aligners	%	Full <12 >11 aligners	%	Full 12-18 >11 aligners	%	Full 18-24 >11 aligners	%
	INVISALIGN												
	Total Fee					5,530.00	100.0%	5,530.00	100.0%	6,930.00	100.0%	7,630.00	100.0%
	Materials												
	Consultation												
	Pans and Ceph	Machine depreciation (20%) / 2,101 exams			10.47	10.47	0.2%	10.47	0.2%	10.47	0.2%	10.47	0.1%
Ink Fleet	Printed Pan	1 box of 50 sheets $16.93	50	2	0.38	0.76	0.0%	0.76	0.0%	0.76	0.0%	0.76	0.0%
	Camera depreciation	$1,300 every 2 years / 2,101 exams times 2			0.33	0.00	0.0%	–	0.0%	0.00	0.0%	0.00	0.0%
Ink Fleet	Ink	8 cartridges per month / (2101/12)		1	2.24	2.24	0.0%	2.24	0.0%	2.24	0.0%	2.24	0.0%
Print	Exit Package	Folder + Information		1	3.44	3.44	0.1%	3.44	0.1%	3.44	0.0%	3.44	0.0%
Budget	Sani Cloth Large	1 bottle $10.25	160	2	0.07	0.14	0.0%	0.14	0.0%	0.14	0.0%	0.14	0.0%
Budget	Mask Blue	1 box of 50 masks $9.00		1	0.19	0.19	0.0%	0.19	0.0%	0.19	0.0%	0.19	0.0%
Wayne	Gloves	1 box Vinyl $3.35	100	2	0.03	0.07	0.0%	0.07	0.0%	0.07	0.0%	0.07	0.0%
Patterson	Sterilization Bag	1 box of 1,000 bags $34.95	1,000	1	0.04	0.04	0.0%	0.04	0.0%	0.04	0.0%	0.04	0.0%
EC Print	Informed Consent	1,000 forms $160.00	1,000	1	0.18	0.18	0.0%	0.18	0.0%	0.18	0.0%	0.18	0.0%
Central Printing	Business card	$0.41 cents per card	500	2	0.41	0.82	0.0%	0.82	0.0%	0.82	0.0%	0.82	0.0%
EC Print	Davis Dollar sheet	2,000 sheets for $180.00	2,000	1	0.10	0.10	0.0%	0.10	0.0%	0.10	0.0%	0.10	0.0%
Central Printing	Letterhead	7000 pieces $2,585	7,000	2	0.41	0.83	0.0%	0.83	0.0%	0.83	0.0%	0.83	0.0%
Postal	Stamp	$0.51 per stamp		2	0.51	1.02	0.0%	1.02	0.0%	1.02	0.0%	1.02	0.0%
Central Printing	Envelope	5,000 envelopes $1,985	5,000	2	0.44	0.89	0.0%	0.89	0.0%	0.89	0.0%	0.89	0.0%
	Pen	*Rainbow Optical Fiber Pen $3 per pen*	1	1	3.35	3.35	0.1%	3.35	0.1%	3.35	0.1%	3.35	0.0%
Central Printing	Magnet	*750 magnets $635*	750	1	1.02	1.02	0.0%	1.02	0.0%	1.02	0.0%	1.02	0.0%
Budget	Tray Cover	1 box $19.95	1,000	2	0.02	0.04	0.0%	0.04	0.0%	0.04	0.0%	0.04	0.0%
	Subtotal Consultation					25.59	0.5%	25.59	0.5%	25.59	0.4%	25.59	0.3%
	Aligners on + Treatment												
Invisalign	Invisalign Trays	Full set of Aligners	One set			862.50	15.6%	1719.25	31.1%	1719.25	24.8%	1719.25	22.5%
Invisalign	Reeboth	Second Stage of Aligners	One set			143.75	2.6%	143.75	2.6%	143.75	2.1%	143.75	1.9%
Patterson	PVS Impression Material	116.95 Aquasil 1 box = 4 impressions	4	2	116.95	233.90	4.2%	233.90	4.2%	233.90	3.4%	233.90	3.1%
Patterson	Wax	1 box $32	100	0.02	32.00	0.64	0.0%	0.64	0.0%	0.64	0.0%	0.64	0.0%
OSC	ARS Burs	1 box $60.95 5 burs	5	1	12.19	12.19	0.2%	12.19	0.2%	12.19	0.2%	12.19	0.2%
3m Unitek	Transbond Light Cure	1 bottle us $45.50 us for 40 patients	1	0.025	52.78	1.32	0.0%	1.32	0.0%	1.32	0.0%	1.32	0.0%
3m Unitek	Transbond LR Paste	$69 us 25 capsules, 3 patients per capsule	25	0.33	3.17	1.05	0.0%	1.05	0.0%	1.05	0.0%	1.05	0.0%

Continued

Exhibit 17.8C, cont'd

Supplier	Product	Description	Units per Box	Qty. per Patient	Unit Cost	Full <12 <10 aligners	%	Full <12 >11 aligners	%	Full 12-18 >11 aligners	%	Full 18-24 >11 aligners	%
Ink Fleet	Record - Pan, Ceph, Photos	1 box of 50 sheets $16.93	50	3	0.38	1.14	0.0%	1.14	0.0%	1.14	0.0%	1.14	0.0%
EC Print	Consent Forms	2,250 forms $190.00	2,250	1	0.09	0.09	0.0%	0.09	0.0%	0.09	0.0%	0.09	0.0%
EC Print	Contract	500 forms $125.00	500	1	0.28	0.28	0.0%	0.28	0.0%	0.28	0.0%	0.28	0.0%
Central Printing	Business card	$0.41 cents per card	500	1	0.41	0.41	0.0%	0.41	0.0%	0.41	0.0%	0.41	0.0%
Central Printing	Progress Report	5,000 cards $225	5,000	1	0.05	0.05	0.0%	0.05	0.0%	0.05	0.0%	0.05	0.0%
Central Printing	Davis Dollars (bills)	7,500 bills $ $360	7,500	3	0.05	0.97	0.0%	0.97	0.0%	0.00	0.0%	0.00	0.0%
	Subtotal Braces On + Treatment					1258.28	22.8%	2115.03	38.2%	2114.07	30.5%	2114.07	27.7%
	Braces off (Deband)												
Patterson	2 Impressions	10 bags of 1lb. $84.81 1lb = 9 patients	10	0.11	8.48	1.88	0.0%	1.88	0.0%	1.88	0.0%	1.88	0.0%
	Lower 3-3	1 unit	1	1	22	22.00	0.4%	22.00	0.4%	22.00	0.3%	22.00	0.3%
	Max Hawley Retainer	1 unit	1	1	61	61.00	1.1%	61.00	1.1%	61.00	0.9%	61.00	0.8%
	2-2	1 unit	1	1	20	20.00	0.4%	20.00	0.4%	20.00	0.3%	20.00	0.3%
Budget	Mask Blue	1 box of 50 masks $9.00	1	1	0.19	0.19	0.0%	0.19	0.0%	0.19	0.0%	0.19	0.0%
Central Printing	Letterhead	7000 pieces $2,585	7,000	2	0.41	0.83	0.0%	0.41	0.0%	0.41	0.0%	0.41	0.0%
Postal	Stamp	$0.51 per stamp		2	0.51	1.02	0.0%	0.51	0.0%	0.51	0.0%	0.51	0.0%
Central Printing	Envelope	5,000 envelopes $1,985	5,000	2	0.44	0.89	0.0%	0.44	0.0%	0.44	0.0%	0.44	0.0%
	Davis Dollars (prize)	40 davis dollars = $10.00 average		10	1.00	10.00	0.2%	1.00	0.0%	1.00	0.0%	1.00	0.0%
Ink Fleet	Smile Certificate	1 box of 50 sheets $16.93	50	1	0.38	0.38	0.0%	0.38	0.0%	0.38	0.0%	0.38	0.0%
	Goody bag (candy or champagne)	Champagne or candy $3.55		1	3.55	3.55	0.1%	3.55	0.1%	3.55	0.1%	3.55	0.0%
	Subtotal Braces Off (Deband)					121.74	2.2%	111.37	2.0%	111.37	1.6%	111.37	1.5%
	Total Materials					1405.61	25.4%	2252.00	40.7%	2251.03	32.5%	2251.03	29.5%
	Labour												
	Doctors					500.00	9.0%	500.00	9.0%	500.00	7.2%	750	9.8%
	Hygiene					213.65	3.9%	213.65	3.9%	251.18	3.6%	288.72	3.8%
	Front Desk					128.01	2.3%	128.01	2.3%	128.01	1.8%	128.01	1.7%
	Repairs & Maintenance					47.90	0.9%	47.90	0.9%	47.90	0.7%	47.90	0.6%
	Financial Coordinators					79.91	1.4%	79.91	1.4%	79.91	1.2%	79.91	1.0%
	Instruments Coordinators					28.41	0.5%	28.41	0.5%	28.41	0.4%	28.41	0.4%

	Value	%	Value	%	Value	%	Value	%
Management	81.52	1.5%	81.52	1.5%	81.52	1.2%	81.52	1.1%
Dental Assistants	67.57	1.2%	67.57	1.2%	67.57	1.0%	67.57	0.9%
Treatment Coordinators	107.70	1.9%	107.70	1.9%	107.70	1.6%	107.70	1.4%
Marketing	35.68	0.6%	35.68	0.6%	35.68	0.5%	35.68	0.5%
Total Labour	1,290.35	23.3%	1,290.35	23.3%	1,327.89	19.2%	1,615.42	21.2%
Total Direct Cost	2,695.97	48.8%	3,542.35	64.1%	3,578.92	51.6%	3,866.45	50.7%
Gross Margin	2,834.03	51.2%	1,987.65	35.9%	3,351.08	48.4%	3,763.55	49.3%
Overhead								
Marketing Doctors	22.78	0.4%	22.78	0.4%	22.78	0.3%	22.78	0.3%
Marketing Patients	58.03	1.0%	58.03	1.0%	58.03	0.8%	58.03	0.8%
Auto Expenses	1.48	0.0%	1.48	0.0%	1.48	0.0%	1.48	0.0%
Bank Charges & Interest	72.49	1.3%	72.49	1.3%	72.49	1.0%	72.49	1.0%
Doctor's Professional Development	16.96	0.3%	16.96	0.3%	16.96	0.2%	16.96	0.2%
Equipment Expense	265.96	4.8%	265.96	4.8%	265.96	3.8%	265.96	3.5%
Facility Expense	334.71	6.1%	334.71	6.1%	334.71	4.8%	334.71	4.4%
Fees & Dues	110.24	2.0%	110.24	2.0%	110.24	1.6%	110.24	1.4%
Professional Fees	118.72	2.1%	118.72	2.1%	118.72	1.7%	118.72	1.6%
Staff Expenses	149.65	2.7%	149.65	2.7%	149.65	2.2%	149.65	2.0%
Bad Debts	8.37	0.2%	8.37	0.2%	8.37	0.1%	8.37	0.1%
Total Overhead	1,159.40	21.0%	1,159.40	21.0%	1,159.40	16.7%	1,159.40	15.2%
Net Profit before Tax	1,674.64	30.3%	828.25	15.0%	2,191.68	31.6%	2,604.15	34.1%
Invisalign + Braces — Full treatment Braces on < 12 Months	191.05	3.5%	191.05	3.5%	191.05	2.8%	191.05	2.5%
Full treatment Braces off < 12 Months	134.81	2.4%	134.81	2.4%	134.81	1.9%	134.81	1.8%
20% of Labour < 12 Months	265.13	4.8%	265.13	4.8%	265.13	3.8%	265.13	3.5%
Subtotal	590.99	10.7%	590.99	10.7%	590.99	8.5%	590.99	7.7%
Net Profit before Tax Invisalign + Braces	1,083.64	19.6%	237.26	4.3%	1,600.69	23.1%	2,013.16	26.4%

Exhibit 17.8D

Description	Hygienist						Doctor		
	Bond Hours	Treatment Hours	Deband Hours	Total Hours	Rate	Cost	Hours	Rate	Cost
Full Treatment and Phase II									
12	1.5	52 weeks / 6 * 20/60 minutes = 2.89	1	5.39	46.19	248.94	2	250	500
18	1.5	78 weeks / 6 * 20/60 minutes = 4.33	1	6.83	46.19	315.66	2	250	500
24	1.5	104 weeks / 6 * 20/60 minutes = 5.78	1	8.28	46.19	382.39	3	250	750
30	1.5	130 weeks / 6 * 20/60 minutes = 7.22	1	9.72	46.19	449.11	3	250	750
Phase I									
LLA				6.00	46.19	277.17	2	250	500
TWINS				3.00	46.19	138.58	1.5	250	375
RPE				3.00	46.19	138.58	1.5	250	375
HWLY				3.00	46.19	138.58	1.5	250	375
CRIB				3.00	46.19	138.58	1.5	250	375
Invisalign	Impression								
12	2	52 weeks / 8 * 15/60 minutes = 1.63	1	4.63	46.19	213.65	2	250	500
18	2	78 weeks / 8 * 15/60 minutes = 2.44	1	5.44	46.19	251.18	2	250	500
24	2	104 weeks / 8 * 15/60 minutes = 3.25	1	6.25	46.19	288.72	3	250	750

Exhibit 17.8E

Employee	Gross Pay	Hours	Average cost per hour	Total No. of Starts	Cost per Patient
Lisa S	46,455.45	1,836.92	25.29		
Corinne	46,059.04	1,857.77	24.79		
Sibel	21,403.00	799.79	26.76		
Nathalie	50,038.83	1,960.87	25.52		
Yana	5,534.22	298.30	18.55		
Total Front Desk	**169,490.54**	**6,753.65**	**25.10**	1324	128.01
Tammy	39,943.28	1,362.15	29.32		
Kim	23,480.10	1,052.06	22.32		
Repairs & Maintenance	**63,423.38**	**2,414.21**	**26.27**	1324	47.90
Danielle	14,430.94	375.39	38.44		
Mojgan (RH)	8,866.00	387.50	22.88		
Mojgan (WB)	27,473.56	1,114.59	24.65		
Tracy	47,139.65	1,612.28	29.24		
Sandra	4,206.26	122.56	34.32		
Manuel	3,681.72	105.19	35.00		
Financial Coordinators	**105,798.13**	**3,717.51**	**28.46**	1324	79.91
Aida	28,979.94	1,634.26	17.73		
Julia	8,634.04	711.13	12.14		
Instruments Coordinators	**37,613.98**	**2,345.39**	**16.04**	1324	28.41
Lisa M.	15,033.56	512.02	29.36		
Lisa M.	33,045.68	983.72	33.59		
Liz	59,854.79	1,791.36	33.41		
Management	**107,934.03**	**3,287.10**	**32.84**	1324	81.52
Donna	24,174.11	1,053.22	22.95		
Bonnie	4,555.56	244.70	18.62		
Mandana	39,818.43	1,676.82	23.75		
Rosanna	1,520.07	69.60	21.84		
Mary	6,569.56	302.65	21.71		
Suzanne	12,823.29	467.26	27.44		
Dental Assistants	**89,461.02**	**3,814.25**	**23.45**	1324	67.57
Cathi	54,887.15	1,482.98	37.01		
Nelida	6,145.68	270.43	22.73		
Gloria	53,203.99	1,749.91	30.40		
Diane	28,359.18	846.24	33.51		
Treatment Coordinators	**142,596.00**	**4,349.56**	**32.78**	1324	107.70
Andrea	72,993.44	1,473.83	49.53		
Nancy	54,079.93	1,106.69	48.87		
Kristen	20,362.24	504.87	40.33		
Kristen (wb)	35,206.67	964.20	36.51		
Melissa (rh)	11,301.79	281.73	40.12		
Melissa (wb)	12,163.63	293.22	41.48		
Debby	5,774.34	138.61	41.66		
Yvonne (RH)	16,053.82	312.57	51.36		
Yvonne (WB)	26,022.38	558.35	46.61		
Tod	58,623.61	1,228.97	47.70		
Samantha	68,401.40	1,439.95	47.50		
Natasha	62,697.07	1,375.80	45.57		
Fatima	68,335.19	1,395.15	48.98		
Patricia (RH)	10,033.39	216.24	46.40		
Patricia (WB)	15,972.96	356.68	44.78		
Hygienist	**538,021.86**	**11,646.86**	**46.19**		

Continued

Exhibit 17.8E

Employee	Gross Pay	Hours	Average cost per hour	Total No. of Starts	Cost per Patient
Elvira					
Marketing	47,240.20	1,495.47	31.59	1324	35.68
Total	1,301,579.14	39,824.00	32.68		

Exhibit 17.8F

Description	Amount			No. of Starts	Cost Patient
	RH	WB	Total		
Marketing Doctors	25,592.30	4,572.09	30,164.39	1,324.00	22.78
Marketing Patients	55,535.22	21,301.44	76,836.66	1,324.00	58.03
Auto Expenses	1,898.09	66.31	1,964.40	1,324.00	1.48
Bank Charges & Interest	64,949.49	31,028.45	95,977.94	1,324.00	72.49
Doctor's Professional Development	22,153.77	297.65	22,451.42	1,324.00	16.96
Equipment Expense	129,596.54	222,539.86	352,136.40	1,324.00	265.96
Facility Expense	245,313.72	197,838.94	443,152.66	1,324.00	334.71
Fees & Dues	8,552.73	137,400.00	145,952.73	1,324.00	110.24
Professional Fees	107,404.36	49,781.47	157,185.83	1,324.00	118.72
Staff Expenses	155,026.59	43,109.68	198,136.27	1,324.00	149.65
Bad Debts	10,647.00	435.00	11,082.00	1,324.00	8.37
Total	826,669.81	708,370.89			1,159.40

CONCLUSION

How do you produce such a great experience for your patients that they will tell everyone they know? Not only it requires technical excellence to produce high-quality orthodontic results in an optimal length of time, but the patients must also receive quality treatment in every other aspect of their relationship with your practice. This chapter has provided an insight into some of the critical elements in managing an ideal orthodontic practice.

It is important for every orthodontic practitioner to understand the principles of efficient patient scheduling, the importance of practice analysis, the factors that significantly contribute to practice building, the patient compliance and the cost containment. One of the practice goals should be to complete patients during their estimated treatment time.

Epilogue

Larry W White

BACK TO THE FUTURE

Since ancient times, predicting the future has held enormous fascination for human beings, often at the expense of the present moment and regrettably to the ignorance of the valuable past. Even though prognosticators of professional progress typically have had no more accuracy than ordinary astrological horoscopes, they sometimes offer tantalizing mind games that excite orthodontists about the near and far future. However, any forecast should keep in mind that life is too complex and baffling for most people to understand even as it happens, much less to predict accurately. With this caveat, I humbly and cautiously address some issues that I see in the future of orthodontics.

THE UNCHANGEABLE

However, before we consider the benefits that are likely to accrue from changes in the future, it might temper our expectations to consider some of the features of our profession that probably will not change. For example, the genetic gift of sensitivity to stimuli, which has helped humans evolve, survive and prosper, will probably not change without some serious, sophisticated and yet unforeseen tinkering with the human genome. This stimuli sensitivity determines how much compliance patients will apply to their therapies.[1-3] For all of the improvements seen in orthodontics over the past 50 years, e.g. bonded appliances, titanium wires, preadjusted appliances, noncompliant therapies, temporary anchorage devices (TADs), etc., orthodontists have not experienced concomitant improvements in modifying patients' behaviours, nor should they expect to experience much relief from this burdensome task in the future.[4]

The inability to obtain reasonable patient compliance will remain the principal deterrent to predictable and successful orthodontic therapy that doctors and patients have with removable invisible appliances, e.g. Invisalign,[5] Essix,[6] Simpli5,[7,8] etc. For this reason, I think effective future management of orthodontic patients will reside with some type of fixed appliance. Nevertheless, rather than despairing about this unchangeable feature of human nature, future mechanotherapies and treatment planning strategies may well develop the capacity to mitigate orthodontic forces to the point that they no longer annoy patients and subsequently encourage greater compliance and consistently improved orthodontic treatments, regardless of the appliance that doctors and patients choose.

SUSTAINING AND DISRUPTIVE TECHNOLOGIES

Clayton Christensen[9] has differentiated technological changes as those that sustain existing products or procedures and those that have a disruptive effect. Sustaining technologies foster improvements and have the purpose of achieving better performance of established articles and methods. Consequently, most advances and improvements have a sustaining character about them and deal with quantitative features.

Disruptive technologies, on the other hand, have qualitative attributes that distinguish them and offer entirely new approaches that soon overpower and displace established products and processes. Radio technology provides a good example of these phenomena. Sustaining technologies concentrated on developing better vacuum tubes, more efficiently and for less cost. Whereas the transistor obsoleted the most sophisticated vacuum tube technology and totally changed the entire radio industry.

Over the past 100 years, orthodontists have seen only a few truly disruptive innovations. The first, of course, was the edgewise bracket introduced by Angle.[10] This bracket gave clinicians the first instrument for controlling teeth in three-dimensions, and nothing has yet superseded it. All of the other innovations in edgewise bracket development, such as the twin bracket design, wing additions, self-ligation types, preadjusted systems, lingual brackets, etc., have merely provided sustaining technologies that, while adding sophistication, have not fundamentally changed the way orthodontists deliver therapy. Neither has the transition from gold wires to stainless steel to nitinol or even plastic filaments offered anything but sustaining procedures.

More recently, Invisalign[5] introduced a disruptive technology that eliminates the use of brackets altogether. Although it fails to have the principal disruptive characteristic of providing a cheaper product, it has other features common to disruptive products, i.e. simpler, smaller and more convenient. Whether mainstream therapists can tweak this technology enough to produce consistently good results that are acceptable to doctors and patients remains to be seen. Nevertheless, without any doubt, this poses a disruptive technology that patients want and for which they will spend more,[11] and orthodontics will have to accommodate to it one way or another.

Orthodontic bonding provides another example of disruptive orthodontic technology that displayed all of the characteristics of disruptive products. First, bonding offered a simple and cheaper product that promised lower margins, not greater profits for manufacturers. Second, bonding in the beginning gave worse product performance than brackets welded to bands. Third, bonding created features that orthodontists valued, i.e. cheaper, simpler, smaller and more convenient ways of attaching brackets to teeth. Within a few years of bonding's introduction, hardly anyone used bands on anterior teeth, and the most profitable product of orthodontic manufacturers went away. Sustaining technologies have improved the delivery of bonding with the implementation of indirect bonding, which after three decades shows much greater growth and acceptance.[11]

THREE-DIMENSIONAL IMAGING

But what can orthodontists expect in the future? Three-dimensional (3D) imaging will continue to have a larger place in the armamentarium of orthodontists. With one image, clinicians will have access to information they could only obtain in the past with multiple imaging procedures, e.g. periapicals, bitewings, occlusal, panoramic, cephalometric, tomograms, CAT scans, etc. While such imaging has obvious clinical advantages, it will result in a never-before-seen consumer sovereignty. The patients will own their records, which will have a universality that will allow them to transfer easily anywhere they wish—electronically. More than ever, patients will drive the outcomes of dental care because of the transparency of the procedures. This will obviously make the delivery of orthodontic therapy more exacting, precise and difficult. Welden Bell,[12] my mentor in orofacial pain management, remarked that unless doctors satisfy the patient's chief complaint, they should consider the therapy a failure. With more patient input and authority, that decades-old admonition will gain new importance.

Up till now, computers have performed primarily clerical tasks in orthodontic offices, and only recently have they assumed tasks of clinical importance, e.g. diagnosis, treatment planning, visualized treatment objectives, indirect bonding, model formation, occlusograms, computer-aided design and manufacturing (CAD CAM) bracket design, robot-manufactured wire forms, etc. At the moment, these tasks remain too costly for most clinicians, but as new sustaining technologies emerge, the cost of these valuable adjuncts will surely diminish and come within the reach of all orthodontists.

Sustaining technology has driven the development of dental impressions and model formation, and accuracy, ease of use, cost and flexibility have continued to improve as dentists progressed from dental compound and impression plaster to hydrocolloid, to alginate, then to polyethers and now to vinyl polysiloxane materials. Some companies have already developed 3D virtual modelling that allows the fabrication of ceramic crowns without the benefit of constructing traditional models of stone. Technology now exists for combining 3D scanning and model construction via stereolithography; but in the case of Invisalign, clinicians must still make real-time vinyl polysiloxane impressions, which the company subsequently scans with computerized tomographic radiographs to develop their virtual and stereolithic models.

A truly disruptive technology and departure from impressions and model formation will occur when information gathered from the patient's 3D cranial image combines with computer technology to produce stereolithic models sans impressions. That technology now exists through SureSmile,[13] but the scarcity of 3D imaging in orthodontic offices makes it impractical to apply. However, I have little doubt that this technology will find extensive use in the near future.

By training and patient expectation, dentists are therapists, not diagnosticians; and that is why mechanotherapies hold so much interest for them. But that will change dramatically in the future because of the disruptive diagnostic and treatment planning technology that will develop. Right now, dentists generally and orthodontists specifically use an iterative model based on personal experiences and their memories of those experiences to help them plan treatment. I continue to doubt that computers will develop human-like artificial intelligence with creative skills, but they do have infinite storage capacity and unrivalled recall capacities that will make them ideal for storing and retrieving collective experiences and weighing treatment options before starting orthodontic therapy.

MASS-PRODUCED CUSTOMIZED ORTHODONTIC APPLIANCES

One development that seems inevitable because it is just now gaining traction is the use of mass-produced, customized orthodontic appliances. Innovations, such as Sure Smile,[13,14] Insignia,[15,16] iBraces and Invisalign,[5] have made such a concept possible as they customize treatment on an individual basis, which, incidentally, the original straight-wire appliance[17] intended to do but couldn't. Nano-particle technology will probably enhance this trend by enabling CAD CAM use within the clinical setting. Heretofore, orthodontists have presided over cottage industries that modelled themselves using a guild mentality. Even as aggressive clinicians discovered ways of effectively and efficiently treating more patients, they began to use an industrial model akin to the manufacturing assembly line. Being therapists first and diagnosticians secondly has driven the profession by therapeutic features, e.g. myriad edgewise brackets, bonding, nitinol wires, preadjusted appliances, etc. This has changed the packaging of orthodontics and caused several clinical adjustments, but has not substantially changed the functionality of our therapeutic delivery model.

TECHNOLOGY, PROCESSES AND BEHAVIOUR

Effective orthodontic management systems require the coalescence of three elements: technology, work processes and behavioural changes. The dismissal of any one or two of these features leaves a fragmented and essentially inefficient model for patient care. Orthodontists have ignored this management principle and achieved success in the past by working with what Chris Anderson, Editor of Wired Magazine, calls a *short-tail model*,[18] which restricted care to a small population that valued their services and could afford a high fee from a limited number of people trained to deliver orthodontic care. Recent evidence indicates that a long-tail model will serve the profession and the public better by providing a larger population with a low-cost, high-quality product.

Technology-driven industries without a labour cartel have a history of lowering costs for customers; e.g. computers, cameras, television, telephones, etc. Orthodontics achieved this price depreciation while practically unconscious of it. For example, in 1952, the average wage earner had to work 432 hours to pay for orthodontic care. In 1997, the number of hours worked to pay for orthodontic care that had considerably more comfort and certainty had dropped to 297 hours. In 2009, the number of hours has dropped to 250. One can only imagine what a coherent orthodontic management system combined with technology could do to lower patient orthodontic investments dramatically and thereby greatly increase the number of people willing to use our services.

For orthodontists to grow and prosper, they must plan on treating more patients, but they cannot do it with traditional methods of management. This will present an imperative for orthodontic professionals to adopt a management style that can optimize available technology, newly designed work processes and behavioural changes needed by doctors, staff and patients to offer therapies that minimize the variables that waste time, decrease efficiency and result in poorer treatment outcomes. A recent study[14] displays the ability of 3D computer-aided treatment design to significantly improve orthodontic therapy in less time and fewer appointments.

Current university graduate systems will provide one of the main obstacles to preparing orthodontists for this new urgency because they still have traditional 2–3-year programs that have minimum interface with the commercial companies that have developed these technologies. This will need to change, but whether orthodontists receive their training in an academic environment or pursue it outside of schools, they should expect a rather steep learning curve. Orthodontists should not expect to add these new skills with any less time, discipline or effort than those traditionally taught in graduate school. At any rate, orthodontists will no longer have the luxury of remaining computer illiterate.

For readers who surmise from this brief look into the future of orthodontics that technology and machines will not only dominate but also direct orthodontic therapy and thereby make orthodontists unnecessary, I offer this rejoinder. Eric Hoffer[19] once said, 'Machines may make people superfluous, but they cannot make them harmless. No matter how many and how ingenious the machines, there will always be people around to mess things up'. He further admonishes us in this same publication, 'For the creative individual, no matter how richly endowed, cannot achieve much without hard work. A learning, creative society is automatically a disciplined society'.

I doubt that technology will obsolete orthodontists for the simple reasons that accurate diagnosis and reasonable treatment planning along with successful patient management will remain the cornerstones of orthodontics, and knowledgeable professionals will need to extend their considerable skill and expertise into the therapeutic equation. The new technologies will augment that need, not diminish it, and orthodontists need to prepare for some intensive and extensive training. In the future, more than ever, orthodontics will require a full-time commitment.

REFERENCES

1. McNamara JA Jr, Trotman CA. Creating the compliant patient. Ann Arbor: Center for Human Growth and Development. University of Michigan; 1997; 33:198.
2. White LW. Behavior modification of orthodontic patients. J Clin Orthod 1974; 9:501–505.
3. White LW. A new paradigm of motivation. PCSO Bulletin 1988:44–45.
4. Chess S, Thomas A. Know your child. New York: Basis Books; 1987.
5. Tuncay OC. The Invisalign system. New Malden: Quintessence; 2006.
6. Sheridan JJ, Ledoux W, McMinn R. Essix appliances: minor tooth movement with divots and windows. J Clin Orthod 1994; 28:659–664.
7. Dischinger W. Red, white and blue aligners. Clin Impressions 2008; 15:36–38.
8. Fuller J. A simple aligner system for minor anterior correction. Clin Impressions 2008; 16:21–22.
9. Christensen CM. The innovator's dilemma. Boston: Harvard Business School Press; 1997.
10. Angle EH. The latest and best in orthodontic mechanism. Dental Cosmos 1929; 71:164–174, 260–270, 409–421.
11. Noble J, Hechter FJ, Karaiskos NE, et al. Future practice plans of orthodotic residents in the United States. Am J Orthod Dentofacial Orthodped 2009; 135:357–360.
12. Bell WE. Orofacial pains. Chicago: Year Book; 1989.
13. Sachdeva R. SureSmile technology in a patient-centered orthodontic practice. J Clin Orthod 2001; 35:245–253.
14. Mah J. Efficacy of the SureSmile Process. W.J. Orthod 2009 [submitted for publication].
15. Andreiko C. JCO interviews Craig Andreiko, DDS, MS, on the Elan and Orthos Systems. J Clin Orthod 1994; 28:459–472.
16. Andreiko C, Smith R. Increasing clinical performance and 3D interactive treatment planning and patient-specific appliances. In: Corp O, ed. Ormco web page. Orange: Ormco Corp; 2008.
17. Andrews LF. Straight wire, the concept and appliance. San Diego: L.A. Wells Company; 1989.
18. Anderson C. The Long Tail. New York: Hyperion Publishers; 2006:168.
19. Hoffer E. Before the Sabbath. New York: Harper and Collins Publisher; 1979.

Index